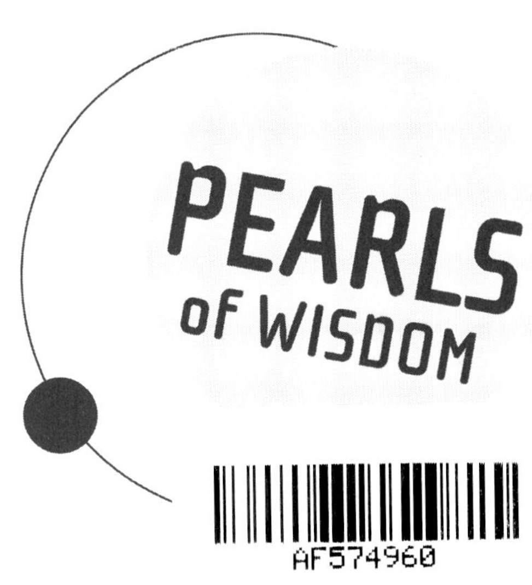

Internal Medicine
BOARD REVIEW

Third Edition

Michael Zevitz
Scott H. Plantz

McGraw-Hill
Medical Publishing Division

New York Chicago San Francisco Lisbon London
Madrid Mexico City Milan New Delhi
San Juan Seoul Singapore
Sydney Toronto

The McGraw-Hill Companies

Internal Medicine Board Review, Third Edition

1 2 3 4 5 6 7 8 9 0 CUS/CUS 0 9 8 7 6 5

ISBN 0-07-146432-8

Notice

Medicine is an ever-changing science. As new research and clinical experience broaden our knowledge, changes in treatment and drug therapy are required. The authors and the publisher of this work have checked with sources believed to be reliable in their efforts to provide information that is complete and generally in accord with the standards accepted at the time of publication. However, in view of the possibility of human error or changes in medical sciences, neither the authors nor the publisher nor any other party who has been involved in the preparation or publication of this work warrants that the information contained herein is in every respect accurate or complete, and they disclaim all responsibility for any errors or omissions or for the results obtained from use of the information contained in this work. Readers are encouraged to confirm the information contained herein with other sources. For example and in particular, readers are advised to check the product information sheet included in the package of each drug they plan to administer to be certain that the information contained in this work is accurate and that changes have not been made in the recommended dose or in the contraindications for administration. This recommendation is of particular importance in connection with new or infrequently used drugs.

The editors were Catherine A. Johnson and Marsha Loeb.
The production supervisor was Phil Galea.
The cover designer was Handel Low.
Von Hoffmann Graphics was printer and binder.

This book is printed on acid-free paper.

Cataloging-in-Publication data for this title is on file at the Library of Congress.

INTERNATIONAL EDITION ISBN: 0-07-110868-8

DEDICATION

To my wife, Joan, the love of my life, and to my children, Erica and Laurel, who have taught me to give it my all in everything that I do.

EDITOR-IN-CHIEF:

Michael Zevitz, M.D.
Assistant Professor
Chicago Medical School
Chicago, IL

ASSOCIATE EDITOR:

Scott H. Plantz, MD
Associate Professor
Chicago Medical School
Mt. Sinai Medical Center
Chicago, IL

CONTRIBUTORS TO PREVIOUS EDITIONS:

Bobby Abrams, M.D.
Attending Physician
Macomb Hospital
Macomb, MI

Jonathan Adler, MD
Instructor of Medicine
Harvard Medical School
Boston, MA

Ishtiaq Ahmad, Ph.D., M.B.B.S.
Research Associate
Laboratory of Cellular and Molecular Cerebral Ischemia
Departments of Neurology and Anatomy & Cell Biology
Center of Molecular Medicine and Genetics
Center of Molecular and Cellular Toxicology
Wayne State University School of Medicine
Detroit, MI

James W. Albers, M.D., Ph.D.
Department of Neurology
University of Michigan
Ann Arbor, MI

W. Michael Alberts, M.D.
Professor and Associate Chair
Department of Internal Medicine
H. Lee Moffitt Cancer Center & Research Institute
University of South Florida
Tampa, FL

Pranav Amin, M.D.
Department of Neurology
Duke University Medical Center
Durham, NC

Linda Anderson, M.D.
Department of Internal Medicine
Pulmonary and Critical Care Medicine Section
University of Nebraska Medical Center
Omaha, NE

Michael L. Ault, M.D.
Instructor in Anesthesiology
Section of Critical Care Medicine
Department of Anesthesiology
Northwestern University Medical School
Chicago, IL

Howard Belzberg, M.D.
Los Angeles County and University of Southern California Medical Center
Los Angeles, CA

Brian Bonanni, M.D.
Duke University Medical Center
Durham, NC

Jon M. Braverman, M.D.
Denver Health Medical Center
University of Colorado School of Medicine
Denver, CO

David F. M. Brown, M.D.
Instructor in Medicine
Harvard Medical School
Massachusetts General Hospital
Boston, MA

Edward Buckley, M.D.
Department of Neurology
Duke University Medical Center
Durham, NC

Leslie S. Carroll, M.D.
Assistant Professor
Chicago Medical School
Toxicology Director
Mt. Sinai medical Center
Chicago, IL

Eduardo Castro, M.D.
Instructor in Medicine
Harvard Medical School
Massachusetts General Hospital
Boston, MA

Seemant Chatruvedi, M.D.
Assistant Professor of Neurology
Wayne State University School of medicine
Co-Director, Harper Hospital Acute Stroke Unit
Detroit, MI

Willie Chen, M.D.
Louisville, KY

Yaoju Chen, MD
Extern
Nephrology Section
Veterans Affairs Medical Center
Milwaukee, WI

Ronald D. Chervin, M.D., MS
Sleep Disorders Center
Department of Neurology
University of Michigan Health System
Ann Arbor, MI

David Chiu, M.D.
Assistant Professor of Neurology
Director, Stroke Center
Baylor College of Medicine
The Methodist Hospital
Houston, TX

Charles H. Cook, M.D.
Assistant Professor of Surgery and Critical Care
The Ohio State University Hospitals
Columbus, OH

Joseph T. Cooke, M.D., FACCP
Associate Professor of Clinical Medicine
Associate Director, Medical Critical Care
The New York Hospital-Cornell Medical Center
New York, NY

William M. Coplin, M.D.
Assistant Professor
Neurology and Neurological Surgery
Wayne State University
Detroit, MI

C. James Corrall, M.D., MPH
Clinical Associate Professor of Pediatrics
Clinical Associate Professor of Emergency Medicine
Indiana University School of Medicine
Indianapolis, IN

Douglas B. Coursin, M.D.
Professor of Anesthesiology and Internal Medicine
Associate Director of the Trauma and
Life Support Center
University of Wisconsin School of Medicine
Madison, WI

Ruben Vargas-Cuba, M.D.
Instructor in Medicine
Chief Medical Resident
Department of Medicine
Tulane University School of Medicine
New Orleans, LA

G. Paul Dabrowski, M.D.
Assistant Professor of Surgery
University of Pennsylvania
Philadelphia, PA

Brian J. Daley, M.D.
Assistant Professor
Division of Trauma and Critical Care
The University of Tennessee Medical Center
Knoxville, TN

Carl W. Decker, M.D.
Madigan Army Medical Center
Fort Lewis, WA

Joshua De Leon, M.D.
Assistant Professor of Medicine
Mount Sinai School of Medicine
New York, NY
Director, Cardiac Catherization and Invasive
Cardiology
Elmhurst Hospital Center
Elmhurst, NY

Peter Emblad, M.D.
Boston City Hospital
Boston, MA

Phillip Fairweather, M.D.
Clinical Assistant Professor
Mount Sinai School of Medicine
New York, NY
Department of Emergency Medicine
Elmhurst Hospital Center
Elmhurst, NY

Craig Feied, M.D.
Clinical Associate Professor
George Washington University
Washington Hospital Center
Washington, D.C.

Eva L. Feldman, M.D., Ph.D.
Department of Neurology
University of Michigan
Ann Arbor, MI

Louis Flancbaum, M.D., FACS, FCCM, FCCP
Associate Professor of Surgery, Anesthesiology, and
Human Nutrition
The Ohio State University Hospitals
Columbus, OH

Mark Franklin, M.D.
Department of Anesthesiology
Northwestern University Medical School
Chicago, IL

Rajesh R. Gandhi, M.D.
Critical Care/Trauma Fellow
University of Pennsylvania
Philadelphia, PA

Judith L. Geidebring, M.D.
Lecturer
University of Michigan
Ann Arbor, MI

Sheree Givre, M.D.
Clinical Assistant Professor
Department of Emergency Medicine
Mount Sinai School of Medicine
New York, NY
Associate Director
Department of Emergency Medicine
Elmhurst Hospital Center
Elmhurst, NY

Bill Gossman, M.D.
Chicago Medical School
Mt. Sinai Medical Center
Chicago, IL

Vicente H. Gracias, M.D.
Instructor of Surgery and Trauma
Surgical Critical Care Fellow
University of Pennsylvania
Philadelphia, PA

L. John Greenfield, Jr., M.D., Ph.D.
Assistant Professor
Department of Neurology
University of Michigan
Ann Arbor, MI

Rajan Gupta, M.D.
Instructor of Surgery and Trauma
Surgical Critical Care Fellow
University of Pennsylvania
Philadelphia, PA

Susan M. Harding, M.D.
Assistant Professor of Medicine
Pulmonary and Critical Care Medicine
University of Alabama
Birmingham, AL

Marilyn T. Haupt, M.D.
Professor, Department of Medicine
Wayne State University School of Medicine
Detroit, MI

Jeffrey W. Hawkins, M.D.
Co-Director, Pulmonary and Critical Care Medicine
Norwood Clinic
Birmingham, AL

Thomas W. Hejkal, M.D.
Department of Ophthalmology
University of Nebraska Medical Center
Omaha, NE

James F. Holmes, M.D.
University of California, Davis
School of Medicine
Sacramento, CA

Eddie Hooker, M.D.
Assistant Professor
University of Louisville
Louisville, KY

Shyam Ivaturi, M.D.
Ridgeland, MS

Cameron Javid, M.D.
Department of Ophthalmology
Tulane University
New Orleans, LA

Mishith Joshi, M.D.
Stroke Fellow
Department of neurology
Wayne State University
Detroit, MI

Marc J. Kahn, M.D.
Assistant Professor of Medicine
Internal Medicine Residency Program Director
Associate Director for Student Programs
Department of Medicine
Section of Hematology/Medical Oncology
Tulane University School of Medicine
New Orleans, LA

Henry J. Kaminski, M.D.
Case Western Reserve University School of Medicine
Department of Veterans Affairs Medical Center
University Hospitals of Cleveland
Cleveland, OH

Stuart Kessler, M.D.
Vice Chairman, Department of Emergency Medicine
Mount Sinai School of Medicine
New York, NY
Director, Department of Emergency Medicine
Elmhurst Hospital Center
Elmhurst, NY

Ali M. Khorrami, M.D., Ph.D.
University Eye Institute
Syracuse, NY

Albert S. Khouri, M.D.
Kentucky Lions Eye Center
Louisville, KY

Lance W. Kreplick, M.D.
Assistant Professor
University of Illinois
EHS Christ Hospital
Oak Lawn, IL

Andrew Lee, M.D.
Department of Ophthalmology
Baylor College of Medicine
Houston, TX

Deborah Anne Lee, M.D., Ph.D.
Assistant Professor
Department of Psychiatry and Neurology
Section of Child Neurology
Clinical Assistant Professor
Department of Pediatrics
Director of the Child Neurology Training Program
Tulane University Medical Center
New Orleans, LA

Kevin R. Lee, M.D.
Chief Resident
Neurological Surgery
Wayne State University
Detroit, MI

Klaus-Dieter K.L. Lessnau, M.D.
New York, NY

Gillian Lewke, P.A., CMA
Physician Assistant
Rockford Memorial Hospital
Rockford, IL

Joseph Lieber, M.D.
Associate Attending in Medicine
Chief, Medical Consult Service
Elmhurst Hospital Center
Elmhurst, NY
Clinical Associate Professor of Medicine
Mount Sinai School of Medicine
New York, NY

Mary W. Lieh-Lai, M.D.
Director, ICU
Associate Professor, Department of Pediatrics
Children's Hospital of Michigan
Wayne State University School of Medicine
Detroit, MI

Marijana Ljubanovic, M.D.
Fellow in Critical Care Medicine
Section of Critical Care Medicine
Department of Anesthesiology
Northwestern University Medical School
Chicago, IL

Lawrence Loo, M.D.
Program Director - Internal Medicine Residency,
Loma Linda University Medical Center;
Chair, Division of General Internal Medicine,
Riverside County Regional Medical Center;
Associate Professor of Medicine, Loma Linda
University School of Medicine;
Loma Linda, CA

Bernard Lopez, M.D.
Assistant Professor
Thomas Jefferson Medical College
Thomas Jefferson University Hospital
Philadelphia, PA

Kenneth Maiese, M.D.
Associate Professor
Laboratory of Cellular and Molecular Cerebral
Ischemia
Departments of Neurology and Anatomy & Cell
Biology
Center of Molecular Medicine and Genetics
Center of Molecular and Cellular Toxicology
Wayne State University School of Medicine
Detroit, MI

John T. Malcynski, M.D.
Instructor of Surgery and Trauma
Surgical Critical Care Fellow
University of Pennsylvania
Philadelphia, PA

Mary Nan S. Mallory, M.D.
Instructor
University of Louisville
Louisville, KY

Sanjeev Maniar, M.D.
Department of Neurology
Wayne State University
Detroit, MI

Gregory P. Marelich, M.D., FACP, FCCP
Assistant Professor of Clinical Internal Medicine
Division of Pulmonary and Critical Care Medicine
University of California Davis Medical Center
Sacramento, CA

Joseph Masci, M.D.
Associate Director of Medicine
Mount Sinai Services
Elmhurst Hospital Center
Elmhurst, NY
Associate Professor of Medicine
Mount Sinai School of Medicine
New York, NY

Terence McGarry, M.D.
Pulmonary and Critical Care Medicine
Elmhurst Hospital Center
Elmhurst, NY
Assistant Professor of Medicine
Mount Sinai School of Medicine
New York, NY

Luis Mejico, M.D.
Department of Neurology
Georgetown University Medical Center
Washington, DC

Kevin Miller, M.D.
Jules Stein Eye Institute
Los Angeles, CA

David Morgan, M.D.
University of Texas
Southwestern Medical Center
Parkland Memorial Hospital
Dallas, TX

Gholam K. Motamedi, M.D.
Department of Neurology
Baylor College of Medicine
Houston, TX

Debasish Mridha, M.D.
Department of Neurology
Wayne State University School of Medicine
Detroit, MI

Anthony M. Murro, M.D.
Associate Professor of Neurology
Department of Neurology
Medical College of Georgia
Augusta, GA

Debra Myers, M.D.
Pulmonary/Critical Care Division
Sleep Disorders Medicine
Assistant Professor
Department of Internal medicine
Wayne State University School of Medicine
Detroit, MI

Sarah T. Nath, M.D.
Sleep Disorders Center
Department of Neurology
University of Michigan Health System
Ann Arbor, MI

Kurt M. Nellhaus, M.D., FCCP
Pulmonary Service, Department of Medicine
Lakes Region General Hospital
Laconia, NH

N. K. Nikhar, M.D., MRCP
Chief Resident
Department of Neurology
University Health Center
Detroit, MI

Scott Olitsky, M.D.
Children's Hospital of Buffalo
Buffalo, NY

Lavi Oud, M.D.
Department of Critical Care Medicine
Wayne State University School of Medicine
Detroit, MI

Igor Ougorets, M.D.
Chief Resident
Department of Neurology
Department of Veterans Affairs Medical Center
University Hospitals of Cleveland
Cleveland, OH

Edward A. Panacek, M.D.
Associate Professor
University of California, Davis
School of Medicine
Sacramento, CA

Deric M. Park, M.D.
Department of Neurology
The University of Chicago
Chicago, IL

Thomas J. Poulton, M.D., FACP, FAAP, FCCM, FCCP
Professor and Chairman
Department of Anesthesiology
Fletcher Allen Health Care
University of Vermont College of Medicine
Burlington, VT

Anthony T. Reder, M.D.
Associate Professor of Neurology
Department of Neurology
The University of Chicago
Chicago, IL

Juan Carlos Restrepo, M.D.
Diplomat of the American Board of Anesthesiology
Board Certified in Critical Care Medicine
VA Medical Center – Jackson Memorial Hospital
University of Miami
Miami, FL

Perry Richardson, M.D.
Department of Neurology
George Washington University Medical Center
Washington, DC

Karen Rhodes, M.D.
University of Chicago Medical Center
Chicago, IL

Luis R. Rodriquez, M.D., F.A.A.P.
Assistant Professor of Pediatrics
Mount Sinai School of Medicine
New York, NY
Elmhurst Hospital Center
Elmhurst, NY

Lisa Rogers, D.O.
Associate Professor of Neurology
Wayne State University School of Medicine
Detroit, MI

Carlo Rosen, M.D.
Instructor in Medicine
Harvard medical School
Massachusetts General Hospital
Boston, MA

Jeffrey Rosenfeld, Ph.D., M.D.
Director Neuromuscular Program
Carolinas Medical Center-Internal Medicine
Charlotte, NC

James A. Rowley, M.D.
Assistant Professor of Medicine
Division of Pulmonary/Critical Care Medicine
Wayne State University School of Medicine
Medical Director
Harper Hospital Sleep Disorders Center
Detroit, MI

Bruce K. Rubin, M.D.
Professor of Pediatrics, Physiology and Pharmacology
Brenner Children's Hospital
Winston-Salem, NC

David Rubenstein, M.D.
Division of Cardiology
Elmhurst Hospital Center
Elmhurst, NY

Robert L. Ruff, M.D., Ph.D.
Departments of Neurology and Neurosciences
Case Western Reserve University School of Medicine
Department of Veterans Affairs Medical Center
University Hospitals of Cleveland
Cleveland, OH

James W. Russell, M.D.
Department of Neurology
University of Michigan
Ann Arbor, MI

Nelson R. Sabates, M.D.
Eye Foundation of Kansas City
University of Missouri, Kansas City School of Medicine
Kansas City, MO

Carla Siegfried, M.D.
Department of Ophthalmology and Visual Sciences
Washington University
St. Louis, MO

Harvey M. Shanies, Ph.D., M.D.
Clinical Associate Professor of Medicine
Mount Sinai School of Medicine
New York, NY
Associate Director of Medicine for Clinical and Academic Pulmonary and Critical Care Medicine
Elmhurst Hospital Center
Elmhurst, NY

Anders A.F. Sima, M.D., Ph.D.
Professor of Pathology and Neurology
Wayne State University School of Medicine
Detroit, MI
Visiting Professor of Pathology
University of Michigan
Ann Arbor, MI
Staff Neuropathologist
Harper Hospital and Detroit Medical Center
Detroit, MI

Sabine Sobek, M.D.
Department of Critical Care Medicine
Wayne State University School of Medicine
Detroit, MI

Dana Stearns, M.D.
Instructor in Medicine
Harvard Medical School
Massachusetts General Hospital

Girish D. Sharma, M.D., FCCP
Assistant Professor of Pediatrics
Section of Pediatric Pulmonology
The University of Chicago Children's Hospital
Chicago, IL

Jack Stump, M.D.
Attending Physician
Rogue Valley Medical Center
Medford, OR

Joan Surdukowski, M.D.
Assistant Professor
Chicago Medical School
Mt. Sinai Hospital
Chicago, IL

Michael J. Taravella, M.D.
University of Colorado
Denver, CO

William O. Tatum, IV, M.D.
Clinical Assistant Professor
Tampa General Hospital Epilepsy Center
Tampa, FL

Menno Terriet, M.D.
Department of Anesthesia
Veterans Affairs Medical Center
Miami, FL

Carlo Tornatore, M.D.
Assistant Professor of Neurology
Department of Neurology
Georgetown University Medical Center
Washington, DC

R. Scott Turner, M.D., Ph.D.
Assistant Professor Department of Neurology
University of Michigan
Ann Arbor, MI

Mythili Venkataraman, M.D.
Attending, Pulmonary Medicine
Director, Bronchology and Invasive Procedures
Elmhurst Hospital Center
Elmhurst, NY
Assistant Professor of Medicine
Mount Sinai School of Medicine
New York, NY

Mladen Vidovich, M.D.
Department of Anesthesiology
Northwestern University Medical School
Chicago, IL

John J. Wald, M.D.
Department of Neurology
University of Michigan
Ann Arbor, MI

Martin Warshawsky, M.D., FACP, FCCP
Director, Respiratory Intensive Care Unit
Elmhurst Hospital Center
Elmhurst, NY
Assistant Professor of Medicine
Mount Sinai School of Medicine
New York, NY

Thais Weibel, M.D.
Department of Neurology
George Washington University Medical Center
Washington, DC

Maria-Carmen B. Wilson, M.D.
Assistant Professor
Department of Neurology
Director, Headache and Pain Program
University of South Florida
School of Medicine
Tampa, FL

Kenneth E. Wood, D.O.
Assistant Professor of Medicine
Director of the Trauma and Life Support Center
University of Wisconsin School of Medicine
Madison, WI

A. Zacharias, M.D.
Department of Neurology
Emory University School of Medicine
Atlanta, GA

Jingwu Zhang, M.D., Ph.D.
Associate Professor of Neurology
Department of Neurology
Baylor College of Medicine
Houston, TX

Kristin Zeller, M.D.
Norfolk, VA

INTRODUCTION

Congratulations! *Internal Medicine Board Review: Pearls of Wisdom* will help you learn some Internal Medicine. Originally designed as a study aid to improve performance on the IM Written Boards/Recertification or IM In-service Examination, this book is full of useful information. While intended for IM specialists, we have learned that Pearls unique format is also useful for house officers and medical students rotating in Internal Medicine. A few words are appropriate discussing intent, format, limitations, and use.

Since *Internal Medicine Board Review* is primarily intended as a study aid, the text is written in rapid-fire question/answer format. This way, readers receive immediate gratification. Moreover, misleading or confusing "foils" are not provided. This eliminates the risk of erroneously assimilating an incorrect piece of information that makes a big impression. Questions themselves often contain a "pearl" intended to reinforce the answer. Additional "hooks" may be attached to the answer in various forms, including mnemonics, visual imagery, repetition, and humor. Additional information not requested in the question may be included in the answer. Emphasis has been placed on distilling trivia and key facts that are easily overlooked, that are quickly forgotten, and that somehow seem to be needed on board examinations.

Many questions have answers without explanations. This enhances ease of reading and rate of learning. Explanations often occur in a later question/answer. Upon reading an answer, the reader may think, "Hmm, why is that?" or, "Are you sure"? If this happens to you, go check! Truly assimilating these disparate facts into a framework of knowledge absolutely requires further reading on the surrounding concepts. Information learned in response to seeking an answer to a particular question is retained better than information that is passively observed. Take advantage of this! Use this book with your preferred source texts handy and open.

The first half of the text is presented in topic areas found on the IM Board Examination. Information presented is mostly limited to straightforward, basic facts. The second section of the book, "Random Pearls", consists of questions grouped into small clusters by topic, presented in no particular order. This section repeats some of the factual information previously covered and builds on this foundation with emphasis on linking information and filling in gaps from the topical chapters.

Internal Medicine Board Review does have limitations. We have found many conflicts between sources of information. We have tried to verify in several references the most accurate information. Some texts have internal discrepancies further confounding clarification.

This book risks accuracy by aggressively pruning complex concepts down to the simplest kernel; the dynamic knowledge base and clinical practice of Internal Medicine is not like that! Furthermore, new research and practice occasionally deviates from that which likely represents the correct answer for test purposes. This text is designed to maximize your score on a test. Refer to your most current sources of information and mentors for direction for practice.

Internal Medicine Board Review is designed to be used, not just read. It is an *interactive* text. Use a 3 x 5 card and cover the answers; attempt all questions. A study method we recommend is oral, group study, preferably over an extended meal or pitchers. The mechanics of this method are simple and no one ever appears stupid. One person holds the book, with answers covered, and reads the question. Each person, including the reader, says "Check" when he or she has an answer in mind. After everyone has "checked" in, someone states his/her answer. If this answer is correct, on to the next one; if not, another person says their answer or the answer can be read. Usually the person who "checks" in first gets the first shot at stating the answer. If this person is being a smarty-pants answer-hog, then others can take turns. Try it, it's almost fun!

This book is also designed to be re-used several times to allow, dare we use the word, memorization. A hollow bullet is provided for any scheme of keeping track of questions answered correctly or incorrectly.

We welcome your comments, suggestions and criticism. Great effort has been made to verify these questions and answers. Some answers may not be the answer you would prefer. Most often this is attributable to variance between original sources. Please make us aware of any errors you find. We hope to make continuous improvements and would greatly appreciate any input with regard to format, organization, content, presentation, or about specific questions. We also are interested in recruiting new contributing authors and publishing new textbooks. We look forward to hearing from you!
Study hard and good luck!

M.E.Z. & S.H.P.

TABLE OF CONTENTS

INTERNAL MEDICINE

Man-a creature made at the end of the week when God was tired.
Mark Twain

CARDIOVASCULAR

Nothing in life is to be feared; it is only to be understood.
Marie Curie

❍ **Are aortic aneurysms more common in men or women?**

Men (10:1). Other risk factors are hypertension, atherosclerosis, diabetes, hyperlipidemia, smoking, alcoholism, syphilis, Marfan's disease, and Ehlers-Danlos disease.

❍ **What is a true aortic aneurysm?**

True aortic aneurysms involve a dilation of all layers of the aorta.

❍ **A patient presents with sudden-onset chest and back pain. Further work-up reveals an ischemic right leg. What is your diagnosis?**

Suspect an acute aortic dissection when chest or back pain is associated with ischemic or neurologic deficits.

❍ **What physical findings suggest an acute aortic dissection?**

Blood pressure differences between arms and/or legs, cardiac tamponade, and aortic insufficiency murmur.

❍ **A 74 year-old male presents with acute-onset testicular pain. Ecchymosis is present in the groin and scrotal sac. What is the diagnosis?**

A ruptured aortic or iliac artery aneurysm.

❍ **What x-ray study should be ordered for a patient with an abdominal mass and a suspected ruptured AAA?**

None. The patient should go to the OR immediately. About 60% of AAA's occur with calcification and appear on a lateral abdominal x-ray.

❍ **What may an x-ray of a patient with an aortic dissection reveal?**

Widening of the superior mediastinum, a hazy or enlarged aortic knob, an irregular aortic contour, separation of the intimal calcification from the outer aortic contour that is greater than 5 mm, a displaced trachea to the right, and cardiomegaly.

❍ **What murmur is expected in patients with substantial aortic stenosis?**

A prolonged, harsh, loud (IV, V, or VI) systolic murmur, crescendo-decrescendo in character.

❍ **Where is the most common site of peripheral aneurysms that develop from arteriosclerosis?**

The popliteal artery. Other sites include the femoral, carotid, and subclavian arteries.

❍ **How long can ST and T changes persist after an episode of pain in unstable angina?**

Several hours.

❍ **What is the most common symptom of thoracic aortic dissection?**

Interscapular back pain.

❍ **Where do aortic dissections most often occur?**

Proximal ascending aorta (60%). Twenty percent of aortic dissections are found between the origin of the left subclavian and the ligamentum arteriosum in the descending aorta, and 10% are found in the aortic arch or the abdominal aorta. Dissection involves intimal tears propagated by hematoma formation.

❍ **What aortic aneurysm diameter is generally considered to be an indication for surgery: a) in the thorax and b) in the abdomen?**

Those with non-dissecting thoracic aneurysm larger than 7 cm in diameter are candidates for surgery. However, surgery should be considered with smaller aneurysms for those with Marfan's syndrome, because of a higher incidence of rupture. Non-dissecting abdominal aortic aneurysms larger than 4 cm in diameter should be considered for surgical repair.

❍ **Describe Debakey's classification of aortic dissections.**

Type I:Dissection of the aortic root, arch, and descending aorta

Type II:Ascending aorta only

Type III:Distal aorta only

❍ **Describe the Stanford classification of aortic dissections.**

Stanford Type A: Involve ascending aorta. (Debakey's Type I and II)

Stanford Type B: Do not involve ascending aorta, distal to the left subclavian artery (Debakey's Type III).

❍ **What dissections can be treated medically?**

Patients with Type B (Debakey's Type III) are eligible for medical, rather than, surgical treatment. Surgical treatment may be required for those with uncontrolable pain, aortic bleeding, hemodynamic instability, increasing hematoma size, or an impending rupture.

❍ **Among those with Marfan's syndrome, at what age does aortic aneurysm become problematic?**

Thirties and forties.

❍ **What is the prognosis for an untreated aortic dissection?**

20% of afflicted individuals die within 24 hours, 60% within 2 weeks, and 90% within 3 months. With surgical treatment, the 10-year survival rate is 50%. Re-dissection occurs in 25% of these patients within 10 years of the original episode.

❍ **Matching:**

1) Quincke's pulse	a) Uvular pulsation during systole
2) Corrigan's pulse	b) Head bobbing
3) de Musset's sign	c) Visible pulsations in nail bed capillaries
4) Muller's sign	d) Femoral artery murmurs during systole if the artery is compressed proximally and during diastole if the artery is compressed distally
5) Duroziez's sign	e) Collapsing pulse
6) Pulsus paradoxus	f) Drop in the systolic blood pressure > 10 mm Hg with inspiration

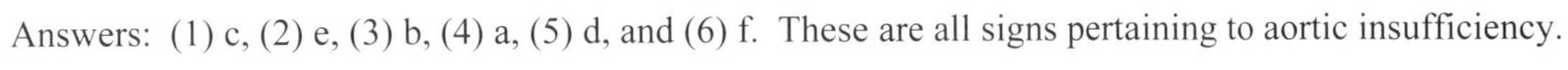
Answers: (1) c, (2) e, (3) b, (4) a, (5) d, and (6) f. These are all signs pertaining to aortic insufficiency.

❍ **What is the most common cause of aortic regurgitation in adults?**

CHF with Aortic root dilation.

Mild aortic regurgitation can also develops as a result of a bicuspid aortic valve, while a severe aortic regurgitation is induced by rheumatic heart disease, syphilis, endocarditis, trauma, an idiopathic degeneration of the aortic valve, a spontaneous rupture of the valve leaflets, or aortic dissection.

❍ **What are the signs and symptoms of acute aortic regurgitation?**

Dyspnea, tachycardia, tachypnea, and chest pain.

❍ **What is the most common cause of aortic stenosis in patients under age 50? Over age 50?**

Under 50: Calcification of congenital bicuspid aortic valves (1% of the population has congenital bicuspid valves)

Over 50: Calcification of degenerating leaflets

❍ **What triad of symptoms characterizes aortic stenosis?**

Syncope, angina, and left heart failure. As the disease progresses, systolic BP decreases and pulse pressure narrows.

❍ **What are the clinical findings in a patient with aortic stenosis?**

Angina, dyspnea on exertion, syncope, sustained apical impulse, narrow pulse pressure, parvus et tardus, systolic ejection crescendo-decrescendo murmur that radiates to the neck, systolic ejection click (not heard in very severe aortic valve stenosis), paradoxically split S1 and soft S2, and audible S4.

❍ **How does a heart murmur reflect the severity of aortic stenosis?**

A longer duration associated with an increasing in intensity indicates severe aortic stenosis. The "loudness" of the murmur is not as important in assessing its severity.

❍ **When should surgery be considered for patients with aortic stenosis?**

Only when symptoms are displayed. The risk of morbidity and mortality associated with the replacement of an aortic valve outweighs any benefit of operating on asymptomatic patients.

❍ **Match the rhythm with the type of SVT.**

1) Wolff-Parkinson-White syndrome
2) Multifocal atrial tachycardia
3) Atrial fibrillation
4) Atrial flutter
5) Accelerated junctional tachycardia
6) Unifocal atrial tachycardia
7) Intra-arterial reentrant tachycardia
8) Nodal tachycardia

a) AV reciprocating tachycardia
b) Automatic tachycardia
c) Reentrant atrial tachycardia
d) AV reentrant nodal tachycardia

Answers: (1) a, (2) b, (3) c, (4) c, (5) d, (6) b, (7) c, and (8) d.

❍ **What are the common causes of multifocal atrial tachycardia?**

COPD, CHF, sepsis, and methylxanthine toxicity. Treat the arrhythmia with magnesium, verapamil, or beta-adrenergic agents.

❍ **How is atrial flutter treated?**

Initiate AV nodal blockade with beta-adrenergic blockers, calcium channel blockers, or digoxin. If necessary, treat a stable patient with chemical cardioversion by using a class IA agent, such as procainamide or quinidine, or a 1C agent, such as propafenone or flecainide, after digitalization. If this treatment fails or if the patient is unstable, electrocardiovert at 25 to 50 J.

❍ **What are some causes of atrial fibrillation?**

Hypertension, rheumatic heart disease, pneumonia, thyrotoxicosis, and an ischemic heart. Pericarditis, ethanol intoxication, PE, CHF and COPD are other causes.

❍ **What are some causes of SVT?**

Digitalis toxicity, pericarditis, MI, COPD, pre-excitation syndromes, mitral valve prolapse, rheumatic heart disease, pneumonia, and ethanol.

❍ **What mechanism most commonly produces SVT?**

AV node. Re-entry. Another common cause is abnormal automaticity, i.e., ectopic foci.

❍ **What is the treatment for SVT caused by digitalis toxicity?**

Stop the digitalis, treat the hypokalemia, and administer magnesium or phenytoin. Provide digoxin-specific antibodies to the unstable patient. Avoid cardioversion, unless the patient is unstable.

❍ **What is the treatment for stable SVT not caused by digitalis toxicity or WPW syndrome?**

Vagal maneuvers, adenosine, verapamil, or beta-blockers.

❍ **Carotid massage or Valsalva maneuver is useful for slowing supraventricular rhythms. When is carotid massage contraindicated?**

With ventricular arrhythmias, dig toxicity, stroke, syncope, or seizures. Carotid massage should be avoided in those with a carotid bruit.

❍ **What are some common vagal maneuvers?**

Breath holding, Valsalva maneuver (bearing down as if having a bowel movement), stimulating of the gag reflex, squatting, pressure on the eyeballs, and immersing the face in cold water.

❍ **Which is more common, premature atrial beats or ventricular beats?**

Premature atrial beats. Palpitations that occur because of premature atrial beats are generally benign and asymptomatic. Reassurance is the only treatment. Less frequent, but more serious, causes of atrial premature beats include pheochromocytoma and thyrotoxicosis. Random PVC's are also benign, but common in the general population. Runs of PVC's, or associated symptoms of dyspnea, angina, or syncope, require investigation and are most likely related to an underlying heart disease.

❍ **What are the diagnostic criteria for a Q wave?**

More than 0.04 seconds and at least one-quarter the size of the R wave in the same lead. Beware, ECG's can be normal in up to 10% of all acute MI's.

❍ **What side effect can occur with a rapid infusion of procainamide?**

Hypotension. Other side effects include QRS/QT prolongation, ventricular fibrillation, and Torsade de pointes.

❍ **What are some adverse drug effects of lidocaine?**

Drowsiness, nausea, vertigo, confusion, ataxia, tinnitus, muscle twitching, respiratory depression, seizures, and psychosis.

❍ **What artery is usually affected by arterial occlusive disease in diabetics?**

The popliteal artery. Because of diabetic neuropathy and the potential for the development of a necrotizing infection in a leg with compromised circulation, it is very important that patients with diabetes are knowledgeable about pedal hygiene.

❍ **What is the Budd-Chiari syndrome?**

Thrombosis in the hepatic vein resulting in abdominal pain, jaundice, and ascites.

❍ **What is the cause of Prinzmetal's angina?**

Coronary artery vasospasm with or without fixed stenotic lesions. Prinzmetal's angina is more often associated with ST segment elevation than with depression. Calcium channel blockers are the drugs of choice to treat this condition. Beta-blockers are relatively contraindicated in patients who have vasospasm without fixed stenotic lesions.

❍ **Eighty to ninety percent of patients who experience sudden non-traumatic cardiac arrest are in what rhythm?**

Ventricular fibrillation. Early defibrillation is the key. In an acute MI, the infarction zone becomes electrically unstable. Ventricular fibrillation is most common during original coronary occlusion or when the coronaries begin to reperfuse.

❍ **In CPR, what is the ventilation to compression ratio for one rescuer? For two rescuers?**

1 rescuer:2 breaths to 15 compressions

2 rescuers:1 breath to 5 compressions

❍ **Which is the most common type of cardiomyopathy?**

Dilated cardiomyopathy. This condition is induced by progression of myocarditis, alcohol, adriamycin, coronary ischemia, diabetes mellitus, pheochromocytoma, thiamine deficiency, thyroid disease, and valvular heart disease. The other types of cardiomyopathies are hypertrophic and restrictive.

❍ **What is the most common discharge diagnosis in patients over 65?**

CHF.

❍ **Which is the most common type of cardiac failure, high or low output?**

Low output failure. Reduced stroke volume, lowered pulse pressure, and peripheral vasoconstriction are all signs of low output failure.

❍ **What is the most common cause of low output heart failure in the world?**

Chagas' disease. In addition to heart failure, patients present with prolonged fever, hepatosplenomegaly, megaesophagus, megacolon, edema, and lymphadenopathy. This disease is most prevalent in Latin America.

❍ **What is the most common cause of low output heart failure in the US?**

CAD. Other causes include congenital heart disease, cor pulmonale, dilated cardiomyopathy, hypertension, hypertrophic cardiomyopathy, infection, toxins, and valvular heart disease.

❍ **Compare the mortality rate from CHF between the sexes.**

Women fair slightly better. The 5-year mortality rate for a female with CHF is 45%, as compared to 60% for males. The majority of deaths from CHF result from ventricular arrhythmias.

❍ **Describe the 3 stages of CXR findings in CHF.**

Stage I:Pulmonary arterial wedge pressure (PAWP) of 12 to 18 mm Hg. Blood flow increases in the upper lung fields (cephalization of pulmonary vessels).

Stage II: PAWP of 18 to 25 mm Hg. Interstitial edema is evident with blurred edges of blood vessels and Kerley B lines.

Stage III:PAWP > 25 mm Hg. Fluid exudes into alveoli with the generation of the classic butterfly pattern of perihilar infiltrates.

❍ **Which do nitrates affect, preload or afterload?**

Predominantly preload.

❍ **Which does hydralazine affect, preload or afterload?**

Afterload.

❍ **Do prazosin, captopril, and nifedipine affect afterload?**

Yes.

❍ **When is dobutamine used in CHF?**

When heart failure is not accompanied with severe hypotension. Dobutamine is a potent inotrope with some vasodilation activity.

❍ **When is dopamine selected in CHF?**

When a patient is in shock. Dopamine is a vasoconstrictor and a positive inotrope.

❍ **What is the most common cause of right ventricular heart failure?**

Left ventricular heart failure.

❍ **Match the sign or symptom with left (L) or right (R) sided heart failure.**

1) Hypotension
2) Hepatomegaly
3) Orthopnea
4) Cough
5) Dyspnea on exertion
6) Abdominal distention
7) Paroxysmal nocturnal dyspnea
8) Hemoptysis
9) S3 gallop
10) Early satiety
11) Jugular venous distention
12) Ascites
13) Rales

Answers : (1) L, (2) R, (3) L, (4) L, (5) L, (6) R, (7) L, (8) L, (9) L, (10) R, (11) R, (12) R, and (13) L.

❍ **What is the rate of restenosis after percutaneous transluminal coronary angioplasty?**

10% to 20% restenose within 6 months. Successful dilation occurs in 90% of the cases, but because of the high rate of restenosis, this option is less attractive than CABG in multi-vessel CAD, in diabetics.

❍ **What is the restenosis rate of coronary vessels following a coronary artery bypass graft (CABG)?**

When using venous grafts, there is a 50% restenosis rate within 5 to 10 years. When the internal mammary artery is used, there is only a 5% restenosis rate at 10 years. Occlusion of the grafts are caused by anastomotic trauma to the vessel, postoperative adhesions, or atherosclerosis.

❍ **How are acute MI, angina pectoralis, and Prinzmetal's angina differentiated?**

The pain is similar but typically differs in radiation, duration, provocation, and palliation. Obtaining an accurate history is the most important tool for diagnosing chest pain!

Angina pectoralis is aggravated by exercise, cold, and excitement, but it is relieved by rest and nitro.

Prinzmetal's angina occurs at rest, during normal activity, and generally at night or in the early morning. It lasts longer than angina pectoralis.

Acute MI's produce pain with a greater radius of radiation that may last for hours.

❍ **A patient presents to the hospital one month after placement of a mechanical prosthetic valve with fever, chills, and a leukocytosis. Endocarditis is suspected. Which type of bacterium is most common?**

Staphylococcus aureus or Staphylococcus epidermidis.

❍ **Which arteries are most commonly involved in giant cell arteritis (chronic inflammation of the large blood vessels)?**

The carotid artery and its branches. Treatment includes high-doses of corticosteroids.

❍ **Atorvastatin (Lipitor) and niacin are used to treat hyperlipoproteinemia. Both of these drugs lower triglycerides and LDL. Which one raises HDL?**

Gemfibrozil and niacin. Atorvastatin has little affect on HDL. However, because niacin often produces significant side effects, such as gastritis, reactivation of peptic ulcers, gout, hyperglycemia, cutaneous flushing, and scaling skin, Atorvastatin remains the first-line drug of choice.

❍ **While taking your boards, why might you become severely annoyed if seated next to a person on ACE inhibitors?**

ACE inhibitors produce a cough in 15% of patients.

❍ **What are the most common side effects of beta-blockers?**

Fatigue and depression.

❍ **What percentage of hypertension is secondary?**

Five percent. Secondary hypertension should be suspected in patients under age 35, patients with a sudden-onset hypertension, and those without a family history for hypertension.

❍ **What is the most common cause of secondary hypertension?**

Renal parenchymal disease. In women, the most common cause is oral contraceptives. In patients over age 50, secondary hypertension can usually be attributed to renal artery stenosis. Other causes include pheochromocytoma, coarctation of the aorta, drugs (cocaine), hyperthyroidism, aldosteronism, and Cushing's syndrome.

❍ **What percentage of patients with aortic dissection are hypertensive?**

70 to 90%. The other risk factors for aortic dissection are trauma, Marfan's syndrome, pregnancy, and coarctation of the aorta.

❍ **What percentage of hypertensive patients are afflicted with left ventricular hypertrophy?**

50%. This is the primary reason that hypertension is a major risk factor for MI, CHF, and sudden death.

❍ **What are the side effects of thiazide diuretics?**

Hyperglycemia, hyperlipidemia, hyperuricemia, hypokalemia, hypomagnesemia, and hyponatremia.

❍ **Which drugs should be administered to lower the BP in a patient with thoracic aortic dissection?**

Sodium nitroprusside and Betablockers

❍ **A patient has a history of episodic blood pressure elevations. She complains of headache, diarrhea, and skin flushing. What is the probable diagnosis?**

Pheochromocytoma.

❍ **A patient, who has a psychiatric history and is taking an MAO inhibitor, has consumed a 12-pack of beer with a meal of pickled herring and a nicely-aged cheese. He now complains of severe headache. Upon examination, his BP is elevated. A diagnosis of acute hypertension is made secondary to hyperstimulation of the adrenergic receptors. What is the treatment?**

An α- and beta-adrenergic antagonist, such as labetalol.

❍ **What is the most common complication of nitroprusside?**

Hypotension. Thiocyanate toxicity, accompanied by blurred vision, tinnitus, change in mental status, muscle weakness, and seizures, is more prevalent in patients with renal failure or prolonged infusions. Cyanide toxicity is uncommon. However, this type of toxicity may occur with hepatic dysfunction, after prolonged infusions, and in rates greater than 10 mg/kg per minute.

❍ **Define a hypertensive emergency.**

Elevated diastolic blood pressure > 115 mm Hg with associated end organ dysfunction or damage.

❍ **How quickly should a patient's blood pressure be lowered in a hypertensive emergency?**

Gradually over 2 to 3 hours to 140 to 160 mm Hg systolic and 90 to 110 mm Hg diastolic. To prevent cerebral hypoperfusion, the blood pressure should not be decreased by more than 25% of the mean arterial pressure.

❍ **What drug can be used for almost all hypertensive emergencies?**

Sodium nitroprusside, except for ecclampsia. It assists in relaxing smooth muscle tissue through the production of c-GMP. As a result, there is decreased preload and afterload, decreased oxygen demand, and a slightly increased heart rate, with no change in myocardial blood flow, cardiac output, or renal blood flow. The duration of action is 1 to 2 minutes. Sometimes, beta-blockade is required to treat rebound tachycardia.

❍ **What is a hypertensive urgency.**

Dangerously elevated diastolic blood pressure > 115 mm Hg without signs of end organ damage. Blood pressure should be gradually reduced over 24 to 48 hours.

❍ **Define uncomplicated hypertension.**

Diastolic blood pressure < 115 mm Hg without symptoms of end organ damage. Uncomplicated hypertension does not require acute treatment.

❍ **What lab findings confirm a hypertensive emergency?**

U/A: RBCs, red cell casts, and proteinuria.
BUN and CR: Elevated.
X-ray: Aortic dissection, pulmonary edema, or coarctation of the aorta.
ECG: LVH and cardiac ischemia.

❍ **What are the signs and symptoms of hypertensive encephalopathy?**

Nausea, vomiting, headache, lethargy, coma, blindness, nerve palsies, hemiparesis, aphasia, retinal hemorrhage, cotton wool spots, exudates, sausage linking, and papilledema. Treat with labetalol or sodium nitroprusside, and lower the mean arterial pressure to approximately 90-110 mm Hg.

❍ **Cardiac hypertrophy will most likely displace the point of maximal impulse to where?**

The normal apical impulse at the medial to midclavicular line in the fourth or fifth intercostal space will be displaced downwards to the sixth intercostal space.

❍ **What maneuvers will increase hypertrophic cardiomyopathy murmurs?**

Valsalva, standing, and amyl nitrate.

❍ **What maneuvers will decrease hypertrophic cardiomyopathy murmurs?**

Handgrip, squatting, and leg elevation in the supine patient.

❍ **Livedo reticularis commonly develops on what body parts?**

The legs. Livedo reticularis is a bluish red discoloration of the skin resulting from vasospasm of the arterioles. This condition is worsened by exposure to cold.

❍ **What is the most common source of acute mesenteric ischemia?**

Arterial embolism (40 to 50%). The source is usually the heart, generally from a mural thrombus. The most common point of obstruction is the superior mesenteric artery.

❍ **What lab results strongly suggest that a patient has mesenteric ischemia?**

Leukocytosis > 15,000, metabolic acidosis (sometimes with anion gap), hemoconcentration, and elevated phosphate and amylase.

❍ **Which type of myocardial infarction is more often associated with thrombosis: transmural or subendocardial?**

Transmural. Thrombolytic therapy increases left ventricle ejection fraction post MI, reduces the development of post infarction CHF, and can reduce early MI mortality by 25%.

❍ **How much aspirin should a post MI patient ingest daily to reduce the incidence of reinfarction?**

81 to 325 mg/day.

❍ **What is the most common cause of death during the first few hours of a MI?**

Cardiac arrhythmias, generally ventricular fibrillation.

❍ **When treating early MI's, beta-blockers decrease the risk of reinfarction. Which patients should not receive beta-blockers?**

Patients with hypotension, diabetes, CHF, severe left ventricular dysfunction, AV block, bradycardia, asthma, or another bronchospastic disease.

❍ **How common are PVC's in post MI patients?**

90% will have PVC's within the first few weeks. Concern arises if the PVC's are complex, which is the case in 20 to 40% of MI patients. Risk of sudden death in post-MI patients with complex PVC's increases 2 to 5 times.

❍ **What percentage of the LV myocardium must to be damaged to induce cardiogenic shock?**

40%. Twenty-five percent or more results in heart failure.

❍ **What percentage of MI's are clinically unrecognized?**

5 to 10%.

❍ **A non-Q wave infarction is usually associated with what?**

Subsequent angina or recurrent infarction. Non-Q wave infarctions also have lower in-hospital mortality rate compared to Q wave MI's.

❍ **Why do T waves invert in an AMI?**

Infarction or ischemia causes a reversal of the sequence of repolarization, i.e., endocardial-to-epicardial as opposed to normal epicardial-to-endocardial.

❍ **What ECG changes arise in a true posterior infarction?**

Large R wave and ST depression in V1 and V2.

❍ **What conduction defects commonly occur in an anterior wall MI?**

The dangerous kind. Damage to the conducting system results in a Mobitz II second or third degree AV block.

❍ **How should PSVT be treated during an AMI?**

Vagal maneuvers, adenosine, or cardioversion. Stable patients may be able to tolerate negative inotropes, such as verapamil or even beta-blockers.

❍ **A patient presents one day after discharge for an AMI with a new, harsh systolic murmur along the left sternal border and pulmonary edema. What is the diagnosis?**

Ventricular septal rupture. Diagnosis is confirmed with Swan-Ganz catheterization or echo. The treatment regime includes nitroprusside, for afterload reduction, and possibly an intra-aortic balloon pump followed by surgical repair.

❍ **When does cardiac rupture usually occur in patients who have suffered acute MI's?**

Fifty percent arise within the first 5 days, and 90% occur within the first 14 days post-MI.

❍ **Which type of infarct commonly leads to papillary muscle dysfunction?**

Inferior wall MI. Signs and symptoms include a mild transient systolic murmur and pulmonary edema.

❍ **A patient presents two weeks post AMI with chest pain, fever, and pleuripericarditis. A pleural effusion is detected by on CXR. What is the diagnosis?**

Dressler's (post-myocardial infarction) syndrome. This syndrome is caused by an immunologic reaction to myocardial antigens.

❍ **What percentage of patients over age 80 experience chest pain with an AMI?**

Only 50%. Twenty percent experience diaphoresis, stroke, syncope, and/or acute confusion.

❍ **Which type of thrombolytic agent is fibrin-specific?**

Tissue plasminogen activator. This agent is a human protein with no antigenic properties.

❍ **What are the most common causes of myocarditis in the US?**

Viruses. Other causes include post-viral myocarditis, an autoimmune response to recent viral infection, bacteria (diphtheria and tuberculosis), fungi, protozoa (Chagas' disease), and spirochetes (Lyme disease).

❍ **What percentage of non-anticoagulated patients with mitral stenosis experience systemic emboli?**

25%. Patients with chronic atrial fibrillation or mitral stenosis should be chronically anticoagulated to prevent atrial mural thrombi.

❍ **What is the most common cause of mitral stenosis?**

Rheumatic heart disease. The most common initial symptom is dyspnea.

❍ **What physical findings may be associated with mitral stenosis?**

Prominent α-wave, early-systolic left parasternal lift, loud and snapping first heart sound, and early-diastolic opening snap with a low-pitched mid-diastolic rumble that crescendos into S1.

❍ **What are the most common causes of acute mitral regurgitation?**

Rupture of the chordae tendinae, rupture of the papillary muscles, and perforation of the valve leaflets. Other causes include AMI and infectious endocarditis.

❍ **A mid-systolic click with a late systolic, crescendo murmur is indicative of what cardiac disease?**

Mitral valve prolapse (MVP).

❍ **Is mitral valve prolapse more common among men or women?**

Women have a stronger genetic link to the disease. However, only 2% to 5% of the entire population has symptomatic MVP.

❍ **What age group typically develops MVP syndrome?**

Patients in their twenties and thirties. Most patients with MVP are asymptomatic. MVP syndrome is symptomatic with chest pain, fatigue, palpitations, postural syncope, and dizziness.

❍ **What is the hallmark sign of MVP?**

A mid-systolic click, sometimes accompanied by a late systolic murmur. MVP, is largely a clinical diagnosis. An echocardiogram is performed to assess the degree of prolapse. Other clinical findings include a laterally displaced, diffuse apical pulse; decreased S1; split S2; and a holosystolic murmur radiating to the axilla.

❍ **What is the most prevalent cause of obstruction of the airway in adults?**

Food, usually meat. Obstruction occurs because the food was poorly chewed.

❍ **You are at a restaurant and the person at the table next to you begins coughing loudly. She stands up and begins wheezing between coughs, but she is still able to eke out a "Help! I'm choking". How should you help?**

Encourage her to cough deeper and keep breathing. Do not interrupt her spontaneous attempts at expulsion if she still has good air exchange, as evidenced by her state of consciousness and the degree of coughing and wheezing. Should she display severe respiratory difficulty with a weakening cough and the inability to talk, perform the Heimlich maneuver.

❍ **What should be done if the above patient is markedly obese and in severe respiratory distress?**

The normal Heimlich maneuver will not be as effective. Instead of positioning your fists above the patient's navel, place your cupped fist on the patient's chest and deliver swift thrusts. This is also the method of choice for pregnant women.

❍ **How do the fixed-rate and demand modes of pacemakers differ?**

Fixed-rate mode produces an impulse at a continuous specific rate, regardless of the patient's own cardiac activity. Demand mode detects the patient's electrical activity and triggers only if the heart is not depolarizing.

❍ **Describe the 3-lettered pacing code used in cardiac pacemakers.**

Letter 1: Chamber paced	Letter 2: Chamber sensed	Letter 3: Pacing function
O:None A:Atrial V:Ventricular D:Dual (A+V)	O:None A:Atrial V:Ventricular D:Dual (A+V)	O:None I:Inhibition T:Triggering D:Dual (I+T)

❍ **What is the treatment for ventricular fibrillation in a patient with a pacemaker?**

Defibrillation, but be sure to keep the paddles away from the pacer generator.

❍ **What is the average life span of a pacemaker?**

8 to 12 years.

❍ **A 25 year-old patient presents with splinted breathing and sharp, precordial chest pain that radiates to the back. The pain increases with inspiration and is mildly relieved by placing the patient in a forward sitting position. What does the ECG indicate?**

The ECG reveals intermittent supraventricular tachycardias, ST-segment elevation in at least seven leads (not counting aVR), PR depression, and T wave inversion may arise. The patient probably has pericarditis.

❍ **What is the most common cause of pericarditis?**

Idiopathic. Other causes are MI, post viral syndrome, aortic dissection that has ruptured into the pericardium, malignancy, radiation, chest trauma, connective tissue disease, uremia, and drugs (i.e., procainamide or hydralazine).

❍ **What physical finding indicates acute pericarditis?**

Pericardial friction rub. The rub is best heard at the left sternal border or apex with the patient in a forward sitting position. Other findings include fever and tachycardia.

❍ **Acute pyogenic pericarditis is most commonly caused by what organisms?**

Staphylococcus and Haemophilus influenza.

❍ **When diagnosing pericardial effusion, how much fluid must be present in the pericardial sac for visualization on an cardiac echocardiography and by x-ray?**

At least 15 ml for an echocardiography and 250 ml for an x-ray.

❍ **What will be the appearance of a pericardial effusion on an x-ray?**

A water-bottle silhouette.

❍ **At what volume does pericardial effusion affect the intrapericardial pressure?**

80 to 200 ml. However, the rate of accumulation is more important than the amount of accumulation. If accumulated slowly, the pericardium can tolerate up to 2000 ml of fluid.

❍ **What is the treatment for idiopathic pericarditis without effusion?**

A two week treatment of 650 mg aspirin every 4 hours, if no contraindications exist and if effusion is not present. Ibuprofen, indomethacin, or colchicine are other alternatives. The use of corticosteroids is controversial, because recurrent pericarditis is common when doses are tapered.

❍ **What is Virchow's triad?**

1) Injury to the endothelium of the vessels

2) Hypercoagulable state

3) Stasis

❍ **What does normal ventilation with mismatched decreased lung perfusion suggest?**

Pulmonary embolus.

❍ **What is the percentage of patients with angiography-proven pulmonary embolus (PE) whose initial ventilation-perfusion scan is reported as low probability?**

12%.

❍ **What are the most common signs and symptoms of PE?**

Tachypnea (92%), CP (88%), dyspnea (84%), anxiety (59%), tachycardia (44%), fever (43%), DVT (32%), hypotension (25%), and syncope (13%).

❍ **Can a patient with a PE have a pO_2 greater than 90 mm Hg?**

Yes, but rarely (5%).

❍ **What is the most common CXR finding in PE?**

Normal. The most common abnormal finding is elevated dome of one hemidiaphragm. This finding is caused by decreased lung volume, which occurs in 50% of patients with PE. Other common findings include a lack of lung markings in the area perfused by the occluded artery, pleural effusions, atelectasis, and pulmonary infiltrates.

❍ **What are two relatively specific CXR findings in PE?**

Hampton's hump: Area of lung consolidation with a rounded border facing the hilum.

Westermark's sign: Dilated pulmonary outflow tract, proximal to the emboli, with decreased perfusion distal to the lesion.

❍ **What test is considered the gold standard for the diagnosis of DVT? For the diagnosis of PE?**

The gold standard test for the diagnosis of DVT is venography. The gold standard for the diagnosis of PE is pulmonary angiography.

❍ **When treating DVT/PE, when should warfarin therapy be initiated?**

On the first or second day after initiation of heparin therapy. Although heparin should be administered immediately, it can be discontinued when the PTT is maintained at 1.5 to 1.8 times normal for at least 3 days.

❍ **How long should chronic warfarin therapy, as a prophylaxis for DVT, be given?**

Warfarin should be administered, for at least 3 to 6 months after a DVT, to maintain an INR at 2 to 3 times normal.

❍ **What historical findings suggest an embolus as opposed to a thrombosis in a lower extremity?**

Embolus: Associated with a history of arrhythmia, valvular disease, MI, no skin changes from chronic arterial insufficiency, and no symptoms in the opposite extremity.

Thrombosis: Opposite extremity shows evidence of chronic arterial occlusive disease with history of rest pain, claudication, etc.

❍ **How is a thrombus distinguished from an embolus on arteriography?**

A thrombus appears as a tapering lumen. An embolus has a sharp cutoff.

❍ **What is the risk factor for PE in a patient with an axillary or subclavian vein thrombus?**

About 15%.

❍ **Rheumatic heart disease is the most common cause of stenosis of what 3 heart valves?**

Mitral, aortic (along with congenital bicuspid valve), and tricuspid.

❍ **What is the 1-year recurrence rate for patients who have been resuscitated from sudden cardiac death?**

30%.

❍ **Describe the Trendelenburg test for varicose veins.**

Raise the leg above the heart, then quickly lower it. If the leg veins become distended immediately after this test is performed, valvular incompetence is evident.

❍ **What is a paradoxical embolus?**

A venous thrombus that goes through a right-to-left intra-cardiac shunt to the arterial side.

❍ **Why is a paradoxical embolus able to cause septic end-organ disease?**

An infected venous thrombus can enter the arterial circulation via the right-to-left intra-cardiac shunt and be sent distal to affect end-organs.

❍ **Splinter hemorrhages, Osler's nodes, Janeway lesions, petechiae, and Roth's spots can be indications of what process?**

They are physical signs associated with infective endocarditis.

❍ **T/F: Osler's nodes are usually nodular and painful.**

True. In contrast, the macular Janeway lesions are painless.

❍ **What other conditions besides infective endocarditis can Osler's nodes be found with?**

Nonbacterial thrombotic endocarditis, gonococcal infections, and hemolytic anemia.

❍ **What percentage of patients with infective endocarditis display peripheral manifestations of the disease?**

50%.

❍ **What is bacterial endocarditis?**

Blood-borne bacteria that attach onto damaged or abnormal heart valves or on the endocardium near anatomic defects.

❍ **How is bacterial endocarditis diagnosed?**

Evidence of valvular vegetations on echocardiogram combined with a positive blood culture.

❍ **If patients have not yet received antibiotics, what percentage of culture negative endocarditis is expected?**

Less than 5%.

❍ **What is the sensitivity rate of two-dimensional transesophageal echocardiograms for detecting vegetations?**

95%.

❍ **Who is at high risk for developing endocarditis?**

People with prosthetic heart valves, previous incidents of endocarditis, complex congenital heart disease, intravenous drug use, and surgically devised systemic pulmonary shunts.

❍ **Who is at moderate risk for developing endocarditis?**

Moderate risk factors include acquired valvular heart disease, hypertrophic cardiomyopathy and uncorrected congenital conditions. These conditions include patent ductus arteriosus, ventricular septal defect, primum atrial septal defect, coarctation of the aorta, and bicuspid aortic valve. It is controversial as to whether mitral valve prolapse with significant regurgitation is a moderate risk factor.

❍ **What are the bacteremia producing procedures that increase the risk for developing bacterial endocarditis?**

Dental and oral procedures increase the risk for developing bacterial endocarditis. Procedures involving the respiratory mucosa, gastrointestinal procedures, genitourinary tract procedures and finally vaginal delivery.

❍ **What is the appropriate prophylaxis for these procedures?**

Depending upon the nature of the procedure, amoxicillin, ampicillin, gentamicin, clindamycin, or a combination of these antibiotics are frequently used.

❍ **What is the most common organism associated with endocarditis?**

Streptococcus viridans, approximately one-third of current cases.

❍ **Fungi cause what percent of prosthetic valve infective endocarditis?**

15%.

❍ **History of contact with mammals and/or birds may suggest infection by what organisms?**

Coxiella burnetii (Q fever), Brucella species, or Chlamydia psittaci.

❍ **A nosocomial cluster of cases postoperatively may be caused by what organisms?**

Legionella species or Mycobacterium species.

❍ **What organism, once accounting for up to a quarter of the cases of endocarditis, is now only responsible for 1-2% of cases?**

Neisseria gonorrhea.

❍ **How is infective endocarditis treated?**

Intravenous antibiotics for 4-6 weeks. Close follow-up is necessary and the patient should have a series of two separate negative blood cultures to demonstrate resolution of the condition. If resolution of the infection does not occur promptly, embolization occurs, or fulminant CHF ensues, surgical valve replacement is indicated. Vegetations over 1 cm in diameter on echocardiogram have a better long-term prognosis with surgical valve replacement rather than medical therapy.

❍ **What are the EKG changes associated with pericarditis?**

Concave upward ST elevation in at least seven leads except V1 and AVR. PR segment depression may also be present.

❍ **Postpericardotomy syndrome, occasionally confused with infectious pericarditis, occurs in what percentage of patients who have undergone pericardotomy?**

10 to 30%.

❍ **What is the most frequently reported bacterial isolate in patients with myocardial abscesses?**

Staphylococcus aureus.

❍ **What is the clinical picture of myocardial abscesses?**

Low-grade fevers, chills, leukocytosis, conduction system abnormalities, nonspecific ECG changes and signs and symptoms of acute MI .

❍ **What is mural endocarditis?**

Inflammation and disruption of the nonvalvular endocardial surface of the cardiac chambers.

❍ **What is the presentation of mural endocarditis?**

Presentation is similar to infective valvular endocarditis.

❍ **What are the risk factors for mural endocarditis?**

Usually, mural endocarditis is from seeding of an abnormal area of endocardium during bacteremia or fungemia. Infectious thrombi from pulmonary veins, ventricular aneurysms, mural thrombi, chordal friction lesions, pacemaker lead insertion sites, idiopathic hypertrophic subaortic stenosis, jet lesions from ventriculoseptal defects, and other congenital defects are other factors. Immunocompromised patients are also at increased risks.

❍ **What is the definitive treatment of an infected atrial myxoma?**

Urgent surgical removal.

❍ **What is the risk for infection of a transvenous pacemaker during the first 3 years after insertion?**

1 to 6%.

❍ **What are the risk factors associated with the development of pacemaker infections?**

Risk factors include: diabetes, malignancy, skin disorders, malnutrition, anticoagulants, steroids, and immunosuppressive medications.

❍ **What are complications of pacemaker insertion?**

Post-insertion hematoma, seroma, or infection.

❍ **What are the infectious complications associated with infected endovascular leads?**

Valvular endocarditis, infected mural thrombi, localized abscesses, and late electrode perforation.

❍ **What is the most common cause of infection early after insertion?**

Staphylococcus aureus.

❍ **What is the most prevalent organism greater than one month after insertion?**

Staphylococcus epidermidis.

❍ **What is a major risk factor for prosthetic vascular graft infection?**

Location. The incidence of infection is 1% to 1.5% for aorto-iliac grafts as opposed to 2% to 7% for femoral-popliteal arterial grafts.

❍ **What is thought to be the cause of this infection?**

95% of the time, contamination at the time of insertion is thought to cause the infection.

❍ **What is the most common organism?**

Staphylococci cause more than 40% of prosthetic vascular graft infections.

❍ **What is the clinical presentation of prosthetic vascular graft infection?**

Erythema, skin breakdown, or purulent drainage. Other symptoms may be thrombosis of the graft, fluid around the graft, or pseudoaneurysm formation.

❍ **What is the treatment for prosthetic vascular graft infection?**

Removal of the graft with debridement of the surrounding tissue. Extra-anatomic bypass may be needed. Often, this is impossible and amputation is required.

❍ **How do you diagnose a line infection?**

Controversial. However, a series of positive blood cultures and/or a positive line tip culture with greater than 15 colony-forming units with the same organism would be considered a line infection. Culturing the distal tip is more sensitive and specific for infection. A warm, tender, erythematous site with purulence is an infected line.

❍ **What time after insertion are pulmonary artery catheters considered to be infected?**

After approximately 72 hours.

❍ **What are complications from arterial catheterization?**

Thrombosis (19-38%), infection (4-23%), pseudoaneurysm, and rupture.

❍ **How should you treat line infections?**

Controversial. Two schools of thought. One is that when a line is removed, the source of infection is removed and the infection is treated. Another school of thought believes antibiotics are required as well.

❍ **What are the most common organisms involved with line infections?**

Staphylococcus epidermidis and Staphylococcus aureus.

❍ **What is the most frequent cause of mitral stenosis?**

Rheumatic fever. Far less common causes include congenital, malignant carcinoid, SLE, rheumatoid arthritis, infective endocarditis with a large vegetation, and the muccopolysaccharidoses of the Hunter-Hurley phenotype.

❍ **What percentage of patients with rheumatic mitral stenosis are female?**

Two-thirds.

❍ **What percentage of patients with rheumatic heart disease have pure mitral stenosis?**

Twenty five percent. An additional 40% have combined MS and MR.

❍ **What is the cross-sectional area of the mitral valve orifice in critical mitral stenosis?**

One cm^2 or less. The normal cross sectional area is between 4-6 cm^2. Mild mitral stenosis begins when the valve is reduced to approximately 2 cm^2.

❍ **What are the principle symptoms in mitral stenosis?**

Dyspnea is most common. Patients with severe mitral stenosis can experience orthopnea, hemoptysis, chest pain, and frank pulmonary edema, often precipitated by exertion, fever, URI, sexual intercourse, pregnancy or the onset of rapid atrial fibrillation.

❍ **What are the two most serious complications of mitral stenosis?**

Thromboembolism, most often occurring in the setting of atrial fibrillation, and pulmonary edema.

❍ **What are the physical findings in patients with mitral stenosis?**

A low-pitched diastolic rumbling murmur, with or without a thrill, at the apex; a diminished S1 heart sound (may be virtually absent in severe MS); an opening snap following the second heart sound; a loud P2 heart sound in patients with pulmonary hypertension; fixed splitting of the second heart sound; a Graham-Steell murmur of pulmonic regurgitation in patients with moderate to severe pulmonary hypertension; and a right parasternal S4 heart sound in patients with right heart failure.

❍ **What maneuvers can one do to differentiate the opening snap of mitral stenosis from a split S2 sound?**

Sudden standing widens the A2-opening snap interval whereas a split S2 narrows on standing. Progressive narrowing of the A2-OS interval on serial examinations suggests an increase in the severity of mitral stenosis.

❍ **What is the most accurate noninvasive technique for quantifying the severity of mitral stenosis?**

Doppler echocardiography.

❍ **What is the medical management strategy of rheumatic mitral stenosis?**

1) Penicillin prophylaxis for beta-hemolytic streptococcal infections and prophylaxis for infective endocarditis; 2) aggressive and prompt treatment of anemia and infections; 3) avoidance of strenuous exertion; 4) oral diuretics and sodium restriction in symptomatic patients; 5) beta-blockers to reduce heart rate; 6) cardioversion of atrial fibrillation, if possible; 7) aggressive slowing of refractory atrial fibrillation; and 8) anticoagulant therapy in patients who have experienced one or more thromboembolic episodes, or who have mechanical prosthetic valves.

❍ **What is the asymptomatic period after an attack of rheumatic fever in patients with mitral stenosis?**

In temperate zones, such as the United States and Europe, about 15-20 years. In tropical and subtropical areas and in underdeveloped areas, about 6-12 years.

❍ **What is the indication for mitral valve surgery or balloon valvuloplasty in patients with mitral stenosis?**

Moderate symptoms (Class II) or greater in a patient with moderate to severe mitral stenosis (mitral valve orifice size less than 1.0 cm^2 per square meter BSA-less than 1.5 to 1.7 cm^2 mitral valve area in normal-sized adults).

❍ **A 28 year-old Hispanic female is referred to you for evaluation of dyspnea and palpitations. She has a diastolic murmur consistent with mitral stenosis. Echocardiography confirms severe, non-calcific mitral stenosis with trivial mitral regurgitation, with a mitral valve area of 0.8 cm^2. EKG reveals atrial fibrillation. She was recently married and would like to start a family. What is the most appropriate course of therapy for this patient?**

Open mitral valvotomy (commisurotomy) followed by cardioversion to normal sinus rhythm. This is palliative, obviates the need for anticoagulation for the immediate future, and results in at least 5-10 years of symptom free life for over half of the patients.

❍ **What is the complication and mortality rates for balloon mitral valvuloplasty?**

The reported mortality rate averages 0.5 %. Complications such as stroke and cardiac perforation occur in 1% of cases, atrial septal defect in 10%, and 2% develop severe mitral regurgitation requiring mitral valve replacement.

❍ **What is the most common cause of mitral regurgitation?**

Rheumatic heart disease. It is more frequent in men than women. Other causes include infective endocarditis, mitral valve prolapse, ischemic heart disease, trauma, SLE, scleroderma, hypertrophic cardiomyopathy, dilated cardiomyopathy involving the left ventricle, and idiopathic degenerative calcification of the mitral annulus.

❍ **What percentage of patients with coronary artery disease considered for CABG have mitral regurgitation?**

Thirty percent. It is secondary to ischemic papillary muscle dysfunction.

❍ **What is the 5-year survival of medically treated patients with severe mitral regurgitation?**

Forty-five percent.

❍ **What are the physical findings of patients with chronic mitral regurgitation?**

Harsh, pansystolic murmur heard best at the apex, radiating to the axilla or the base. The murmur is diminished by maneuvers that decrease preload or afterload, such as amyl nitrate inhalation, Valsalva or standing and increases with maneuvers that increase preload or afterload, such as squatting, handgrip or phenylephrine administration.

❍ **What are the most common causes of acute mitral regurgitation?**

Acute myocardial infarction with papillary muscle dysfunction (15% of acute MI results in acute mitral regurgitation) or papillary muscle rupture (.3% of acute MI), infective endocarditis, chordae tendinae rupture secondary to chest trauma, rheumatic fever, mitral valve prolapse, and hypertrophic cardiomyopathy with rupture of chordae tendinae.

❍ **What are the physical findings in patients with severe, chronic mitral regurgitation?**

Diminished S1 heart sound with wide splitting of S2, a loud P2 in patients with pulmonary hypertension, an S3 gallop at the apex, and a harsh pansystolic murmur at the apex with a thrill.

❍ **Which is the best test to assess the detailed anatomy of rheumatic mitral valve disease and determine whether mitral valve replacement is necessary or whether reconstruction is feasible?**

Transesophageal echocardiography.

❍ **What is the appropriate medical management of mitral regurgitation?**

Vasodilator therapy with ACE inhibitors is the hallmark of therapy, even in patients who are asymptomatic. Diuretics are used in patients with severe MR. Cardiac glycosides, such as digoxin, are indicated in patients with severe MR and clinical evidence of heart failure. Endocarditis prophylaxis is indicated in all patients with MR. Anticoagulation should be given to all patients in atrial fibrillation.

❍ **A 33 year-old female comes to you for a physical and you notice a harsh systolic murmur at the apex that is also heard at the base. The murmur increases on standing and Valsalva and decreases with handgrip. What is the most likely finding on echocardiography?**

Mitral valve prolapse. The murmur of pure mitral regurgitation decreases with Valsalva and standing and increases with handgrip or squatting.

❍ **A 46 year-old male with a history of rheumatic fever at age 12 is admitted with an acute myocardial infarction. The patient's post-MI course is complicated by congestive heart failure. Echocardiogram reveals severe mitral regurgitation with rupture of one of the papillary muscles, prolapse of the posterior mitral valve leaflet without apparent calcification. Systolic function by echocardiogram is mildly reduced. What is the appropriate course of action in this patient?**

Mitral valve reconstruction and repair of the papillary muscle.

❍ **What are the indications for operation in patients with severe, chronic mitral regurgitation?**

Patients with NYHA class II symptoms with end-systolic LV diameter of >45mm by echocardiography. Asymptomatic patients with severe MR under the age of 70 with ejection fractions less than 70% and end-systolic LV diameter >40mm by echocardiography who are likely to be candidates for mitral valve repair should also be strongly considered for surgery.

❍ **What is the classic triad of symptoms of aortic stenosis?**

Syncope (often exertional), angina, and heart failure.

❍ **What is the most common cause of aortic stenosis in patients under age 65?**

Calcification of congenitally bicuspid aortic valves (50%) followed by rheumatic heart disease (25%)

❍ **What is the most common cause of aortic stenosis in patients over age 65?**

Calcific degeneration of the aortic leaflets.

❍ **Once patients with aortic stenosis become symptomatic, what is their average survival without valve replacement?**

From the onset of syncope or angina, the mean survival is 2-3 years. From the onset of congestive heart failure, the mean survival is 1.5 years.

❍ **A 72 year-old gentleman is referred to you by a general surgeon because of a systolic heart murmur. On examination, you hear a mid-systolic crescendo-decrescendo murmur at the right parasternal second ICS, radiating to the carotids. Carotid upstroke is delayed. The patient is asymptomatic without any history of angina or syncope. Echocardiography reveals an aortic valve area of 0.85 cm^2. He is not in need of elective surgery. What should you advise the patient to do?**

Surgery is not necessary at this point, but the patient should be told that he must report any symptoms of angina, dyspnea, or syncope. At that point, he should be promptly referred for left heart catheterization and coronary angiography in preparation for surgical replacement of the valve. In the meantime, repeat echocardiography should be carried out every 6-12 months.

❍ **What is the operative risk for aortic valve replacement?**

In patients without frank CHF, the operative risk ranges from 2-8%. It is not appreciably higher in patients requiring concomitant myocardial revascularization.

❍ **What is the strongest predictor of postoperative LV dysfunction following aortic valve replacement?**

Preoperative LV dysfunction.

❍ **How does a heart murmur reflect the severity of aortic stenosis?**

The longer the duration of the murmur and the greater the increase in intensity of the murmur, the more severe the aortic stenosis. The degree of loudness of the murmur is not as important in assessing severity.

❍ **What is the best pharmacologic agent for patients with asymptomatic aortic stenosis?**

Without contraindications, beta-blockers are the best agents as they are the most useful in treating the left ventricular hypertrophy and its sequelae that develop as a result of aortic stenosis.

❍ **A 68 year-old female with severe asymptomatic aortic stenosis suddenly complains of dyspnea and palpitations. On EKG, she is found to be in atrial fibrillation with a ventricular rate of 130 beats per minute. What is the most appropriate action to be taken?**

Immediate DC cardioversion, followed by a search for previously unrecognized mitral valve disease. Once stabilized, the patient should be referred for cardiac catheterization and aortic valve replacement.

❍ **What percentage of patients with mitral valve prolapse, who develop severe mitral regurgitation or infective endocarditis, require mitral valve surgery?**

About 5%, mostly men over the age of 50.

❍ **What is the most common sustained tachyarrhythmia in patients with mitral valve prolapse?**

Paroxysmal supraventricular tachycardia.

❍ **What do patients with mitral valve prolapse have in common with patients with recognized heritable disorders of connective tissue?**

Mitral valve prolapse may be inherited as an autosomal dominant phenotype and a large proportion of patients with mitral valve prolapse have systemic features such as anterior chest deformity, scoliosis, kyphosis, hypermobile joints and arm span greater than height. In addition, mitral valve prolapse is common in patients with Marfan's syndrome, the Ehlers-Danlos syndrome and adult polycystic kidney disease.

❍ **What is mitral valve prolapse syndrome?**

A symptom complex consisting of palpitations, chest pain, easy fatigability, exercise intolerance, dyspnea, orthostatic phenomena, and syncope or pre-syncope in patients with mitral valve prolapse, predominantly related to autonomic dysfunction.

❍ **What disorders are seen with increased frequency in patients with MVP syndrome?**

Graves' disease, asthma, migraine headaches, sleep disorders, fibromyositis, and functional gastrointestinal syndromes.

❍ **What are the most beneficial therapies in patients with mitral valve prolapse?**

Daily exercise, beta-blockers, adequate intravascular volume and reassurance.

❍ **What infrequent cause of mitral regurgitation is associated with an increased risk of stroke, independent of other factors?**

Mitral annular calcification.

❍ **A 28 year-old black female comes to you with pain and stiffness in her shoulders, knees, elbows and wrists for three days. She is acutely febrile, but denies cough, shortness of breath, dysuria, diarrhea, abdominal pain. On auscultation, you notice a harsh pansystolic murmur at the apex radiating to the axilla. Prior to her symptoms, she felt well, but states that she has frequent episodes of joint pain which last a couple of days, then disappear. She denies any vaginal discharge and denies any sexual intercourse for the last 6 weeks. Her mother has rheumatoid arthritis. Her sedimentation rate is 50. What should you suspect and test for in this patient?**

The primary anti-phospholipid syndrome of SLE.

❍ **What is the most common cause of isolated severe aortic regurgitation?**

Aortic root dilatation resulting from medial disease. Other common causes include congenital (bicuspid) aortic valve, previous infective endocarditis, and rheumatic heart disease.

❍ **A 64 year-old gentleman who is three weeks post-cholecystectomy suffers from moderate malnutrition. He has been on TPN for 10 days and for the last four days, has spiked a fever of 102° F. The patient is noticeably dyspneic with a respiratory rate of 26 and a HR of 110, in sinus rhythm by ECG. Blood cultures grow Candida albicans. CXR reveals moderate pulmonary congestion. An S3 gallop is heard at the apex and a low-pitched decrescendo diastolic murmur is heard at the LSB. An echocardiogram reveals a 17 mm diameter vegetation on the non-coronary cusp of the aortic valve and Doppler echo reveals severe aortic regurgitation. What is the best course of action for this patient?**

IV Amphotericin, IV vasodilators such as Nitroprusside, IV Dobutamine followed by urgent AV replacement. Vegetation larger than 10 mm in diameter, particularly fungal, are rarely controlled with pharmacologic therapy alone, and surgery is almost always needed, even if the aortic regurgitation is mild or moderate.

❍ **What murmur may be mistaken for mitral stenosis?**

The Austin-Flint murmur of severe aortic regurgitation, which occurs from a powerful regurgitant jet from the aorta, imparted to the anterior leaflet of the mitral valve, limiting the opening of the anterior leaflet of the mitral valve.

❍ **What is the survival of chronic aortic regurgitation after diagnosis?**

The five-year survival, after diagnosis, is 75%. The ten-year survival is 50%. Once symptoms begin, without surgical treatment, death occurs within 4 years after the development of angina, 2 years after the development of CHF.

❍ **What percentage of patients with asymptomatic severe aortic regurgitation develop LV systolic dysfunction, sudden death or symptoms within 10 years?**

40%.

❍ **What is the 5 and 10 year mortality of symptomatic severe aortic regurgitation without surgical valve replacement?**

25% and 50%, respectively.

❍ **What are the indications for aortic valve replacement in patients with chronic aortic regurgitation?**

LV end-systolic dimension of >50mm, LVEF < 50%, and the onset of symptoms of angina or CHF.

❍ **What is the preferred pharmacologic agent in patients with asymptomatic chronic aortic regurgitation?**

Nifedipine, or ACE inhibitors. Both have shown major improvements in LVEF and major reduction in LV end-diastolic volume and mass with significantly lower incidence of the need for aortic valve replacement at 5 years.

❍ **What is the most common acquired abnormality that produces clinically significant tricuspid regurgitation?**

Dilatation of the tricuspid annulus related to right ventricular dilatation.

❍ **What is the most common congenital abnormality producing tricuspid regurgitation?**

Tricuspid valve prolapse. Less common is Ebstein's anomaly.

❍ **What is the most common cause of acute tricuspid regurgitation and what is the preferred management of this situation?**

Tricuspid valve endocarditis, often as a result of intravenous drug abuse. The preferred management is complete removal of the valve with immediate or eventual replacement of the valve. Antibiotic therapy usually is futile in preventing valve surgery.

❍ **A 38 year-old Hispanic female with known mitral valve prolapse is scheduled for dental cleaning. Her dentist calls you asking for recommendations for endocarditis prophylaxis. She is not allergic to penicillin. What are your recommendations?**

Amoxicillin 3.0 gm po one hour before the procedure followed by 1.5 gm po six hours after the initial dose.

❍ **What is the incidence of culture-negative endocarditis?**

About 5%.

❍ **How does the sensitivity of transthoracic echocardiography compare with transesophageal echocardiography in the diagnosis of infective endocarditis?**

Transthoracic echocardiography carries a diagnostic sensitivity of 30-40%, whereas transesophageal echocardiography carries a diagnostic sensitivity between 90-100%.

❍ **A 55 year-old gentleman who underwent a 4 vessel CABG three years ago has mild mitral and tricuspid regurgitation is scheduled for colonoscopy for rectal bleeding. What recommendations regarding endocarditis prophylaxis would you give the surgeon?**

No antibiotic prophylaxis is needed in this setting.

❍ **How much myocardial damage from an acute myocardial infarction is necessary to result in congestive heart failure?**

Congestive heart failure is usually evident clinically if more than 25% of the left ventricle is infarcted.

❍ **What three secondary processes resulting in myocardial deterioration occur following acute myocardial infarction?**

Ventricular remodeling, typically following Q-wave infarctions; infarct expansion, occurring most frequently from anterior-apical infarctions and results in thinning of the left ventricular wall; and ventricular dilatation, an early and progressive response to acute myocardial infarction that is an important predictor of increased mortality following myocardial infarction.

❍ **What factors play a role in the peak incidence of myocardial infarction being from 6 AM to noon?**

Blood pressure, coronary arterial tone, blood viscosity, circulating catecholamines and platelet aggregability increase on awakening and assumption of an erect posture.

❍ **What is the most common cause of death related to acute myocardial infarction?**

Ventricular fibrillation, occurring within the first hour following symptoms.

❍ **What percentage of patients with acute myocardial infarction develop cardiogenic shock?**

10%.

❍ **What percentage of patients who are found to have myocardial infarction by other objective means, such as cardiac enzymes or radionuclide imaging studies, have normal initial ECG's?**

10%.

❍ **What is the mortality among patients with their first myocardial infarction?**

2-3% in patients under 40 years of age, 7-10% in patients between 70-80 years of age, and 32% in patients older than 80 years of age.

❍ **What percentage of arteries successfully opened with thrombolytic therapy for acute myocardial infarction, reocclude?**

15% of arteries successfully opened reocclude during the first few days following thrombolytic therapy.

❍ **What is the mortality benefit from aspirin alone in acute myocardial infarction with thrombolytic therapy and in subsequent reinfarction?**

Aspirin reduced mortality from acute myocardial infarction by 23% and reduced non-fatal reinfarction by 49%. When used with thrombolytic therapy, there was a 40-50% reduction in mortality from acute myocardial infarction.

❍ **A 63 year-old gentleman presents to the Emergency department with moderate substernal chest pressure and lightheadedness for 90 minutes. His BP on admission is 80/40 and his HR is 110/min and regular. Physical exam reveals JVD to the angle of the jaw, a right parasternal S3 gallop, an apical S4 gallop and clear lungs on auscultation. ECG reveals 2 mm ST elevation in leads II, III, and aVF with reciprocal ST depression in V1-V3. What is the most likely diagnosis and what is the most appropriate initial therapy?**

Inferior myocardial infarction with right ventricular infarction. Following 160-325 mg of aspirin administration, thrombolytic therapy, and a large bolus of intravenous saline followed by a moderately high infusion rate of saline are indicated. If the patient remains hypotensive despite adequate intravenous saline, as measured by the development of lung congestion on auscultation, intravenous Dobutamine is indicated.

❍ **A 47 year-old woman is admitted to you with substernal chest pressure for 1 hour. Serial ECG's and CK measurements confirm a non-Q wave anterior wall myocardial infarction. She has no arrhythmias, no evidence of heart failure and no recurrent chest pain while in the hospital. You discharge her on Diltiazem and aspirin on the fifth hospital day after she had a normal pre-discharge low-level treadmill exercise test. You schedule her for a symptom-limited treadmill test in two weeks. Three days after discharge, she reports a ten-minute episode of substernal chest pressure, while walking across the room, relieved with one sublingual nitroglycerin. What should you advise her to do?**

Readmit her to the hospital, place her on intravenous heparin and nitroglycerin and perform cardiac catheterization with coronary angiography the following morning.

❍ **A 56 year-old gentleman presents to your office three weeks after suffering an inferior wall myocardial infarction, treated successfully with r-TPA . He has non-insulin dependent diabetes mellitus. He denies any post-infarct symptoms. You supervise a symptom-limited treadmill exercise test which reveals 2 mm horizontal ST depression in the inferior and lateral leads after three minutes of exercise on Bruce protocol. On your recommendation, he undergoes a coronary angiogram and cardiac catheterization which reveals >70% stenosis of the proximal LAD, mid-RCA and first obtuse marginal branch of the circumflex. The LVEF on ventriculogram is 44%. What should you advise your patient at this time?**

Undergo 3-vessel coronary artery bypass graft surgery.

❍ **A 70 year-old man is admitted to the hospital with chest pain of 3 hours duration. ECG demonstrates anterior ST elevation for which he is given aspirin, r-TPA, heparin and intravenous nitroglycerin. His symptoms resolve. Serum chemistries reveal a peak CPK of 1800 and a CK-MB fraction of 15%. He is eventually transferred out of the CCU and his hospitalization is uneventful until day 5, when he develops sudden, severe shortness of breath. BP is 110/75 and his pulse is 125 and regular. Examination reveals a new systolic murmur. What would the most appropriate therapeutic intervention be?**

Intravenous sodium nitroprusside. This patient is most likely suffering from rupture of the left ventricular septum and subsequent defect, a not uncommon complication of MI. Afterload reduction is key to stabilization until surgical repair of the VSD can be performed, usually in about 8-12 weeks, after the infarct has healed. If nitroprusside fails to stabilize the patient, intra-aortic balloon counterpulsation and intravenous nitroglycerin should be employed.

❍ **A 60 year-old patient suffers an acute inferior myocardial infarction. Three hours after he arrives in the hospital, he develops ventricular fibrillation and is successfully defibrillated back to normal sinus rhythm within 30 seconds. He makes a full recovery and has no further post-MI**

complications. What does his ventricular fibrillation episode indicate with regard to his subsequent risk of sudden death?

This episode has no bearing on his subsequent risk of sudden death. Ventricular fibrillation in the immediate setting of an acute myocardial infarction has no prognostic significance.

❍ **A 65 year old female presents to the hospital with sudden crushing chest discomfort and moderate shortness of breath. Her initial ECG reveals 2mm ST depression in leads V1-V4 with inverted T waves. She has bibasilar rales in the lower half of both lungs on auscultation. CXR reveals moderate pulmonary edema. Serial ECG's and CPK's confirm a non-Q wave myocardial infarction. With diuretics, her pulmonary edema resolves within 24 hours. What is the most appropriate management strategy at this point?**

Cardiac catheterization with coronary angiography. A non-Q wave MI that results in pulmonary edema signifies a large amount of myocardium at risk for reinfarction within the next year.

❍ **What arrhythmias that occur in patients with acute myocardial infarction require temporary pacing?**

Complete heart block (3° AV block); new LBBB; new bifascicular block; marked sinus bradycardia with ischemic pain, hypotension, CHF, frequent PVC's or syncope despite atropine; and Mobitz II type 2° AV block.

❍ **A 54 year-old gentleman, admitted two days ago with an acute anterolateral myocardial infarction, suddenly develops atrial fibrillation with a ventricular rate of 135/min. He subsequently complains of substernal chest discomfort. His BP is 135/70. What is the most appropriate immediate action to be taken?**

Synchronized DC cardioversion.

❍ **What percentage of patients with acute myocardial infarction develop paroxysmal atrial fibrillation?**

10-15%.

❍ **T/F: The presence of occasional PVC's is a reliable predictor of ventricular fibrillation following acute myocardial infarction.**

False.

❍ **A 58 year-old gentleman is admitted with an acute anteroseptal myocardial infarction. He is in pulmonary edema clinically, confirmed by CXR. His blood pressure is 122/76, his HR is 122. Despite two doses of 80 mg of intravenous furosemide, he remains in pulmonary edema. A Swan-Ganz pulmonary artery catheter is inserted and his initial hemodynamics reveal a cardiac output of 3.1 L/min and a pulmonary capillary wedge pressure of 27 mm Hg. What is the most appropriate pharmacologic agent in this setting?**

Intravenous Dobutamine, at a dose of 5 to 20 mcg/kg/min.

❍ **What is the mortality of cardiogenic shock in acute myocardial infarction?**

>70%.

❍ **What is the incidence of rupture of the free wall of the left ventricle in patients with acute myocardial infarction who do not survive?**

10%. It is almost always fatal, occurring between 1 and 5 days following infarction.

❍ **What percentage of patients with acute myocardial infarction develop left ventricular aneurysms?**

10%. 80% of LV aneurysms are located in the anterior-apical segment and result from occlusion of the left anterior descending artery.

❍ **What are the major complications of left ventricular aneurysms?**

LV thrombus formation (with the subsequent risk of thromboembolic events), CHF, and ventricular arrhythmias.

❍ **What percentage of patients with acute anterior-apical Q wave infarctions develop LV mural thrombi?**

50%. Over half develop mural thrombi within the first 24 hours.

❍ **What percentage of patients with acute myocardial infarction have a clinically evident embolic event?**

4%, most within the first week following infarction.

❍ **What is the current recommended therapy for patients with large anterior myocardial infarctions?**

Reperfusion therapy with thrombolytics, beta-blockers, intravenous nitroglycerin, and ACE inhibitors to limit and retard ventricular remodeling. Intravenous heparin in a sufficient dose to prolong the APTT to 1.5 to 2.0 times control should be started on admission and continued to discharge. In patients with large akinetic apical segments or mural thrombi, oral anticoagulation with warfarin is indicated for 3-6 months.

❍ **What is the significance of pericarditis following acute myocardial infarction?**

Pericarditis occurs in about 20% of patients with acute myocardial infarction, more likely in Q-wave infarcts than non-Q wave infarcts. Patients with pericarditis usually have significantly larger infarcts, lower ejection fractions, and a higher incidence of congestive heart failure. The presence of pericarditis and/or pericardial effusion following acute myocardial infarction is associated with a higher mortality.

❍ **A previously healthy 65 year-old man is admitted with an acute inferior myocardial infarction. Within several hours, he is hypotensive (BP 90/60), and oliguric. Insertion of a pulmonary artery catheter reveals the following pressures: pulmonary artery wedge pressure, 3 mm Hg; pulmonary artery, 21/3 mm Hg; and mean right atrial pressure, 11 mm Hg. What is the best treatment for this man?**

Fluids until his wedge pressure is between 16-20 mm Hg.

❍ **A 60 year-old man with a recent syncopal episode is hospitalized with congestive heart failure and chest pain. His BP is 165/85 mm Hg, his pulse is 85/min and there is a grade III/VI harsh systolic murmur at the apex and aortic area. An echocardiogram reveals a disproportionately thickened septum and anterior systolic motion of the mitral valve. What is this patient's diagnosis and what physical findings would most likely be present?**

Obstructive hypertrophic cardiomyopathy (IHSS). The murmur typically decreases with handgrip and squatting, and increases with Valsalva vasodilators, standing, nitroglycerin, diuretics and digoxin. Mitral regurgitation is frequent as a result of anterior systolic motion of the mitral valve. Congestive heart failure is present because of diastolic dysfunction, thus an S4 gallop is common.

❍ **A 68 year-old male with diabetes and a 60 pack-year history of smoking presents with sudden, severe substernal chest discomfort, radiating through to the interscapular area. BP is 150/80 mm Hg in the right arm and 135/65 mm Hg in the left arm. He complains of right arm numbness and weakness and you hear a II/IV diastolic murmur along the left sternal border. ECG reveals 1.5 mm ST elevation in the inferior leads. What is the diagnosis?**

Acute proximal thoracic aortic dissection, with involvement of the right coronary artery and brachiocephalic artery, as well as acute aortic regurgitation.

❍ **In the patient described in the last question, what other life-threatening complication must one look for, both on auscultation and on CXR?**

Pericardial effusion with cardiac tamponade. Look for pericardial rub on auscultation and marked cardiomegaly on CXR. Pulsus paradoxus of >10 mm Hg is virtually diagnostic of cardiac tamponade in this setting.

❍ **What CXR findings occur with a dissecting thoracic aortic aneurysm?**

Tortuosity of the proximal aorta with an enlarged aortic knob, mediastinal widening, pleural effusion (most common on the left), extension of the aortic shadow, displaced trachea to the right, cardiomegaly, and separation of the intimal calcification from the outer contour that is greater than 5 mm.

❍ **Where is an aortic dissection most likely to occur?**

Dissection involves intimal tears that are propagated by hematoma formation. Tears most commonly occur in the proximal ascending aorta (60%). 20% are found between the origin of the left subclavian and the ligamentum arteriosum in the descending aorta, 10% are found in the aortic arch, and 10% are found in the abdominal aorta distal to the renal arteries.

❍ **What is the definitive diagnostic procedure of choice for dissecting aortic aneurysms?**

Aortography.

❍ **When should surgery be advised for a non-dissecting thoracic aneurysm? For a non-dissecting abdominal aneurysm?**

A non-dissecting thoracic aneurysm should be resected if it is larger than 6 cm in diameter or has symptoms attributable to the aneurysm. Thoracic aneurysm enlarging under observation should also be resected. Non-dissecting abdominal aneurysms should be surgically resected if it is larger than 4 cm in diameter.

❍ **What is the prognosis for an untreated dissecting aortic aneurysm?**

Twenty five percent die within 24 hours, 50% die within one week, 75% percent die within one month and 90% die within 3 months. With surgical treatment, the 10 year survival is 50%, the five year survival is 75-80%. Redissection occurs in 25% within 10 years of the original dissection.

❍ **Which age group is typically afflicted with Marfan's syndrome accompanied by aortic dissection?**

Individuals between 30-50. Aortic aneurysms, in general, occur most frequently in individuals between 60-80.

❍ **What are the most common causes of MAT (multifocal atrial tachycardia)?**

COPD with exacerbation is the most common cause, followed by CHF, sepsis and methylxanthine toxicity. Treatment consists of treatment of the underlying disorder as well as the use of verapamil, magnesium, or digoxin for slowing the arrhythmia.

❍ **How is atrial flutter treated?**

Initiate A-V nodal blockade with beta-adrenergic blocking agents, calcium channel blockers or digoxin to slow the rate. Once this is accomplished, treat a stable patient with chemical cardioversion using a class 1A agent, such as quinidine or procainamide. If this fails to convert the patient, or the patient is unstable, synchronized electrocardioversion should be attempted starting at 25-50 Joules.

❍ **What are the most common causes of atrial fibrillation?**

Coronary artery disease, with myocardial ischemia, and hypertensive heart disease are the most common causes. Mitral or aortic valvular heart disease, cor pulmonale, dilated cardiomyopathy, hypertrophic cardiomyopathy (particularly the obstructive type), alcohol intoxication "holiday heart syndrome", hypo- or hyperthyroidism, pulmonary embolism, sepsis, hypoxia, pre-excitation syndrome and pericarditis are also common causes.

❍ How is atrial fibrillation treated?

The treatment of atrial fibrillation consists of three major considerations: 1) control of ventricular rate, 2) conversion, if possible or feasible, to sinus rhythm, and 3) prevention of thromboembolic events, particularly CVA. Rate control is best managed with beta-adrenergic blockers or calcium channel blockers (diltiazem or verapamil), or less desirable, digoxin. Digoxin should be used in patients with poor LV systolic function and those with a contraindication to beta-blockers and calcium channel blockers. Digoxin provides good rate control at rest, but often suboptimal rate control during exertion. Conversion to sinus rhythm, in the stable patient, is best managed, initially, with antiarrhythmic agents, such as 1A agents like quinidine or procainamide, 1C agents such as propafenone or Class III agents like amiodarone or sotalol. In the unstable patient or the patient with acute ischemia, hypotension or pulmonary edema, immediate synchronized electrical cardioversion, starting at 200 joules should be performed. If, in the stable patient, cardioversion with antiarrhythmic agents is unsuccessful, synchronized electrical cardioversion should be performed without interruption of antiarrhythmic therapy. Patients with atrial fibrillation of 1 year duration or longer, or those with left atrial size of >5.0 cm on echocardiography should not be cardioverted because of the extremely low success rate. Patients with recent atrial fibrillation >3 days duration should be started on Warfarin and anticoagulated to an INR between 2-3.5 for at least three weeks, before any attempt to cardiovert to sinus rhythm, because of the significant risk of embolic CVA. Those patients with chronic atrial fibrillation should be on lifelong Warfarin, unless an absolute contraindication to Warfarin exists or the patient cannot reliably take Warfarin.

❍ What percentage of patients with atrial fibrillation converted to sinus rhythm will revert back into atrial fibrillation?

50% will revert back to atrial fibrillation within one year of cardioversion, regardless of medical therapy.

❍ What is the risk of CVA in patients with atrial fibrillation, with and without anticoagulation?

Patients with atrial fibrillation, not anticoagulated with warfarin, have a 25% incidence of CVA within 5 years (5% per year). Those patients anticoagulated to therapeutic levels have a 4% incidence of CVA within 5 years (0.8% per year). Aspirin is a clearly inferior substitute to warfarin, but is much more preferable to no anticoagulant or antithrombotic therapy.

❍ What is the most common mechanism responsible for supraventricular tachycardia (SVT)?

AV node re-entry.

❍ What are the common causes of SVT?

Myocardial ischemia, myocardial infarction, congestive heart failure, pericarditis, rheumatic heart disease, mitral valve prolapse, pre-excitation syndromes, COPD, ethanol intoxication, hypoxia, pneumonia, sepsis and digoxin toxicity.

❍ What is the treatment of paroxysmal SVT?

In a hemodynamically stable patient, intravenous adenosine. If unsuccessful, then intravenous verapamil, beta-blockers or procainamide. In the unstable patient with hypotension, angina, or heart failure, immediate synchronized cardiversion should be performed.

❍ What is the key feature of Mobitz I 2° AV block (Wenkebach)?

A progressive prolongation of the PR interval until the atrial impulse is no longer conducted through to the ventricle, resulting in a dropped QRS. Almost always transient, atropine and transcutaneous/transvenous pacing is required for the rare instances of symptoms or cardiac instability.

❍ What is the feature of Mobitz II 2° AV block?

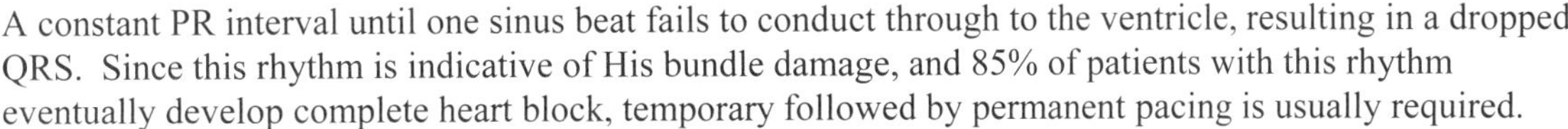

A constant PR interval until one sinus beat fails to conduct through to the ventricle, resulting in a dropped QRS. Since this rhythm is indicative of His bundle damage, and 85% of patients with this rhythm eventually develop complete heart block, temporary followed by permanent pacing is usually required.

❍ **A 57 year-old male is scheduled for a total colectomy for ulcerative colitis. He has stable angina for several years and has hypertension. His pre-op ECG reveals NSR, LVH and 1° AV block. What is the likelihood of high degree AV block occurring in the perioperative period?**

Patients with 1° AV block have an extremely low incidence of developing high degree AV block in the perioperative period or any other period. Thus, no temporary pacing in the perioperative period is required.

❍ **A 26 year-old male present to your clinic for an insurance physical. An ECG reveals Wolff-Parkinson-White syndrome. He is asymptomatic and has no history of palpitations or arrhythmia. What is the most appropriate management of this patient?**

No therapy or work-up is required at this time since there is no evidence that the risk of sudden death can be safely mitigated or that individuals with asymptomatic WPW can be reliably risk stratified with regard to sudden death.

❍ **What is the most commonly occurring form of ventricular tachycardia?**

Ventricular tachycardia (VT) occurring in patients with healed myocardial infarction. Other causes include bundle branch reentry VT, VT of right ventricular outflow tract origin, idiopathic left ventricular tachycardia, drug-induced VT (proarrhythmia), and VT due to right ventricular dysplasia. Rare causes include long QT syndrome and lymphocytic myocarditis.

❍ **A 48 year old male with no history of angina, MI or other cardiac symptoms is referred to you for evaluation of palpitations. A 24-hour Holter monitor reveals four three-beat runs of ventricular tachycardia without any symptoms. The patient has no risk factors for coronary artery disease, is a non-smoker, and has a normal resting ECG. His echocardiogram is normal. What is the best management strategy for this patient?**

No therapy or further work-up is required. The patient should be reassured that the risk of sudden death is very low and that medical therapy will either worsen his arrhythmia or be of no significant benefit.

❍ **A 28 year-old male with two previous episodes of palpitations and shortness of breath in the last year is brought in to the Emergency Department by paramedics with severe palpitations, hypotension and shortness of breath. His BP is 90/55 and his HR is 195/minute. A rhythm strip reveals narrow complex QRS tachycardia. A 12-lead ECG reveals what appears to be atrial fibrillation. Synchronized cardioversion is successful in terminating the arrhythmia, and the post-cardioversion ECG reveals Wolff-Parkinson-White syndrome. What is the most appropriate management strategy in this patient?**

Electrophysiology testing with intracardiac mapping, followed by catheter ablation of the accessory conduction pathway.

❍ **A 67 year-old woman with severe 3-vessel coronary artery disease with very small distal vessels, deemed inoperable, is brought into the Emergency Department following a syncopal episode. The paramedics caught the final beats of what looked like a wide-complex QRS tachycardia on a rhythm strip and you confirm this on inspection of the tracing. She is now awake, alert and breathing comfortably. An echocardiogram performed one month ago revealed a dilated left ventricle with poor systolic function (estimated ejection fraction ~ 20-25%). What is the most appropriate management strategy for this patient?**

Empiric therapy with Amiodarone.

❍ **What percentage of patients treated with long-term Amiodarone for ventricular tachycardia will develop bradycardia that requires permanent pacing?**

15%.

❍ **In patients with coronary artery disease, which patients have been shown to benefit from revascularization with bypass grafting?**

Patients with left main coronary artery disease (>50% stenosis) and those with three vessel coronary artery disease (>70% stenosis) with depressed LV systolic function (<40% LVEF).

❍ **What is the first-line pharmacologic therapy for a forty year-old obese white female with uncomplicated mild hypertension?**

Beta-blockers or a thiazide diuretic.

❍ **What is the preferred choice of anti-hypertensive therapy for a 58 year-old white male with severe COPD and mild hypertension?**

Long-acting calcium channel blockers, such as verapamil or nifedipine. These agents are particularly useful in patients with a likelihood of pulmonary hypertension.

❍ **What is the agent of choice in diabetic patients with hypertension?**

ACE inhibitors.

❍ **What drugs have been shown to regress LV hypertrophy and reduce LV mass?**

Beta-blockers, verapamil, alpha-methyldopa (Aldomet), ACE inhibitors, and thiazide diuretics.

❍ **Which agent is more likely to cause bradycardia, verapamil or diltiazem?**

Diltiazem. Diltiazem blocks conduction through both the SA and AV node, whereas verapamil blocks only the AV node.

❍ **Which drugs can increase serum digoxin levels?**

Quinidine, procainamide, verapamil, and amiodarone.

❍ **What is the most frequent side effect of verapamil?**

Constipation.

❍ **What are the most frequent side effects of nifedipine?**

Lower extremity edema, dizziness, and headache.

❍ **What pharmacologic agent should be avoided in a patient with paroxysmal atrial fibrillation who is presently in sinus rhythm?**

Dihydropyridine calcium channel blockers, such as nifedipine. They predispose patients to relapse back into atrial fibrillation.

❍ **What medications, used to maintain sinus rhythm in a patient recently cardioverted from atrial fibrillation, should be avoided in patients with stress-test proven myocardial ischemia?**

Class 1C antiarrhythmics, such as flecainide and propafenone and class 1A agents, such as quinidine and procainamide. They can lead to lethal proarrhythmia in patients with active myocardial ischemia. Amiodarone, an agent that has anti-ischemic properties, is the preferred agent.

❍ **What antihypertensive agents are preferred agents to use in a 63 year-old obese, African-American male?**

Diuretics and/or ACE inhibitors.

❍ **Non-traumatic cardiac arrest patients are most likely to be successfully resuscitated from what abnormal rhythm?**

Ventricular fibrillation. Success is time dependent, generally declining at a rate of 2-10% per minute.

❍ **What is the affect of a dopamine infusion greater than 5 ug/kg/min?**

Peripheral arterial vasoconstriction.

❍ **What are the end-points in procainamide loading infusion for patient with unstable VT?**

Hypotension, QRS widened more than 50% of pre-treatment width, arrhythmia suppression, or a total of 17 mg/kg.

❍ **How many deaths per year in the U.S. are due to cardiovascular disease?**

930,000, 43% of all deaths per year. More than 1/2 of all deaths occur in women. 2/3 of sudden deaths, due to CAD, take place outside the hospital, and most occur within 2 hours of the onset of symptoms.

❍ **In a patient with ventricular fibrillation, what regimen should be used in the administration of bretylium?**

5 mg/kg IV bolus followed by 10 mg/kg IV bolus. The maximum dose is 30-35 mg/kg.

❍ **What drug is used in the treatment of verapamil overdose?**

Calcium chloride

❍ **If a defibrillator is available, what is the immediate treatment of a patient with ventricular fibrillation?**

Unsynchronized countershock at 200J.

❍ **What is the differential diagnosis of pulseless electrical activity?**

Tension pneumothorax, acidosis, MI, PE, OD, cardiac tamponade, hypoxia, hypovolemia, hyperkalemia, and hypothermia (TAMPOT plus 4H is the pnemonic).

❍ **What is the differential diagnosis of asystole?**

Drug overdose, acidosis, hyperkalemia, hypothermia, hypokalemia, hypoxia.

❍ **What is the treatment for unstable supraventricular tachycardia?**

Synchronized cardioversion.

❍ **A patient in the ED suddenly demonstrates ventricular fibrillation on the monitor. The patient is alert and has a pulse. What should you do?**

Check the monitor leads.

❍ **Inferior wall MI's commonly lead to what two types of heart block (via mechanism of damage to autonomic fibers in the atrial septum giving increased vagal tone impairing AV node conduction)?**

First degree AV block and Mobitz Type I (Wenckebach) second degree AV block. Sinus bradycardia can also occur. Progression to complete AV block is not common.

❍ **Anterior wall MI's may directly damage intracardiac conduction. This may lead to which type of arrhythmias?**

The dangerous type! A Mobitz II second degree AV block can suddenly progress to complete AV block.

❍ **What are the potential, often rare, complications of Mycoplasma pneumonia?**

Non-pulmonary: Hemolytic anemia, aseptic meningitis, encephalitis, Guillain-Barre syndrome, pericarditis, and myocarditis

❍ **What is the most common cause of multifocal atrial tachycardia?**

COPD.

❍ **What is the treatment for verapamil-induced hypotension?**

Calcium gluconate, 1 gram IV over several minutes.

❍ **Which type of drug is contraindicated for the treatment of Torsade de pointes?**

Any drug that prolongs repolarization (QT interval). For example, class Ia antiarrhythmics, such as quinidine and procainamide, are contraindicated for treating Torsade de pointes. Other drugs that share this effect include TCA's, disopyramide, and phenothiazine.

❍ **What are the classic ECG results associated with posterior MI?**

A large R wave in leads V1 and V2, ST depression in leads V1 and V2, Q waves in the inferior leads and, occasionally, ST elevation in the inferior leads.

❍ **What are the classic ECG finding for Wolff-Parkinson-White syndrome?**

A change in the upstroke of QRS, the delta wave.

❍ **What cardiovascular injury is commonly associated with a sternal fracture?**

Myocardial contusions (blunt myocardial injury).

❍ **Which valve is most commonly injured during blunt trauma?**

Aortic valve.

❍ **What is the most likely cause of a new systolic murmur and ECG infarct pattern in a patient with chest trauma?**

Ventricular septal defect.

❍ **What is the most common complication of extracorporeal circulation?**

Stroke occurs in 1 to 2% of patients after open-heart operations. Other postoperative complications are arrhythmias, bleeding, renal failure, and respiratory complications.

❍ **What drug is used to reverse heparin after open-heart surgery?**

Protamine.

❍ **In 90% of the population, the right coronary artery terminates as:**

The posterior descending artery.

❍ **The left main coronary artery gives rise to which two coronary arteries?**

The left anterior descending artery and the left circumflex coronary artery.

❍ **What is the vessel of preference in coronary bypass grafting?**

The internal mammary artery. This artery has a much higher rate of patency at 10 years than venous grafts (95% versus 50%). Also, venous grafts tend to be more prone to atherosclerosis.

❍ **Which nerve should be located and avoided during pericardiotomy?**

Phrenic nerve. The phrenic nerve runs along the superolateral aspect of the pericardium.

❍ **A radial pulse on examination indicates a BP of at least what level?**

80 mm Hg.

❍ **A femoral pulse on examination indicates a BP of at least what level?**

70 mm Hg.

❍ **A carotid pulse indicates a BP of at least what level?**

60 mm Hg.

❍ **Where is the most common location of left ventricular aneurysms?**

Anterolateral left ventricle (80%). Left ventricular aneurysms result from transmural infarctions and subsequent replacement of muscle with fibrous tissue. Unlike atherosclerotic aneurysms, these aneurysms progressively enlarge but rarely rupture.

❍ **What is the cardiac arrhythmia?**

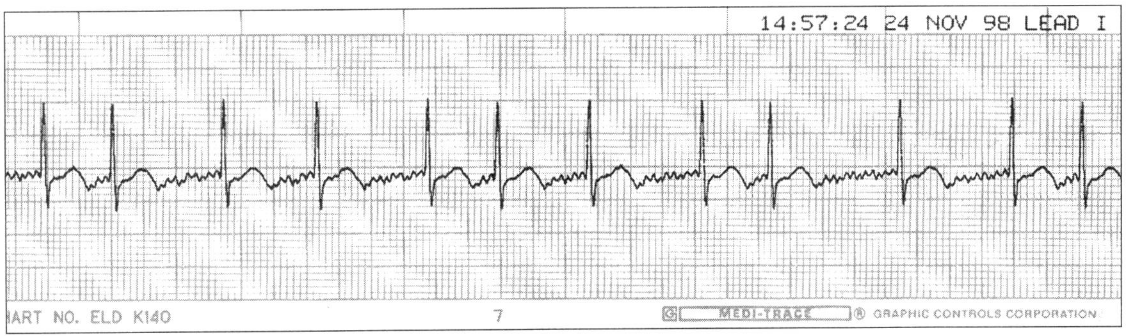

Atrial fibrillation.

❍ **What is the cardiac arrhythmia?**

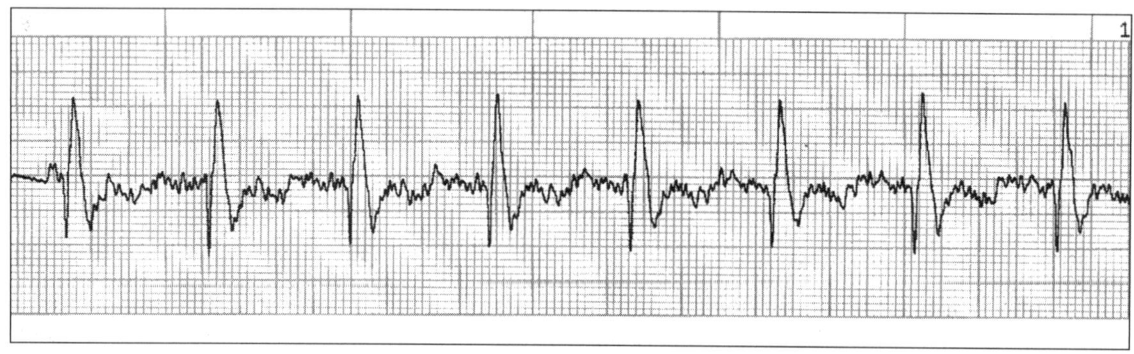

Ventricular paced rhythm with artifact.

❍ **What is the cardiac arrhythmia?**

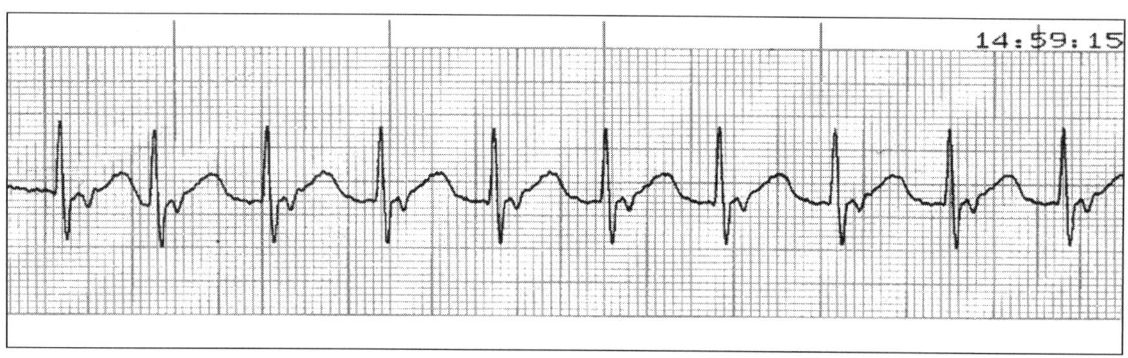

Accelerated junctional rhythm with retrograde P waves.

❍ **What is the cardiac rhythm seen below?**

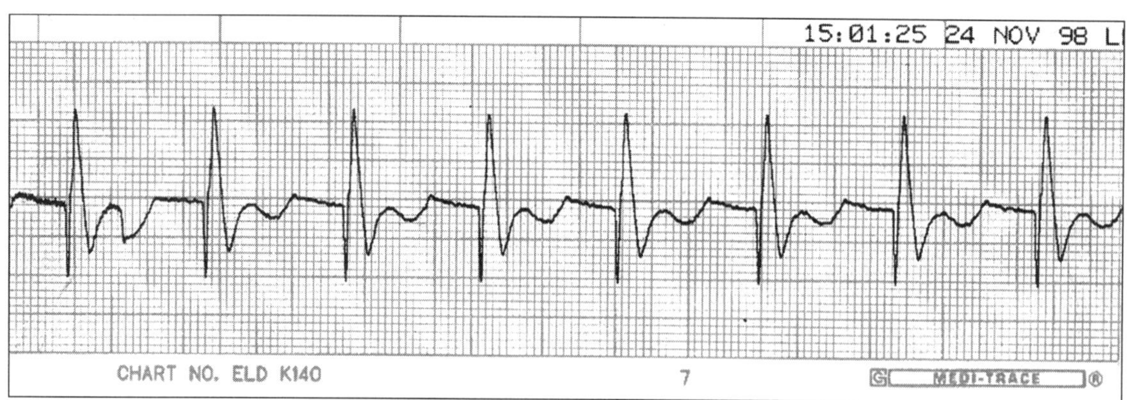

Ventricular pacemaker rhythm.

❍ **What is the ECG rhythm abnormality seen below?**

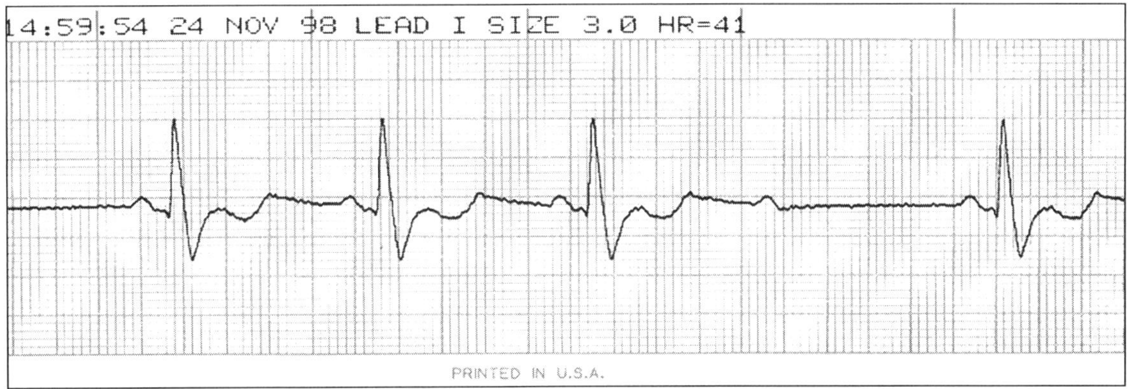

Mobitz II 2nd degree AV block.

❍ **What is the ECG rhythm abnormality seen below?**

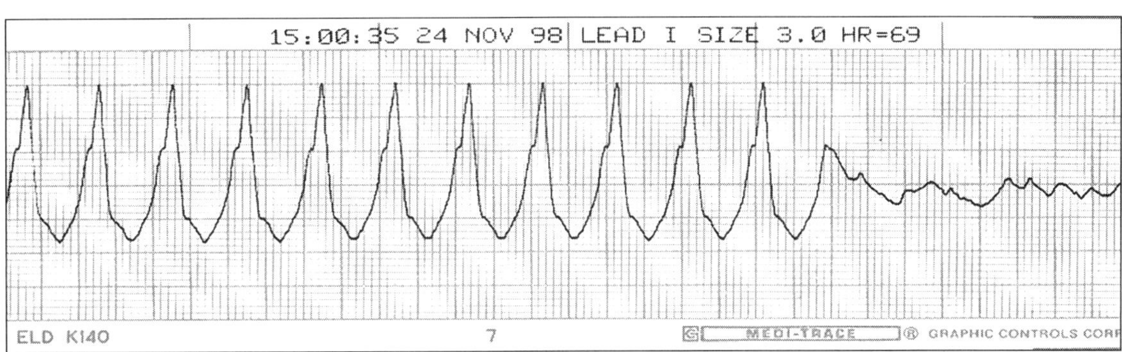

Ventricular tachycardia evolving into ventricular fibrillation.

❍ **What is the cardiac arrhythmia below?**

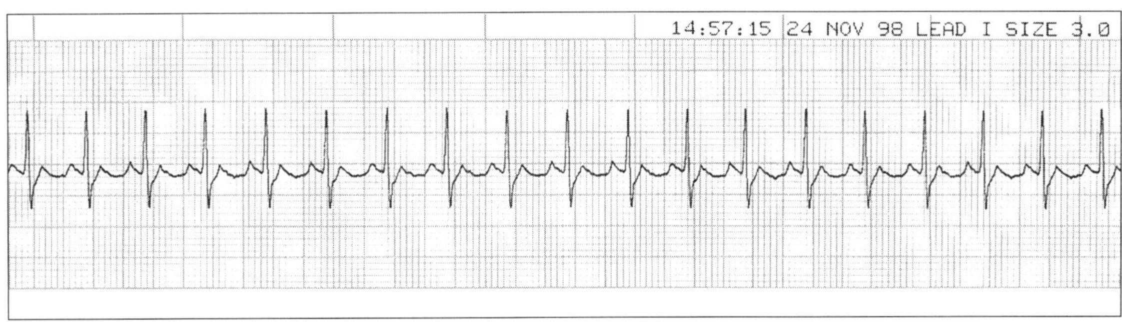

Atrial tachycardia with 2:1 conduction.

❍ **What is the abnormality in the ECG seen below?**

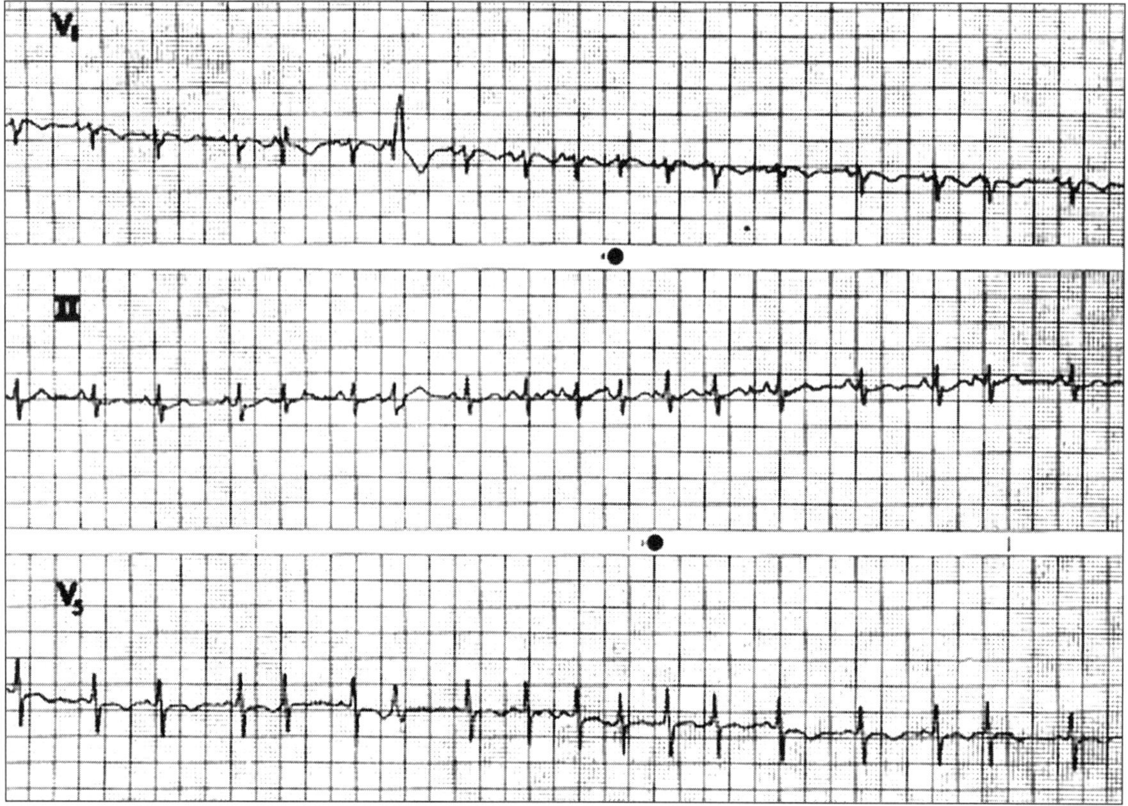

Multifocal atrial tachycardia.

❍ **What is the abnormality seen in the rhythm below?**

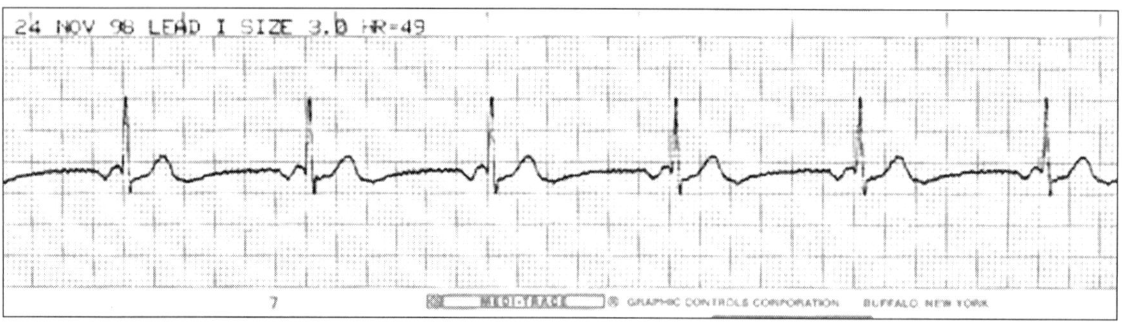

Junctional rhythm.

❍ **What is the abnormality seen in the rhythm below?**

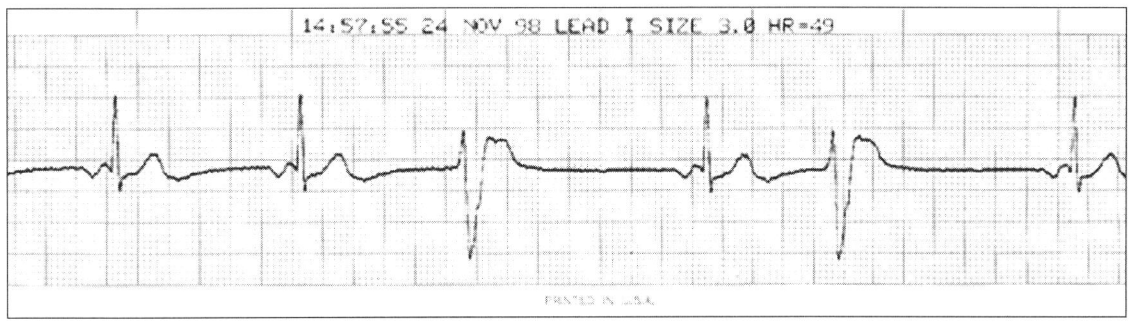

Junctional rhythm with escape ventricular beats.

❍ **What is the abnormality seen in the rhythm below?**

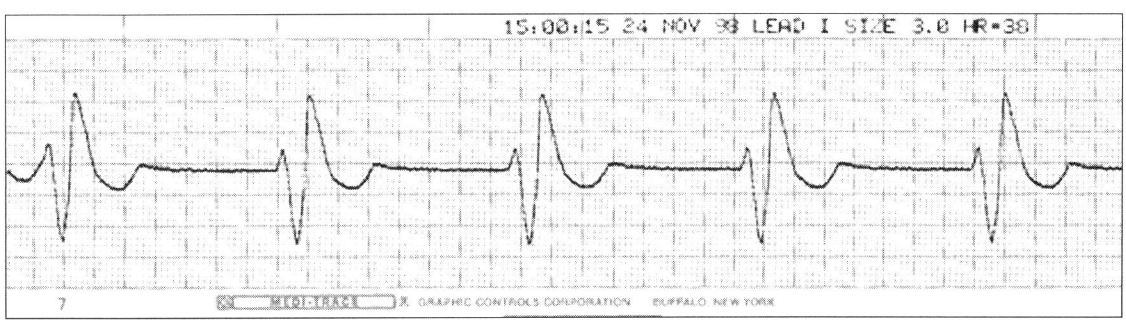

Idioventricular rhythm.

What is the abnormality seen in the rhythm below?

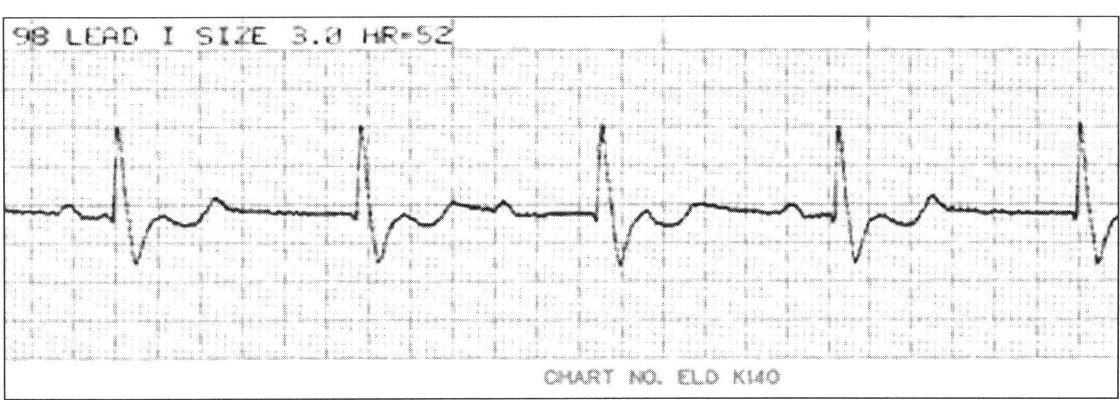

2:1 AV block.

❍ **What is the abnormality seen in the rhythm below?**

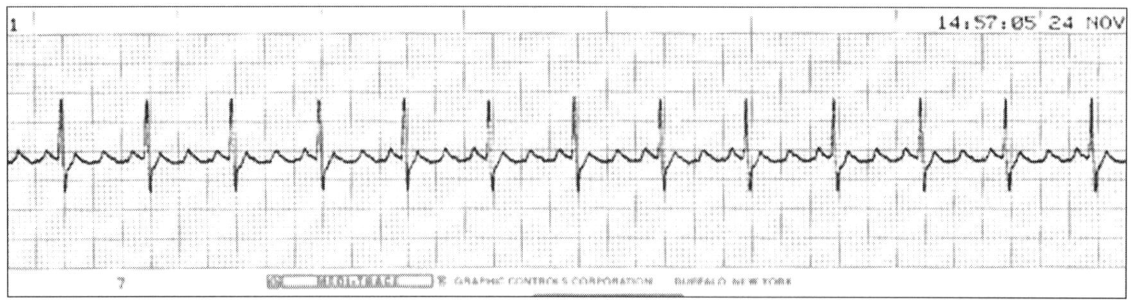

Atrial flutter.

❍ **What is the abnormality seen in the rhythm below?**

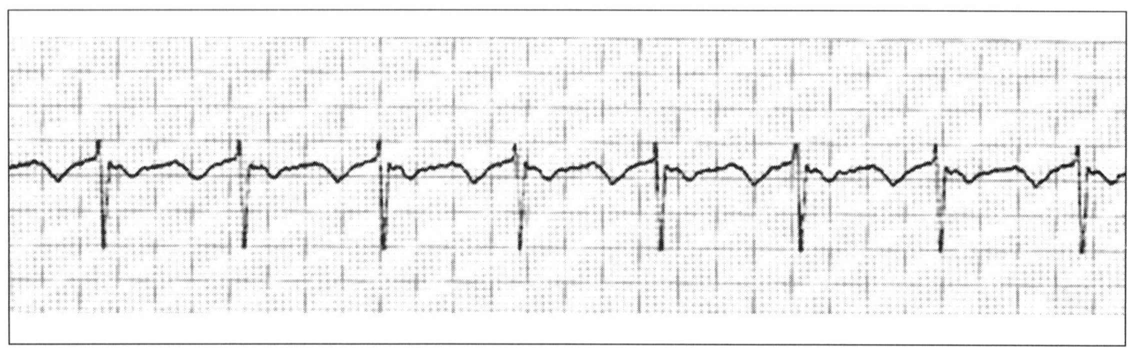

Rhythm strip erroneously mounted upside down. When viewed right-side up, it shows normal sinus rhythm.

❍ **What is the rhythm abnormality seen below?**

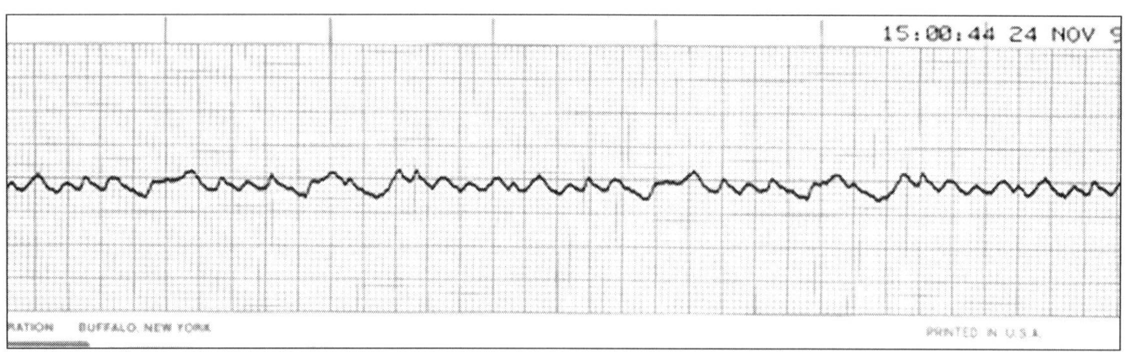

Ventricular fibrillation.

❍ What is the rhythm abnormality seen below?

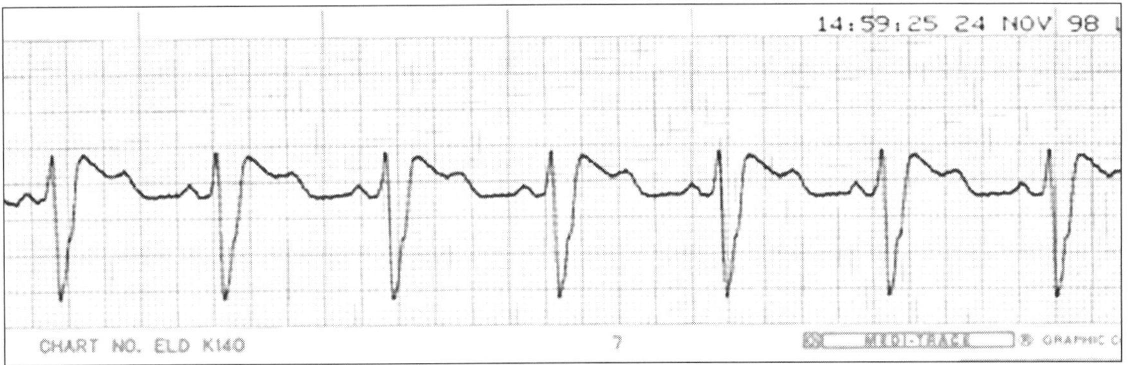

Complete heart block.

❍ What does the Doppler echocardiogram below show?

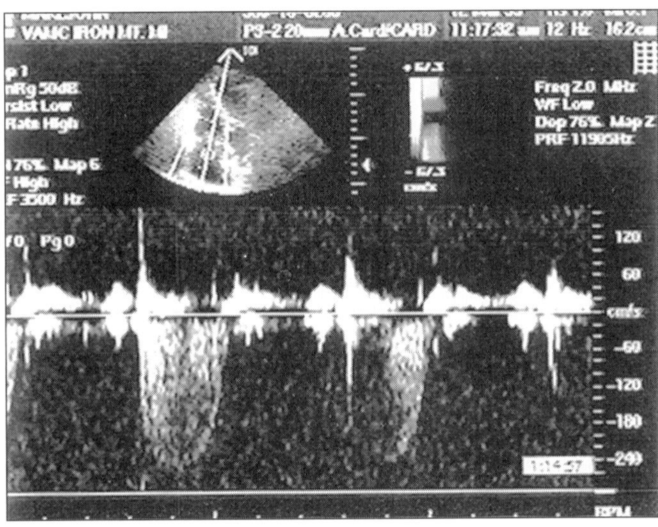

Mild tricuspid regurgitation with mild pulmonary hypertension, as evidenced by a 25 mm peak gradient across the tricuspid valve.

❍ **What is the interpretation of this ECG shown below?**

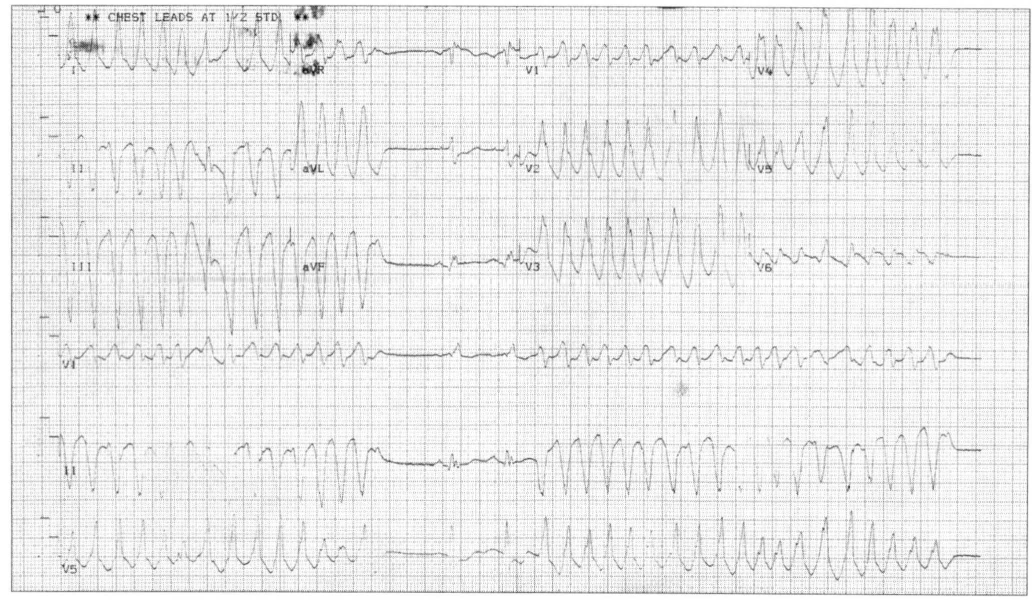

Ventricular tachycardia, most likely originating from the left ventricle.

❍ **What is the interpretation of this ECG shown below?**

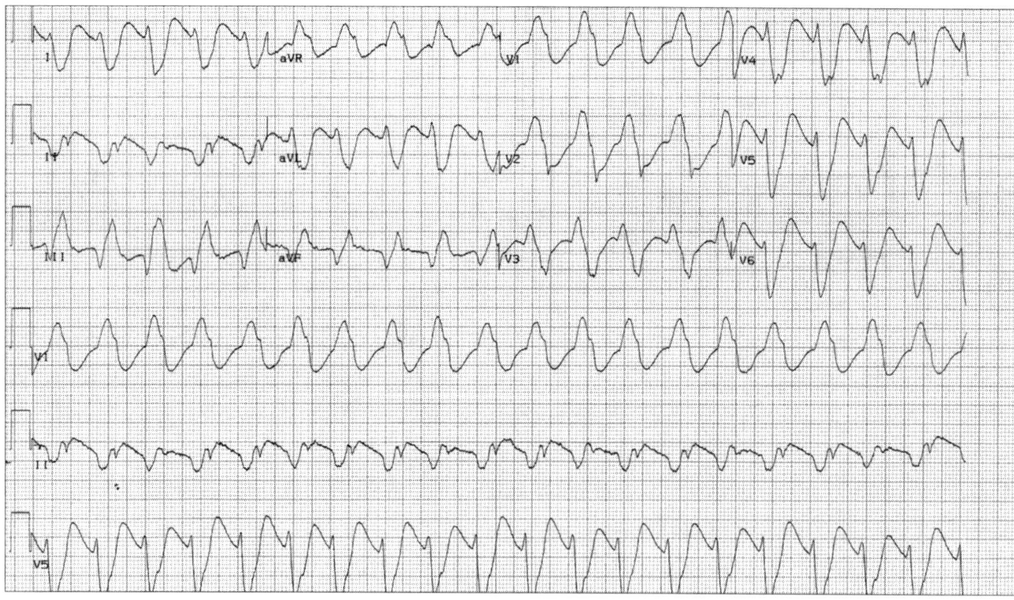

Ventricular tachycardia with hyperkalemia. Note the very wide QRS complex with the early stages of a "sine wave".

❍ What is the interpretation of the ECG shown below?

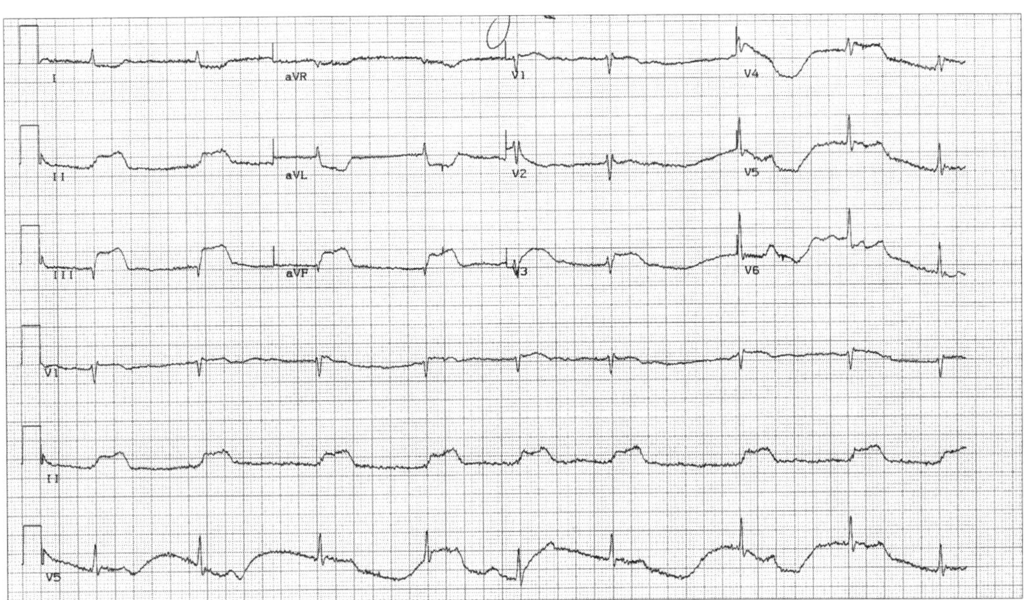

Acute inferior myocardial infarction with posterior wall involvement, atrial fibrillation with slow ventricular rate.

❍ What is the interpretation of the ECG shown below?

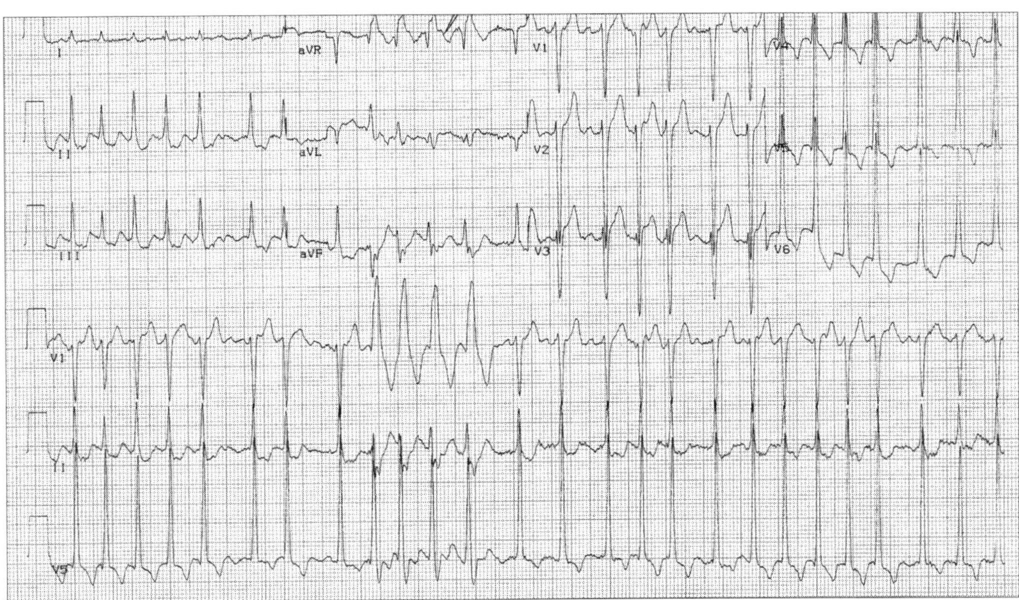

Atrial fibrillation with rapid ventricular rate of 155, LVH, and ischemic-type ST depression in the inferior and lateral leads.

❍ In the above ECG, does this patient absolutely have myocardial ischemia?

Not necessarily. Patients with supraventricular tachycardia of any type with ST depression can have "ischemic" appearing ST depression without having myocardial ischemia. The ST depression can be as a result of abnormal repolarization that occurs in any tachyarrhythmia. Nonetheless, it would be incorrect to automatically assume that this patient's ST depression is not due to myocardial ischemia.

○ What is the interpretation of the ECG shown below?

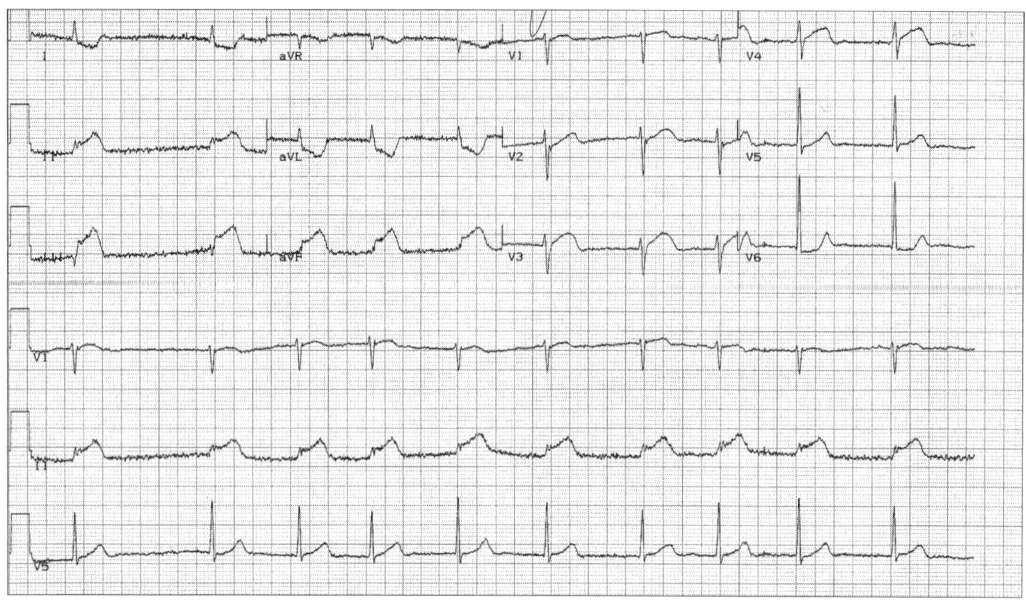

Acute inferior myocardial infarction, atrial fibrillation with slow ventricular rate.

○ This ECG is from a patient who received intravenous dipyridamole as part of a pharmacological stress test. Eight minutes into the test, the patient developed substernal chest tightness. The ECG at that time is shown below. What is the result of his stress test? (His resting ECG is normal)

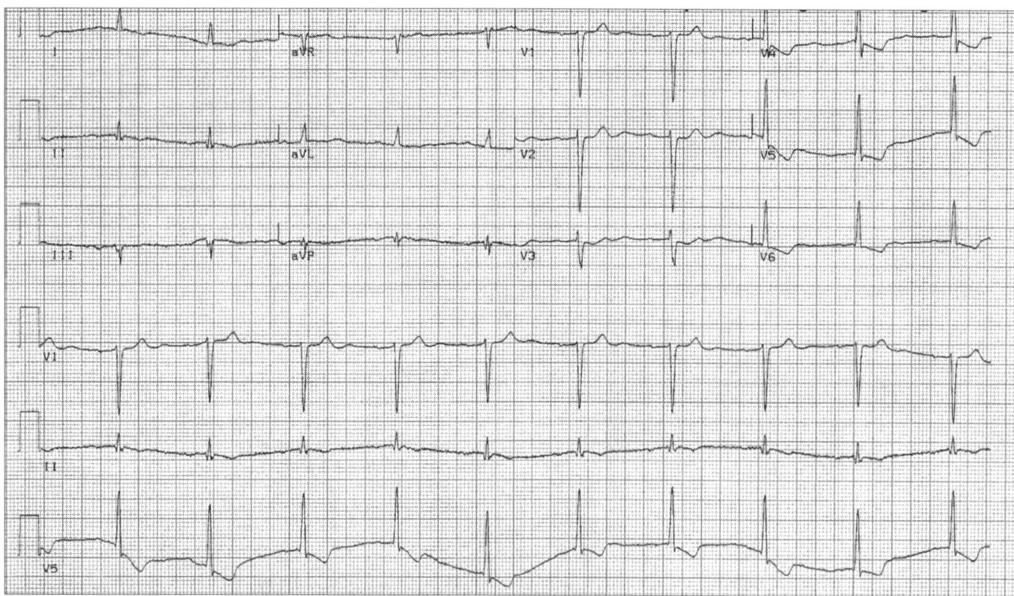

This ECG shows 1-1.5 mm ST depression in the inferior and lateral leads, consistent with myocardial ischemia from a critical stenosis in one or more coronary arteries.

❍ What is the interpretation of the ECG shown below?

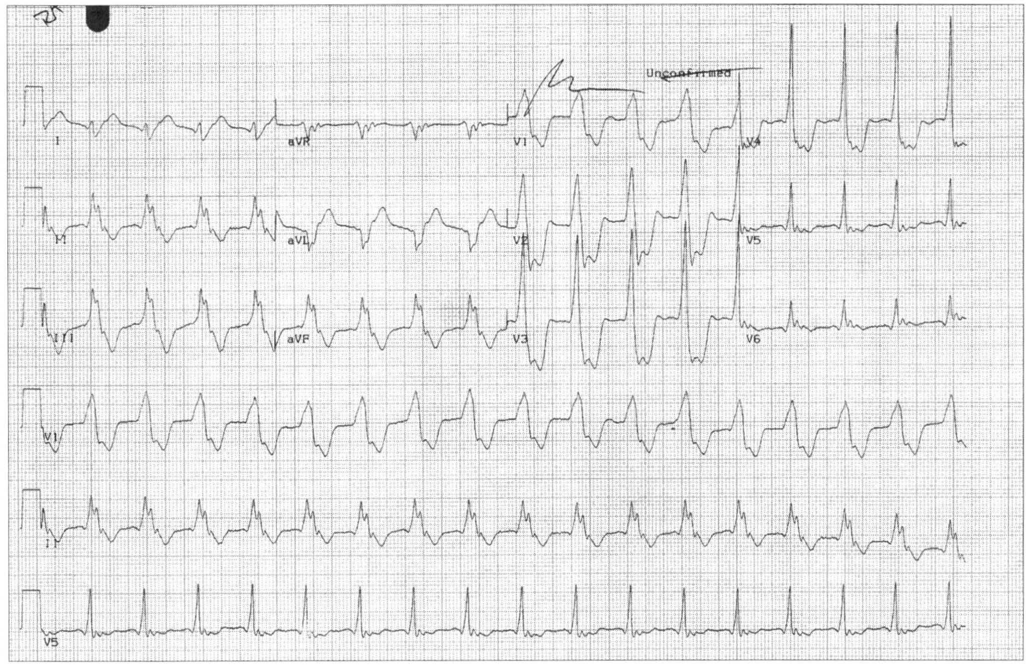

Ventricular tachycardia with a ventricular rate of 103. Note the VA conduction evidenced by the retrograde P waves, which occur in the early part of the ST segment.

❍ What is the abnormality in the M-mode echocardiogram shown below?

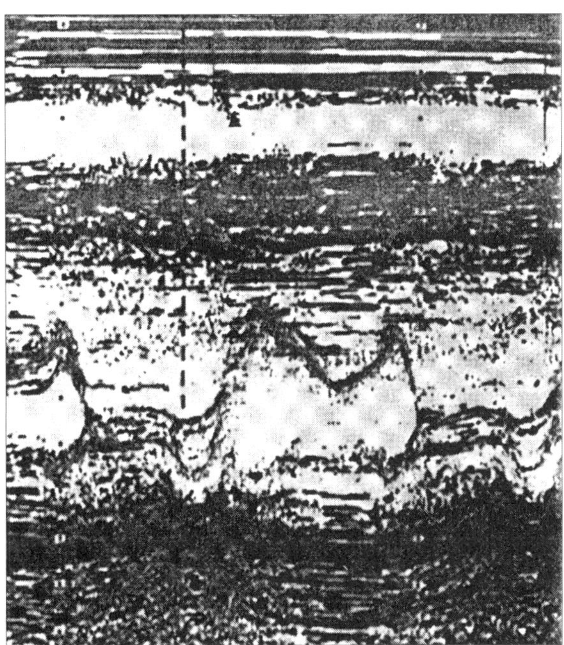

Prolapse of the posterior leaflet of the mitral valve.

O What is the abnormality in the echocardiogram shown below?

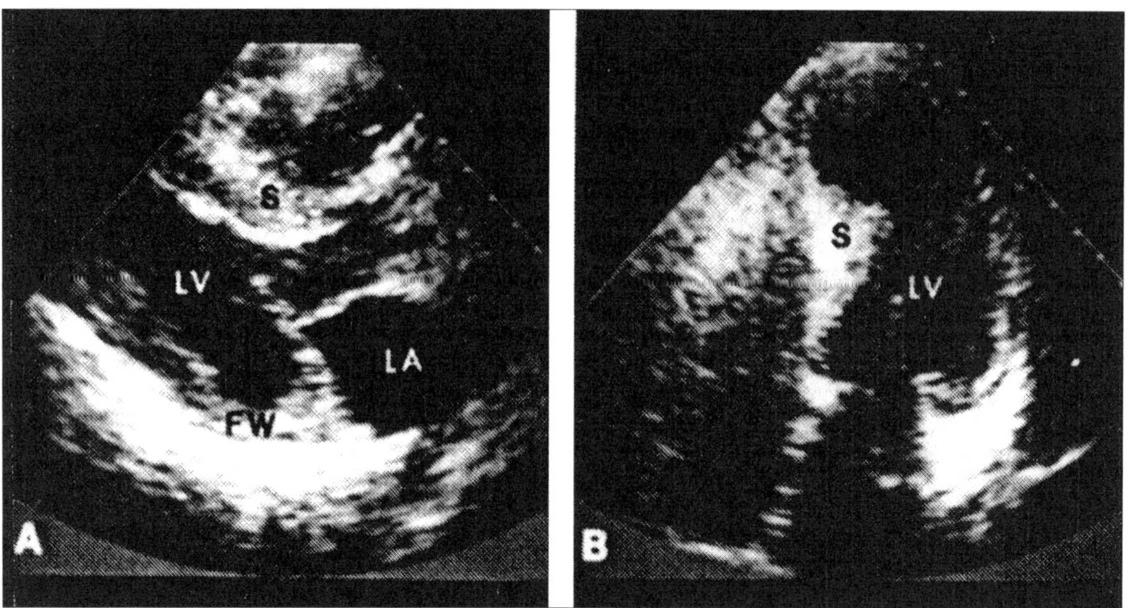

Hypertrophic cardiomyopathy. Note the very thickened septum and anterior systolic motion of the mitral valve.

O What is the interpretation of the ECG seen below?

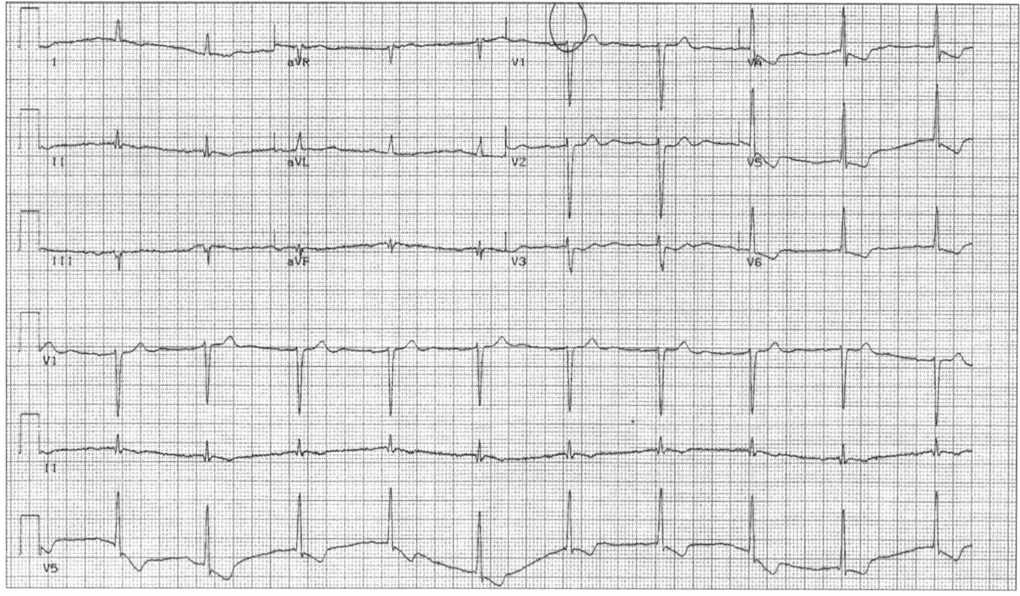

Ectopic atrial rhythm with an old inferior infarction and non-specific ST-T abnormality.

❍ **What is the interpretation of the ECG seen below?**

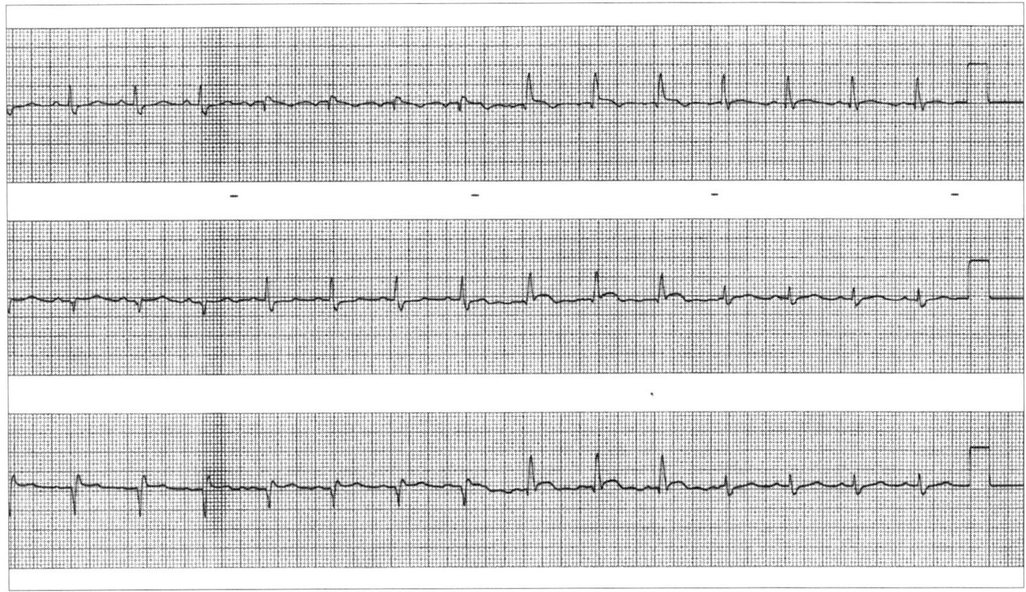

Normal sinus rhythm, RBBB, left anterior fascicular block and an acute anterior myocardial infarction.

❍ **What is the interpretation of the ECG seen below?**

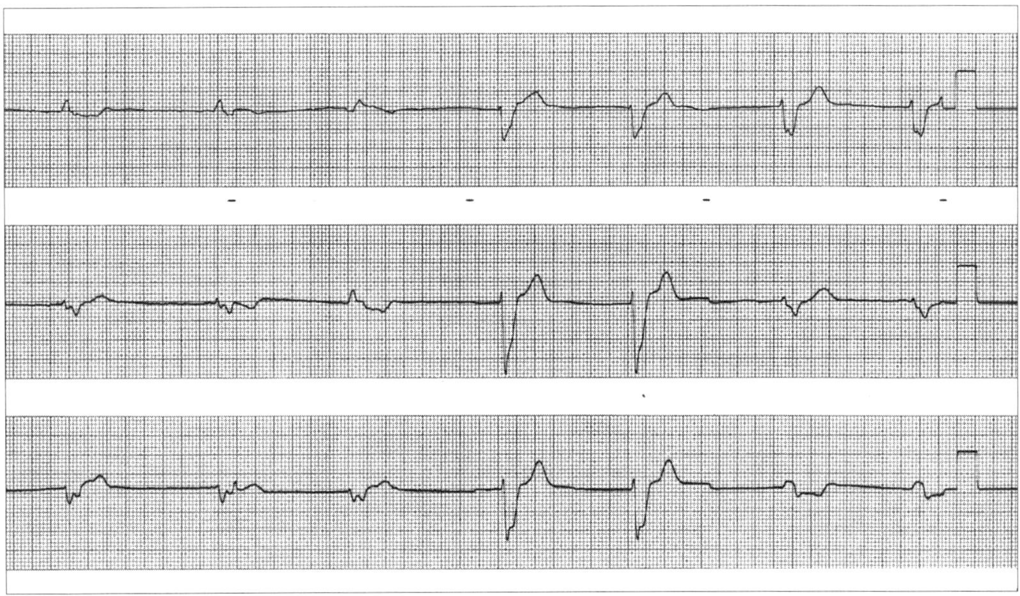

Idioventricular rhythm, rate of 40/min.

❍ **What is the interpretation of the ECG seen below?**

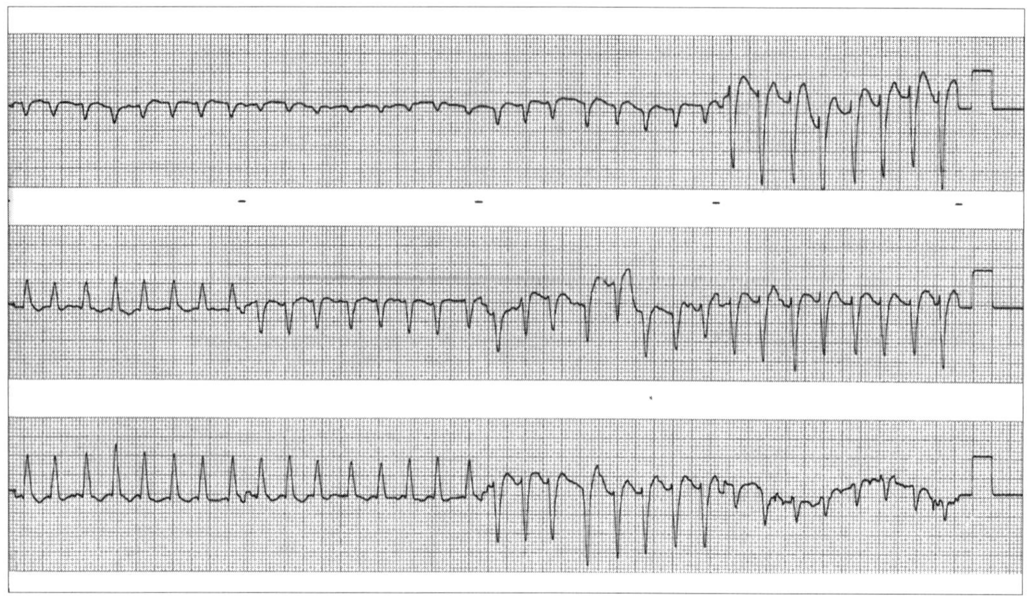

Supraventricular tachycardia.

PULMONARY

The best way to stop smoking is to carry wet matches.
Anonymous

❍ **What should be suspected if a very young, non-smoking patient has symptoms similar to those associated with emphysema?**

Alpha-1-antitrypsin deficiency. Without α-1-antitrypsin, excess elastase accumulates, resulting in lung damage. Treatment for this condition is the same as that emphysema. An α-1 proteinase inhibitor may also be useful.

❍ **What two drugs can cause ARDS?**

Heroin and aspirin.

❍ **How long after an initial insult does ARDS usually occur?**

12 to 72 hours.

❍ **A 14 year-old boy was exposed to asbestos for three days and has a non-productive cough and chest pain. Does this boy have asbestosis?**

No. Although a non-productive cough and pleurisy are symptoms of asbestosis, other signs, such as exertional dyspnea, malaise, clubbed fingers, crackles, cyanosis, pleural effusion and pulmonary hypertension, should be displayed before making a diagnosis of asbestosis. In addition, asbestosis does not develop until 10 to 15 years after the beginning of consistent, regular exposure to asbestos.

❍ **Asbestosis increases the risk of what two diseases?**

Lung cancer and malignant mesothelioma.

❍ **What procedures should be performed to confine aspiration in a patient who is continuously vomiting and at risk for aspiration pneumonia?**

Lie the patient on his right side in Trendelenburg. This will help confine the aspirate to the right upper lobe.

❍ **How can aspiration be prevented when intubating?**

By avoiding unnecessary increase in intragastric pressure from overzealous bag-valve-mask ventilation, and by applying cricoid pressure during intubation.

❍ **When is aspiration most likely to occur during surgery?**

During the induction of anesthesia.

❍ **Where does aspiration generally occur as revealed by chest x-ray?**

The lower lobe of the right lung. This is the most direct path for foreign bodies into the lung.

❍ **What is the pH of aspirated fluid that suggests a poor prognosis?**

$pH < 2.5$.

❍ **A 29 year-old triathlete develops wheezing when exercising. What would be a reasonable treatment program?**

A sodium cromoglycate (cromolyn sodium) inhaler. Sodium cromoglycate stabilizes mast cells that are involved in the early and late phase bronchoconstrictive reactions of asthma. Sodium cromoglycate is only a prophylactic treatment for exercise-induced asthma and is not effective once the attack has begun.

❍ **What x-ray markings may be observed in a patient with a long history of bronchial asthma?**

Increased bronchial wall markings and flattening of the diaphragm. The bronchial wall markings are caused by epithelial inflammation and thickening of the bronchial walls.

❍ **What is the "best" pulmonary function test for the diagnosis of asthma?**

FEV_1/FVC. This test determines the amount of air exhaled in 1 minute compared to the total amount of air in the lung that can be expressed. A ratio under 80% is diagnostic of asthma. Peak flow monitors are helpful in monitoring asthma at home, or during an acute exacerbation.

❍ **Is wheezing an integral part of asthma?**

No. Thirty-three percent of children with asthma will only have cough variant asthma with no wheezing.

❍ **Which is more effective for relieving an acute exacerbation of bronchial asthma in a conscious patient: nebulized albuterol or albuterol MDI administered via an aerosol chamber?**

They are both equally effective.

❍ **What treatment should be initiated for a patient with acute asthma who does not improve with humidified O_2, albuterol nebulizers, steroids, and anticholinergics?**

Subcutaneous epinephrine, 0.3 cc administered every 5 minutes.

❍ **Asthmatics will most likely have a family history of what?**

Asthma, allergies, or atopic dermatitis.

❍ **Which type of exercise usually triggers an asthmatic episode in patients with exercise-induced asthma?**

High intensity exercise for more than 5 to 6 minutes.

❍ **What are the recommended therapeutic serum theophylline levels?**

10 to 15 mg/L.

❍ **What medications should be avoided for a pregnant patient with asthma?**

Epinephrine and parenteral beta-adrenergic agonists.

❍ **What is the role of methylprednisolone (Solu-Medrol) in asthmatic patients?**

Long-term management. Because of its long half-life, it may be ideal for chronic use in nocturnal breakthrough exacerbations. It is not useful in the acute setting.

❍ **What is a normal peak expiratory flow rate in adults?**

Males: 550 to 600 L/minute. Females: 450 to 500 L/minute. However, this varies somewhat with body size and age.

❍ **Sympathomimetic agents are used to treat asthma. What enzyme do they activate?**

Adenyl cyclase.

❍ **What reaction is catalyzed by adenyl cyclase?**

Adenyl cyclase catalyzes ATP to cyclic AMP.

❍ **What effects do increased levels of c-AMP have on bronchial smooth muscle and the release of chemical mediators, such as histamine, proteases, platelet activation and chemotactic factors, from airway mast cells?**

Smooth muscles are relaxed and release of mediators is decreased. Recall that the effects of c-AMP are opposed by c-GMP. Thus, another treatment approach can be provided by decreasing the levels of cyclic GMP via the use of anticholinergic (antimuscarinic) agents, such as ipratropium bromide.

❍ **Right upper lobe cavitation with parenchymal involvement is a classic indicator for what?**

TB. Lower lung infiltrates, hilar adenopathy, atelectasis, and pleural effusion are also common.

❍ **Which beta-adrenergic receptors primarily control bronchiolar and arterial smooth muscle tone?**

Beta-2-adrenergic receptors.

❍ **Terbutaline is administered subcutaneously for asthma in what dose?**

0.01 ml/kg of 1 mg/ml terbutaline up to 0.25 ml (i.e., 0.25 mg, which may be repeated once in 20 to 30 minutes).

❍ **Is theophylline useful in the emergency management of a severely asthmatic patient?**

No. It has not been shown to affect further bronchodilatation in patients fully treated with beta-adrenergic agents. However, theophylline can be used successfully for inpatient management of asthma and may be started in the hospital.

❍ **If corticosteroids are prescribed, how should prednisone be dosed?**

1 to 2 mg/kg/day in 2 divided doses. Tapering is not necessary if the duration of therapy is 5 days or less.

❍ **What effect does pre-existing acidosis have on the efficacy of treatment with beta-adrenergic agonists?**

Decreased efficacy.

❍ **If one prefers the most simplified algorithm for determining loading dose of theophylline, what are the appropriate doses for a patient who has not recently been given theophylline? A patient who has recently been given theophylline?**

No recent dose: load with 7 mg/kg theophylline. Recent dose: load with 5 mg/kg theophylline.

❍ **What is the appropriate parenteral dose of methylprednisolone (Solu-Medrol) to administer to a pediatric patient with status asthmaticus?**

1 to 2 mg/kg every 6 hours.

❍ **If mechanical ventilation is required for such a patient, what is an appropriate setting for the initial tidal volume?**

10 ml/kg.

❍ **What is the most common postoperative respiratory complication?**

Atelectasis. Respiratory failure and aspiration pneumonia are other postoperative complications.

❍ **What percentage of patients who have had abdominal surgery also develop atelectasis?**

> 25%.

❍ **Atelectasis accounts for what percentage of postoperative fevers?**

90%.

❍ **Why do we care about postoperative atelectasis?**

If it persists for more than 72 hours, pneumonia may develop. Perioperative mortality rates are then 20%. Incentive spirometry is an important therapy for the prevention of atelectasis.

❍ **A chest x-ray shows honeycombing, atelectasis, and increased bronchial markings. What is the diagnosis?**

Bronchiectasis, an irreversible dilation of the bronchi that is generally associated with infection. Bronchography shows dilations of the bronchial tree, but this method of diagnosis is not recommended for routine use.

❍ **Bronchiectasis occurs most frequently in patients with what conditions?**

Cystic fibrosis, immunodeficiencies, lung infections, or foreign body aspirations.

❍ **Which organisms are most commonly associated with acute exacerbations of bronchitis in smokers? In non-smokers?**

Smokers: Streptococcus pneumoniae and H. influenzae

Non-smokers: Mycoplasma pneumoniae

❍ **Which organisms commonly cause exacerbations of chronic bronchitis?**

Streptococcus pneumoniae and H. influenzae.

❍ **Where in the US is coccidioidomycosis most prevalent?**

The Southwest. If severe, treat the afflicted patient with amphotericin B.

❍ **Which populations are predisposed to progressive infection with coccidioidomycosis?**

African Americans and diabetics.

❍ **What is the hallmark symptom of COPD?**

Exertional dyspnea.

❍ **What pulmonary function test correlates best with day to day function, morbidity, and mortality in COPD patients?**

FEV_1/FVC.

❍ **What parameters should make you consider initiating "home oxygen" therapy for a patient with COPD?**

If the patient has a resting pO_2 less than 55 mm Hg, or if the patient has a pO_2 of less than 60 mm Hg with evidence of tissue hypoxia. O_2 desaturation with exercise may also require home O_2. Home O_2 therapy, at least 18 hours/day, may increase the life span of a patient with COPD by 6 to 7 years.

❍ **What percentage of cigarette smokers develop chronic bronchitis?**

10 to 15%. Chronic bronchitis generally develops after 10 to 12 years of smoking.

❍ **Other than smoking, what are the risk factors for COPD?**

Environmental pollutants, recurrent URI (especially in infancy), eosinophilia or increased serum IgE, bronchial hyperresponsiveness, a family history of COPD, and protease deficiencies.

❍ **Is there any hope for patients with COPD who quit smoking?**

Yes. Symptomatically speaking, coughing stops in up to 80% of these patients. Fifty-four percent of COPD patients find relief from coughing within a month of quitting.

❍ **If a patient with chronic bronchitis suffers an acute exacerbation of his illness, such as dyspnea, cough, or purulent sputum, what type of O_2 therapy should be initiated?**

We have forever been warned against overriding the COPD patient's drive to breathe by over-oxygenating him. Patients with COPD are no longer prompted to breathe by hypercarbia, but by hypoxia alone. However, in the case of acute exacerbation of bronchitis, oxygen therapy should be guided by pO_2 levels. Adequate oxygen must be maintained at a pO_2 above 60 mm Hg. This should be accomplished with the minimal amount of oxygen necessary. The pO_2 must be kept above 60 mm Hg even if the patient loses the drive to breathe.

❍ **Which pulmonary function test shows an increase in COPD?**

Residual volume. All other tests (FEV_1, FEV_1/FVC, and $FEV_{25\%ñ75\%}$,) indicate decreases and diffusion capacity.

❍ **Which part of the lung is affected by emphysema? By chronic bronchitis?**

Emphysema:Terminal bronchi

Chronic bronchitis:Large airways

❍ **What is the risk of placing a patient with COPD on a high FIO_2?**

Suppression of the hypoxic ventilatory drive.

❍ **What is the definition of chronic bronchitis?**

A productive cough for 3 months out of each year for 2 years straight.

❍ **In treating a patient with a common cold, you prescribe an oral decongestant. Is it necessary to also suggest an antitussant?**

No. Most coughs, arising from a common cold, are caused by the irritation of the tracheobronchial receptors in the posterior pharynx as a result of postnasal drip. Postnasal drip can be relieved with decongestant therapy, thus eliminating the need for cough suppressant therapy.

❍ **What are the most common etiologies of a chronic cough?**

Postnasal drip (40%), asthma (25%), and gastroesophageal reflux (20%). Other etiologies include bronchitis, bronchiectasis, bronchogenic carcinoma, esophageal diverticuli, sarcoidosis, viruses, and drugs.

❍ **What drugs can induce a chronic cough?**

ACE inhibitors cause chronic cough as a result of the accumulation of prostaglandins, kinins, or substances that excite the cough receptors (Remember that ACE sitting next to you at the boards!!). Beta-blockers evoke bronchoconstriction, and thus, coughing by blocking beta-2 receptors. Never give beta-blockers to asthmatics or other patients with an airway disease.

❍ **Hoarseness can herald far greater problems than viral laryngitis. At what point is a more thorough workup indicated?**

If hoarseness persists for over 6 to 8 weeks or is accompanied by a mass, chest pain, weight loss, aspiration dyspnea, or any other signs of malignancy. You should be suspicious of smokers with chronic cough or hoarseness if there is a change in either.

❍ **Your vitamin-crazed father insists that his "vitamin C a day" regime has helped him avoid colds for the past 53 years. Is there any validity to this statement?**

No. Studies have failed to show a prophylactic effect of vitamin C. However, it has been shown that consuming 1 g of vitamin C per day decreases the severity and duration of symptoms associated with the common cold by 23%.

❍ **What is the duration of a common cold?**

3 to 10 days (self-limited).

❍ **What result from the sweat test is considered positive for cystic fibrosis?**

> 60 mEq/L.

❍ **What is the classic triad of cystic fibrosis?**

1) COPD
2) Pancreatic enzyme deficiency
3) Abnormally high concentration of sweat electrolytes

❍ **What is the most common presentation of newborns with cystic fibrosis?**

GI obstruction due to meconium ileus.

❍ **Empyema is most often caused by what organism?**

Staphylococcus aureus. Gram-negative organisms and anaerobic bacteria may also cause empyema.

❍ **What percentage of effusions are associated with malignancy?**

25%.

❍ **What is the "thumb print sign"?**

A soft tissue inflammation of the epiglottis on a lateral x-ray of the neck.

❍ **Hantavirus occurs most commonly in what geographic location?**

Southwestern US, especially in areas with deer mice.

❍ **What is the definition for massive hemoptysis?**

Coughing of more than 600 ml of blood in 24 hours.

❍ **What are the most common causes of hemoptysis in non-hospitalized patients?**

Bronchitis, bronchogenic carcinoma, and idiopathic causes.

❍ **What systemic illnesses cause hemoptysis?**

Lung cancer, amyloidosis, CHF, mitral stenosis, sarcoidosis, SLE, vasculitis, coagulation disorders, and pulmonary-renal syndromes.

❍ **Life threatening hemoptysis should be suspected when there is:**

1) A large volume of blood
2) Appearance of a fungus ball in a pulmonary cavity on chest x-ray
3) Hypoxemia

❍ **What percentage of people in the Ohio and the Mississippi valleys are infected with histoplasmosis?**

100% in endemic areas. However, only 1% of these individuals develop the active disease. The spores of H. capsulatum can remain active for 10 years. For unknown reasons, bird and bat feces promote the growth of the actual fungus. The disease is transmitted when the spores are released and inhaled.

❍ **What is Pancoast syndrome?**

Tumor of the apex of the lung that gives rise to Horner's syndrome and shoulder pain. The tumor invades the brachial plexus.

❍ **What is Horner's syndrome?**

Miosis, ptosis, and anhydrosis (lack of sweat).

❍ **What antibiotic is the most effective for treating uncomplicated lung abscess?**

Clindamycin.

❍ **T/F: Flora of lung abscesses are usually polymicrobial.**

True.

❍ **What is the most common cancer, excluding skin cancer, in the US?**

Lung cancer.

❍ **What cancer is the leading cause of cancer death?**

Lung cancer.

❍ **What cancers generally metastasize to the lungs?**

Breast, colon, prostate, renal, and cervical cancers.

❍ **What routine program is recommended for screening lung cancer in the adult population?**

None. Screening programs for lung cancer have not demonstrated a decrease in morbidity or mortality. Practitioners must be aware of the signs and symptoms associated with lung cancer, including chronic non-productive cough, increased sputum production, hemoptysis, dyspnea, recurrent pneumonia, hoarseness, pleurisy, weight loss, shoulder pain, SVC syndrome, exercise fatigue, and anemia. Incidental findings on a chest x-ray should also be investigated.

❍ **Where do the following cancers most commonly develop within the lung: adenocarcinoma, large cell, squamous cell and small cell?**

Adenocarcinoma and large cell carcinomas are usually located peripherally, while squamous and small cell carcinomas are located centrally.

❍ **Which form of lung cancer is the most common?**

Squamous cell carcinoma (40 to 50%), followed by adenocarcinoma (35%) and small-cell (oat cell) carcinoma (25%).

❍ **Name 5 HIV-related pulmonary infections.**

PCP, TB, histoplasmosis, cryptococcus, and CMV.

❍ **What diagnostic test is helpful for the identification of a sub-clinical PCP infection?**

Exertional pulse oximetry is positive for PCP if after 3 minutes of exercise the O_2 saturation decreases by 3% or the A-a gradient increases by 10 mm Hg from rest.

❍ **What laboratory tests aid in the diagnosis of PCP?**

A rising LDH or a LDH > 450 and an ESR > 50. A low albumin implies a poor prognosis.

❍ **The initial therapy for PCP includes what antibiotics?**

Trimethoprim-sulfamethoxazole (Bactrim) or pentamidine.

❍ **What other medication should be prescribed to a patient with PCP?**

Corticosteroids when the pO_2 is < 70 mm Hg or an A-a gradient > 35 mm Hg.

❍ **What two drugs are used as prophylactic treatment to prevent PCP in HIV patients?**

Aerosolized pentamidine (Pentam) or trimethoprim/sulfamethoxazole (Bactrim).

❍ **Where does pain from pleurisy radiate?**

The shoulder, as a result of diaphragmatic irritation.

❍ **Currant jelly sputum is indicative of what kind of pneumonia?**

Klebsiella. Currant jelly stools are associated with intussusception.

❍ **What are the most common causes of Staphylococcal pneumonias?**

Drug use and endocarditis. This pneumonia produces high fever, chills, and a purulent productive cough.

❍ **A 23 year-old male presents with a dry cough, malaise, fever, and a sore throat that have developed in the past two weeks. What is the diagnosis?**

Mycoplasma pneumonia. This condition usually has a slow onset and occurs in the young. Treat the patient with erythromycin or tetracycline.

❍ **What are the extrapulmonary manifestations of mycoplasma?**

Erythema multiforme, pericarditis, and CNS disease.

❍ **What is the most frequent etiology of nosocomial pneumonia?**

Pseudomonas auruginosa. There is a high mortality associated with pneumonia caused by Pseudomonas. It most frequently occurs in immunocompromised patients or patients on mechanical ventilation.

❍ **A 67 year-old alcoholic was found in an alley, covered in his own vomit and beer. Upon examination, he is shaking, has a fever of 103.5^{o} F, and is coughing up currant jelly sputum. What is the diagnosis?**

Pneumonia induced by Klebsiella pneumoniae. This is the most likely etiology in alcoholics, the elderly, the very young, and immunocompromised patients. Other gram-negative bacteria, such as E. coli and other Enterobacteriaceae, may cause pneumonia in alcoholics who have aspirated.

❍ **A 46-year-old smoker comes to your office bragging about a three day business convention he attended last week in Las Vegas. He is nauseated and coughing; he has chills and a fever of 103. 5° F, his pulse is 68. Should you be concerned about your own health, as he has just given a mighty cough in your direction?**

No. This patient probably has Legionnaires' disease. Unless you attended the same convention in Las Vegas, you are unlikely to catch pneumonia from him. Legionella pneumophila contaminates the water in air conditioning towers and moist soil. It is not easily transmitted from person to person.

❍ **Match the pneumonia with the treatment.**

1) Klebsiella pneumoniae	a) Erythromycin, tetracycline, or doxycycline
2) Streptococcal pneumoniae	b) Penicillin G

3) Legionella pneumophila
4) Haemophilus influenza
5) Mycoplasma sp.

c) Cefuroxime and clarithromycin
d) Erythromycin and rifampin

Answers: (1) c, (2) b, (3) d, (4) c, and (5) a.

❍ **What are the classic chest x-ray findings in a patient with mycoplasma pneumonia.**

Patchy diffuse densities involving the entire lung. Pneumatoceles, cavities, abscesses, and pleural effusions can occur, but are uncommon. Treat the patient with erythromycin.

❍ **What are the classic chest x-ray finding associated with Legionella pneumonia.**

Dense consolidation and bulging fissures. Expect elevated liver enzymes and hypophosphatemia. Patient with Legionella pneumonia classically presents with a relative bradycardia.

❍ **A 43 year-old male presents of pleurisy, sudden onset of fever and chills, and rust colored sputum. What is the diagnosis?**

Pneumococcal pneumonia caused by Streptococcus pneumoniae, the most common community-acquired pneumonia. It is a consolidating lobar pneumonia and can be treated with penicillin G or erythromycin.

❍ **A 20 year-old college student is home for winter break and presents complaining of a 10-day history of a non-productive dry hacking cough, malaise, a mild fever, and no chills. What is the diagnosis?**

Mycoplasma pneumoniae, also known as walking pneumonia. Although this is the one of the most common pneumonia that develops in teenagers and young adults, it is an atypical pneumonia and is most frequently occurs in close contact populations, i.e., schools and military barracks.

❍ **A 56 year-old smoker with COPD presents with chills, fever, green sputum, and extreme shortness of breath. An x-ray shows a right lower lobe pneumonia. What is expected from the sputum culture?**

Haemophilus influenza. This organism is generally found in pneumonia and bronchitis patients with COPD. The next most common organism detected in this patient population is Moraxella catarrhalis. Ampicillin/clavulanate (Augmentin) is the drug of choice, but patients at high risk should have yearly influenza vaccinations.

❍ **Describe the different presentations of bacterial and viral pneumonia.**

Bacterial pneumonia is typified by a sudden onset of symptoms, including pleurisy, fever, chills, productive cough, tachypnea, and tachycardia. The most common bacterial pneumonia is Streptococcus pneumoniae.

Viral pneumonia is characterized by gradual onset of symptoms, no pleurisy, chills or high fever, general malaise, and a non-productive cough.

❍ **What two antimicrobial agents are broadly effective against organisms that cause both typical and atypical pneumonias?**

Azithromycin and clarithromycin.

❍ **What percent of upper-respiratory infectious agents are non-bacterial?**

Non-bacterial agents account for over 90% of pharyngitis, laryngitis, tracheal bronchitis, and bronchitis.

❍ **Name two anti-viral medications that are useful for viral pneumonia.**

Amantadine, for influenza A, and aerosolized Ribavirin, for RSV.

❍ **If a patient has a patchy infiltrate on a chest x-ray and bullous myringitis, what antibiotic should be prescribed?**

Erythromycin for mycoplasma.

❍ **What kind of pneumonia occurs in alcoholics and persons with aspiration pneumonia?**

Pneumonia resulting from either Gram-negative or anaerobic bacterium.

❍ **What secondary bacterial infection often occurs following a viral pneumonia?**

Staphylococcal pneumonia.

❍ **What three findings should be present to consider a sputum sample adequate?**

1) > 25 PMN's
2) < 10 squamous epithelial cells per low-powered field
3) A predominant bacterial organism

❍ **In what season does Legionella pneumonia most commonly occur?**

Summer. Legionella pneumophila thrive in environments such as the water cooling towers that are used in large buildings and hotels. Staphylococcal pneumonias also occur more frequently in summer.

❍ **An older patient with GI symptoms, hyponatremia, and a relative bradycardia probably has which type of pneumonia?**

Legionella.

❍ **Should steroids be used in aspiration pneumonia?**

No.

❍ **What is the indication for a chest tube in pneumothorax?**

Over 15% pneumothorax or a clinical indication, such as respiratory distress or enlarging pneumothorax.

❍ **What therapy may increase the body's absorption of a pneumothorax or pneumomediastinum?**

A high FiO_2.

❍ **What is the profile of a classic patient with a spontaneous pneumothorax?**

Male, athletic, tall, slim and 15 to 35 years of age.

❍ **What is the recurrence rate of spontaneous pneumothorax?**

30 to 50%.

❍ **What special chest x-rays may be useful for diagnosing pneumothorax?**

Expiratory film and lateral decubitus film on the affected side.

❍ **Which types of pneumonia are commonly associated with pneumothorax?**

Staphylococcal, TB, Klebsiella, and PCP.

❍ **What is the anticoagulant treatment schedule for a PE?**

IV heparin until PTT is 2 to 2.5 times normal. After a day, warfarin is added until the INR is greater than 2.0. If clots recur, consider a Greenfield filter in the IVC. Pulmonary embolectomy is only necessary in cases of massive embolisms.

❍ **What three syndromes are associated with the various degrees of pulmonary embolism?**

- Acute cor pulmonale: Occurs with massive embolism that obstructs over 60% of the pulmonary circulation.
- Pulmonary infarction: Occurs with embolization to the distal branches of the pulmonary circulation.
- Acute dyspnea: Milder obstruction not enough to warrant infarction.

❍ **What is the equation for the A-a gradient?**

A-a $= [(713 \text{ mm Hg} \times FiO_2\%)-pCO_2-pO_2/.8)]$

The normal A-a gradient is 5 to 15 mm Hg. The A-a gradient increases with PE and diffusion defects (i.e., pulmonary edema and right to left cardiac shunts).

❍ **Most pulmonary embolisms arise from what veins?**

The iliac and femoral veins.

❍ **Primary pulmonary hypertension is most common in what population?**

Young females. PPH is rapidly fatal within a few years.

❍ **What heart sounds accompany pulmonary hypertension?**

A narrowed second heart sound split and a louder P2.

❍ **What is the major etiology of pulmonary hypertension?**

Chronic hypoxia.

❍ **T/F: Pulse oximetry is a reliable method for estimating oxyhemoglobin saturation in a patient suffering from CO poisoning.**

False. COHb has light absorbance that can lead to a falsely elevated pulse oximeter transduced saturation level. The calculated value from a standard ABG may also be falsely elevated. The oxygen saturation should be determined by using a co-oximeter that measures the amounts of unsaturated O_2Hb, COHb, and metHb.

❍ **Sarcoidosis is most common in what race and age group?**

African Americans between 20 and 40 years of age.

❍ **What will the chest x-ray of a patient with sarcoidosis classically reveal?**

Bilateral hilar and paratracheal adenopathy with diffuse nodular appearing infiltrate. Sarcoidosis can be staged by the chest x-ray:

Stage 0: Normal
Stage 1: Hilar adenopathy
Stage 2: Hilar adenopathy and parenchymal infiltrates
Stage 3: Parenchymal infiltrates only
Stage 4: Pulmonary fibrosis

❍ **What other systems can be affected by sarcoidosis?**

The cardiovascular, gastrointestinal, immunological, integumental, lymphatics, and the ocular systems.

❍ **Upper lobe nodules and eggshell hilar node calcification are displayed on x-rays of an individual with what disease?**

Silicosis.

❍ **What occupations are most commonly associated with silicosis?**

Sandblasting and mining.

❍ **Is there a higher risk of lung cancer for patients with silicosis?**

No.

❍ **What is the average exposure time necessary for the development of silicosis following silicon dioxide inhalation?**

20 to 30 years. Employees in mining, pottery, soap production, and granite quarrying are at risk. This population also has a higher chance of acquiring TB.

❍ **What is the indication for long-term tracheostomy?**

When intubation is expected to exceed 3 weeks.

❍ **Differentiate between transudate and exudate.**

Transudate: Serum protein is < 0.5 and LDH is < 0.6. Most common with CHF, renal disease, and liver disease.

Exudate: Serum protein > 0.5, LDH > 0.6. Most common with infections, malignancy, and trauma.

❍ **What are the side effects of INH?**

Neuropathy, pyridoxine loss, lupus-like syndrome, anion-gap acidosis and hepatitis.

❍ **What percentage of tuberculosis cases are drug resistant?**

About 15%. The rate is highly dependent upon geographic location.

❍ **What are the classic signs and symptoms of TB?**

Night sweats, fever, weight loss, malaise, cough, and a greenish yellow sputum most commonly observed in the mornings.

❍ **What are some common extrapulmonary TB sites?**

The lymph nodes, bone, GI tract, GU tract, meninges, liver, and the pericardium.

❍ **T/F: Patients under 35 years of age with positive TB skin tests should undergo at least 6 months of isoniazid chemoprophylaxis.**

True.

❍ **Is a URI accompanied by a high fever usually caused by a bacterial or a viral source?**

Bacterial. However, most URI's are viral in origin.

❍ **A patient presents with cough, lethargy, dyspnea, conjunctivitis, glomerulonephritis, fever, and purulent sinusitis. What is the probable diagnosis?**

Wegener's granulomatosis. This is a necrotizing vasculitis and pulmonary granulomatosis that attacks the small artery and veins. Treat the patient with corticosteroids and cyclophosphamide.

❍ **What serological test is diagnostic for Wegener's granulomatosis?**

c-ANCA in association with appropriate clinical evidence. A renal, lung, or sinus biopsy may also be helpful in making the diagnosis.

❍ **Are sedatives beneficial for anxious asthmatic patients?**

No. However, sedatives are appropriate for use during rapid sequence intubation (RSI).

❍ **Speaking of RSI, discuss some agents that may be used to induce unconsciousness.**

Agent	Trade name	Class	Onset	Duration	Dose
Thiopental	Pentothal	Barbiturate	~ 30 seconds	2 to 30 minutes, depending on source	2.0 to 5.0 mg/kg at 40 mg/minute
Methohexital	Brevital	Barbiturate	Fast	Very short	5 to 12 ml of 1% solution at 1 ml/5 seconds
Fentanyl	Sublimaze	Opiate	2 minutes	~ 20 minutes	20 to 150 mg/kg
Midazolam	Versed	Benzodiazepine	~ 5 minutes	~ 30 minutes	0.1 mg/kg
Etomidate	Amidate	Benzoderiv.	1 minutes	3 to 12 minutes	0.2 to 0.4 mg/kg

❍ **What is the mechanism of alveolar hypoventilation (manifested by high PCO2) in myxedema?**

Depression of the hypoxic and hypercapnic respiratory drive. Respiratory muscle myopathy and phrenic neuropathy are uncommon.

❍ **Should all individuals with chronic unexplained alveolar hypoventilation be tested for hypothyroidism?**

Yes.

❍ **Is obstructive sleep apnea common in hypothyroidism?**

Yes. Contributing factors include enlarged tongue and myopathy. Hypothyroidism should be excluded in most patients with sleep apnea.

❍ **What other endocrine disorder is associated with an increased frequency of sleep apnea?**

Acromegaly. Sleep apnea may be central or obstructive in origin.

❍ **What is the appearance of flow volume loop in large goiter?**

Flattening of inspiratory loop suggestive of variable extrathoracic upper airway obstruction.

❍ **Which adjunctive therapy for chronic cough could precipitate thyroid storm?**

SSKI.

❍ **What is the common location of ectopic parathyroids?**

The mediastinum.

❍ **Can beta-adrenergic agonists result in tolerance?**

Yes. Repeated administration of beta agonist bronchodilators can result in hyposensitization of the receptors, but this should not preclude their use. Glucocorticoids have been shown to restore the depressed receptor responsiveness.

❍ **Prior steroid administration can precipitate adrenal insufficiency under conditions of stress. How long can this effect last?**

Up to one year.

❍ **Which pulmonary infection is a common cause of adrenal insufficiency, especially in third world countries?**

Tuberculosis.

❍ **What is the common mechanism of hyponatremia in pulmonary tumors and infections?**

SIADH.

❍ **What type of lung cancer is commonly associated with hypercalcemia?**

Squamous cell carcinoma. The production of parathormone related peptide can produce hypercalcemia even without bony metastases.

❍ **Which non-neoplastic pulmonary disease is often associated with hypercalcemia and hypercalciuria?**

Sarcoidosis.

❍ **What type of lung tumors can cause excessive ACTH production and Cushing's syndrome?**

Small cell carcinoma and carcinoid tumors.

❍ **What are the neuroendocrine tumors of the lung?**

Typical carcinoid, atypical carcinoid and small cell carcinoma.

❍ **Is carcinoid syndrome common with pulmonary carcinoid?**

No. It is rare, with incidence ranging from 2 to 7%.

❍ **Does diabetes predispose to the development of pulmonary tuberculosis?**

Yes, especially when poorly controlled.

❍ **In thyroid carcinoma, what factors favor metastasis to the lung?**

Follicular subtype, inadequate treatment of the primary cancer, and cervical lymph node involvement.

❍ **What are the pulmonary manifestations in Paget's Disease?**

High output cardiac failure with pulmonary edema, impaired respiratory control from bony involvement at base of skull, vertebral fractures leading to kyphosis and restrictive lung disease.

❍ **What is acute chest syndrome in sickle cell lung disease?**

The syndrome includes fever, chest pain, leukocytosis and pulmonary infiltrate. The major dilemma is in distinguishing infarction from pneumonia. It can also be caused by fat embolism and pulmonary edema.

❍ **What is sickle cell chronic lung disease?**

It is thought to be the result of years of uncontrolled and often asymptomatic sickling and characterized by pulmonary hypertension, cor pulmonale and ventilatory defects.

❍ **What is the commonest cause of pneumonia in sickle cell disease?**

Streptococcus pneumoniae.

❍ **What are the preventive measures commonly employed in sickle cell disease?**

Pneumococcal vaccine, Hemophilus influenza b vaccine and yearly influenza vaccine in those with chronic pulmonary symptoms.

❍ **Which type of pneumonia is often associated with cold agglutinins?**

Mycoplasma pneumoniae.

❍ **Name some of the hypercoagulable states predisposing to thrombosis and pulmonary embolism.**

Deficiencies of protein C, protein S and antithrombin III; factor V mutation; antiphospholipid syndrome; malignancy particularly adenocarcinoma; Nephrotic syndrome, protein losing enteropathy, extensive burns; Paroxysmal nocturnal hemoglobinuria; and oral contraceptives.

❍ **What are the pulmonary manifestations of polycythemia?**

Pulmonary embolism related to hyperviscosity and pulmonary hemorrhage related to an increased bleeding tendency.

❍ **What is the differential diagnosis of pulmonary infiltrates in patients with hematological malignancies?**

Infections, treatment related (radiation, chemotherapy), hemorrhage, malignant infiltration and hyperleukocytosis.

❍ **What is pseudohypoxemia?**

Hypoxemia from consumption of oxygen by cells in blood during transport, as can occur in hyperleukocytosis.

❍ **Which interstitial lung disease may be associated with diabetes insipidus?**

Eosinophilic granuloma or histiocytosis X.

❍ **What is the typical time period during which acute radiation pneumonitis develops?**

Within the first eight weeks after radiation.

❍ **What are the factors that increase the bleeding complications after transbronchial lung biopsy?**

Renal failure, hemorrhagic diathesis, and lymphoma.

❍ **T/F: Most episodes of transfusion associated acute lung injury (TRALI) are caused by donor antibodies reacting with recipient neutrophil or HLA antigens.**

True.

❍ **What is the predominant change in the lung volumes in pregnancy?**

Decrease in functional residual capacity by as much as 15-25%.

❍ **T/F: The elevated diaphragm depresses tidal breathing.**

False. The tidal volume actually increases and accounts for much of the increased minute ventilation and mild respiratory alkalosis.

❍ **Does the decreased functional residual capacity result in early airway closure in pregnancy?**

No.

❍ **Why is the incidence of thromboembolism increased in pregnancy?**

Venous stasis from the uterine pressure on the inferior vena cava, increase in clotting factors, increased fibrinogen and decreased fibrinolysis.

❍ **What are some of the risk factors for thromboembolism in pregnancy?**

C-Section, multiparity, bed rest, obesity, increased maternal age, and surgical procedures.

❍ **What are the predisposing factors for amniotic fluid embolism?**

Older maternal age, multiparity, C-Section, amniotomy, and insertion of intrauterine fetal monitoring devices.

❍ **How does amniotic fluid enter maternal circulation?**

Through uterine tears or injury, or endocervical veins.

❍ **What are the major consequences of amniotic fluid embolism?**

Cardiorespiratory collapse and DIC.

❍ **What are the potential mechanisms of cardiorespiratory collapse?**

Mechanical obstruction of pulmonary vasculature, alveolar capillary leak, pulmonary edema from LV failure, anaphylaxis.

❍ **How can amniotic fluid embolism be diagnosed?**

By demonstrating fetal squames in sputum or buffy coat preparations of blood. Pulmonary microvascular cytology of the blood drawn from the distal lumen of the PA catheter.

❍ **What is the treatment of amniotic fluid embolism?**

Supportive.

❍ **What is the mortality rate in amniotic fluid embolism?**

About 80%.

❍ **What is the classic presentation of venous air embolism?**

Sudden hypotension with a mill wheel murmur audible over the precordium.

❍ **What is the preferred patient position in suspected venous air embolism?**

Left lateral decubitus.

❍ **What are the factors in pregnancy increasing the risk of aspiration of stomach contents?**

Increased intragastric pressure from the gravid uterus, progesterone induced relaxation of the lower esophageal sphincter, delayed gastric emptying in labor and depressed mental status from analgesia.

❍ **What are some of the common misconceptions about the management of asthma during pregnancy?**

That dyspnea is common in pregnancy and that medications should be sparsely used. Uncontrolled asthma causes more fetal harm than medications.

❍ **Should immunotherapy be used in pregnant asthmatics?**

Immunotherapy may be continued if felt to be useful but should not be initiated during pregnancy.

❍ **T/F: An arterial PCO2 of 35 mm Hg does not represent severe asthma.**

False. This may represent pseudonormalization since there is chronic mild hyperventilation in pregnancy.

❍ **What is the pulmonary complication of tocolytic therapy?**

Tocolytic induced pulmonary edema.

❍ **Which agents are associated with this syndrome?**

Terbutaline, ritadrine and magnesium sulfate.

❍ **What are some of the proposed mechanisms for tocolytic induced pulmonary edema?**

Fluid overload, myocardial toxicity, reduced oncotic pressure and increased capillary permeability.

❍ **What is the therapy of this syndrome?**

Stop the tocolytics and supportive care.

❍ **What factors should be taken into account during intubation in pregnancy?**

Upper airway hyperemia may require smaller endotracheal tube and the decreased FRC may lower oxygen reserve and therefore patients should be adequately preoxygenated with 100% followed by a quick apnea time during intubation.

❍ **Name the anticoagulant safe in pregnancy.**

Heparin. Warfarin is contraindicated.

❍ **Name the antibiotics that should be avoided in pregnancy.**

Tetracyclines, aminoglycosides, chloramphenicol and sulfonamides.

❍ **Can influenza vaccine be used in pregnancy?**

Yes.

❍ **Name the antituberculous drugs that should be avoided in pregnancy.**

Streptomycin and ethionamide.

❍ **Should therapy of active tuberculosis in pregnancy be postponed till after delivery?**

No.

❍ **An unusual manifestation of bleomycin lung toxicity is nodular lesions mimicking pulmonary metastases. What is found pathologically?**

Bronchiolitis obliterans organizing pneumonia.

❍ **What are the proven risk factors for the development of bleomycin lung toxicity?**

1) Total accumulative dose, 2) older age (rare<70), 3) radiation therapy, 4) multidrug regimens, 5) high FiO2.

❍ **What is the most characteristic presentation of bleomycin lung toxicity?**

Pulmonary fibrosis

❍ **T/F: The return of pulmonary function abnormalities to normal after withdrawal of bleomycin is the rule.**

False.

❍ **What are four distinct presentations of bleomycin lung toxicity?**

Chronic pulmonary fibrosis, hypersensitivity lung reaction, acute pneumonitis, acute chest pain syndrome.

❍ **What dose of radiation is generally required to cause the synergistic effect of bleomycin and radiotherapy on the incidence of bleomycin lung toxicity?**

5000-6000 rads.

❍ **An acute chest pain syndrome can occur with which chemotherapeutic agents?**

Methotrexate and bleomycin.

❍ **What are the risk factors for methotrexate (MTX) pulmonary toxicity?**

Primary biliary cirrhosis, frequency of administration, adrenalectomy, tapering of corticosteroid therapy and use in multi-drug regimens.

❍ **What drug will produce hilar and mediastinal adenopathy as a toxic reaction?**

Methotrexate.

❍ **Hemolytic-Uremic syndrome has been associated with which chemotherapeutic agent?**

Mitomycin. This complication has a high mortality and can cause a microangiopathic hemolytic anemia, renal failure, cerebrovascular events and other manifestations of a vasculopathy. Blood transfusions are often associated with this disorder.

❍ **What is the most common presentation for lung toxicity caused by cytosine arabinoside?**

Non-cardiogenic pulmonary edema. Fever, dyspnea and cough typically appear within 4 weeks of completing drug therapy. Acute pulmonary disease with diffuse alveolar infiltrates and pleural effusions occur, mechanical ventilation is often required and mortality approaches 50%.

❍ **Chronic interstitial pneumonitis can be caused by cyclophosphamide. What physical finding is more common with cyclophosphamide-induced lung injury than other chemotherapy-related lung injuries?**

Fever.

❍ **Radiation therapy is a potent risk factor for the development of pulmonary toxicity due to which chemotherapy agents?**

Cyclophosphamide, busulfan and bleomycin.

❍ **What is the nature of the lung toxicity associated with the cytokine, interleukin-2?**

Massive fluid retention and pulmonary edema.

❍ **What toxicity has been observed with the use of all-transretinoic acid for the treatment of acute leukemia?**

Acute lung disease associated with massive fluid retention.

❍ **What is the incidence of cough induced by captopril?**

1-2%.

❍ **What is the incidence of enalapril-induced cough?**

24.7%.

❍ **T/F: Generally the cough related to ACE inhibitors resolves within a few days of withdrawal of the drug.**

False. The resolution of cough may be slow, taking several weeks.

❍ **Is ACE inhibitor cough more common in men or women?**

Male : female = 1:2.

❍ **What is the usual time course for lung toxicity with gold salts?**

Several days of fever, cough and dyspnea.

❍ **What are the bronchoalveolar lavage findings in patients with gold salt induced hypersensitivity pulmonary disease?**

Increased numbers of lymphocytes.

❍ **What are four syndromes of penicillamine induced lung toxicity?**

Chronic pneumonitis, hypersensitivity lung disease, bronchiolitis obliterans and pulmonary-renal syndrome.

❍ **A syndrome similar to Goodpasture's disease has been reported with which drug?**

Penicillamine.

❍ **Name at least 5 drugs known to have caused bronchiolitis obliterans organizing pneumonia**

Bleomycin, penicillamine, amiodarone, cocaine, cyclophosphamide, mitomycin C, methotrexate, sulfasalazine and gold.

❍ **What acute pulmonary reaction might one encounter at the time of a persantine-thallium study for cardiac ischemia?**

Bronchospasm due to dipyridamole.

❍ **After removal from cardiopulmonary bypass during coronary revascularization surgery, a patient develops severe wheezing. What drug might be responsible?**

Protamine.

❍ **Alveolar proteinosis has been described in association with the use of what drug?**

Busulfan.

❍ **A sarcoidosis-like lesion has been described with use of which chemotherapeutic agent?**

Nitrosoureas.

❍ **A mid-inspiratory squeak while non-specific may be auscultated with what pathologic lesion occasionally seen as an adverse effect of certain drugs?**

Bronchiolitis obliterans, e.g. penicillamine.

❍ **T/F: Clubbing is very unusual with drug-induced interstitial lung disease.**

True.

❍ **Which of the following drugs have dose dependent lung toxicity: cyclophosphamide, bleomycin or BCNU?**

Bleomycin and BCNU.

❍ **What are the historical findings in patients with an acute pleuripulmonary reaction to nitrofurantoin?**

Fever, dyspnea, cough, and pleuritic pain, typically within hours or several days of starting the drug.

❍ **T/F: Untreated acute nitrofurantoin lung toxicity will progress to the chronic form within several months.**

False. There seems to be no overlap between the acute and the chronic forms.

❍ **Acute respiratory failure occurring in patients taking amiodarone is associated with which two procedures?**

Cardiovascular surgery and angiography.

❍ **What are the risk factors that predispose to a higher incidence of pulmonary injury by amiodarone?**

1) A maintenance dose of amiodarone in excess of 400 mg/day, 2) use of angiography, 3) cardiac or lung surgery, 4) concomitant lung disease.

❍ **The presence of foamy appearing macrophages and infiltration of inflammatory cells including lymphocytes, plasma cells, histiocytes and neutrophils suggests lung injury from what drug?**

Amiodarone.

❍ **What laboratory and radiological findings help distinguish amiodarone lung toxicity from CHF?**

1) Elevated ESR, 2) reduced DLCO, 3) abnormal gallium-67 uptake 4) high attenuation of infiltrates on CT scan of lungs.

❍ **Pulmonary reactions often occur when drugs or agents combine synergistically with each other. Fill in the associated agent causing the pulmonary lesion listed to the right.**

Bleomycin	+	a	=	NCPE (non-cardiogenic pulmonary edema)
Mitomycin	+	b	=	NCPE
Mitomycin	+	c	=	NCPE
Amphotericin B	+	d	=	NCPE
Vinblastine	+	e	=	Asthma
Nitrofurantoin	+	f	=	Pulmonary granulomas
Amiodarone	+	g	=	NCPE

a-oxygen, b-5-fluorouracil, c-leukocyte transfusion, d-leukocyte transfusion, e-mitomycin, f-low dose methotrexate, g-oxygen.

❍ **What chemotherapeutic agents have been associated with pulmonary veno-occlusive disease?**

Bleomycin, mitomycin-3C, BCNU, etoposide and cyclophosphamide.

❍ **What is the incidence of aspirin-induced bronchospasm in patients with nasal polyps?**

Up to 75%.

❍ **T/F: In aspirin-induced bronchospasm, there can be cross-reactivity with non-steroidal anti-inflammatory drugs.**

True.

❍ **What are the risk factors for the development of tocolytic-induced pulmonary edema?**

Use of corticosteroids, fluid overload, twin gestation, multiparous state, anemia, and silent cardiac disease.

❍ **A lymphocytic interstitial pneumonitis has been associated with which antiarrhythmic?**

Flecainide.

❍ **Mediastinal lipomatosis is associated with what drug class?**

Corticosteroids.

❍ **What laboratory finding distinguishes patients with primary SLE and drug-induced lupus?**

Drug- induced lupus has a positive ANA, but a negative ds-DNA.

❍ **T/F: Beta-adrenergic antagonists in massive overdose may cause severe bronchospasm in normal individuals.**

False.

❍ **T/F: Cardioselective beta-blockers avoid precipitation of bronchospasm in asthmatic individuals.**

False.

❍ **What is the therapeutic drug of choice for beta-blocker-induced bronchospasm?**

Inhaled ipratropium bromide.

❍ **What is the pulmonary lesion associated with overdosage of phenothiazine?**

Non-cardiogenic pulmonary edema.

❍ **T/F: Anaerobic lung infections do not occur in edentulous patients.**

False.

❍ **Hematogenous embolization from a septic jugular thrombophlebitis is a rare cause of anaerobic lung infection. What is the incriminated organism?**

Fusobacterium necrophorum (Lemiere's Syndrome).

❍ **The three most common bacterial genera known to cause anarobic lung infection are:**

Peptostreptococcus, fusobacterium and bacteroides.

❍ **Name 4 antibiotics known to have in vitro activity against anaerobic bacteria in virtually all cases.**

Metronidazole, chloramphenicol, imipenem and beta-lactam/beta-lactamase inhibitors.

❍ **When should bronchoscopy be used in the setting of a lung abcess?**

Perform in atypical presentations, failure to respond to therapy or in situations where there is no apparent risk factor for aspiration.

❍ **Which gram-negative aerobes are known to cause lung abscess?**

Pseudomonas and Klebsiella.

❍ **What are the two major risk factors for the development of anaerobic lung infection?**

Periodontal disease and predisposition to aspiration.

❍ **T/F: The presence of a cuffed endotracheal tube makes aspiration pneumonia an unlikely cause of new pulmonary infiltrates.**

False.

❍ **T/F: Retrospective reviews indicate that antibiotic therapy for aspiration pneumonia will hasten the resolution of pulmonary infiltrates.**

False.

❍ **With aspiration pneumonias manifesting as lobar infiltrates, which are the most common sites?**

Superior segments of lower lobes and posterior segments of the upper lobes.

❍ **What is the drug of choice for pneumonias acquired in the outpatient setting due to anaerobic bacteria?**

Clindamycin.

❍ **What are the predominant organisms that complicate aspiration in a hospital setting?**

S. aureus, E. coli, Ps. aeruginosa, Klebsiella sp. or Proteus sp.

❍ **Why is clindamycin superior to penicillin in the treatment of anaerobic lung abcess?**

The presence of penicillin-resistant bacteroides melaninogenicus.

❍ **What factor determines the magnitude of injury in gastric acid aspiration?**

The gastric pH. A pH of less than 3 produces the most severe injury.

❍ **Empyema in the absence of parenchymal lung infiltrate suggests what underlying process?**

Subphrenic or other intra-abdominal abcess.

❍ **What is the incidence of Bacteroides fragilis in anaerobic lung infections?**

5-7%.

❍ **What is the recommended duration of antibiotic therapy for necrotizing anaerobic pneumonia, lung abcess or empyema?**

4 - 8 weeks.

❍ **Under what circumstances is aspiration of vomitus, oral secretions or foreign material likely?**

Anything producing an altered level of consciousness (e.g. alcohol, overdose, general anesthesia, stroke), impaired swallowing or abnormal gastro-intestinal motility, or disruption of the esophageal sphincters predisposes to aspiration.

❍ **T/F: Nasogastric and gastric tubes increase the risk of aspiration.**

True.

❍ **T/F: Normals may aspirate small amounts of oral contents without developing clinical complications.**

True.

❍ **What determines the likelihood of pulmonary complications from aspiration?**

Frequency of aspiration, volume of aspirate, and character of aspirate.

❍ **What are the signs of a large obstructing foreign body in the larynx or trachea?**

Respiratory distress, stridor, inability to speak, cyanosis, loss of consciousness, and death.

❍ **What are the symptoms of a smaller (distally lodged) foreign body?**

Cough, dyspnea, wheezing, chest pain and fever.

❍ **What is the procedure of choice for foreign body removal?**

Rigid bronchoscopy. Fiberoptic bronchoscopy is an alternate procedure in adults, not in children. If bronchoscopy fails, thoracotomy may be required.

❍ **What are the common radiographic findings in foreign body aspiration?**

Normal film, atelectasis, pneumonia, contralateral mediastinal shift (more marked during expiration), and visualization of the foreign body.

❍ **What are the common directly toxic (non-infected) respiratory tract aspirates?**

Gastric contents, alcohol, hydrocarbons, mineral oil, animal and vegetable fats. All of these produce an inflammatory response and pneumonia. Gastric contents are the commonest offender.

❍ **What are the consequences of aspirating acid?**

The response is rapid, with near immediate bronchitis, bronchiolitis, atelectasis, shunting and hypoxemia. Pulmonary edema may occur within 4 hours. The clinical manifestations are dyspnea, wheezing, cough, cyanosis, fever and shock.

❍ **What is the antibiotic choice for gastric acid aspiration?**

None.

❍ **What is the role of corticosteroids in gastric acid aspiration?**

None.

❍ **What is the main priority in treating gastric acid aspiration?**

Maintenance of oxygenation. Intubation, ventilation, and PEEP (positive end expiratory pressure) may be required.

❍ **What are the radiographic manifestations of acid aspiration?**

Varied, may be bilateral diffuse infiltrates, irregular "patchy" infiltrates, or lobar infiltrates.

❍ **What outcomes occur in patients who do not rapidly resolve gastric acid aspiration pneumonitis?**

ARDS (adult respiratory distress syndrome), progressive respiratory failure and death; bacterial superinfection.

❍ **Under what circumstances are antibiotics used in aspiration?**

Aspiration of infected material, intestinal obstruction, immune compromised host, and evidence of bacterial superinfection after a non-infected aspirate (new fever, infiltrates, or purulence after the initial 2 to 3 days).

❍ **What is the usual source of infected aspirated material?**

The oropharynx.

❍ **What pleuripulmonary infections may occur after aspirating infected oropharyngeal material?**

Necrotizing pneumonia, lung abscess, "typical" pneumonia, and empyema.

❍ **What is the predominant oropharyngeal flora in outpatients?**

Anaerobes. Community acquired aspiration is usually anaerobic. The most common aerobes involved are streptococcus species.

❍ **What is the antibiotic of choice for outpatient acquired infectious aspiration pneumonia?**

Either clindamycin or high-dose penicillin.

❍ **What is the bacteriology of inpatient acquired infectious aspiration pneumonia?**

Mixed aerobic and anaerobic organisms. Unlike outpatients, Staphylococcus aureus, Escherichia coli, Pseudomonas aeruginosa, and Proteus species are common.

❍ **What antibiotics treat inpatient acquired infectious aspiration pneumonia?**

Beta-lactamase resistant penicillins, cephalosprins, or clindamycin plus an aminoglycoside. Imipenem may also be used, especially in the immunocompromised.

❍ **How long after aspiration is lung abscess usually detected?**

Two weeks or more.

❍ **What is the duration of treatment for lung abscess?**

Until radiographic resolution or stabilization with a small residual scar or cyst. This may take 6 weeks or more.

❍ **What are the clinical consequences of aspiration of liquid gastric contents with pH greater than 2.5?**

Hypoxemia, bronchospasm and atelectasis may develop, but usually resolve within 24 hours.

❍ **Lipoid pneumonia is associated with chronic aspiration of what substance?**

Mineral oil. Also animal or vegetable oils and oil-based nose drops.

❍ **What is the preferred antibiotic for near drowning in polluted (high coliform counts) water?**

None.

❍ **What is the priority in treatment of near drowning?**

Maintenance of oxygenation.

❍ **What are the indications for intubation and ventilation after near drowning?**

Apnea, pulselessness, altered mental status, severe hypoxemia, and respiratory acidosis.

❍ **What is the frequency of ARDS (adult respiratory distress syndrome) after near drowning?**

40%.

❍ **What are the major causes of massive hemoptysis?**

Tuberculosis, bronchiectasis and lung cancer.

❍ **What causes hemoptysis in patients with tuberculosis (either active or healed)?**

Pulmonary artery (Rasmussen's) aneurysm, bronchiolar ulceration and necrosis, bronchiectasis, broncholithiasis, lung cancer and mycetoma (fungus ball).

❍ **What is the purpose of bronchoscopy in hemoptysis?**

Localization and diagnosis.

❍ **What are the invasive therapies for massive hemoptysis?**

Thoracotomy, embolization, balloon tamponade (via bronchoscopy), double-lumen tube for lung separation and independent ventilation, and laser bronchoscopy.

❍ **What is the most feared complication of bronchial artery embolization?**

Anterior spinal artery embolization.

❍ **When is surgery indicated for massive hemoptysis?**

Localized massive hemoptysis unresponsive to other therapy; or electively, after stabilization, for long term control of localized bleeding.

❍ **What is the most common cause of hemoptysis in the United States?**

Bronchitis.

❍ **What percent of patients with an endobronchial neoplasm and a normal chest x-ray present with hemoptysis?**

15%.

❍ **Which metastatic tumors can produce hemoptysis?**

Breast, colon, kidney, malignant melanomas.

❍ **What benign tumor (or low-grade malignancy) is likely to cause hemoptysis?**

Bronchial carcinoid (adenoma).

❍ **What is the commonest cause of hemoptysis in patients with leukemia?**

Fungal infections, often aspergillus.

❍ **Which bacterial pneumonias frequently cause frank hemoptysis?**

Pseudomonas aeruginosa, Klebsiella pneumoniae, and Staphylococcus aureus.

❍ **What are the major cardiovascular causes of hemoptysis?**

Mitral stenosis, pulmonary hypertension, Eisenmenger's complex.

❍ **How does pulmonary artery catheterization produce hemoptysis?**

By pulmonary artery rupture, aneurysm formation or pulmonary infarct.

❍ **What is the frequency of hemoptysis in pulmonary embolization?**

20%.

❍ **Calculate the alveolar-arterial oxygen (A-aO_2) gradient given the following arterial blood gas obtained at sea level: pH 7.24, PaCO_2 60 PaO_2 45.**

30 mmHg.

To calculate the alveolar-arterial oxygen gradient, first calculate the expected alveolar partial pressure of oxygen (PAO_2) using the alveolar gas equation: PAO_2 = PIO_2 - PaCO_2/R, where PIO_2 is the partial pressure of oxygen in the inspired gas and R is the respiratory exchange ratio, commonly estimated at 0.8. PIO_2 is calculated as follows: PIO_2 = FIO_2 (P_B-P_{H2O}) where FIO_2 is the inspired concentration of oxygen (0.21 at sea level), P_B is the atmospheric pressure (760 mm Hg at sea level) and P_{H2O} is the partial pressure of water (47 mmHg). At sea level, PIO_2 is equal to 150 mmHg. Thus, for this example, PAO_2 = 150 - 60/0.8 or 75 mmHg.

The A-aO2 gradient is PAO_2 - PaO_2. Therefore, in this example, the A-aO_2 gradient is 75 - 45 or 30 mmHg.

❍ **What is the normal A-aO_2 gradient?**

10 mmHg in a 20 year-old.

❍ **What is the age related decline in PaCO_2?**

The PaO_2 declines by 2.5 mmHg per decade. Given that a PaO_2 of 95-100 mmHg is normal for a 20 year-old, a PaO_2 of 75-80 would be normal for a 80 year-old. This decline is secondary to an increase in the A-aO_2 gradient, which increases from about 10 mmHg in a 20 year-old to 20-25 mmHg in an 80 year-old.

❍ **What are the four principal mechanisms that lead to hypoxemia?**

Hypoventilation, diffusion limitation, shunt and ventilation-perfusion inequality. A fifth mechanism, low inspired oxygen concentration, is important only at altitudes above 8000 feet..

❍ **Which of the four above mechanisms is the most common?**

Ventilation-perfusion inequality.

❍ **What are the 3 major mechanisms of hypoventilation and what clinical conditions are associated with each?**

1. Failure of the central nervous system ventilatory centers - drugs (narcotics, barbiturates), stroke.
2. Failure of the chest bellows - chest wall diseases (kyphoscoliosis), neuromuscular diseases (amyotrophic lateral sclerosis), diaphragm weakness.
3. Obstruction of the airways - asthma, chronic obstructive pulmonary disease.

❍ **How can hypoxemia secondary to hypoventilation alone be distinguished from the other causes of hypoxemia?**

If the hypoxemia is from hypoventilation alone, the A-aO_2 gradient is normal. It is elevated in all other causes.

❍ **What are the most common clinical conditions in which shunt is the primary mechanism for hypoxemia?**

Alveolar filling with fluid (pulmonary edema) and pus (pneumonia) are the most commonly seen clinically. Any condition that fills or closes the alveoli preventing gas exchange can lead to shunt.

❍ **How can shunt be distinguished from the other causes of hypoxemia?**

If given 100% oxygen, the hypoxemia patient with shunt will not have a significant increase in their PaO_2. There will be a significant increase in PaO_2 when 100% oxygen is given to patients with hypoventilation or ventilation-perfusion inequality.

❍ **A leftward shift in the oxyhemoglobin dissociation curve indicates an increased or decreased hemoglobin affinity for oxygen?**

Increased.

❍ **Changes in temperature, $PaCO_2$ or pH, or the level of 2,3-diphosphoglycerate (2,3-DPG) cause a shift in the oxyhemoglobin dissociation curve. To cause a rightward shift, what are the changes that must occur?**

Increased temperature, increased $PaCO_2$, decreased pH, and increased 2,3-DPG level. An easy way to remember this is that these conditions are often associated with decreased tissue oxygen levels. By right-shifting the curve, more oxygen is released from the hemoglobin to the tissues.

❍ **What is the Bohr effect?**

The rightward shift of the oxyhemoglobin desaturation curve, secondary to decreased pH, is known as the Bohr effect.

❍ **Which types of hemoglobin are associated with an leftward shift of the oxyhemoglobin dissociation curve?**

Hemoglobin F (fetal hemoglobin), carboxyhemoglobin, and methemoglobin.

❍ **Which drugs cause methemoglobinemia?**

Oxidant drugs, such as antimalarials, dapsone, nitrites/nitrates (nitroprusside) and local anesthetics (lidocaine). Methemoglobinemia occurs when the iron moiety of hemoglobin is oxidated from the ferrous to the ferric state.

❍ **Which common enzyme deficiency predisposes to the development of methemoglobinemia in the presence of the above drugs?**

G-6-PD deficiency.

❍ **What is the treatment of methemoglobinemia?**

Methylene blue.

❍ **What are the determinants of the oxygen content of blood?**

Hemoglobin concentration, the PaO_2 and SaO_2. The equation to determine the oxygen content of blood is: $CaO_2 = (1.34 \times [Hgb] \times SaO_2) + (PaO_2 \times 0.003)$. The first term is the hemoglobin bound oxygen and the second is the dissolved oxygen. Dissolved oxygen content is a minor portion of total oxygen content unless PaO_2 is very high.

❍ **How does the shape of the oxyhemoglobin dissociation curve effect the oxygen content of blood?**

Since SaO_2 does not increase significantly if the $PaO_2 > 60$ mmHg, the oxygen content of blood will increase significantly above this level only by increasing the hemoglobin concentration.

❍ **What are the determinants of oxygen delivery to the peripheral tissues?**

Oxygen content of the blood (CaO_2) and cardiac output. An increase in either will increase oxygen delivery to the tissues.

❍ **What is orthodeoxia?**

A decrease in PaO_2, occurring when the patient moves from the supine to the upright position.

❍ **What is the normal tidal volume and minute ventilation in an average 70-kg subject?**

The normal tidal volume (V_T) is 500-600 ml and the normal minute ventilation (V_E) is 5-6 L/min.

❍ **What is the difference between anatomic and physiologic dead space?**

Dead space refers to areas of lung that are ventilated but not perfused. Anatomic dead space refers to the conducting airways (trachea, bronchi and bronchioles) where there is no gas exchange because there are no alveoli. Physiologic dead space includes the anatomic dead space and any diseased lung in which there is ventilation but no perfusion.

❍ **What is the normal dead space in an average 70-kg subject?**

150 ml.

❍ **Which pulmonary diseases are most associated with an increased physiologic dead space?**

Asthma and chronic obstructive pulmonary disease (COPD).

❍ **How is the minute ventilation related to alveolar and dead space ventilation?**

Minute ventilation (V_E) is the product of tidal volume multiplied by breathing frequency

($V_E = V_T \times f$). Alveolar ventilation (V_A) is that portion of the minute ventilation that contributes to gas exchange while dead space ventilation (V_D) is that portion that does not contribute to gas exchange. Thus, $V_E = V_A + V_D$.

❍ **What is the effect of increased alveolar ventilation (V_A) on $PaCO_2$?**

$PaCO_2$ will decrease as V_A increases.

❍ **What is the relationship between alveolar ventilation, minute ventilation and the dead space ratio (V_D/V_T)?**

Alveolar ventilation is proportional to both minute ventilation and the term ($1-V_D/V_T$). Any process that decreases minute ventilation or increases the dead space will decrease alveolar ventilation.

❍ **Why do asthmatics eventually have an increased $PaCO_2$ if untreated?**

As the asthma attack continues untreated, the work of breathing will continue to increase. Eventually, the diaphragm fatigues and the patient hypoventilates. The hypoventilation, in association with the increased dead space and increased CO_2 production, increases the $PaCO_2$.

❍ **What is the normal $PaCO_2$ and does it vary with age?**

Normal $PaCO_2$ is 35-45 mmHg and does not vary with age.

❍ **What is the Haldane effect?**

The decrease in carbon dioxide content with increases in hemoglobin oxygen saturation.

❍ **What is the normal expected change in pH if there is an acute change in the $PaCO_2$?**

The pH will increase or decrease 0.8 units for every 10 mmHg decrease or increase (respectively) in $PaCO_2$.

❍ **In chronic respiratory acidosis or alkalosis, what is the expected change in pH?**

The pH will increase or decrease 0.3 units for every 10 mmHg decrease or increase, respectively, in $PaCO_2$.

❍ **What is the expected change in serum bicarbonate in chronic respiratory acidosis or alkalosis?**

Bicarbonate increases by approximately 3 mEq/l for each 10 mmHg increase in $PaCO_2$ in chronic respiratory acidosis. Bicarbonate decreases by 4-5 mEq/l for each 10 mmHg decrease in $PaCO_2$ in chronic respiratory alkalosis.

❍ **What are the consequences of hypercapnia?**

Acute hypercapnia has physiologic consequences due to the increased $PaCO_2$ itself and the decreased pH. Physiologic effects of the $PaCO_2$ increase include:

1. Increases in cerebral blood flow.
2. Confusion, headache ($PaCO_2 > 60$mmHg), obtundation and seizures ($PaCO_2 > 70$mmHg).
3. Depression of diaphragmatic contractility.

The primary consequences of the decreased pH are on the cardiovascular system with changes in cardiac contractility (decreased), the fibrillation threshold (decreased), and vascular tone (predominantly vasodilatation).

❍ **What are the consequences of hypocapnia?**

Acute hypocapnia has physiologic consequences due to the decreased $PaCO_2$ itself and the increased pH.

Physiologic effects of the $PaCO_2$ decrease include:

1. Decreases in cerebral blood flow. This reflex is used in the management of neurologic disorders with high intracranial pressures as a short-term measure to decrease the increased intracranial pressure.
2. Confusion, myclonus, asterixis, loss of consciousness and seizures.

The primary consequences of the increased pH are, again, primarily on the cardiovascular system with increased cardiac contractility and vasodilatation.

❍ **A 25 year-old male presents to the emergency room obtunded. Examination is significant for a respiratory rate of 8/min and pinpoint pupils. An arterial blood gas reveals a pH of 7.28, a $PaCO_2$ of 55, and a PaO_2 of 60. What is the cause of the hypoxemia and hypercapnia?**

Acute narcotic overdose leading to hypoventilation.

❍ **A 30 year-old female presents with dyspnea and signs of right-sided heart failure. The PaO_2 on room air is 55 mmHg and on 100% oxygen is 70 mmHg. What is the cause of the hypoxemia?**

Shunt, as there is no significant increase in the PaO_2 on 100% oxygen.

❍ **The chest x-ray reveals no pulmonary parenchymal lesions but does show prominent hila and an enlarged right ventricle. What diagnostic test should be performed?**

The patient has no pulmonary parenchymal lesions to cause a shunt; therefore, she most likely has an intracardiac right-to-left shunt (most likely a previously undiagnosed atrial septal defect). An echocardiogram should be performed.

❍ **A 45 year-old obese male presents with dyspnea, peripheral edema, snoring, and excessive daytime sleepiness. A room air arterial blood gas in drawn and the pH is 7.34, $PaCO_2$ 60 mmHg, the PaO_2 is 58 mmHg, and the calculated HCO_3^- is 28 mEq/l. What is acid-base disturbance?**

Chronic, compensated respiratory acidosis. If this was acute respiratory acidosis, the pH would be 7.24 with a normal HCO_3^-.

❍ **What is the cause of the hypoxemia?**

Hypoventilation is one cause. However, since the A-aO_2 gradient is elevated, there is another cause in addition to the hypoventilation. In an obese patient, both ventilation-perfusion inequality and shunt (secondary to atelectasis) can contribute to the development of hypoxemia.

❍ **What is the cause of the hypoventilation?**

Obesity-hypoventilation syndrome.

❍ **A 50 year-old woman presents with a pneumonia in the right lower and middle lobes. On 50% oxygen by face mask, her PaO_2 is 75 mmHg. Should the patient be positioned right side down or up?**

Up. Blood flow is gravity dependent. If the patient is positioned right side down, blood flow will preferentially go to the right side. However, because of the pneumonia, this will increase the amount of shunt, lowering the PaO_2 further.

❍ **A 65 year-old male presents with dyspnea and dry cough. Chest x-ray reveals bilateral interstitial infiltrates and biopsy reveals idiopathic pulmonary fibrosis. Room air PaO_2 is 60 mmHg. What is the mechanism of hypoxemia?**

Ventilation-perfusion inequality. It is a common mistake to attribute the hypoxemia as secondary to diffusion impairment because of the pulmonary fibrosis. Diffusion impairment is a rare cause of hypoxemia.

❍ **T/F: If a patient presents with a $PaCO_2$ of 75, he/she should be emergently intubated.**

False. There is no $PaCO_2$ level at which a patient must be intubated. Intubation is based upon the total clinical condition of a patient, not just upon a blood gas result.

❍ **A 45 year-old presents to the ER after being rescued from a fire. He is dyspneic and cyanotic. SaO_2 on 50% mask is 84%. The blood gas, however, reveals a PaO_2 of 125 mmHg. Why the discrepancy?**

A fire victim is likely to have carbon monoxide poisoning. The carbon monoxide has converted the hemoglobin to carboxyhemoglobin, which decreases the binding of oxygen to hemoglobin and prevents an accurate pulse oximetry reading. However, carbon monoxide does not affect dissolved oxygen, which is what is measured in the arterial blood gas.

❍ **What is the treatment for carbon monoxide poisoning?**

100% oxygen, which increases carbon monoxide clearance by competing for binding to hemoglobin. If there is no significant response to 100% oxygen, hyperbaric oxygen (oxygen provided at higher than atmospheric pressure) is an alternative therapy.

❍ **A 25 year-old woman with a history of mitral valve prolapse presents with 'nervousness', chest tightness, hand numbness and mild confusion. Arterial blood gas reveals: pH 7.52, $PaCO_2$ 25 mmHg, PaO_2 108 mmHg. What is the diagnosis?**

Acute anxiety attack.

❍ **Why is the PaO_2 elevated?**

Because the lower $PaCO_2$ means a higher P_AO_2 (see alveolar gas equation above).

❍ **What is the treatment?**

The acute hyperventilation can be terminated by having the patient breathe in and out of a bag. Anxiolytics can also be provided.

❍ **T/F: A normal $PaCO_2$ in a patient with an asthma exacerbation is a good sign.**

Maybe. A normal $PaCO_2$ in an asthmatic is good if the patient is feeling improved and less dyspneic. However, it can be a sign of impending respiratory failure if the patient continues to feel dyspneic and is working hard to breathe.

❍ **T/F: Oxygen should never be given to a hypoxemic patient with COPD who has chronic CO_2 retention.**

False. Oxygen should always be given to a patient who is hypoxemic.

❍ **But I was taught that patients with chronic CO_2 retention given oxygen will have their drive to breathe blunted. Why should I give them oxygen?**

It has been shown that giving oxygen to a chronic CO_2 retainer does not result in a significant decrease in minute ventilation. The $PaCO_2$ will go up, but the rise is probably a result of changes in the ventilation-perfusion inequalities.

It is important to give these patients oxygen because a patient is more likely to die of hypoxemia than of hypercapnia. However, oxygen should be given judiciously with repeat $PaCO_2$ determinations to ensure that the $PaCO_2$ does not rise precipitously.

❍ **What are the indications for chronic oxygen therapy?**

1. Resting $PaO_2 < 55$ mmHg or $SaO_2 < 88\%$.
2. Resting PaO_2 56-59 mmHg or SaO_2 89% in presence of evidence of cor pulmonale and/or polycythemia.
3. During exercise if the PaO_2 falls below 55 mmHg or the SaO_2 below 88% with a low level of exertion.

❍ **How is chronic bronchitis defined?**

Daily expectoration of sputum for a minimum of three months a year for at least two years in a smoker or ex-smoker, without other underlying pulmonary disease.

❍ **What is the major side effect associated with the inhalation of N-acetylcysteine?**

Cough and bronchospasm , most likely due to irritation from the low pH (2.2) of the aerosol solution.

❍ **What are the contraindications to the use of chest physical therapy?**

Gastroesophageal reflux can be exacerbated by postural drainage or by chest percussion. Chest physical therapy does not appear to be effective in patients with end stage lung disease.

❍ **What is the effect of macrolide antibiotics (erythromycin, clarithromycin) on mucus hypersecretion?**

Some macrolide antibiotics have the ability to down regulate mucus secretion by an unknown mechanism. This is thought to be due to an anti-inflammatory activity.

❍ **What effect do the beta agonist bronchodilators have on mucus clearance?**

Variable. Although the beta agonists can increase ciliary beat frequency, clearance does not seem to improve. Beta agonists are also mucin secretagogues. Documented improvement in airflow with the use of beta agonists, as in asthma, indicates a predictable improvement in cough clearance.

❍ **What are the 4 major cell types of primary bronchogenic carcinoma.**

Small cell undifferentiated, large cell undifferentiated, squamous cell, and adenocarcinoma.

❍ **Differentiating which of these from the others is most important in planning the therapeutic approach?**

Small cell undifferentiated.

❍ **Exposure to what mineral, used as insulation, greatly enhances the carcinogenic potential of exposure to cigarette smoke?**

Asbestos.

❍ **Second hand cigarette smoke exposure is a risk factor for the development of what two major lung diseases?**

Lung cancer and COPD.

❍ **Which primary lung cancer is most frequently associated with paraneoplastic syndromes?**

Small cell undifferentiated carcinoma.

❍ **What other exposures are also factors contributing to the development of bronchogenic carcinoma?**

Radon, uranium, nickel, arsenic, bis (chloromethyl) ether, ionizing radiation, vinyl chloride, mustard gas, polycyclic aromatic hydrocarbons, and chromium.

❍ **The incidence of lung cancer is increasing in the USA among members of which gender?**

Females.

❍ **What accounts for this increase?**

Increased cigarette smoking prevalence.

❍ **Which vitamin has been associated with a protective effect against the development of lung cancer?**

Vitamin A.

❍ **What organs are frequently involved with metastases from primary lung cancer?**

Adrenal, brain, liver, and bone.

❍ **Hypercalcemia in the absence of bony metastases is associated with which lung cancer?**

Squamous cell carcinoma (a paraneoplastic syndrome associated with tumor elaboration of a PTH-like substance).

❍ **The syndrome of inappropriate secretion of antidiuretic hormone is associated with which cell type?**

Small cell undifferentiated carcinoma.

❍ **Bilateral periostitis, typically affecting the long bones and associated with lung cancer, is known as what other disease?**

Hypertrophic osteoarthropathy (HPO).

❍ **This finding is most frequently associated with which type of lung cancer?**

Adenocarcinoma.

❍ **Does the presence of HPO alone contraindicate a surgical approach in the treatment of lung cancer?**

No.

❍ **What myopathic syndrome is associated with lung cancer?**

Eaton-Lambert Syndrome.

❍ **What finding on physical examination can be used to differentiate Eaton-Lambert Syndrome from Myasthenia Gravis?**

Muscle function improves with repeated activity in the former, but degrades in the latter.

❍ **Tumor involvement in which lymph node location most clearly contraindicates a surgical approach to the therapy of non-small cell lung cancer? Hilar, contralateral mediastinal, infrapulmonary, or subcarinal?**

Contralateral mediastinal.

❍ **Is routine preoperative head CT scanning and nuclear scanning of liver and bone advocated in patients with lung cancer?**

No.

❍ **Of the following, which pattern of calcification of a solitary pulmonary nodule is most likely to be associated with a malignant lesion: lamellar (onion skin), popcorn, eccentric, or central?**

Eccentric.

❍ **Radiographic stability for what period is assumed to indicate benign origin of a solitary pulmonary nodule?**

Two years.

❍ **Doubling of the volume of a solitary pulmonary nodule is associated with what percentage increase in its diameter?**

Twenty-six percent?

❍ **What is the initial diagnostic test in a clinically stable patient suspected of having lung cancer?**

Sputum cytologic examination.

❍ **Should patients who smoke >1 pack of cigarettes per day be screened yearly with sputum cytology examinations?**

No.

❍ **Should patients who smoke >2 packs of cigarettes per day be screened annually with a PA radiograph of the chest?**

No.

❍ **Does local tumor invasion of the chest wall always contraindicate a surgical approach to lung cancer therapy?**

No.

❍ **Does a malignant pleural effusion always contraindicate a surgical approach to lung cancer therapy?**

Yes.

❍ **Is pre-operative radiotherapy indicated in the treatment of malignant tumors of the superior pulmonary sulcus?**

Yes.

❍ **What finding indicates emergent radiation therapy for superior vena cava syndrome?**

Cerebral edema.

❍ **What is the major indication for laser bronchoscopy in the treatment of bronchogenic carcinoma?**

Tumor obstruction of large airways.

❍ **What predicted post-operative FEV1 contraindicates surgical therapy for lung cancer?**

<750-800 cc.

❍ **Which of the following is the preferred method to predict post-operative FEV1 in patients whose pre-operative FEV1 is <2 liters: Quantitative perfusion lung scanning, quantitative ventilation lung scanning, split lung function utilizing a Carlens tube, or the lateral position test?**

Quantitative perfusion lung scanning.

❍ **Which of the following is an alternative method of assessing operability in patients with lung cancer: Stress echocardiography, cardiopulmonary exercise testing, weighing the patient while submerged, or the helium mixing time?**

Cardiopulmonary exercise testing.

❍ **Which method of mediastinal lymph node sampling is least likely to be useful in the pre-operative assessment of patients with lung cancer: Mediastinoscopy, mediastinotomy (Chamberlain procedure), sternotomy or transbronchial needle aspiration?**

Sternotomy.

❍ **Which radiographic finding is least likely to be associated with lung cancer: Linear density, rat tail bronchus, deep sulcus sign, or starburst appearance?**

Deep sulcus sign.

❍ **What is the 5 year survival all patients diagnosed with primary lung cancer?**

<15%.

❍ **Which primary lung cancer is most likely to cavitate?**

Squamous cell carcinoma.

❍ **Which primary lung cancer is least likely to present as a solitary pulmonary nodule?**

Small cell undifferentiated carcinoma.

❍ **What is the 5 year survival of non-small cell carcinoma of the lung treated with combination chemotherapy?**

<10%.

❍ **The best 5-year survival for non-small cell carcinoma of the lung is achieved by what therapy modality?**

Surgical resection.

❍ **What is the surgical 5-year survival for stage 1 non-small cell carcinoma of the lung?**

50-60%.

❍ **Are curative doses of radiotherapy in inoperable lung cancer effective in resultant long-term survival?**

No.

❍ **In the absence of trauma, which of the following is most likely to be the etiology of a bloody pleural effusion: a leaking thoracic aortic aneurysm, pneumonia, tuberculosis, lung cancer or a pulmonary infarction?**

Lung cancer.

❍ **The increase in death rate from lung cancer among smokers, as opposed to non-smokers, is how high?**

8 to 20-fold.

❍ **Bronchorrhea can be the presenting symptom in which subtype of adenocarcinoma of the lung?**

Bronchoalveolar cell carcinoma.

❍ **Do low tar cigarettes decrease the risk of lung cancer?**

No.

❍ **The risk of lung cancer following smoking cessation approaches that of lifelong non-smokers after how many years?**

15.

❍ **Is the incidence of lung cancer among urban residents is >5 fold higher than among rural residents?**

No, it is about 1.5 times higher than in rural residents.

❍ **The most common malignancy associated with asbestos exposure is which of the following: esophageal carcinoma, primary lung cancer, mesothelioma, or gastric carcinoma?**

Primary lung cancer.

❍ **Is alpha-1 antitrypsin deficiency associated with an increased risk of lung cancer?**

No.

❍ **Which of the following physical findings is most specifically associated with lung cancer: cachexia, localized wheezing, acanthosis nigricans, or alopecia areata?**

Localized wheezing.

❍ **Does a superior performance status have an association with improved survival among patients with non-small cell lung cancer?**

Yes.

❍ **Is an ipsilateral pleural effusion in a patient with a malignant lung tumor always assumed to represent tumor spread, and thus contraindicate a surgical therapeutic approach?**

No.

❍ **Can a patient with lung cancer be declared inoperable solely based on functional status?**

Yes.

❍ **Which of the following can fill the vacated hemithorax following pneumonectomy: organized fluid, contralateral shifted lung parenchyma, mediastinal contents, elevated hemi-diaphragm or intra-abdominal contents?**

All of the above.

❍ **Should one assume that two coexistent solitary pulmonary nodules represent metastases?**

No.

❍ **What percentage of solitary pulmonary nodules, in patients with a previous diagnosis of extrathoracic malignancy, represent metastatic disease?**

50%.

❍ **Are the majority of solitary pulmonary nodules seen on routine chest x-ray malignant?**

No.

❍ **A solitary pulmonary nodule in an HIV-infected patient may represent which of the following: PCP, histoplasmosis, cryptococcosis, or bronchogenic carcinoma?**

All of the above.

❍ **What is the ratio of CO_2 produced to O_2 consumed called?**

Respiratory quotient.

❍ **What is the point where exercising muscle begins anaerobic metabolism?**

Anaerobic threshold (AT).

❍ **What happens to $PaCO_2$ in exercise?**

Below AT it is normal. It is reduced above AT due to the ventilatory response to lactic acidosis. In COPD, $PaCO_2$ may rise with exercise.

❍ **What happens to PaO_2 in exercise?**

Usually normal, but may decrease in patients with lung disease.

❍ **What is the maximal O_2 consumption?**

The O_2 consumption at which O_2 consumption plateaus despite increased power. This is the most important measure of fitness, but may be difficult to achieve. The peak O_2 consumption at maximal exercise is often used instead.

❍ **What are the criteria for peak O_2 consumption?**

The patient should appear tired, or be near predicted maximal heart rate or predicted maximal minute volume. A lactate level over 8 mEq/L, or RQ over 1.15 are other criteria.

❍ **How does interstitial lung disease (ILD) affect maximal work rate and O_2 consumption?**

Both are reduced.

❍ **What happens to minute ventilation at submaximal work rates in ILD?**

Increased due to increased dead space ventilation. Respiratory rate increases, tidal volume decreases.

❍ **What happens to maximal voluntary ventilation and breathing reserve in ILD?**

Both are reduced.

❍ **Do patients with ILD desaturate during exercise?**

Yes.

❍ **T/F: Anaerobic threshold less than 40% in COPD suggests concomitant cardiovascular disease.**

True.

❍ **What is the best test of impairment in disability testing?**

Peak or maximal O_2 consumption. Anaerobic threshold my also be used. If maximal consumption is less than 15 ml/kg/min, the patient is unable to do most jobs. 15 to 25 correlates with moderate work. Over 25, the patient can do most jobs.

❍ **What improvements can be expected from pulmonary rehabilitation?**

Increased peak oxygen consumption and maximum work capacity, improved efficiency (decreased O_2 consumption for a given task) and improved motivation.

❍ **Does incentive spirometry prevent post operative pulmonary function abnormalities?**

No, however complications are reduced.

❍ **What are the common pulmonary complications after upper abdominal surgery?**

Atelectasis, bronchitis, cough, pneumonia, pleural effusion, and respiratory failure.

❍ **What is the incidence of post-operative respiratory complications in patients with COPD?**

50% or more.

❍ **Are pulmonary complications reduced after laparoscopic cholecystectomy compared to standard cholecystectomy?**

Yes, pulmonary function abnormalities are also reduced.

❍ **What studies best predict the risk of post operative pulmonary complications?**

Arterial blood gases and spirometry. CO_2 retention, FEV1 less than 70% of predicted, FVC less than 70% of predicted, and MVV less than 50% of predicted indicate high risk.

❍ **Is regional anesthesia preferred in patients with COPD?**

No.

❍ **Is cessation of smoking 24 hours pre-operatively beneficial?**

Yes, by reduction in pulse, blood pressure, and carboxyhemoglobin level.

❍ **What is the pre-operative therapy for patients with COPD?**

Bronchodilators, hydration, chest physiotherapy/incentive spirometry, and antibiotics if sputum is purulent. For maximum benefit, smoking cessation 4 to 8 weeks prior to surgery (if possible).

❍ **Which produces more hypoxemia - intravenous or inhalation anesthesia?**

Inhalation.

❍ **What is the purpose of the pre-operative assessment of lung function prior to pulmonary resection?**

Prediction of long term respiratory status.

❍ **How is lung function assessed prior to lung resection?**

Spirometry, diffusion capacity, and blood gases. If FEV1is greater than 2L, or >60% of predicted, and/or diffusion capacity is greater than 60% of predicted, and arterial CO_2 is less than or equal to 45 mm Hg, no further testing is required.

❍ **What is the further assessment of patients with operable lung cancer who fail to meet the blood gas and spirometric (or diffusion capacity) criteria for resection?**

Quantitative lung scanning, to assess the relative contribution of each lung to overall function.

❍ **What is the minimum postoperative FEV1 following resection?**

800cc or 40% of predicted normal FEV1.

❍ **What is the further assessment of patients with operable lung cancer who do not meet the minimum predicted postoperative FEV1criteria after lung scanning?**

Cardiopulmonary exercise testing.

❍ **What is the criteria for pulmonary resection by exercise testing?**

Maximal oxygen consumption more than 15 ml/kg/min.

❍ **What are some infection syndromes which can lead to ventilatory insufficiency.**

Botulism, tetanus, Campylobacter, polio, diphtheria, Guillain-Barré syndrome.

❍ **Which neuromuscular diseases and spinal diseases can lead to ventilatory insufficiency?**

Muscular dystrophy, polymyositis, myotonic dystrophy, polyneuritis, Eaton-Lambert syndrome, myasthenia gravis, amyotrophic lateral sclerosis, injury, Guillain-Barré syndrome, multiple sclerosis, Parkinson's disease and stroke.

❍ **By what mechanism do intravenous aminoglycosides potentially contribute to respiratory insufficiency?**

Non-depolarizing neuromuscular blockade.

❍ **Respiratory muscle function, and thus the likelihood of ventilator weaning, can be assessed at the bedside by which parameters?**

Negative inspiratory force (NIF - actually a pressure) > -20 to -30 cm H_2O absolute value, Vital capacity > 10 cm H_2O.

❍ **Adequacy of alveolar ventilation is reflected by which component of arterial blood gas analysis?**

$PaCO_2$.

❍ **Patients on mechanical ventilation can develop hypoventilation based on what factors?**

Increased dead space (including length of ventilator circuit proximal to the "Y" piece separating the inspiratory and expiratory limbs), decreased tidal volume, overdistention of lung, air leaks, and massive pulmonary embolism.

❍ **What are some factors that can interfere with the bellows function of the test?**

Abdominal binding, massive obesity, trauma with flail chest, massive effusion, massive ascites, pneumothorax, thoracic burn with eschar, neuromuscular blockade, and strapping of ribs.

❍ **What combination of medications, often used in the treatment of status asthmaticus requiring mechanical ventilation, may result in prolonged weakness?**

Steroids and neuromuscular blocking agents.

❍ **What is the principle mechanism of increased $PaCO_2$ with increased FiO_2?**

Worsening V/Q mismatch and the Haldane effect.

❍ **How does malnutrition contribute to respiratory failure?**

Increase in the oxygen cost of breathing, respiratory muscle weakness.

❍ **What conditions or commonly used medications result in an increase in serum theophylline concentration?**

Cimetidine, macrolides, quinolones, verapamil, fever, congestive heart failure, and liver failure.

❍ **What conditions or commonly used medications result in a decrease in serum theophylline concentration?**

Barbiturates, phenytoin, carbamazepine, rifampin, smoking, barbecued or smoked food consumption.

❍ **What effect does intrinsic PEEP have on the work of breathing of patients receiving mechanical ventilation?**

Increased elastic work, increased work to trigger assisted breaths.

❍ **How can the work of breathing with mechanical ventilation associated with intrinsic PEEP be reduced?**

Add CPAP, reduce tidal volume, reduce inspiratory time, and increase expiratory time.

❍ **What are complications associated with mask ventilation?**

Skin breakdown, aspiration pneumonia, aerophagia. pneumothorax, and barotrauma (volutrauma).

❍ **Through what mechanism does PEEP decrease cardiac output?**

Reduced preload.

❍ **Through what mechanism does positive pressure ventilation increase cardiac output?**

Decreased afterload.

❍ **How can compliance of the lung/chest wall be approximated from airway pressure measurements during mechanical ventilation?**

Tidal volume/(Inspiratory plateau pressure - End expiratory pressure).

❍ **What evidence of barotrauma can be observed on chest x-ray?**

Pneumomediastinum, pneumothorax, pneumopericardium, subcutaneous emphysema, and pulmonary interstitial emphysema.

❍ **What are the primary determinants of the work of breathing?**

Minute ventilation, lung/chest wall compliance, and presence of intrinsic PEEP.

❍ **What are the determinants of $PaCO_2$?**

Carbon dioxide production and alveolar ventilation.

❍ **What are some conditions under which CO_2 production is increased?**

Lipogenesis, fever, and hyperthyroidism.

❍ **What is the preferred FiO_2 for patients with ARDS?**

The lowest that will maintain a hemoglobin oxygen saturation of about 90%.

❍ **What is the goal when attempting to determine the optimum level of PEEP for a patient with ARDS undergoing mechanical ventilation?**

Determine the level of PEEP that produces the maximum oxygen delivery.

❍ **How is oxygen delivery calculated?**

Cardiac Output x Arterial Blood Oxygen Content.

❍ **What is the primary determinant of the oxygen content of arterial blood?**

The product of hemoglobin concentration and the % hemoglobin oxygen saturation of arterial blood. The amount of oxygen dissolved in the plasma (a function of the PaO_2) is negligible at one atmosphere of pressure.

❍ **How long does it take to demonstrate the earliest manifestations of oxygen toxicity while breathing 100% oxygen?**

1-2 hours.

❍ **How can adequate tidal volume be delivered to a patient undergoing volume cycled mechanical ventilation whose endotracheal tube cuff is failing to maintain an adequate seal without changing the tube?**

Increase the mandatory tidal volume.

❍ **What is the maximum acceptable endotracheal tube cuff pressure?**

Approximately 26 cm H_2O at the end of expiration.

❍ **What is the potential harm of excess endotracheal tube cuff pressure?**

Excess pressure can induce ischemia and necrosis of the underlying tissue resulting in tracheomalacia and tracheal stenosis.

❍ **What are indications for stress ulcer prophylaxis in critically ill patients?**

Mechanical ventilation and coagulopathy.

❍ **What position is preferred for patients suspected of having an air embolism?**

Left lateral decubitus.

❍ **What is bronchiectasis?**

Bronchiectasis is an abnormal dilatation of the proximal medium sized bronchi greater than 2 mm in diameter. It is due to the destruction of the muscular and elastic components of their walls, usually associated with chronic bacterial infection and fowl smelling sputum.

❍ **Is bronchiectasis always associated with purulent expectoration?**

No, especially when it involves the dependent zones of the lung such as upper lobes, as in tuberculosis.

❍ **Which lung segments are most frequently involved in bronchiectasis?**

Posterior basal segments of the left or right lower lobes.

❍ **What are the most common causes of upper lobe bronchiectasis?**

Tuberculous endobronchitis.

Allergic bronchopulmonary aspergillosis (ABPA).

❍ **What is the most important functional impairment of the bronchiectatic airway?**

Impaired tracheobronchial clearance, which predisposes to airway colonization and infection with pathogenic organisms.

❍ **What physiologic and anatomic alterations have been described in patients with bronchiectasis?**

Impaired tracheobronchial clearance.

Enlargement of the bronchial arteries and extensive anastamosis between these vessels and the pulmonary arteries.

Diminished total pulmonary arterial blood flow.

Functional decrease in the cross sectional- area of the pulmonary vasculature with hypoxia.

Left to right intrapulmonary shunting.

Decreased ventilation of bronchographically abnormal areas.

❍ **What are the major pulmonary function abnormalities in bronchiectasis?**

Most patients have some amount of airflow obstruction. Restriction may be noted in patients with bronchiectasis associated with restrictive lung diseases.

❍ **What are the symptoms of bronchiectasis?**

Chronic cough, purulent sputum, fever, weakness, weight loss, dyspnea in some patients, and hemoptysis. Hemoptysis is generally mild, originates from bronchial arteries, and is not a common cause of death (< 10% of deaths attributed to hemoptysis).

❍ **What are the most common complications of bronchiectasis?**

Recurrent attacks of pneumonia, empyema, pneumothorax, and lung abscess.

❍ **What are the less common complications that can be seen in bronchiectasis?**

Brain abscess, amyloidosis, and cor pulmonale.

❍ **What is the primary indication for bronchography?**

For pre-surgical evaluation of patients with focal bronchiectasis.

❍ **What is the sensitivity of a CT scan in detecting bronchiectasis?**

80-85%.

❍ **What is the specificity of CT scan in detecting bronchiectasis?**

~ 85%.

❍ **What laboratory investigations aid in the evaluation of idiopathic bronchiectasis?**

Serum protein electrophoresis to r/o alpha-1-anti-trypsin deficiency.

Immunoglobulin levels with IgG subclass.

Pilocarpine iontophoresis sweat test.

Serum precipitins for Aspergillus.

Electron microscopy of sperm or respiratory epithelium for primary ciliary dyskinesia (PCD).

❍ **What is the mainstay of treatment of bronchiectasis?**

Antibiotics.

❍ **How should the choice of antibiotic treatment be guided?**

Sputum culture for aerobes and mycobacteria.

❍ **What is an acceptable cost- effective choice of empirical antibiotic in bronchiectasis with mixed flora?**

Amoxicillin + Clavulanic acid or Trimethoprim-Sulfamethoxazole.

❍ **What are the adjunctive treatment measures that may be beneficial in patients with bronchiectasis?**

Chest Physiotherapy.

Nutritional support.

Inhaled Indomethacin - Shown to decrease bronchial hypersecretion, by inhibiting neutrophil recruitment.

Bronchodilators.

Supplemental oxygen.

Immunoglobulin administration for Immunoglobulin deficiency.

Replacement treatment for patients with alpha-1-anti-trypsin deficiency.

Recombinant DNAase to reduce sputum viscosity in patients with Cystic fibrosis (CF).

❍ **What are the indications for surgery in bronchiectasis?**

Patients with focal bronchiectasis who fail medical management.

Patients who are noncompliant with medical management.

Patients with massive, life threatening hemoptysis.

❍ **What are the treatment options for massive, life-threatening hemoptysis?**

Endobronchial bronchoscopic tamponade with a Fogarty balloon catheter.

Bronchial arteriography and embolization - may cause serious neurologic deficits from inadvertent obstruction of the spinal arteries.

Surgical resection of the involved lobe.

❍ **What is Middle lobe syndrome?**

Bronchiectasis and chronic recurrent pneumonia of the right middle lobe.

❍ **What are the causes of the Middle lobe syndrome?**

Angulation at the origin of the right middle lobe bronchus.

Extrinsic compression of the right middle lobe bronchus by enlarged lymph nodes combined with an absence of collateral ventilation.

❍ **What is Kartagener's syndrome?**

Triad of: (1) Situs inversus, (2) Bronchiectasis, and (3) Nasal polyps or recurrent sinusitis.

❍ **What are the major diagnostic criteria for allergic bronchopulmonary aspergillosis (ABPA)?**

History of asthma.

Increased IgE levels.

Peripheral blood eosinophilia.

Precipitating antibodies against Aspergillus.

Central bronchiectasis.

❍ **What is the most characteristic pattern of bronchiectasis in ABPA?**

Saccular proximal bronchiectasis of the upper lobes.

❍ **What immunodeficiency states have been shown to be associated with bronchiectasis?**

Abnormal B-lymphocyte function.

Congenital or acquired hypogammaglobulinemia with decreased circulating IgG levels.

IgG subclass deficiency in the presence of normal total IgG levels.

❍ **What is the most common immunoglobulin (Ig) deficiency?**

Selective IgA deficiency is the most common immunoglobulin deficiency, affecting 1 in 800 individuals. It is usually associated with IgG subclass deficiency and presents as recurrent sinopulmonary infections.

❍ **What are the possible manifestations of alpha-1-anti-trypsin deficiency?**

Panlobular emphysema.

Bronchiectasis.

Hepatic cirrhosis.

❍ **What is cystic fibrosis (CF)?**

CF is a multisystem disorder affecting children and young adults, characterized by chronic obstruction and infection of airways, and exocrine pancreatic insufficiency.

❍ **What is the incidence of CF?**

1 in 2500 live births among whites, and 1 in 17,000 live births among blacks.

❍ **What is the inheritance pattern of CF?**

Autosomal recessive.

❍ **What is the site of mutation?**

At a single gene locus on the long arm of chromosome 7. This locus codes for a large protein (Cystic fibrosis transmembrane regulator- CFTR protein) that has several transmembrane domains and phosphorylation sites and two cytoplasmic ATP binding sites.

❍ **What is the chance of an unaffected sibling of a patient with CF to be a carrier?**

66%.

❍ **What is the chance of having a child with CF, when one parent is a carrier and the other is heterozygous for the CF gene?**

25%.

❍ **Pathology in CF is confined predominantly to what part of the lung?**

Mucous obstruction and infection in the lungs are confined mostly to the conducting airways.

❍ **Why is a pneumothorax more common in advanced CF?**

Subpleural cysts often occur on the mediastinal surfaces of the upper lobes and are thought to contribute to pneumothorax in patients with advanced disease.

❍ **What is the most common site of non-pulmonary pathology in CF?**

GI tract, with striking changes seen in the exocrine pancreas. Islets of Langerhans are spared.

❍ **What are the reproductive abnormalities in CF?**

In males: The vas deferens, tail and body of the epididymis and the seminal vesicles are either absent or rudimentary.

In females: Uterine cervical glands are distended with mucous and cervical canal is plugged with tenacious mucous secretions. Endocervicitis also seen.

❍ **What are the most frequent respiratory pathogens in patients with CF?**

Staphylococcus aureus and Pseudomonas aeruginosa.

❍ **What are the immunological defects in CF?**

CF patients have low levels of serum IgG in the first decade of life which increase dramatically once chronic infection is established. T-lymphocyte numbers are adequate. With advancing severity of pulmonary disease, lymphocytes of CF patients proliferate less briskly in response to P. aeruginosa and other gram-negative organisms. Deficient opsonic activity of alveolar macrophages are seen in patients with established P. aeruginosa infection. Major IgG subclass in serum and lungs in CF patients is IgG.

❍ **T/F: Patients with CF have a higher incidence of atopy and asthma when compared to the general population.**

True. The presence of atopy or asthma does not affect the severity, natural course or prognosis compared to non-atopic or non-asthmatic patients with CF.

❍ **What is the earliest manifestation of CF lung disease?**

Cough, later associated with greenish, tenacious, purulent sputum, reflecting Pseudomonas aeruginosa infection.

❍ **What are the respiratory symptoms of CF?**

Cough with greenish sputum and wheezing.

❍ **What are the earliest organisms to be detected in airway of patients with CF?**

S. aureus and H. influenza. P. aeruginosa is typically cultured from respiratory secretions months to years later.

❍ **What is the most common organism to be detected from the airways of patients with advanced CF?**

Pseudomonas aeruginosa.

❍ **T/F: The recovery of P. aeruginosa, particularly the mucoid form, from the lower respiratory tract of a child or young adult with chronic lung symptoms is virtually diagnostic of CF.**

True.

❍ **What other organisms have been found to colonize the respiratory tract of patients with CF?**

Pseudomonas cepacia, Escherichia coli, Xanthomonas maltophilia, Klebsiella, Proteus and anaerobes.

❍ **What is the earliest radiographic change in CF?**

Hyperinflation of the lung, reflecting obstruction of small airways.

❍ **Where are the earliest and most severe radiographic changes located?**

Right upper lobe.

❍ **What are the initial lung function abnormalities in CF?**

Small airway obstruction as evidenced by decreased maximum mid expiratory flow.

Reduced flow at low lung volumes.

Elevation of RV/TLC ratio.

Decreased diffusion capacity.

❍ **What are the various radiographic manifestations of CF?**

Hyperinflation.

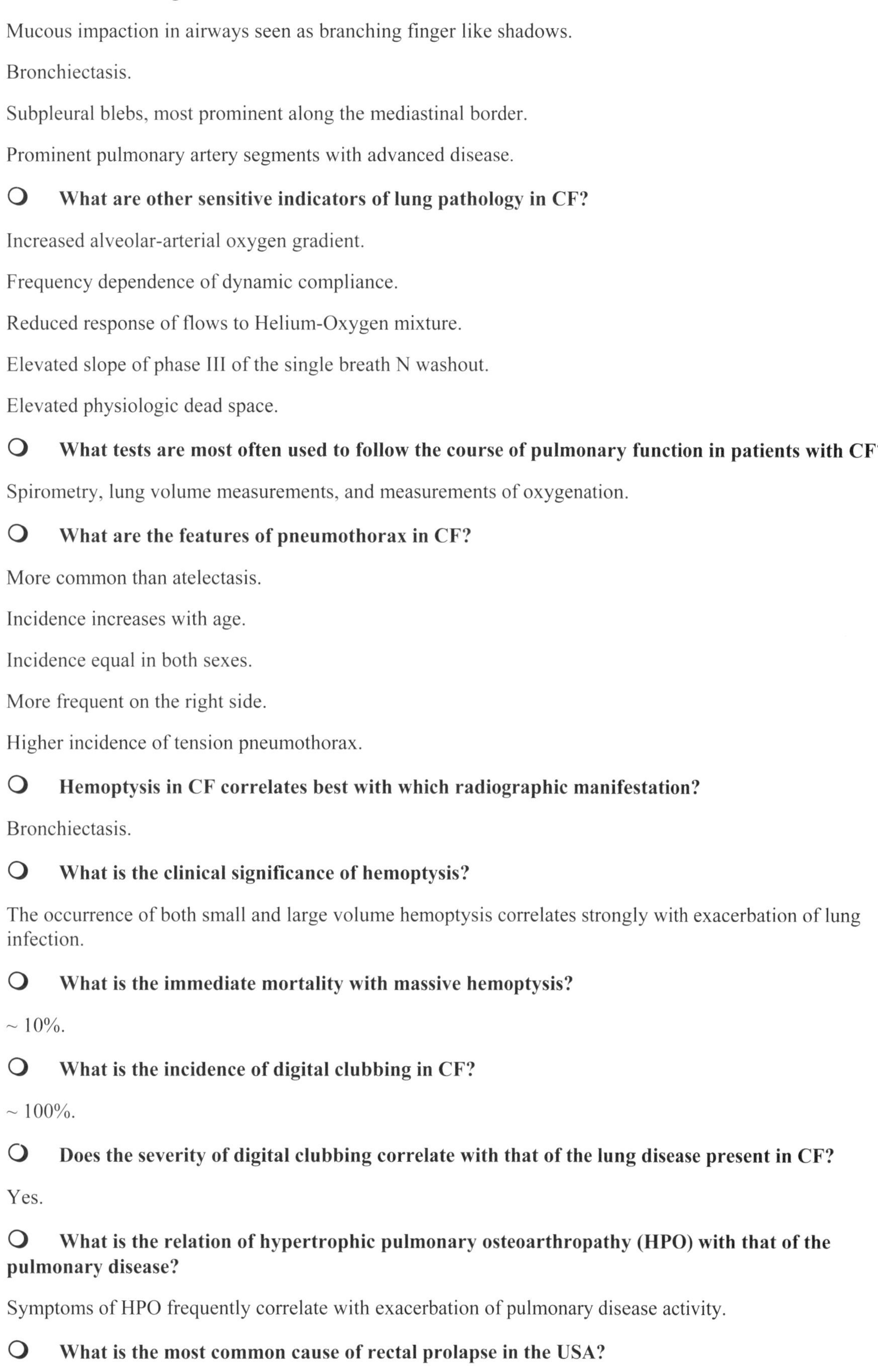

Peribronchial cuffing.

Mucous impaction in airways seen as branching finger like shadows.

Bronchiectasis.

Subpleural blebs, most prominent along the mediastinal border.

Prominent pulmonary artery segments with advanced disease.

❍ **What are other sensitive indicators of lung pathology in CF?**

Increased alveolar-arterial oxygen gradient.

Frequency dependence of dynamic compliance.

Reduced response of flows to Helium-Oxygen mixture.

Elevated slope of phase III of the single breath N washout.

Elevated physiologic dead space.

❍ **What tests are most often used to follow the course of pulmonary function in patients with CF?**

Spirometry, lung volume measurements, and measurements of oxygenation.

❍ **What are the features of pneumothorax in CF?**

More common than atelectasis.

Incidence increases with age.

Incidence equal in both sexes.

More frequent on the right side.

Higher incidence of tension pneumothorax.

❍ **Hemoptysis in CF correlates best with which radiographic manifestation?**

Bronchiectasis.

❍ **What is the clinical significance of hemoptysis?**

The occurrence of both small and large volume hemoptysis correlates strongly with exacerbation of lung infection.

❍ **What is the immediate mortality with massive hemoptysis?**

~ 10%.

❍ **What is the incidence of digital clubbing in CF?**

~ 100%.

❍ **Does the severity of digital clubbing correlate with that of the lung disease present in CF?**

Yes.

❍ **What is the relation of hypertrophic pulmonary osteoarthropathy (HPO) with that of the pulmonary disease?**

Symptoms of HPO frequently correlate with exacerbation of pulmonary disease activity.

❍ **What is the most common cause of rectal prolapse in the USA?**

CF.

❍ **What is the incidence of exocrine pancreatic insufficiency in CF?**

90-95%.

❍ **What is the incidence of symptomatic biliary cirrhosis in patients with CF?**

2-5%.

❍ **What is the most characteristic pattern of hepatobiliary disease in CF?**

Focal biliary cirrhosis.

❍ **What are the diagnostic criteria for CF?**

Primary:
Characteristic pulmonary manifestations and/or,
Characteristic gastrointestinal manifestations and/or,
A family history of CF

Plus
Sweat Cl (concentration > 60 mEq/L) [repeat measurement if sweat Cl is 50 - 60 mEq/ L].

Secondary Criteria:
Documentation of dual CFTR mutations, and
Evidence of one or more characteristic manifestations.

❍ **What are the conditions associated with an elevated sweat chloride?**

CF, Hypothyroidism, Pseudohypoaldosteronism, Hypoparathyroidism, Nephrogenic Diabetes Insipidus, Type I glycogen storage disease, Mucopolysaccharidosis, Malnutrition, PGE administration, Hypogammaglobulinemia, and Pancreatitis.

❍ **What is the test recognized by the CF foundation to be the definitive diagnostic test for CF?**

Collection of sweat (at least 50 mg in a 45 minute period) by pilocarpine iontophoresis, coupled with chemical determination of the chloride concentration (> 60 mEq/L, >80 mEq/L in adults).

❍ **What is the sensitivity and specificity of pilocarpine iontophoresis sweat test in detecting CF?**

Sensitivity = 100%

Specificity > 90%

❍ **What are the advantages of chest physical therapy?**

Clears secretions.

Improves flow rates and lung function.

❍ **What is the effect of nutritional supplementation on the disease?**

Patients with adequate nutrition experience a slower rate of decline of lung function.

❍ **What is the 2-year survival after a double lung transplant?**

50%.

❍ **How do you manage pulmonary complications of CF?**

PULMONARY COMPLICATION	MANAGEMENT
Right heart failure	Improve oxygenation through intensive pulmonary therapy.
Respiratory failure	Vigorous medical therapy of the underlying lung disease and infection.
Atelectasis	Aggressive antibiotic therapy and frequent chest physiotherapy.
Pneumothorax	Conservative if < 10% and patient asymptomatic. Pleurodesis to avoid recurrence.
Small volume hemoptysis	Aggressive treatment of lung infection.
Persistent massive hemoptysis	Bronchial artery embolization along with aggressive treatment of the lung infection.

❍ **What is the life expectancy in CF?**

50% patients survive to 28 - 30 years of age.

❍ **What factors improve survival in CF?**

Better survival in patients living in northern climates.

Males.

Blacks.

Patients followed at established care centers.

Patients with better pancreatic function.

❍ **What is stridor due to?**

With extrathoracic airway obstruction, the pressure inside the extrathoracic part of the airway is much more negative relative to atmospheric pressure. This results in further narrowing of the larynx during inspiration and therefore, stridor.

❍ **Grunting is observed during what phase of respiration?**

Expiratory-exhalation against a closed glottis.

❍ **What type of airway obstruction would most likely be observed with this arterial blood gas while breathing 50% oxygen: pH 7.12, PCO_2 80 Torr, PO_2 250 Torr?**

Extrathoracic and central intrathoracic airway obstruction.

❍ **What is the most common organism isolated from patients with bacterial tracheitis?**

Staphylococcus aureus.

❍ **How do retropharyngeal abscesses arise?**

Lymphatic spread of infections in the nasopharynx, oropharynx, or external auditory canal.

❍ **What is the most common type of tracheo-esophageal fistula?**

Blind esophageal pouch with a fistulous connection of the trachea to the distal esophagus.

❍ **What is the preliminary test most helpful in establishing the presence of a vascular ring?**

Contrast esophagram.

❍ **What is the narrowest part of the adult airway?**

The glottic opening.

❍ **What is the time constant?**

The product of compliance and resistance.

❍ **A 22-year-old with cerebral palsy and vegetative state was intubated for 10 days because of aspiration pneumonia. She is weaned from mechanical ventilation, extubated, and one hour later, develops stridor and severe retractions. She is appropriately suctioned and given three aerosol treatments of racemic epinephrine. Her arterial blood gas is pH 7.20, PCO_2 80, PO_2 80 on 100% oxygen. What should be done next?**

Intubation.

❍ **A 17 year-old male complains of dysphagia and fever. Tonsillar exudates and anterior cervical adenitis are noted. What sign differentiates Group A Strep from other causes of pharyngitis?**

A sandpaper-like rash.

❍ **A 24 year-old female has a high fever, hoarseness, and increased stridor of 3 hours duration. She also has a low fever and sore throat. Examination shows an ill appearing woman with a temperature of 40° C, inspiratory stridor, drooling and mild intercostal retractions. She prefers to sit up. The most likely diagnosis is:**

Epiglottitis.

❍ **The predominant auscultatory finding in a patient with a foreign body lodged in the right mainstem bronchus:**

Expiratory wheezing.

❍ **In the diagnosis of a radioluscent foreign body lodged in the right mainstem bronchus, producing incomplete obstruction, inspiratory and expiratory films will show air-trapping and increased luscency of the lung on the involved side. This phenomenon is due to:**

Ball-valve airtrapping. Air enters around the foreign body during inspiration, but is trapped as the airway closes around the foreign body during expiration, preventing emptying of that side.

❍ **Cor pulmonale, resulting from chronic airway obstruction, is thought to be due what?**

Chronic alveolar hypoventilation and the resulting increase in pulmonary vascular resistance.

❍ **The total work of breathing is divided into what to purposes?**

1. To overcome lung and chest wall compliance.

2. To overcome airway and tissue resistance.

❍ **What are the main characteristics of a transudate?**

Protein <3 g/dl; Pleural fluid protein-Plasma protein ratio <0.5; Pleural fluid LDH <2/3 upper level of serum LDH (<200 IU); Pleural fluid LDH-Plasma LDH ratio <0.6.

❍ **What are the main characteristics of an exudate?**

Protein 3 g/dl; Pleural fluid protein-Plasma protein ratio 0.5; Pleural fluid LDH >2/3 of upper level of serum LDH (>200 IU); Pleural fluid LDH-Plasma LDH ratio 0.6.

❍ **What is the usual specific gravity of an exudate?**

1.020 or greater on a refractometer.

❍ **What are some clinical disorders associated with increased capillary permeability causing exudative pleural effusion?**

Pleuripulmonary infections, circulating toxins, systemic lupus erythematosus, rheumatoid arthritis, sarcoidosis, tumor, pulmonary infarction, viral hepatitis.

❍ **What are the clinical features associated with pleural effusion?**

A pleural rub (may be the only finding in the early stages), pleuritic chest pain due to involvement and inflammation of parietal pleura, cough (distortion of lung), dyspnea (mechanical inefficiency of respiratory muscles stretched by outward movement of chest wall and downward movement of diaphragm), diminished chest wall movements, dull percussion, decreased tactile and vocal fremitus, decreased breath sounds and whispering pectoriloquy. With large amounts, there may be contralateral shift of the mediastinum.

❍ **What is the minimum amount of pleural liquid that can be detected roentgenographically?**

Approximately 400 ml in upright views of the chest. Lateral decubitus film taken with the patient lying on the affected side can detect as little as 50 ml of liquid.

❍ **Is there a role of a lateral decubitus film with the suspected side being superior?**

In this position the fluid gravitates towards the mediastinum. This facilitates the evaluation of the underlying lung for infiltrates or atelectasis.

❍ **What is the most common cause of exudative effusion?**

Parapneumonic effusion is the most common cause of exudative effusion.

❍ **What is a parapneumonic effusion?**

Pleural effusion associated with pneumonia, lung abscess, bronchiectasis.

❍ **What are the common organisms causing empyema?**

Anaerobes are the most common organisms found in culture positive empyema, followed by staphylococcus, Gram negative aerobes and Pneumococcus.

❍ **What are the clinical features of parapneumonic pleural effusion?**

Effusion, associated with aerobic organism, is associated with acute illness, such as fever, chest pain, sputum production and leukocytosis, while parapneumonic effusion, due to anaerobes, usually presents as sub-acute illness over 7-10 days.

❍ **What features indicate development of complicated parapneumonic effusion?**

Presence of persistent fever or chest pain on appropriate antibiotics suggest a complicated effusion, which on roentgenography, is seen as moderate to large ipsilateral loculated effusion or a reverse D-sign on lateral view.

❍ **How does the presence or absence of a complicated parapneumonic effusion affect the treatment strategies?**

An uncomplicated parapneumonic effusion responds to the antibiotics directed at pneumonia. A complicated effusion needs to be treated with antibiotics and a procedure should be performed to drain the purulent effusion with or without a fibrinolytic agent.

❍ **What are the surgical strategies to treat a complicated parapneumonic effusion?**

The surgical approach varies with the stage of complicated effusion and it may be in the form of chest tube or radiologically guided catheter, with or without fibrinolytic agents, empyemectomy and decortication, thoracoscopy or thoracotomy, or open drainage.

❍ **What are the indications for the chest tube placement in parapneumonic effusion?**

Presence of a complicated parapneumonic effusion, as evidenced by presence of fever, presence of loculations, gross appearance of fluid purulent (pus), increased WBC count and low glucose (usually <40 mg/dl), a decreased pH (less than 7.0 or 0.15 less than the arterial pH), and elevated LDH (>1000 IU/L) are usually considered indications for placement of chest tube for drainage.

❍ **What are the fibrinolytic agents and the regimens for the treatment of complicated effusions?**

Streptokinase in doses of 250,000-units/ 30-60 ml of normal saline, administered via a chest tube which is kept clamped for 1-2 hours. Urokinase, 1000 units, administered in a similar fashion, is also considered equally effective. Streptokinase is cheaper.

❍ **How long should a chest tube be left in after it has been placed for the treatment of parapneumonic pleural effusion?**

The chest tube should be left in place until the volume of the pleural drainage per 24 hours is under 50 ml and the draining fluid becomes serous.

❍ **What factors predict whether closed tube drainage will be sufficient for the treatment of complicated parapneumonic effusion?**

More than 80% of class I parapneumonic effusions (pleural fluid pH < 7.2, negative cultures) can be managed successfully with a chest tube drainage for 4-7 days. All patients in class II (empyema, positive cultures and without loculations) require chest tube drainage. While 80% of class III parapneumonic effusions (multiple loculations or trapped lungs) require thoracotomy, a small percentage can be managed by multiple chest tubes.

❍ **What are the typical roentgenographic features of a tuberculous pleural effusion?**

These are usually unilateral, small to moderate and more commonly on the right side. Two thirds of these can be associated with coexisting parenchymal disease (which may not be apparent on chest radiograph). They are commonly associated with primary disease. The incidence of loculations may be up to 30%.

❍ **What are the characteristic features of a tuberculous pleural effusion?**

Pleural fluid is exudative with a protein content > 0.5 g/L, >90-95% lymphocytes (in the acute phase, there may be a polymorphonuclear response).

❍ **What is the typical eosinophil count of a tuberculous pleural effusion?**

An eosinophil count of greater than 10% usually excludes tubercular effusion. The eosinophil count in pleural fluid can be elevated after pneumothorax and thoracentesis.

❍ **What are the diagnostic features of a tuberculous pleural effusion?**

90-95% of cases can be diagnosed by a combination of histology and culture of pleural biopsy tissue. Pleural fluid culture, sputum culture, AFB smear of pleural fluid and pleural biopsy material can provide additional diagnostic yield. Measurement of adenosine deaminase, lysozyme, and gamma interferon may be helpful, but are not diagnostic.

❍ **What is the typical response to treatment in a case with tuberculous pleural effusion?**

Patient usually becomes afebrile in 2 weeks. The effusion usually resolves in 4-6 weeks. The resorption will occur with or without treatment. The recurrence rate may be as high as 62% at five years.

❍ **What is the treatment of tuberculous pleural effusion?**

A 9 month course of Isoniazid 300 mg and Rifampin 600 mg, daily. Therapeutic thoracentesis is recommended only to relieve dyspnea. Corticosteroids can decrease the duration of fever and time required for fluid absorption, but they do not decrease the amount of pleural thickening at 12 months after treatment is initiated. Therefore, they are recommended only for patients who are markedly symptomatic and only after institution of appropriate antimicrobial therapy.

❍ **What is the incidence of pleural involvement in patients with thoracic actinomycosis?**

Fifty percent.

❍ **What is the most common cause of transudate pleural effusion?**

Congestive heart failure.

❍ **What are the common features of pleural effusion associated with congestive heart failure?**

Bilateral effusion, more commonly right-sided, associated with cardiomegaly. Fluid is transudate, serous, <1000 mononuclear cells, pH >7.4, pleural fluid glucose levels same as serum.

❍ **What are the radiological features of pleural effusion associated with cirrhosis?**

Small to massive right-sided effusion in 70%, left sided in 15%, bilateral in 15% with normal heart size.

❍ **What is the mechanism of a pleural effusion associated with atelectasis?**

Atelectasis leads to decreased perimicrovascular pressure, resulting in a pressure gradient. Fluid moves from the parietal pleural interstitium into the pleural space due to decreased perimicrovascular pressure.

❍ **How common is atelectasis-associated pleural effusion in intensive care units (ICU) and what are the common conditions associated with it?**

Atelectasis is a common cause of pleural effusion in the ICU. Pleural effusion is seen with postoperative atelectasis associated with thoraco-abdominal surgery, such as upper abdominal surgery, thoracotomy, open heart surgery (phrenic nerve injury), after pulmonary embolism, and with other abdominal conditions such as pancreatitis, splenic infarction, subphrenic or hepatic abscess.

❍ **What is the mainstay of treatment for pleural effusion associated with atelectasis?**

Treatment of underlying condition and chest physiotherapy.

❍ **What is the incidence pleural effusion associated with nephrotic syndrome?**

Approximately 20%.

❍ **What is the primary mechanism of pleural effusion in nephrotic syndrome?**

Decreased plasma oncotic pressure due to hypoalbuminemia.

❍ **What are the roentgenographic features of the pleural effusion seen with nephrotic syndrome?**

Small, bilateral effusions, frequently sub-pulmonic. Presence of unilateral, much larger effusions, which are hemorrhagic or exudative, suggests the presence of a pulmonary embolism. There may be a polymorphonuclear predominance in these cases.

❍ **What is the incidence of pleural effusion associated with malignancy?**

Malignant pleural effusions are second most common exudative effusions after parapneumonic effusions. The most common malignancies are lung and breast cancer.

❍ **What are the conditions associated with malignant transudative effusions?**

Lymphatic obstruction, endobronchial obstruction, and hypoalbuminemia due to the primary malignancy.

❍ **What is the typical chest radiographic findings in pleural effusion associated with lung cancer?**

Ipsilateral massive effusion with mass, with or without adenopathy.

❍ **When do you suspect malignancy?**

Massive effusion, large effusion without contralateral mediastinal shift or bilateral effusions with normal heart size suggest malignancy.

❍ **In a case with malignant effusion, what is the yield of various diagnostic procedures?**

Positive cytology in 60-95%, positive pleural biopsy in 50%, and positive thoracoscopy in 95% cases.

❍ **What type of pleural effusion is associated with malignant mesothelioma?**

Large unilateral effusion. Contralateral pleural plaques are present in 20% of the cases. Loculated pleural masses may be evident after thoracentesis.

❍ **What factors play a role in the pathogenesis of pleural effusion associated with pulmonary embolism?**

Effusions are present in 40-50% of cases of pulmonary embolism. Increased capillary permeability, due to ischemia and leak of protein rich fluid into pleural space, are the main factors. Atelectasis may contribute to transudate and lung necrosis can lead to hemorrhage.

❍ **What are the conditions causing amylase rich pleural effusion?**

Acute and chronic pancreatitis, adenocarcinoma of lung and ovary, lymphoma, esophageal rupture, chronic lymphatic leukemia, pneumonia and ruptured ectopic pregnancy.

❍ **What are the characteristics of a pleural effusion associated with chronic pancreatitis?**

Large or massive unilateral effusion that occurs rapidly after thoracentesis. The pleural fluid can have very high amylase content (>200,000 IU/L). Direct fistulous communications from the pancreatic bed are responsible. Failure of conservative treatment is an indication for the surgical intervention, such as drainage (up to 50%)

❍ **What factors differentiate acute pancreatitis associated pleural effusion from that associated with chronic pancreatitis?**

Pleural effusion is more commonly associated with acute pancreatitis. The reported incidence is 15%. It is rare in chronic pancreatitis. This is usually a small, left sided pleural effusion formed due to increased capillary permeability and usually does not require specific treatment.

❍ **What is the incidence of pleural involvement in systemic lupus erythematosus?**

50% to 75% of patients with systemic lupus erythematosus develop pleural effusion or pleuritic pain during the course of their disease.

❍ **What are the clinical features of lupus pleuritis?**

Pleuritic chest pain is the most common presentation. Other features are cough, dyspnea, pleural rub, and fever. An episode of pleuritis usually indicates exacerbation of lupus.

❍ **What are the radiological features of lupus pleuritis?**

Small to moderate bilateral effusions are most common. Unilateral and massive effusion can occur. Other radiographic abnormalities such as alveolar infiltrates, atelectasis, and increasing cardiac silhouette can occur.

❍ **What are the characteristic features of pleural fluid in patients with lupus?**

LE cells in the pleural fluid. A ratio of pleural fluid/serum ANA of >1.0 is suggestive of lupus.

❍ **What kind of pleural effusion is associated with lymphangiomyomatosis?**

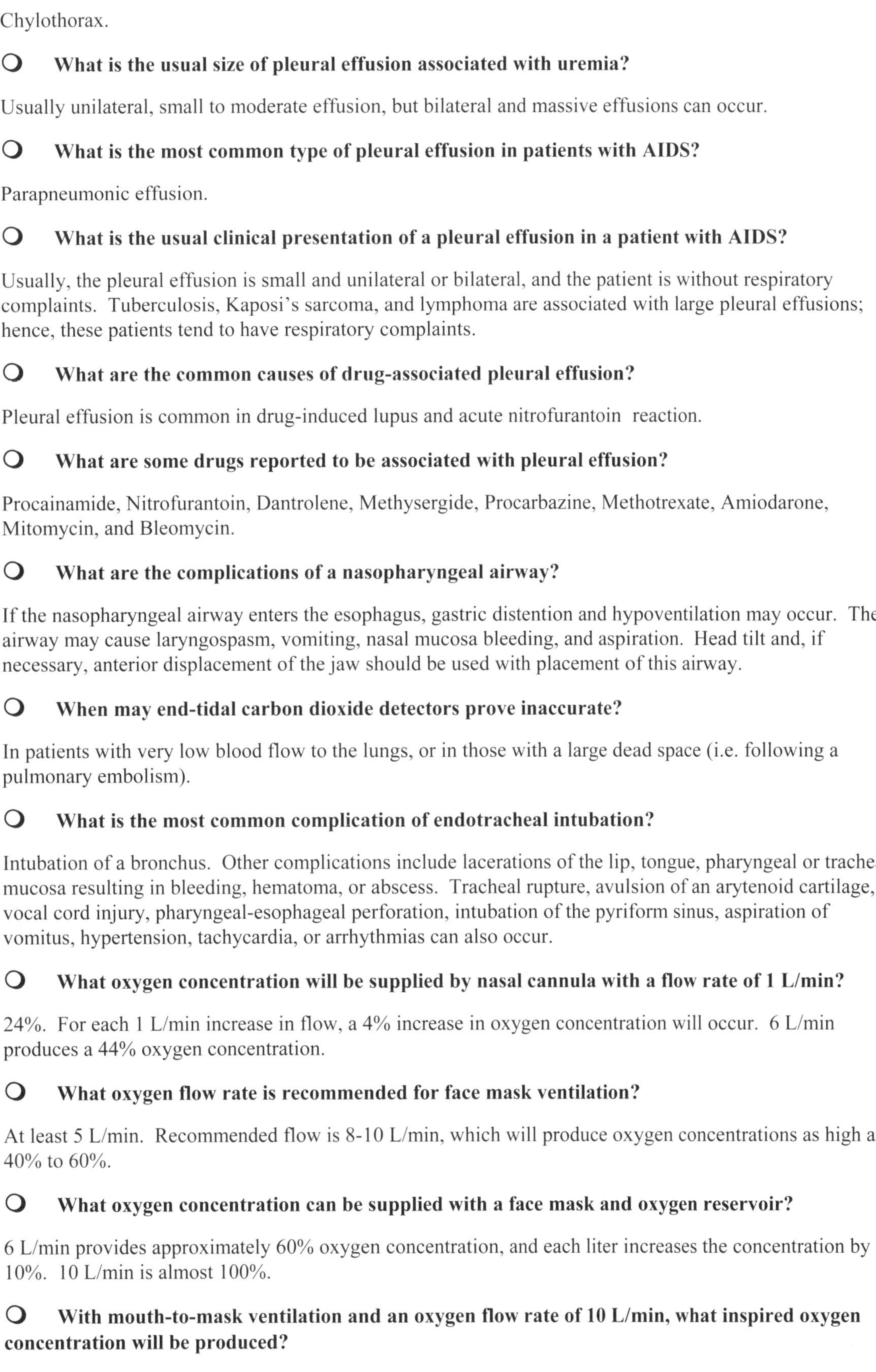

Chylothorax.

❍ **What is the usual size of pleural effusion associated with uremia?**

Usually unilateral, small to moderate effusion, but bilateral and massive effusions can occur.

❍ **What is the most common type of pleural effusion in patients with AIDS?**

Parapneumonic effusion.

❍ **What is the usual clinical presentation of a pleural effusion in a patient with AIDS?**

Usually, the pleural effusion is small and unilateral or bilateral, and the patient is without respiratory complaints. Tuberculosis, Kaposi's sarcoma, and lymphoma are associated with large pleural effusions; hence, these patients tend to have respiratory complaints.

❍ **What are the common causes of drug-associated pleural effusion?**

Pleural effusion is common in drug-induced lupus and acute nitrofurantoin reaction.

❍ **What are some drugs reported to be associated with pleural effusion?**

Procainamide, Nitrofurantoin, Dantrolene, Methysergide, Procarbazine, Methotrexate, Amiodarone, Mitomycin, and Bleomycin.

❍ **What are the complications of a nasopharyngeal airway?**

If the nasopharyngeal airway enters the esophagus, gastric distention and hypoventilation may occur. The airway may cause laryngospasm, vomiting, nasal mucosa bleeding, and aspiration. Head tilt and, if necessary, anterior displacement of the jaw should be used with placement of this airway.

❍ **When may end-tidal carbon dioxide detectors prove inaccurate?**

In patients with very low blood flow to the lungs, or in those with a large dead space (i.e. following a pulmonary embolism).

❍ **What is the most common complication of endotracheal intubation?**

Intubation of a bronchus. Other complications include lacerations of the lip, tongue, pharyngeal or tracheal mucosa resulting in bleeding, hematoma, or abscess. Tracheal rupture, avulsion of an arytenoid cartilage, vocal cord injury, pharyngeal-esophageal perforation, intubation of the pyriform sinus, aspiration of vomitus, hypertension, tachycardia, or arrhythmias can also occur.

❍ **What oxygen concentration will be supplied by nasal cannula with a flow rate of 1 L/min?**

24%. For each 1 L/min increase in flow, a 4% increase in oxygen concentration will occur. 6 L/min produces a 44% oxygen concentration.

❍ **What oxygen flow rate is recommended for face mask ventilation?**

At least 5 L/min. Recommended flow is 8-10 L/min, which will produce oxygen concentrations as high as 40% to 60%.

❍ **What oxygen concentration can be supplied with a face mask and oxygen reservoir?**

6 L/min provides approximately 60% oxygen concentration, and each liter increases the concentration by 10%. 10 L/min is almost 100%.

❍ **With mouth-to-mask ventilation and an oxygen flow rate of 10 L/min, what inspired oxygen concentration will be produced?**

About 50%.

❍ **What are the risks of use of the transtracheal catheter ventilation?**

Pneumothorax, hemorrhage, and esophageal or thyroid perforation.

❍ **Among patients with cystic fibrosis, what bacteria are seen with increased frequency as causes of pneumonia?**

Pseudomonas aeruginosa and Staphylococcus aureus.

❍ **What is the most common cause of community-acquired pneumonia among alcoholic patients?**

Streptococcus pneumoniae.

❍ **Which other bacteria are seen with increased frequency as causes of pneumonia among alcoholic patients?**

Klebsiella pneumoniae and Hemophilus influenza.

❍ **What pathophysiologic process is suggested by infiltrates in the right upper lobe or the apical segment of the lower lobe?**

Aspiration.

❍ **The number of epithelial cells seen on microscopic examination of sputum smears is indicative of the presence or absence of significant contamination of the specimen with oral secretions. How many epithelial cells per high power field are considered indicative of such contamination?**

Ten or more.

❍ **What degree of leukocytosis is considered a risk factor for poor outcome among patients with bacterial pneumonia?**

Greater than 30,000 cells/mm^3.

❍ **What degree of leukopenia is considered a risk factor for poor outcome among patients with bacterial pneumonia?**

Less than 4000 cells/mm^3.

❍ **What bacteria are associated with pneumonia following influenza?**

Streptococcus pneumoniae, Staphylococcus pneumoniae, and Hemophilus influenza.

❍ **What is the leading identifiable cause of acute community-acquired pneumonia in adults?**

Streptococcus pneumoniae.

❍ **In addition to Streptococcus pneumoniae, what other bacteria are associated with acute, lobar pneumonia in adults?**

Hemophilus influenza, Staphylococcus aureus, Klebsiella pneumoniae, and Streptococcus pyogenes.

❍ **How long before elective splenectomy should the pneumococcal vaccine be administered in order to achieve an adequate antibody response?**

Two weeks or more.

❍ **What two underlying medical conditions are associated with Hemophilus influenzae pneumonia?**

Chronic obstructive lung disease and HIV infection.

❍ **What is the treatment of choice (antibiotic and dose) for Legionella pneumoniae?**

Erythromycin 1 gram intravenously, every six hours.

❍ **What second antibiotic should be added in severe cases?**

Rifampin 600 mg every twelve hours.

❍ **Can the pneumococcal vaccine be given simultaneously with influenza vaccine?**

Yes.

❍ **How many of the more than 80 antigenic capsular types of Streptococcus pneumoniae are included in the current pneumococcal vaccine?**

23.

❍ **At what age should the pneumococcal vaccine be administered among healthy adults with no comorbid conditions?**

Age 65 or greater.

❍ **Should patients who received the prior 14-valent vaccine be given the 23-valent vaccine now available?**

Yes.

❍ **Are any extrapulmonary manifestations specific for the diagnosis of Legionnaire's disease?**

No.

❍ **What category of bacteria is most important in community-acquired aspiration pneumonia?**

Anaerobic.

❍ **What two categories of bacteria are most important in hospital-acquired aspiration pneumonia?**

Gram negative bacilli and Staphylococcus aureus.

❍ **What is the antibiotic of choice for penicillin-allergic patients with community-acquired aspiration pneumonia?**

Clindamycin.

❍ **What antibiotic has been consistently effective against highly penicillin-resistant Streptococcus pneumoniae?**

Vancomycin.

❍ **Can infection with penicillin-resistant Streptococcus pneumoniae be recognized on clinical grounds?**

No.

❍ **Is the pneumococcal vaccine equally effective against penicillin-resistant and penicillin-sensitive strains of Streptococcus pneumoniae?**

Yes.

❍ **What is the most important risk factor for Moraxella catarrhalis pneumonia?**

Chronic obstructive lung disease.

❍ **Is penicillin effective in the treatment of pneumonia due to Moraxella catarrhalis?**

No.

❍ **What two new macrolide antibiotics offer broad coverage of the following common causes of community-acquired pneumonia: Streptococcus pneumoniae, Hemophilus influenzae, Legionella pneumoniae, Moraxella catarrhalis, and Mycoplasma pneumoniae?**

Azithromycin and clarithromycin.

❍ **What common type of community-acquired pneumonia is typically spread by aspiration of microdroplets from common water supplies?**

Legionnaire's disease.

❍ **What is the most common etiologic agent of atypical pneumonia?**

Myocplasma pneumoniae.

❍ **What is considered to be the second most common cause of atypical pneumonia?**

Chlamydia pneumoniae.

❍ **Of the following organisms, which is commonly spread by person-to-person contact: Legionella pneumoniae or Mycoplasma pneumoniae?**

Mycoplasma pneumoniae.

❍ **What class of antibiotics are the drugs of choice for the treatment of Klebsiella pneumoniae pneumonia?**

The cephalosporins.

❍ **Is single antibiotic therapy typically effective in the treatment of Klebsiella pneumoniae pneumonia?**

Yes.

❍ **What is the most common cause of community-acquired bacterial pneumonia among patients infected with HIV?**

Streptococcus pneumoniae.

❍ **What other forms of bacterial pneumonia appear to occur with increased frequency among patients infected with HIV?**

Hemophilus influenzae and Pseudomonas aeruginosa.

❍ **What three x-ray findings are associated with a poor outcome in patients with pneumonia?**

Multi-lobe involvement, pleural effusion, and cavitation.

❍ **What is the single most important risk factor for hospital-acquired bacterial pneumonia?**

Endotracheal intubation.

❍ **What are the two most important risk factors for the development of anaerobic lung abscess?**

Poor oral hygiene and a predisposition toward aspiration.

❍ **Which lung is most often the site of anaerobic lung abscess formation?**

The right lung.

❍ **Which lung segments are most often the site of lung abscess formation?**

The posterior segments of the upper lobe and the superior segments of the lower lobes.

❍ **What are the characteristic findings on sputum gram stain in cases of anaerobic lung abscess?**

Numerous polymorphonuclear cells and both gram-positive and gram-negative bacteria of various morphologies.

❍ **What is the antibiotic of choice for the treatment of anaerobic lung abscess?**

Clindamycin.

❍ **What anaerobic respiratory infection is associated with slowly enlarging pulmonary infiltrates, pleural effusions, rib destruction and fistula formation?**

Actinomycosis.

❍ **What are the most important anatomical defenses of the lower respiratory tract?**

The vocal cords and the epiglottis.

❍ **What proportion of the patients with pneumonia develop pleural effusions?**

40%.

❍ **What are the four indications for drainage of a pleural effusion associated with pneumonia?**

Positive gram stain or culture, the presence of gross pus, pleural fluid glucose less than 40 mg/dl or fluid pH less than 7.0.

❍ **What pathological process is suggested by an air-fluid level in the pleural space?**

Bronchopleural fistula.

❍ **What is the definition of nosocomial pneumonia?**

Pneumonia occurring in patients who have been hospitalized for at least 72 hours.

❍ **What are the two most important routes of transmission of nosocomial bacterial pneumonia?**

Person-to-person transmission via healthcare workers and contaminated ventilator tubing.

❍ **How may stress ulcer prophylaxis in ICU patients contribute to the development of nosocomial pneumonia?**

By raising the gastric pH and increasing bacterial colonization.

❍ **What agent used for the prevention of stress ulcers in ICU patients is associated with the lowest risk of nosocomial pneumonia?**

Sucralfate.

❍ **What is the overall mortality rate of nosocomial pneumonia?**

40%.

❍ **What proportion of hospitalized patients develop nosocomial pneumonia?**

1%.

❍ **Which broad spectrum antibiotics have been shown to be effective in monotherapy of moderate to severe nosocomial pneumonia of uncertain etiology?**

Ceftazidime, cefotaxime, and imipenem.

❍ **What common nosocomial respiratory pathogens would not be adequately covered by any of these agents?**

Methicillin-resistant Staphylococcus aureus, enterococcus, and highly resistant gram negative bacilli.

CRITICAL CARE

The human mind makes progress, but it is a progress in spirals.
Madame de Stael

❍ **What factors are responsible for total ventricular output (cardiac output)?**

Heart rate, myocardial contractility, preload, and afterload

❍ **What are the ventilation and perfusion relationship between Zone 1, Zone 2 and Zone 3 of the lung?**

Zone 1 represents dead space (ventilation occurs without perfusion); zone 2 contains high V/Q units (ventilation occurs in excess of perfusion); zone 3 represents areas of optimal V/Q matching.

❍ **What is the equation for determining a patient's oxygen extraction ratio?**

Oxygen extraction ratio=$C(a\text{-}v)O_2/CaO_2$ where CaO_2 is arterial blood oxygen content and CvO_2 is the mixed venous blood oxygen content

❍ **What is a normal oxygen extraction ratio in a healthy adult?**

25%.

❍ **What is the normal whole lung V/Q ratio?**

4 liters of ventilation to 5 liters of blood flow or 0.8.

❍ **Blood drawn from the tip of a pulmonary artery catheter wedged in zone III will reflect PO_2 from what source?**

Pulmonary capillary.

❍ **Which mitral valve abnormalities can lead to large v waves on the pulmonary artery wedge tracing?**

Both mitral stenosis and mitral regurgitation can lead to large v waves because of overfilling of the left atrium.

❍ **How do increases in heart rate alter the systolic and diastolic components of the cardiac cycle?**

As heart rate increases and cardiac cycle time decreases, systolic time remains relatively constant while diastolic time decreases, thereby, increasing the ratio of systole/diastole.

❍ **What information regarding flow is obtained from a Reynolds number?**

The Reynolds number is calculated from the equation Re=2rvd/n, where r=radius, v=average velocity, d=density and n=viscosity. When the Reynolds number exceeds 2000, turbulent flow is probable; less than 2000 indicates probable laminar flow.

❍ **What property of helium allows less turbulence in a high flow system?**

Density. The low density of helium yields a lower Reynolds number when compared with a gas of higher density (air or oxygen) in the same system.

❍ **What is Boyle's law of gases?**

$P_1V_1 = P_2V_2$ where P is pressure, V is volume and temperature is constant.

❍ **What is the calculation for mean arterial pressure (MAP) based on systolic (SBP) and diastolic pressure (DBP)?**

MAP = DBP + 1/3(SBP-DBP).

❍ **What is the hemodynamic response to an acute complete spinal cord injury at the C7 level?**

Initially there is hypertension and tachycardia secondary to increased circulating catecholamines at the time of the injury followed shortly thereafter by hypotension due to vasodilatation and bradycardia secondary to loss of cardiac accelerator input.

❍ **During the first minute of apnea, how much would you expect $PaCO_2$ will rise?**

During apnea, the $PaCO_2$ will increase approximately 6 mmHg during the first minute and then 3-4 mmHg each minute thereafter.

❍ **Which pulmonary function test is least dependent on patient effort?**

Forced expiratory flow 25-75% is obtained from the mid-expiratory portion of the flow-volume loop and the least dependent on patient effort.

❍ **In the resting healthy adult what percentage of total body oxygen consumption is spent on the work of breathing?**

In the resting healthy adult, 2-3% of total oxygen consumption is spent on the work of breathing.

❍ **What is the most important factor in control of ventilation under normal conditions?**

Under normal conditions, $PaCO_2$ of the arterial blood is the most important factor in control of ventilation.

❍ **What do peripheral chemoreceptors located in the carotid and aortic bodies respond to?**

The peripheral chemoreceptors respond to decreases in arterial PO_2 and pH, and increases in arterial PCO_2.

❍ **What is functional residual capacity (FRC).**

The volume of gas in the lung after a normal expiration is the FRC and is comprised of residual volume and expiratory reserve volume.

❍ **What are the two most important determinants of coronary perfusion pressure?**

The two most important determinants of coronary perfusion pressure are diastolic blood pressure and left ventricular end-diastolic pressure, their relationship being:

CPP = DBP - LVEDP.

❍ **What are the determinants of stroke volume?**

Preload, contractility and afterload are important determinants of stroke volume.

❍ **How would you calculate systemic vascular resistance (SVR)?**

$$SVR = \frac{MAP - CVP}{C.O.} \times 80 \left[\frac{dyne - sec}{cm^5}\right]$$

❍ **How would you calculate pulmonary vascular resistance (PVR)?**

$$PVR = \frac{PAP - PAOP}{C.O.} \times 80 \left[\frac{dyne - sec}{cm^5}\right]$$

❍ **What is the closing capacity of the lungs?**

Closing capacity (closing volume plus residual volume) is the lung volume at which small airways close. Closing capacity is normally well below FRC (Functional Residual Capacity) but rises steadily with age.

❍ **What are the four major forms of cellular hypoxia?**

Anemic hypoxia, hypoxemic hypoxia, circulatory hypoxia, histotoxic hypoxia.

❍ **What are the four major causes of arterial hypoxemia?**

Hypoventilation, ventilation/perfusion inequality, shunt and diffusion impairment.

❍ **How does one assess oxygenation?**

Skin color pulse oximetry and blood gas analysis.

❍ **How does one assess ventilation?**

End tidal CO2 monitoring and blood gas analysis.

❍ **What is a tension pneumothorax?**

An injury to the lung allowing intrapleural air to collect without escaping out the chest wall or trachea. This accumulation of air compresses the lung, and shifts the mediastinum, leading to impaired venous return and hypotension.

❍ **What are the physical findings for tension pneumothorax?**

Distended neck veins, hypotension, tracheal deviation, and hyperresonant hemithorax.

❍ **What is the treatment for tension pneumothorax?**

Immediate decompression of the hyperresonant hemithorax is instituted, based on clinical suspicion. Radiography should not be used to confirm tension pneumothorax..

❍ **What is adequate urinary output to gauge resuscitation?**

For adults 0.5 cc/kg/hr or about 50 cc/hr.

❍ **What is the most common intracranial bleeding?**

Subdural hematomas, in about a third of head injuries with positive CT findings.

❍ **How does one determine need for transfer?**

Transfer of the patient is needed for definitive care and is dependent on the resources available at the initial treatment area, i. e. availability of surgical care, need for monitoring, need for other specialized care. Such determinations can be made with information during the initial evaluation and resuscitation.

❍ **T/F: A splenectomy is usually necessary.**

False. Immediate surgery and repair can salvage Ninety-eight percent (98%) of injured spleens.

❍ **Primary or spontaneous bacterial peritonitis is more frequently seen in patients with which underlying conditions?**

Nephrotic Syndrome, chronic liver disease and systemic lupus erythematosus.

❍ **What are the MRI findings suggestive of herpes simplex encephalitis?**

Edema or hemorrhage in the temporal lobes.

❍ **If herpes simplex encephalitis is suspected, how can the diagnosis be confirmed?**

Brain biopsy and culture.

❍ **What is the most common cause of fulminant hepatic failure in the U.S.?**

Acute viral hepatitis.

❍ **What characterizes liver dysfunction in fulminant hepatic failure ?**

Uncorrectable coagulopathy, jaundice and encephalopathy. All three occur together in an illness of less than eight-week's duration.

❍ **What are the risks and complications of pericardiocentesis ?**

Cardiac tamponade, myocardial infarction, intra-abdominal injuries and pneumothorax.

❍ **What are the indications for calcium therapy?**

Documented or suspected hypocalcemia, hyperkalemia, hypermagnesemia, and calcium channel blocker overdose.

❍ **What are the arterial blood gas findings of a salicylate overdose?**

Respiratory alkalosis and an increased anion gap metabolic acidosis.

❍ **What are the indications for using digoxin immune F antibody?**

The occurrence of a life-threatening dysrhythmias, due to digoxin over dose, or digoxin serum levels that are associated with a risk for developing a life-threatening dysrhythmia.

❍ **Tumor lysis syndrome is characterized by what lab findings?**

Hyperuricemia, hyperkalemia, and hyperphosphatemia.

❍ **What is the major goal of therapy for tumor lysis syndrome ?**

Prevention of acute renal failure. The principles for treatment include alkalinization of the urine, vigorous hydration and diuresis, and prevention of the formation of toxic metabolites.

❍ **What is the blood gas analysis characteristic of a patient with malignant hyperthermia?**

Metabolic and respiratory acidosis.

❍ **Treatment for malignant hyperthermia should include?**

A change in the anesthetic agent to remove possible triggers, administration of Dantrolene and the procedure should be terminated.

❍ **A twenty two-year-old sickle cell patient presents with pallor, weakness, tachycardia and abdominal fullness. What should you suspect first?**

Acute splenic sequestration.

❍ **The treatment for this patient should include?**

Colloid and whole blood transfusions for correction of hypovolemia, anemia and prevention of circulatory failure.

❍ **Subsequent episodes of acute splenic sequestration may be avoided by what treatment?**

Splenectomy or chronic transfusions.

❍ **What infectious agents are associated with necrotizing enterocolitis?**

Gram negative enteric bacilli; E. coli, Klebsiella pneumonia, and Enterococcus.

❍ **What conditions do both intracranial calcifications and skin lesions present with?**

Toxoplasmosis, Cytomegalovirus and Sturge-Weber Syndrome.

❍ **What are the most common presenting findings in ARDS?**

Tachypnea and hypoxemia.

❍ **What are the NIH criteria for the diagnosis of ARDS?**

PaO_2/FiO_2 ratio < 200, bilateral infiltrates, wedge pressure < 18.

❍ **What is the cause of hypoxemia in ARDS?**

An increase in alveolar fluid causing reduced diffusion of oxygen into capillaries, thus increasing the shunt.

❍ **What is the mortality of ARDS?**

Most series show a mortality of 40-60%. Some research protocols have shown a reduction to 25-30%.

❍ **What are the major risk factors for ARDS?**

Sepsis, trauma, aspiration, multiple transfusions, shock, and pulmonary contusions; however, many other systemic and local insults may trigger ARDS.

❍ **Why is the pulmonary artery wedge pressure an important feature in the diagnosis of ARDS?**

The presence of a significantly elevated wedge pressure implies that the pulmonary edema may be hydrostatic, and therefore due to left ventricular dysfunction rather than alveolar or pulmonary dysfunction.

❍ **Does PEEP improve ARDS?**

PEEP commonly improves oxygenation. However, it does not reduce the amount of total lung water, which is the marker for the amount of pulmonary edema present.

❍ **What is the distribution of pulmonary edema in ARDS?**

Routine chest x-ray appears to show a diffuse distribution. However, CT scan studies reveal an increased involvement in the dependent portions of the lung fields.

❍ **What are the x-ray findings in ARDS?**

Diffuse ground-glass-like infiltrates that do not follow anatomical boundaries, more commonly bilateral.

❍ **What complications are associated with ARDS?**

Barotrauma leading to pneumothorax, pulmonary infection, pulmonary hypertension, and multisystem organ failure.

❍ **What is the advantage of pressure controlled ventilation in ARDS?**

It often allows for higher mean airway pressures, and therefore better oxygenation with relatively lower peak airway pressures.

❍ **Is surfactant therapy helpful in ARDS?**

While there is some evidence that exogenous surfactant is helpful in some pediatric cases of respiratory failure, the studies in adults have failed to show a benefit so far.

❍ **What are the three phases of ARDS?**

Acute or exudative (up to 6 days), proliferative phase (4 to 10 days), and chronic or fibrotic phase (after 7 days).

❍ **What is the role of PEEP in ARDS?**

To maintain alveolar inflation and functional residual capacity.

❍ **What is compliance and how is it calculated?**

Compliance is the measure of the elasticity of the lungs. It is calculated by measuring the change in volume for the change in pressure.

❍ **What are the changes in compliance in ARDS?**

Due to increased fluid and debris in the alveoli, there is a decrease in the compliance in ARDS.

❍ **What are the negative effects of PEEP on cardiovascular function?**

PEEP may reduce cardiac output by reducing venous return, by increasing pulmonary vascular resistance, and by shifting the interventricular septum to the left, thus reducing the left ventricular end diastolic volume.

❍ **What are three ways that the optimal level of PEEP can be determined?**

Compliance, oxygenation, and cardiac output.

❍ **What is the role of corticosteriods in ARDS?**

Several studies have failed to show any benefit for the use of steroids in ARDS. There is some evidence that there may be a danger in using steroids in ARDS associated with sepsis. There is some evidence to suggest that in certain cases, in the late phases of ARDS steroids may reduce the fibrosis associated with late ARDS.

❍ **What interventions have been shown to reduce the mortality of ARDS?**

Although a great number of studies have been done to reduce the mortality of ARDS, to date the only strong evidence for reduced mortality is in the computerized protocol for management of ventilator support. Other studies on a variety of interventions in the inflammatory cascade including prostaglandins and steroids have failed to show benefit. There is recent interest in the use of prone positioning for patients with ARDS.

GASTROINTESTINAL

Death is nature's way of saying, "Your table is ready".
Robin Williams

❍ **Where are carcinoid tumors usually located?**

The appendix (50%). The second most common location is the small bowel, i.e., the ileum.

❍ **What are the most common cancers of the small bowel?**

Adenocarcinoma, followed by carcinoid, lymphoma, and leiomyosarcoma. The small bowel is not a common site for malignancy and accounts for only 2% of all GI malignancies.

❍ **Where are the majority of benign tumors of the small bowel located?**

60% are in the ileum, 25% in the jejunum, and 15% in the duodenum.

❍ **What carcinoid tumors have the highest rate of metastasis?**

Ileal carcinoids. Malignancy is highly dependent on the size of the tumor: only 2% of tumors under 1 cm in diameter are malignant, while 80 to 90% of tumors > 2 cm are malignant.

❍ **Kultschitzsky cells are the precursors to what tumor?**

Carcinoid. A carcinoid tumor can arise anywhere in the GI tract, but its most frequent site of involvement is the appendix.

❍ **A patient complains of severe pain when defecating. He is constipated, has blood-streaked stools and a bloody discharge following bowel movements. What is the diagnosis?**

Anal fissure. Ninety percent of anal fissures are located in the posterior midline. If fissures are found elsewhere in the anal canal, then anal intercourse, TB, carcinoma, Crohn's disease, and syphilis should be considered.

❍ **Which are more painful, internal or external hemorrhoids?**

External. The nerves above the pectinate or dentate line are supplied by the autonomic nervous system and have no sensory fibers. The nerves below the pectinate line are supplied by the inferior rectal nerve and have sensory fibers.

❍ **Differentiate between first, second, third, and fourth degree hemorrhoids.**

First degree: Appear in the rectal lumen, but do not protrude past the anus

Second degree: Protrude into the anal canal if the patient strains only

Third degree: Protrude into the anal canal, but can be manually reduced

Fourth degree: Protrude into the canal and cannot be manually reduced

Treatment for degrees one and two is a high-fiber diet, Sitz baths, and good hygiene. The treatment of choice for third or fourth degree hemorrhoids is rubber band ligation. Other treatments are photocoagulation, electrocauterization, and cryosurgery.

❍ **Diverticular disease is most common in which part of the colon?**

The sigmoid colon, which accounts for 95% of diverticular disease.

❍ **What percentage of patients with diverticula are symptomatic?**

20%.

❍ **Ulcerative colitis has two peaks of incidence. When do they occur?**

The second and sixth decades.

❍ **What are some extraintestinal manifestations of ulcerative colitis?**

Ankylosing spondylitis, sclerosing cholangitis, arthralgias, ocular complications, erythema nodosum, aphthous ulcers in the mouth, thromboembolic disease, pyoderma gangrenous, nephrolithiasis, and cirrhosis of the liver.

❍ **If blood is recovered from the stomach after an NG tube is inserted, where is the most likely location of the bleed?**

Above the ligament of Treitz.

❍ **Where do the majority of Mallory-Weiss tears occur?**

In the stomach (75%), gastroesophageal junction (20%), and distal esophagus (5%).

❍ **Where is angiodysplasia most frequently found?**

In the cecum and proximal ascending colon. Lesions are generally singular; bleeding is intermittent and seldom massive.

❍ **Are tumors located in the jejunum and ileum more likely malignant or benign?**

Benign. Tumors of the jejunum and ileum comprise only 5% of all GI tumors. The majority are asymptomatic.

❍ **What is the most common remnant of the omphalomesenteric duct?**

Meckel's diverticulum.

❍ **What is the Meckel's diverticulum rule of 2's?**

2% of the population has it, it is 2 inches long, 2 feet from the ileocecal valve, occurs most commonly in children under 2, and is symptomatic in 2% of patients.

❍ **What is the most likely cause of rectal bleeding in a patient with Meckel's diverticulum?**

Ulceration of ileal mucosa adjacent to the diverticulum lined with gastric mucosa.

❍ **What is the difference in the prognosis between familial polyposis and Gardner's disease?**

Although both are inheritable conditions of colonic polyps, Gardner's disease rarely results in malignancy, while familial polyposis virtually always results in malignancy.

❍ **How much blood must be lost in the GI tract to cause melena?**

50 ml. Healthy patients normally lose 2.5 ml/day.

❍ **What are the most common causes of upper GI bleeding?**

PUD (45%), esophageal varices (20%), gastritis (20%), and Mallory-Weiss syndrome (10%).

❍ **What percentage of patients with upper GI bleeds will stop bleeding within hours of hospitalization?**

85%. About 25% of these patients will re-bleed within the first 2 days of hospitalization. If no re-bleeding occurs in five days, the chance of re-bleeding is only 2%.

❍ **What are the most common causes of re-bleeding in patients with upper GI bleeds?**

PUD or esophageal varices.

❍ **What percentage of patients with PUD bleed from their ulcers?**

20%.

❍ **Bleeding ulcers are more predominant in patients with which blood type?**

Type O. The reason is not known.

❍ **Where are bleeding duodenal ulcers most commonly located?**

On the posterior surface of the duodenal bulb.

❍ **How soon after an episode of bleeding has occurred can an ulcer patient be fed?**

12 to 24 hours after the bleeding has stopped.

❍ **List in decreasing order of frequency the top 3 causes of upper GI bleed?**

Duodenal (45%), gastric (20%), and Varices (10%).

❍ **Which type of ulcer is more likely to re-bleed?**

Gastric ulcers are three times more likely to re-bleed compared to duodenal ulcers.

❍ **Where is the most common site of duodenal ulcers?**

The duodenal bulb (95%). Surgery is indicated only if perforation, gastric outlet obstruction, intractable disease, or uncontrollable hemorrhage occur.

❍ **What is the most common site for gastric ulcers?**

The lesser curvature of the stomach. Surgery is considered earlier in gastric ulcers because of the higher recurrence rate after medical treatment, and because of the higher potential for malignancy.

❍ **What is the most common cause of portal hypertension?**

Intrahepatic obstruction (90%), which is most often due to cirrhosis. Other causes of portal hypertension are increased hepatic flow without obstruction, i.e., fistulas, and extrahepatic outflow obstruction.

❍ **What organism causes amebic liver abscesses?**

Entamoeba histolytica. Amebic liver abscesses are primarily found in middle-aged men living in, or who have traveled to, tropical areas. Ninety percent occur in the right lobe of the liver. Treatment is with oral metronidazole.

❍ **What are the most commonly isolated organisms in pyogenic hepatic abscesses?**

E. coli and other gram-negative bacteria. The source of such bacteria is most likely an infection in the biliary system.

❍ **Which has a higher mortality rate, amebic or pyogenic liver abscesses?**

Pyogenic. The mortality rate for a singular pyogenic abscess is 25%, and for multiple abscesses up to 70%. Amebic abscesses have mortality rates of only 7% if uncomplicated by superinfection. Amebic abscesses are more likely to be singular in nature, while pyogenic abscesses can be singular or multiple.

❍ **What clinical sign can assist in the diagnosis of cholecystitis?**

Murphy's sign--pain on inspiration with palpation of the RUQ. As the patient breaths in, the gallbladder is lowered in the abdomen and comes in contact with the peritoneum just below the examiner's hand. This will aggravate an inflamed gallbladder, causing the patient to discontinue breathing deeply.

❍ **What is the difference between cholelithiasis, cholangitis, cholecystitis, and choledocholithiasis?**

Cholelithiasis: Gallstones in the gallbladder

Cholangitis: Inflammation of the common bile duct, often secondary to bacterial infection or choledocholithiasis

Cholecystitis: Inflammation of the gallbladder secondary to gallstones

Choledocholithiasis: Gallstones, which have migrated from the gallbladder to the common bile duct

❍ **What percentage of people with asymptomatic gallstones will develop symptoms?**

Only 50%.

❍ **Which ethnic group has the largest proportion of people with symptomatic gallstones?**

Native Americans. By the age of 60, 80% of Native Americans with previously asymptomatic gallstones will develop symptoms, as compared to only 30% of Caucasian Americans and 20% of African Americans.

❍ **What percentage of patients with cholangitis are also septic?**

50%. Chills, fever, and shock can occur.

❍ **What percentage of gallstones can be visualized on ultrasound?**

95%. Ultrasound is the diagnostic procedure of choice in patients with suspected cholecystitis.

❍ **How much bile can held within a distended gallbladder?**

50 ml.

❍ **What is Charcot's triad?**

1) Fever
2) Jaundice
3) Abdominal pain

This is the hallmark of acute cholangitis.

❍ **What is Reynolds' pentad?**

Charcot's triad plus shock and mental status changes. This is the hallmark of acute toxic ascending cholangitis.

❍ **What are the majority of gallstones composed of?**

Cholesterol (75 to 95%). The rest are made of pigment.

❍ **What percentage of gallstones will be visualized by an x-ray?**

20%.

❍ **What percentage of patients with cancer of the gallbladder will also have cholelithiasis?**

90%.

❍ **What is the diagnostic test of choice for acute cholecystitis?**

HIDA scan (technetium-99-labeled N-substituted iminodiacetic acid scan). The HIDA scan uses a gamma-ray-emitting isotope that is selectively extracted by the liver into bile. The labeled bile can then be used to determine if there is cystic duct obstruction or extrahepatic bile duct obstruction, which is based whether the bile fills the gall bladder or enters the intestine. For practical reasons, the diagnosis is frequently make using clinical impressions, CBC and ultrasound.

❍ **How effective is oral dissolution therapy with bile acids for those with symptomatic gallstones?**

Oral therapy with bile acids can dissolve up to 90% of stones. However, therapy works only on stones smaller than 0.5 mm, made of cholesterol, and floating in a functioning gallbladder. Patients are then treated for 6 to 12 months and 50% have recurrence of gallstones within 5 years.

❍ **What are the contraindications to lithotripsy?**

Stones > 2.5 cm, more than 3 stones, calcified stones, stones in the bile duct, and poor overall condition of the patient.

❍ **What electrolyte disturbances are associated with acute pancreatitis?**

Hypocalcemia and hypomagnesemia.

❍ **Serum amylase is frequently elevated in acute pancreatitis. What other conditions can cause a similar rise in amylase?**

Bowel infarction, cholecystitis, mumps, perforated ulcer, and renal failure. Lipase is more specific. A two-hour urine amylase is a more accurate test in pancreatitis.

❍ **What are the most common causes of acute pancreatitis?**

Alcoholism (40%) and gallstone disease (40%). The remaining cases of acute pancreatitis are due to familial pancreatitis, hypoparathyroidism, hyperlipidemia, iatrogenic pancreatitis, and protein deficiency.

❍ **What are some abdominal x-ray findings associated with acute pancreatitis?**

A sentinel loop (either of the jejunum, transverse colon, or duodenum); a colon cutoff sign, which is an abrupt cessation of gas in the mid or left transverse colon due to inflammation of the adjacent pancreas; or calcification of the pancreas. About two-thirds of patients with acute pancreatitis will have x-ray abnormalities.

❍ **What is the most common cause of pancreatic pseudocysts in adults?**

Chronic pancreatitis. Pseudocysts are generally filled with pancreatic enzymes and are sterile. They present about 1 week after the patient has a bout with acute pancreatitis displayed as upper abdominal pain with anorexia and weight loss. Forty percent will regress spontaneously.

❍ **What is the treatment for pancreatic pseudocysts?**

Initial therapy is to wait for regression (4 to 6 weeks). If no improvement occurs, or if superinfection occurs, surgical drainage or excision is required.

❍ **What are Ranson's criteria?**

A means of estimating prognosis for patients with pancreatitis.

At initial presentation	Developing within 24 hours
Age > 55	Hematocrit falling > 10%
WBC > 16,000/mm^3	Increase in BUN > 8 mg/dl
AST > 250 UI/L	Serum Ca$^+$ < 8 mg/dl
Serum glucose > 200 mg/dl	Arterial PO_2 < 60 mm Hg

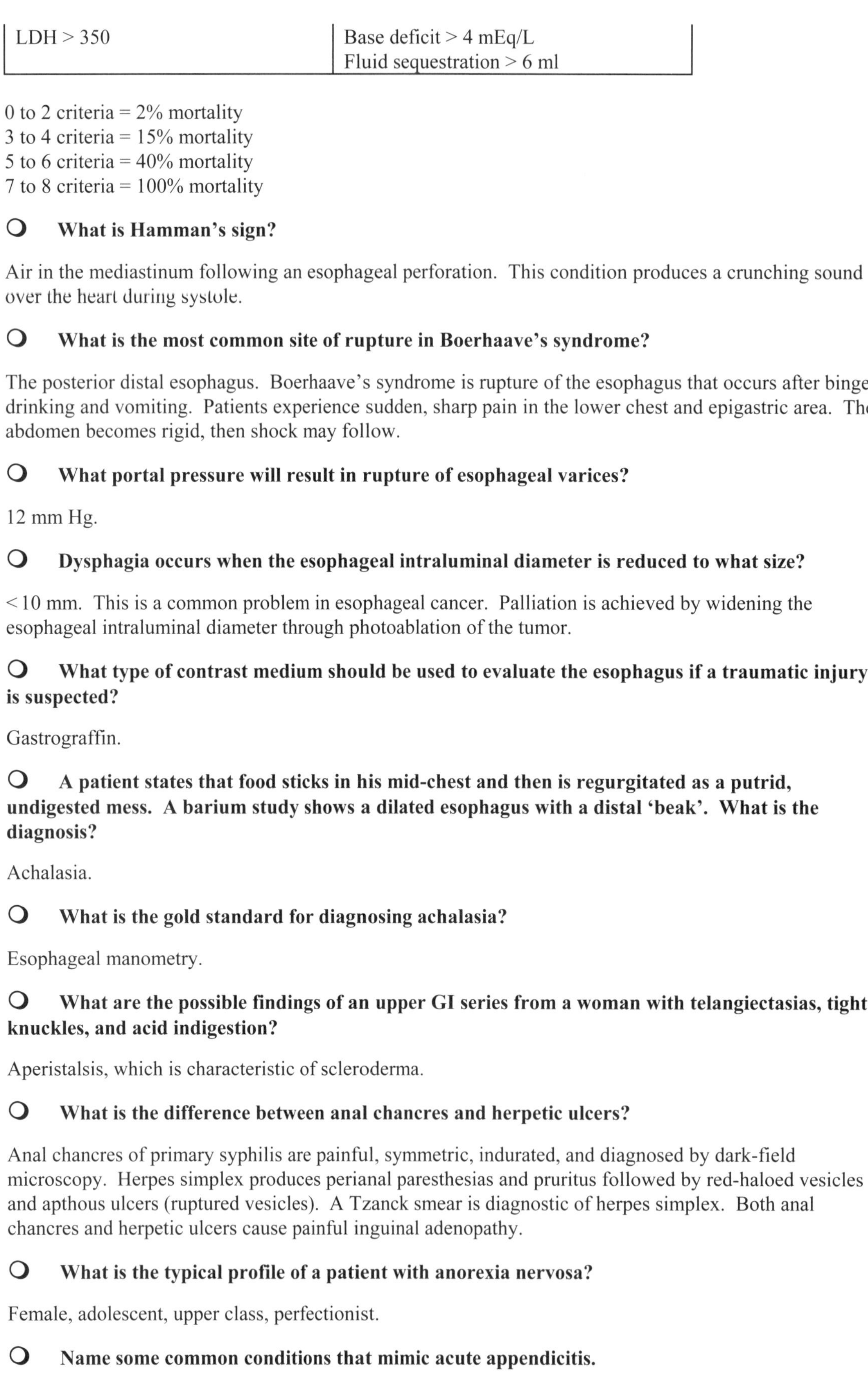

LDH > 350	Base deficit > 4 mEq/L Fluid sequestration > 6 ml

0 to 2 criteria = 2% mortality
3 to 4 criteria = 15% mortality
5 to 6 criteria = 40% mortality
7 to 8 criteria = 100% mortality

❍ **What is Hamman's sign?**

Air in the mediastinum following an esophageal perforation. This condition produces a crunching sound over the heart during systole.

❍ **What is the most common site of rupture in Boerhaave's syndrome?**

The posterior distal esophagus. Boerhaave's syndrome is rupture of the esophagus that occurs after binge drinking and vomiting. Patients experience sudden, sharp pain in the lower chest and epigastric area. The abdomen becomes rigid, then shock may follow.

❍ **What portal pressure will result in rupture of esophageal varices?**

12 mm Hg.

❍ **Dysphagia occurs when the esophageal intraluminal diameter is reduced to what size?**

< 10 mm. This is a common problem in esophageal cancer. Palliation is achieved by widening the esophageal intraluminal diameter through photoablation of the tumor.

❍ **What type of contrast medium should be used to evaluate the esophagus if a traumatic injury is suspected?**

Gastrograffin.

❍ **A patient states that food sticks in his mid-chest and then is regurgitated as a putrid, undigested mess. A barium study shows a dilated esophagus with a distal 'beak'. What is the diagnosis?**

Achalasia.

❍ **What is the gold standard for diagnosing achalasia?**

Esophageal manometry.

❍ **What are the possible findings of an upper GI series from a woman with telangiectasias, tight knuckles, and acid indigestion?**

Aperistalsis, which is characteristic of scleroderma.

❍ **What is the difference between anal chancres and herpetic ulcers?**

Anal chancres of primary syphilis are painful, symmetric, indurated, and diagnosed by dark-field microscopy. Herpes simplex produces perianal paresthesias and pruritus followed by red-haloed vesicles and apthous ulcers (ruptured vesicles). A Tzanck smear is diagnostic of herpes simplex. Both anal chancres and herpetic ulcers cause painful inguinal adenopathy.

❍ **What is the typical profile of a patient with anorexia nervosa?**

Female, adolescent, upper class, perfectionist.

❍ **Name some common conditions that mimic acute appendicitis.**

Mesenteric lymphadenitis, PID, Mittlesmertz, gastroenteritis, and Crohn's disease.

❍ **What conditions are associated with an atypical presentation of acute appendicitis?**

Situs inversus viscerum, malrotation, hypermobile cecum, long pelvic appendix, and pregnancy (1/2200).

❍ **What are the most frequent symptoms of acute appendicitis?**

Anorexia and pain. The classical presentations of anorexia and periumbilical pain with progression to constant RLQ pain are present in only 60% of the cases.

❍ **What percentage of patients with acute appendicitis cases have an elevated WBC count?**

An elevated leukocyte count and an elevated absolute neutrophil count are present in 85% of the cases.

❍ **Until discounted, what intra-abdominal pathology should be assumed for a pregnant woman with right upper quadrant pain?**

Acute appendicitis.

❍ **Rovsing's, psoas, and obturator signs can all indicate an inflamed posterior appendix. What are these signs?**

Rovsing's sign: RLQ pain with palpation over the LLQ

Psoas sign: RLQ pain with right thigh extension

Obturator sign: RLQ pain with internal rotation of the flexed right thigh

❍ **What does an ultrasound show in acute appendicitis?**

Fixed, tender, non-compressible mass, but only in 75 to 90% of cases.

❍ **What does abdominal CT scanning show in acute appendicitis?**

Not much in early appendicitis. However, the study is useful to determine the causes of a right lower quadrant mass, such as late appendicitis, perforation/abscess, carcinoma, and pseudomyxoma. Newer scanning techniques are increasing the utility of CT for evaluation of suspected appedicitis.

❍ **What does laparoscopy show in acute appendicitis?**

Appendicitis, if you're lucky. Unfortunately, determining that the appendix is inflamed does not prove appendicitis. However, finding another cause of the abdominal pain does not rule out appendicitis either.

❍ **Barrett's esophagitis is associated with which type of cancer?**

Esophageal adenocarcinoma. Squamous cell carcinoma is the predominant cancer of the upper esophagus.

❍ **Which method is more sensitive for locating the source of GI bleeding, a radioactive Tc-labeled red cell scan or angiography?**

A bleeding scan can detect a site bleeding at a rate as low as 0.12 ml/minute, while angiography requires rapid bleeding, i.e., greater than 0.5 ml/min.

❍ **A patient with an "acid stomach" develops melena and vomits bright red blood. Is esophagitis a feasible cause?**

No. Capillary bleeding rarely causes impressive acute blood loss. Arterial bleeding from a complicated ulcer, foreign body, or Mallory-Weiss tear or bleeding from esophageal varices are much more probable.

❍ **Repeated violent bouts of vomiting can result in both Mallory-Weiss tears and Boerhaave's syndrome. What is the difference between the two?**

Mallory-Weiss tears: Involve the submucosa and mucosa, typically in the right posterolateral wall of the gastroesophageal junction.

Boerhaave's syndrome: A full-thickness tear, usually in the unsupported left posterolateral wall of the abdominal esophagus.

❍ **Recurrent pneumonias, especially in the right middle lobe or the superior segments of the bilateral upper lobes, are indicative of what syndrome?**

Aspiration associated with motor diseases and gastroesophageal reflux.

❍ **What is the antidote for botulism poisoning?**

Trivalent A-B-E antitoxin.

❍ **What is the most frequent complication of choledocholithiasis?**

Cholangitis (60%). Other complications are bile duct obstruction, pancreatitis, biliary enteric fistula, and hemobilia.

❍ **Gallbladder stones are generally formed of what material?**

Cholesterol. The diagnostic test of choice is ultrasound. This technique may show stones, sludge, bile plugging, or dilated bile ducts.

❍ **Acalculous cholecystitis commonly occurs in what conditions?**

Postoperative, posttraumatic and burn patients secondary to dehydration, and hemolysis secondary to blood transfusions.

❍ **A patient with a history of gallstones presents with acute, postprandial right upper quadrant pain. What's the KUB likely to show?**

Nothing specific. Only about 10% of gallstones are radiopaque. Complications of cholelithiasis, such as emphysematous cholecystitis, perforation, and pneumobilia, are uncommon but useful findings.

❍ **A 22 year-old female with sickle-cell disease presents with fever, shaking chills, and jaundice. What is the diagnosis?**

Charcot's triad suggests ascending cholangitis. The precipitating cause is probably pigment stones resulting from chronic hemolysis.

❍ **A postoperative patient develops right upper quadrant pain, nausea, and low-grade fevers. According to his surgeon, the gallbladder did not contain stones. What is the probable diagnosis?**

Acalculous cholecystitis.

❍ **Eight years after her cholecystectomy, a woman develops right upper quadrant pain and jaundice. What is the chance of recurrent biliary tract stones developing?**

At least 10%, due either to retained stones or in-situ formation by biliary epithelium.

❍ **List the ultrasound findings that are suggestive of acute cholecystitis.**

Formation of gallstones or sludge in acalculous cholecystitis, thickening of the wall of the gallbladder by more than 5 mm, and the presence of pericholecystic fluid. A dilated common bile duct, i.e., > 10 mm suggests common duct obstruction.

❍ **What two findings in acute cholecystitis mandate an emergency laparotomy?**

Emphysematous cholecystitis and perforation. Otherwise, timing of surgery is somewhat dependent upon the institution and the surgeon.

❍ **Can non-gallstone cholecystitis perforate?**

Yes. Up to 40% of gallbladder perforations are associated with acalculous cholecystitis.

❍ **A 24 year-old male complains that he has endured two days of rice-water stools, muscle cramps and extreme fatigue. He looks pale, dehydrated, and very ill. The patient states that he has just returned from India. What is the diagnosis?**

Cholera. The incidence of cholera in the US is 1/10,000,000. This disease usually develops in persons that have traveled to endemic areas, such as India, Africa, Southeast Asia, southern Europe, Central and South America, and the Middle East. Infection occurs by consuming unpurified water, raw fruits and vegetables, and under cooked seafood.

❍ **A patient presents with palmar erythema, spider angiomas, testicular atrophy, and asterixis. What other signs and symptoms may be exhibited?**

Hematemesis, encephalopathy, hepatomegaly, splenomegaly, jaundice, caput medusa, ascites, and gynecomastia may also occur. This patient has cirrhosis.

❍ **A cirrhotic patient vomits bright red blood and has a systolic blood pressure of 90 mm Hg. After aggressive fluid resuscitation with 4 units of packed RBCs and a gastric lavage, his pressure is still 90 mm Hg. What's next?**

Assume a coagulopathy. Transfuse fresh frozen plasma, start a vasopressin or octreotide drip, and arrange for an emergency endoscopic evaluation/intervention, usually for sclerotherapy or banding.

❍ **How does the pathology of Crohn's disease differ from that of ulcerative colitis?**

Crohn's is a transmucosal, segmental, granulomatous process, while ulcerative colitis is a mucosal, juxtapositioned, ulcerative process.

❍ **A young man with atraumatic chronic back pain, eye trouble, and painful red lumps on his shins develops bloody diarrhea. What is the point of this question?**

To remind you of the extraintestinal manifestations of inflammatory bowel disease, such as ankylosing spondylitis, uveitis, and erythema nodosum, not to mention kidney stones.

❍ **At least one-third of the patients with Crohn's disease develop kidney stones. Why?**

Dietary oxalate is usually bound to calcium and then excreted. When terminal ileal disease leads to decreased bile salt absorption, the resulting fattier intestinal contents bind calcium by saponification. Free oxalate is 'hyper-absorbed' in the colon, resulting in hyperoxaluria and calcium oxalate nephrolithiasis.

❍ **Complications of Crohn's disease include perirectal abscesses, anal fissures, rectovaginal fistulas, and rectal prolapse. What percentage of patients with Crohn's disease have perirectal involvement?**

Approximately 90%.

❍ **What are the odds that a patient with severe ileal disease will be cured by surgery?**

Virtually zero. Crohn's disease invariably recurs in the remaining GI tract. In contrast, total proctocolectomy with ileostomy is curative procedure for ulcerative colitis.

❍ **What hereditary diseases evident in infancy may cause cirrhosis?**

Glycogen storage disease, cystic fibrosis, galactosemia, fructose intolerance, tyrosinemia, and acid cholesterol esterhydrolase deficiency.

❍ **A cirrhotic patient presents with weakness and edema. What electrolyte imbalances might be present?**

Hyponatremia (dilutional or diuretic-induced), hypokalemia (from GI losses, secondary hyperaldosteronism, or diuretics), and hypomagnesemia.

❍ **What diuretic is the optimal choice for treating most cirrhotics with ascites?**

Potassium-sparing agents. Treat the hyperaldosterone state specifically.

❍ **A confused cirrhotic patient enters the hospital. She is afebrile and has asterixis. What should your examination include to determine the precipitant of hepatic encephalopathy?**

Assess her mental status and examine her for localizing neurologic signs suggestive of an occult head injury. Look for dry mucous membranes and a low jugular venous pressure, which are indicative of hypovolemia and azotemia. In addition, check a stool guiac for GI bleeding. Focused lab testing can pinpoint other causes, including diuretic overuse and hypokalemia, hypoglycemia, anemia, hypoxia, and infection. Administer thiamine and folate.

❍ **Aside from fixing the above, what therapy is useful?**

Lactulose. This synthetic disaccharide produces an acidic diarrhea which traps nitrogenous wastes in the gut.

❍ **Are there any useful therapies for the rapid renal failure that can accompany cirrhosis?**

Unfortunately there is not. The hepatorenal syndrome still has a mortality rate that approaches 100%.

❍ **What is the most common neoplasm of the GI tract?**

Colon cancer. It is also the second most common cause of cancer death in the US.

❍ **What are the current recommendations from the American Cancer Society for screening colon cancer?**

An annual digital examination for patients over 40 and an annual testing for occult blood in patients over 50. A flexible sigmoidoscopy should be performed every 3 to 5 years on individuals older than 50 years. Earlier screening is required in patients with familial polyposis.

❍ **Which is the most common type of colon cancer?**

Adenocarcinoma (95%).

❍ **Which is the most common type of rectal cancer?**

Adenocarcinoma (95%).

❍ **To where on the body does colon cancer most commonly spread?**

The regional lymph nodes. Hematogenous spread occurs most often to the liver or lungs.

❍ **Where is the most common site of colorectal cancer?**

For adenocarcinoma, 60 to 65% of cases occur in the distal colon or the rectum, and 35 to 40% occur in the proximal colon. The typical sites for carcinoid, squamous, and melanoma are the appendix or the rectum, the anal area, and the area adjacent to the dentate line, respectively.

❍ **Adenocarcinoma of the colon is associated with a ras oncogene mutations in 40 to 50% of patients. These mutations typically involve what chromosomes?**

Chromosomes 17 and 18.

❍ **Clinically, what are the differences between right-sided and left-sided adenocarcinoma of the colon?**

Right-sided: Pain and/or mass in RLQ, occult blood in stool, dyspepsia, fatigue secondary to anemia; stool appearance rarely changes.

Left-sided: Change in bowel habits, red blood in stool, reduced caliber of stool, and pencil thin stools.

❍ **T/F: Serum CEA is a proficient screening tool for colorectal cancer.**

False. Although 70% of patients with colorectal cancer will have an elevated CEA, it is not specific for colorectal cancer. It is however, a good measure of recurrent colon cancer.

❍ **It has been conclusively determined that a 72 year-old female has cancer of the colon with involvement of the regional lymph nodes. What Duke's stage is this?**

Duke's stage C.

❍ **Describe the Duke's stages.**

Duke's stage A:	Mucosal involvement, which may involve the submucosa
Duke's stage B1:	Cancer extends to muscularis propria but not through the serosa
Duke's stage B2:	Cancer extends beyond the serosa
Duke's stage C:	Regional lymph node involvement
Duke's stage D:	Distant metastases

❍ **What is the typical five-year survival rate for a colon cancer Duke's stage A?**

95%. Duke's B1 is 85 to 90%, B2 is 60 to 70%, C is 15 to 25%, and D is 5%.

❍ **What stool studies are crucial for evaluating acute diarrhea?**

None. Most cases require no testing, just oral rehydration. In patients at risk for complications, i.e., at the extremes of age, recently hospitalized, or immunocompromised, enteroinvasive infection should be ruled out with a stool guiac and fecal leukocyte test. Also consider checking for ova and parasites.

❍ **Which diarrheal illnesses cause fecal leukocytes?**

The usual culprits are Shigella, Campylobacter, and enteroinvasive E. coli. Others include Salmonella, Yersinia, Vibrio parahaemolyticus, and C. difficile. Fecal WBC's are absent in toxigenic and enteropathogenic infection, even with such a virulent organism as Vibrio cholera. Viral and parasitic infections rarely produce fecal WBC's.

❍ **What is the most common cause of bacterial diarrhea?**

E. coli (enteroinvasive, enteropathogenic, enterotoxigenic).

❍ **Which is the most common form of acute diarrhea?**

Viral diarrhea. It is generally self-limited, lasting only 1 to 3 days.

❍ **Diarrhea that develops within 12 hours of a meal is most probably caused by what?**

An ingested pre-formed toxin.

❍ **When does traveler's diarrhea typically occur?**

3 to 7 days after arrival in a foreign land.

❍ **What is the treatment for traveler's diarrhea?**

Traveler's diarrhea is usually caused by E. Coli; the preferable treatment is with Bactrim.

❍ **What is the definition of chronic diarrhea?**

Passage of > 200 g of loose stool per day for over three weeks.

❍ **A 73 year-old women with no prior medical history presents with fever, chills, vomiting, nausea, and an acute onset of pain in her left lower quadrant. Her pain becomes worse after she eats and is mildly relieved after a bowel movement. Upon physical examination, you note that she has guarding, rebound tenderness, and a tender, firm, non-mobile mass in the left lower quadrant. What is the diagnosis?**

Diverticulitis.

❍ **Where in the colon are diverticula most commonly found?**

The sigmoid and distal colon.

❍ **If there is associated bleeding with the diverticulitis, where is the most likely etiology?**

The right side of the colon. Fifty percent of the bleeds originate in this area even though diverticulitis is more common in the left side.

❍ **T/F: A barium enema is not a good diagnostic test if diverticulitis is suspected.**

True. If a patient is having an acute attack of diverticulitis, the risk of perforation is too great.

❍ **Why is pentazocine, not morphine, the analgesic of choice for the treatment of diverticulitis?**

Morphine increases colonic pressure.

❍ **What would be the preferred choice for an outpatient antibiotic regimen for uncomplicated diverticulitis?**

Ciprofloxacin plus metronidazole.

❍ **Is diverticulitis the probable diagnosis for a patient with low abdominal pain and bright red blood per rectum?**

No. Typically diverticulosis bleeds, while diverticulitis doesn't. Diverticular bleeding is usually painless.

❍ **What barium findings distinguish colonic obstruction caused by acute diverticulitis from that caused by colon cancer?**

Diverticulitis is extraluminal. Thus, the mucosa appears intact and involved bowel segments are longer. Adenocarcinoma distorts the mucosa, involves a short segment of bowel, and has overhanging edges.

❍ **What is the most common cause of oropharyngeal dysphagia?**

CVA. Other causes include Alzheimer's, bulbar and pseudobulbar palsy, myasthenia gravis, skeletal myopathies, and cranial nerve palsies.

❍ **What symptoms are usually associated with neuromuscular dysphagia?**

Nasopharyngeal regurgitation and hoarseness.

❍ **A 40 year-old smoker describes an acute crescendo substernal chest tightness penetrating to his back. The pain is not relieved by antacids. An ECG shows ST changes, and his pain resolves 7 to 10 minutes after a nitroglycerin tablet. Is this angina?**

Maybe, although the delayed response to nitrates characterizes "esophageal colic" which is caused by segmental esophageal spasm and is often triggered by reflux.

❍ **An elderly woman has trouble swallowing solids and later develops difficulty with liquids. She presents with sudden drooling after dinner. What is the concern?**

A peptic stricture or esophageal cancer complicated by bolus obstruction.

❍ **What is the most common symptom of esophageal disease?**

Pyrosis (heartburn).

❍ **What classical features distinguish chest pain of esophageal origin from cardiac ischemia?**

None. Exertional pain and palliation with rest or NTG occur in both groups. Pain relief in the GI group usually takes 7 to 10 minutes, while ischemic pain usually responds in 2 to 3 minutes.

❍ **What is the most common benign esophageal neoplasm?**

Leiomyoma. Papilloma and fibrovascular polyps also occur, but benign esophageal neoplasms are rare.

❍ **What percentage of patients with esophageal cancer are also afflicted with distant metastasis?**

80%. The 5 year survival rate is 5%. If the cancer is squamous and there is no lymph node involvement, the survival rate is 15 to 20%.

❍ **What is the most common location of esophageal cancer?**

The lower third (50%), followed by the upper third (20%) and the middle third (30%).

❍ **Objects bigger than what size rarely pass the stomach?**

5 cm × 2 cm.

❍ **What is the appropriate management for an ingested button battery that is in the stomach?**

In asymptomatic patients, repeat radiographs. Endoscopic retrieval is required if symptoms occur or if the battery does not pass the pylorus after 48 hours.

❍ **Most objects, even sharp ones, pass through the GI tract without incident. When should such objects be removed?**

Remove if they obstruct or perforate, if longer than 5 cm × 2 cm, and if they are toxic (such as batteries). Sharp or pointed objects, including sewing needles and razor blades, should be removed if they haven't yet passed the pylorus.

❍ **What is the best way to remove a meat bolus causing esophageal obstruction?**

Endoscopy. However, IV glucagon, 1 mg IV push after a small test dose, then repeated as a 2 mg dose at 20 minutes if there is no relief, or sublingual nifedipine, 10 mg, may resolve the problem. Both medications relax esophageal smooth muscle. Meat tenderizer should be avoided because perforation has occurred.

❍ **What test must be performed after the food bolus is cleared?**

Either a barium study or endoscopy. This confirms the passage or removal of the foreign body and checks for underlying pathology, which is present in most adults with obstructing food boluses.

❍ **Gastric carcinoma is most prevalent in people with which blood type?**

Type A.

❍ **People who live in what countries are at greatest risk for gastric carcinoma?**

Japan, Chile, and Hispanic countries. Risk factors include a diet high in additives, achlorhydria, intestinal metaplasia, polyps or dysplasia, H. pylori infection (disputed), familial polyposis, and pernicious anemia.

❍ **What is the most common type of gastric carcinoma? What percentage of these are ulcerative, polypoid or linitis plastica?**

Adenocarcinomas account for 90% of gastric carcinomas. Of these, 75% are ulcerative, 10% are polypoid, and 15% are diffuse infiltrative scirrhous (linitis plastica).

❍ **What percentage of gastric carcinomas produce a positive hemoccult test?**

50%.

❍ **What percentage of gastric carcinomas are associated with a palpable mass?**

25%.

❍ **What is a Krukenberg tumor?**

A gastric carcinoma that has metastasized to the ovary.

❍ **Stomach cancer is associated with the enlargement of what lymph nodes?**

Supraclavicular nodes. These are called Virchow's nodes.

❍ **What is the treatment of choice for gastric carcinoma?**

A radical subtotal gastrectomy with gastrojejunostomy or gastroduodenostomy. Chemotherapy is not very effective and can only be used for some palliation.

❍ **Which type of hepatitis is characterized by an SPGT greater than the SGOT?**

Viral hepatitis. The SGPT is usually greater than 1,000.

❍ **Which type of hepatitis is usually contracted through blood transfusions?**

Hepatitis C accounts for 85% of hepatitis infections via this route.

❍ **A poor prognosis is associated with which two LFT's in acute viral hepatitis?**

A total bilirubin > 20 mg/dl and a prolongation of the prothrombin time > 3 seconds. The extent of transaminase elevation is not a useful marker.

❍ **Match the following hepatitis serologies with the correct clinical description.**

1) HBsAg (-) and anti-HBs (+)a) Ongoing viral replication, z
4) HBeAg (+)d) Prior infection or vaccination, not infectious

Answers: (1) d, (2) c, (3) b, and (4) a.

❍ **T/F: The d-agent can cause hepatitis D in a patient without active hepatitis B.**

False. The d-agent is an incomplete, 'defective" RNA virus that is responsible for hepatitis D. It is an obligate co-virus and requires hepatitis B for replication.

❍ **You stick yourself with a needle withdrawn from a chronic hepatitis B carrier. You've been vaccinated but have never had your antibody status checked. What is the appropriate post-exposure prophylaxis?**

Measure your anti-HB titer. If it's adequate (> 10 mIU), treatment is not required. If it is inadequate, you need a single dose of HBIG as soon as possible and a vaccine booster.

❍ **List three types of internal hernias.**

1) Diaphragmatic hernia
2) Lesser sac hernia, i.e., through the foramen of Winslow
3) Omental or mesenteric hernia

❍ **Are small or large hernias more dangerous?**

Small, because incarceration is more likely.

❍ **What are the borders of Hesselbach's triangle?**

The inguinal ligament, the inferior epigastric vessels, and the lateral border of the rectus abdominis.

❍ **Which type of hernia passes through Hesselbach's triangle?**

Direct hernias.

❍ **Among women, which is more common, inguinal or femoral hernia?**

Inguinal. Femoral hernias occur more commonly among women than in men, but inguinal hernias are the most common type of hernia in women.

❍ **Distinguish between a groin hernia, a hydrocele, and a lymph node.**

Hydroceles transilluminate and are not tender. Lymph nodes are freely moving and firm. Hernias don't transilluminate and may produce bowel sounds.

❍ **A patient's groin bulged two days ago. He then developed severe pain with progressive nausea and vomiting. He has a tender mass in his groin. What should you NOT do?**

Don't try to reduce a long-standing, tender, incarcerated hernia! The abdomen is no place for dead bowel.

❍ **What simple test can distinguish between conjugated and unconjugated hyperbilirubinemia?**

A dipstick test for urobilinogen, which reflects conjugated (water soluble) hyperbilirubinemia.

❍ **In addition to conjugated hyperbilirubinemia, what liver function abnormalities suggest biliary tract disease?**

Elevated alkaline phosphatase levels that are out of proportion to transaminases.

❍ **Portal hypertension produces internal hemorrhoids through what veins?**

The superior rectal and inferior mesenteric veins. Internal hemorrhoids are proximal to the fabled dentate line in the 2, 5, and 9 o'clock positions in the prone patient and are typically not palpable on rectal examination.

❍ **What is the treatment for intussusception?**

A barium enema is both a diagnostic tool and often curative, i.e., it can reduce the intussusception. If the barium enema is unsuccessful, surgical reduction may be required.

❍ **Crampy abdominal pain with mucus in the stool indicates what syndrome?**

Irritable bowel syndrome. Patients are afebrile and often improve after passing flatus.

❍ **List four contraindications to the introduction of a nasogastric tube.**

1) Suspected esophageal laceration or perforation
2) Near obstruction due to stricture
3) Esophageal foreign body
4) Severe head trauma with rhinorrhea

❍ **What test should be performed when an elderly patient is suffering from pain that is out of proportion to the physical examination?**

Angiography. This test is the gold standard for diagnosing mesenteric ischemia.

❍ **What is the most common form of mesenteric ischemia?**

Strangulation due to obstruction.

❍ **What is the defining characteristic for obesity?**

A weight 20% above the height/weight recommendation.

❍ **What is the body mass index (BMI) of a 150 kg individual who is 1.5 meters tall?**

100 kg/m. The normal range is 20 to 25 kg/m.

❍ **In order of prevalence, what are the three most common causes of colonic obstruction?**

Cancer, diverticulitis, and volvulus.

❍ **An elderly man is constipated but does not have tenesmus, abdominal pain, nausea, or vomiting. A rectal examination determines that he has hard stool in the vault. A KUB shows a colon "full of stool". Is an enema all he needs?**

No. Fecal impaction with "obstipation" is both common and benign; however, it is usually associated with tenesmus. The patient must also be evaluated for a colorectal tumor.

❍ **A KUB suggests a large bowel obstruction. What are the next steps in this examination?**

An unprepped sigmoidoscopy to confirm obstruction, followed by a barium study to determine the cause. If a pseudo-obstruction is suspected, don't order a barium study because of the possibility of concretion and obstruction. Colonoscopy can be diagnostic as well as therapeutic.

❍ **Pseudo-obstruction is typically caused by medications. What are three classes of drugs that give rise to pseudo-obstruction?**

Anticholinergics, anti-parkinsonian drugs, and tricyclic antidepressants.

❍ **What is the most frequent cause of small bowel obstruction?**

Adhesions, followed by incarcerated hernias, are the most common causes of extraluminal obstruction. Gallstones and bezoars are the most common causes of intraluminal obstruction.

❍ **An elderly woman has a recurrent small bowel obstruction with a unilateral pain in one thigh. What occult process may be present?**

An obturator hernia incarceration. This condition often presents with pain down the medial thigh to the knee.

❍ **What are the major causes of acute pancreatitis?**

Alcohol and biliary gallstone disease.

❍ **What disease is indicated by epigastric pain that radiates to the back and is relieved, to some extent, by sitting up?**

Pancreatitis.

❍ **A non-drinker presents with acute pancreatitis. What conditions may underlie this acute process?**

Biliary tract disease, blunt or penetrating trauma, a posterior penetrating duodenal ulcer, diabetes (ketoacidosis), and hypertriglyceridemia.

❍ **Is a serum amylase test or a lipase test more sensitive for pancreatitis?**

A lipase test is 75 to 100% sensitive, while an amylase test is 70 to 90% sensitive. The two tests in combination are up to 95 to 97% sensitive. Remember that up to 10% of patients with severe acute pancreatitis may have a normal amylase, and in chronic pancreatitis, up to 30% of cases will have normal amylase levels.

❍ **Is a nasogastric tube always required for acute pancreatitis?**

No, only if nausea and vomiting are severe. In fact, one study showed that NG tubes contributed to more complications, including aspiration.

❍ **When are antibiotics useful in acute pancreatitis?**

Because pancreatitis is a chemical disease, antibiotics are only useful for treating complications, such as abscess or sepsis, and those cases that are associated with choledocholithiasis.

❍ **Are plain films a useful diagnostic tool for pancreatitis?**

Yes. The plain films of patients with gallstone pancreatitis, abscess pancreatitis, and chronic pancreatitis show upper quadrant calcifications, air in the region of the pancreas, and calcific stripling in the epigastrium, respectively.

❍ **Where is the most common site of pancreatic cancer?**

The pancreatic duct system (90 to 95%). If an ultrasound and CT are negative, an ERCP may still verify the presence of cancer.

❍ **With regards to pancreatic cancer, distinguish between periampullary lesions and lesions of the body and tail.**

Periampullary lesions most commonly develop at the head of the pancreas. These lesions are usually adenocarcinomas and are associated with jaundice, weight loss, and abdominal pain.

Lesions of the body and tail tend to be much larger at presentation because of their retroperitoneal location and their distance from the common bile duct. Weight loss and pain are typical.

❍ **What is the most common cause of lower GI perforation?**

Diverticulitis, followed by tumor, colitis, foreign bodies, and instrumentation.

❍ **Which types of patients are at risk for gallbladder perforation?**

The elderly, diabetics, and those with recurrent cholecystitis.

❍ **What does burning epigastric pain shooting to the back, hypovolemic shock, and a high amylase level suggest?**

A posterior perforation of a duodenal ulcer.

❍ **Enteric coated potassium tablets, typhoid, tuberculosis, tumors, and a strangulated hernia can all cause what rare process?**

Non-traumatic small bowel perforation.

❍ **What percentage of patients with a perforated viscous also have radiographic evidence of a pneumoperitoneum?**

60 to 70%. Therefore, one-third of patients will not have this sign. Maintain the patient in either the upright or the left lateral decubitus position for at least 10 minutes prior to taking x-rays.

❍ **After a high-speed motor vehicle accident, an unrestrained driver develops abdominal and chest pain radiating to the neck. An upper chest film shows left-sided pleural fluid. What gastroesophageal catastrophe might have occurred?**

Impact against a steering wheel can result in Boerhaave's syndrome with esophageal perforation and mediastinitis.

❍ **What test should be ordered if a perforated esophagus is suspected?**

A water-soluble contrast study. In the mean time, start broad-spectrum antibiotics and consult a surgeon immediately.

❍ **A patient's sore throat worsened after a week. She appears ill and complains of spiking fevers and central chest burning. What is the diagnosis?**

A retropharyngeal or parapharyngeal abscess with extension to the superior mediastinum.

❍ **A former IV drug user with sickle-cell disease and a history of splenectomy presents with unremitting fever, crampy abdominal pain, and meningismus. He has no diarrhea but has recently purchased a pet turtle. What bacteria may be the culprit?**

Salmonella typhi, the causative agent of typhoid fever. The infection rate is remarkably high for HIV, asplenic, and sickle-cell disease patients. Rose spots occur in 10 to 20% of these cases. Relative bradycardia with a high fever and a low to normal WBC with a pronounced left shift are suggestive findings.

❍ **What is the treatment for the above patient?**

IV fluoroquinolone, ceftriaxone, or chloramphenicol. Check blood cultures for the presence of bacteremia. Avoid anti-motility agents.

❍ **Is peptic ulcer disease more common in males or in females?**

Males, (3:1).

❍ **What percentage of PUD patients are afflicted with duodenal ulcers? Gastric ulcers?**

75% and 25%, respectively.

❍ **Are patients with duodenal PUD usually younger or older?**

Younger. Duodenal PUD is more often associated with H. pylori. Older people tend to develop gastric ulcers as a result of NSAID use.

❍ **In what percentage of patients will a visible vessel in the base of an ulcer result in a re-bleed?**

50%. A clean ulcer base will re-bleed in only 1% of patients.

❍ **What are some indications for surgery in a bleeding ulcer?**

A visible vessel in the ulcer bed, more than 6 units of blood transfused in 24 hours, or more than 3 to 4 units transfused per day for three days.

❍ **Do gastric or duodenal ulcers heal faster?**

Duodenal.

❍ **Are "stress ulcers" a surgical problem?**

Typically not. The diffuse gastric bleeding that results from CNS tumors, head trauma, burns, sepsis, shock, steroids, aspirin, or alcohol is usually mucosal and can be life-threatening. However, this condition can usually be managed medically. Endoscopic diagnosis is key.

❍ **Are gastric and duodenal perforations associated with malignant ulcers or with benign ulcers?**

Benign ulcers.

❍ **What medical conditions are related to an increased incidence of PUD?**

COPD, cirrhosis, and chronic renal failure.

❍ **Where is the most common location of a perforated peptic ulcer?**

The anterior surface of the duodenum or pylorus and the lesser curvature of the stomach.

❍ **Is a person with massive upper GI bleeding likely to have a perforated ulcer?**

No.

❍ **After the fluid and blood resuscitation of a bleeding ulcer, what is the most useful diagnostic test?**

Endoscopy, which can also be therapeutic, with cryo- or electrocautery of an arterial bleeder.

❍ **What clinical finding essentially eliminates a gastric outlet obstruction in a patient with early satiety and ulcer symptoms?**

Bilious vomitus.

❍ **What are two endocrine problems that can cause peptic ulcer disease?**

Zollinger-Ellison syndrome and hyperparathyroidism (hypercalcemia).

❍ **A postprandial mid-abdominal pain indicates what ectopic syndrome?**

Peptic ulcer in a Meckel's diverticulum.

❍ **T/F: H_2-blockers decrease the risk of perforation and re-bleeding in peptic ulcer disease.**

False. However, cimetidine reduces the need for surgery, improves the rate of ulcer healing, and lowers the mortality rate from the initial bleeding episode.

❍ **Should you be concerned when administering cimetidine to a wheezing, anticoagulated patient with a seizure disorder?**

Sure. By decreasing blood flow to the liver and competing with the drug-eliminating cytochrome P-450 system, cimetidine can increase the levels of theophylline, warfarin, and phenytoin, not to mention diazepam, propranolol, and lidocaine.

❍ **A patient with "half a stomach", as a result of a bleeding ulcer, presents with weight loss, epigastric burning, and diarrhea. What are potential reasons?**

An obstructed afferent loop (Billroth II), bile reflux gastritis, dumping syndrome, malabsorption, remnant carcinoma. Anemia (from B_{12}, iron, and folate malabsorption) and osteoporosis (from vitamin D and calcium malabsorption) are also common.

❍ **T/F: Antibiotics are not required after an uncomplicated perirectal abscess is incised and drained.**

True, assuming the patient has no underlying immunoincompetence, such as HIV, diabetes, or malignancy. Primary aftercare includes Sitz baths beginning the next day.

❍ **Do pilonidal abscesses communicate with the anal canal?**

No. They are virtually always midline and overlie the lower sacrum. Posterior-opening, horseshoe-type anorectal fistulas can find their way to the lower sacrum but are rarely in the midline. Remember Goodsall's rule.

❍ **Should pilonidal cysts be excised in the office?**

Probably not. Incision and drainage are okay, followed by a bulky dressing, analgesics, and hot Sitz baths, which should be initiated the next day. Antibiotics are not typically necessary. Excision should be completed in the OR once the acute infection clears up.

❍ **A patient with new diarrhea and abdominal pain has been on antibiotics for sinusitis for two weeks. What might be revealed by sigmoidoscopy?**

Yellowish superficial plaques. This finding is indicative of pseudomembranous colitis. Stool studies will implicate the C. difficile toxin.

❍ **What is the treatment for pseudomembranous colitis?**

Oral vancomycin, 125 mg QID, or oral metronidazole, 500 mg QID. Either regimen should be administered for 7 to 10 days. Cholestyramine, which binds the toxin, can help relieve the diarrhea. Perform follow-up stool studies to confirm clearance of the toxin.

❍ **Procidentia in adults mandates what intervention?**

Proctosigmoidoscopy and surgical repair.

❍ **Is it better to have cancer of the anal margin or of the anal canal?**

Anal margin cancer. This cancer is usually low-grade and does not metastasize until the late stages. Anal canal cancer is more aggressive and metastasizes early.

❍ **What is the most common presenting symptom of rectal cancer?**

Persistent hematochezia. Other symptoms include tenesmus and the feeling of incomplete voiding after a bowel movement.

❍ **An ascitic patient has a with fever but no localizing signs or symptoms of infection. He also has a normal WBC. Because you know that spontaneous bacterial peritonitis (SBP) can be an occult disease, you perform an abdominal paracentesis. What WBC in the ascitic fluid suggests SBP?**

WBC > 250/mm^3. Also perform a Gram's stain on the fluid and obtain at least 10 cc of fluid in culture bottles. Test the fluid for aerobic and anaerobic organisms.

❍ **What organism is usually responsible for causing SBP.**

E. coli. Streptococcus pneumoniae is second.

❍ **What is the best therapy for SBP?**

Intravenous ampicillin. An aminoglycoside is a reasonable empiric therapy pending culture results.

❍ **What two therapies can reduce the risk of recurrence of SBP?**

Diuretics, which decrease ascitic fluid, and nonabsorbable oral antibiotics, which decrease the gut bacterial load thereby limiting bacterial translocation. Both treatments reduce the risk of recurrence in compliant patients.

❍ **A patient with chronic and occasionally bloody diarrhea develops severe diarrhea and abdominal pain with marked distention. What "can't miss" diagnosis is confirmed by these signs?**

Toxic megacolon. This condition is a life-threatening complication of ulcerative colitis.

❍ **What are the peak ages for the onset of ulcerative colitis?**

15 to 35 years, with a smaller incident rate in the seventh decade.

❍ **What percentage of ulcerative colitis cases have rectal involvement?**

95%. The inflammation extends proximally and continuously.

❍ **Watery diarrhea with profuse rectal discharge and weakness might suggest which type of "uncommon" tumor?**

Villous adenoma.

❍ **A double bubble on an x-ray or a 'bird's beak" and dilated colon on a barium enema are indicative of what?**

Volvulus.

❍ **A patient presents with tremor, ataxia, dementia, cirrhosis, and grey-green rings around the edge of his cornea. What is the diagnosis?**

Wilson's disease. Kaiser-Fleischer rings, i.e., golden brown or grey-green pigmentation around the cornea, CNS disturbances, chronic hepatitis, and cirrhosis are all caused by copper retention as a result of impaired copper excretion.

❍ **In Wilson's disease, what are the levels of copper in the urine and serum?**

Serum copper levels are low because there is a deficiency in ceruloplasmin, the copper-binding protein. However, urine copper is high. Treatment for this disease is penicillamine, which chelates copper.

❍ **What are the commonest causes of acute pancreatitis?**

Alcohol and gallstones.

❍ **What are some other causes of pancreatitis?**

Surgery, trauma, ERCP, viral and mycoplasma infections, hypertriglyceridemia, vasculitis, drugs, penetrating peptic ulcer, anatomic abnormalities about the ampulla of Vater, hyperparathyroidism, end stage renal disease and organ transplantation.

❍ **What are some of the drugs known to cause pancreatitis?**

Sulfonamides, estrogens, tetracyclines, pentamidine, azathioprine, thiazides, furosemide and valproic acid.

❍ **What are some of the infectious causes of pancreatitis?**

Mumps, viral hepatitis, Coxsackie virus group B, and mycoplasma.

❍ **What are the common symptoms of acute pancreatitis?**

Epigastric or diffuse abdominal pain radiating to the back, nausea and vomiting.

❍ **What are the common signs of acute pancreatitis?**

Fever, tachycardia, hypotension, distended abdomen, guarding with diminished or absent bowel sounds. Rarely seen signs include tender subcutaneous nodules from fat necrosis, and hypocalcemic tetany.

❍ **What is the mechanism of hypotension in severe cases of acute pancreatitis?**

Fluid sequestration in the intestine and retroperitoneum, systemic vascular effects of kinins, vomiting and bleeding.

❍ **What is Cullen's sign?**

Periumbilical ecchymosis.

❍ **Does acute pancreatitis commonly progress to chronic pancreatitis?**

No. Only rarely.

❍ **What are the pathological spectra in acute pancreatitis?**

Edematous pancreatitis (mild cases), and necrotizing pancreatitis (severe cases). Hemorrhagic pancreatitis may evolve from either of them.

❍ **T/F: Idiopathic acute pancreatitis may be the result of occult biliary microlithiasis or biliary sludge.**

True.

❍ **What is the commonest lipid profile that may result in pancreatitis?**

Type V lipid profile. Marked hypertriglyceridemia (usually levels > 1000 mg/dl).

❍ **How does this promote pancreatitis?**

Toxic action of fatty acids released by lipase in the pancreas.

❍ **What is the mechanism of necrosis and vascular damage in acute pancreatitis?**

Autodigestion of the pancreas by various proteolytic and lipolytic enzymes.

❍ **What are the laboratory abnormalities in pancreatitis?**

Leukocytosis, hemoconcentration followed by anemia, hyperglycemia, prerenal azotemia, hypoxemia, hyperamylasemia, LFT abnormalities.

❍ **Hyperamylasemia still remains central to the diagnosis of pancreatitis. Why?**

Widespread availability, low cost. Sensitivity 89% and specificity 86%.

❍ **T/F: Normal amylase levels rule out pancreatitis.**

False. Amylase peaks within a few hours of an attack and decline.

❍ **What are some other causes of hyperamylasemia besides pancreatitis?**

Pancreatic pseudocyst, pancreatic trauma, pancreatic carcinoma, ERCP, perforated duodenal ulcer, mesenteric infarction, renal failure, intestinal obstruction, salivary gland origin, ovarian disorders, prostate tumors, DKA, macroamylasemia.

❍ **Does the level of amylase elevation correlate with severity?**

No. Higher levels are seen in biliary pancreatitis.

❍ **What is the role of serum lipase determinations?**

Slightly less sensitive but much more specific. Also elevated in renal failure, non-pancreatic acute abdominal conditions. Lipase levels are elevated longer.

❍ **What are the findings on abdominal x-ray?**

Generalized ileus, sentinel loops and colon cutoff sign. Biliary and pancreatic calcifications may be seen.

❍ **What is the role of abdominal ultrasound in pancreatitis?**

Less sensitive than CT. Useful for detection of biliary obstruction and progression of pseudocysts.

❍ **What is the role of CT scanning?**

Useful in diagnosis, assess severity, detection of complications, a guide to aspiration and drainage of collections.

❍ **Is ERCP useful in pancreatitis?**

ERCP can establish ductal disruption in traumatic pancreatitis. It may also be useful in some early cases of acute biliary pancreatitis.

❍ **What are the criteria for severity in biliary pancreatitis on admission?**

Age > 70 years, WBC's > 18x109/l, glucose > 220 mg/dl, LDH > 400 U/l, and AST > 250 U/l.

❍ **What are the criteria for severity in biliary pancreatitis at 48 hours?**

Fall in hematocrit > 10, rise in BUN > 2 mg/dl, calcium < 8 mg/dl, base deficit > 5 mEq/l, fluid sequestration > 4 l.

❍ **What are the simplified Glasgow Prognostic criteria in pancreatitis?**

Age > 55 years, WBC's > 15x109/l, glucose > 180 mg/dl, LDH > 600 U/l, BUN > 45 mg/dl, calcium < 8 mg/dl, albumin < 32 gm/l, arterial PO2 < 60 mm Hg.

❍ **What is the preferred analgesic for pancreatitis?**

Meperidine is preferred over morphine.

❍ **How is the pancreas treated in acute pancreatitis?**

NPO until near complete resolution of pain and tenderness.

❍ **What are the septic complications of pancreatitis?**

Pancreatic abscess, infected pseudocyst, infected fluid collections.

❍ **When should they be suspected?**

Persistent fever, leukocytosis, pain, tenderness and overall clinical deterioration.

❍ **How can they be confirmed?**

CT scanning and CT guided percutaneous aspiration of collections.

❍ **When is surgery indicated in pancreatitis?**

Infected pancreatic necrosis or abscess that cannot be adequately drained and treated.

❍ **Should immediate surgery be performed in gallstone pancreatitis?**

No. It should be performed after the pancreatitis is subsided.

❍ **When should ERCP and endoscopic sphincterotomy be performed in patients with gallstone pancreatitis?**

In those with severe disease or those with mild disease that worsen with medical treatment.

❍ **What is the mortality in acute pancreatitis?**

1% for those with 2 or less factors by the Ranson's criteria, 16% for those with three or four factors, 40% for 5 or 6, 100% for 7 or 8 factors.

❍ **What pleuripulmonary abnormalities may be seen in pancreatitis?**

Elevated hemidiaphragm, atelectasis, pleural reaction or effusion, hypoxemia and acute lung injury including ARDS.

❍ **What is the nature of pleural fluid in pancreatitis?**

Exudate with high amylase levels.

❍ **Does pleuripulmonary complications indicate severe disease?**

Yes.

❍ **What is the mortality rate in those requiring mechanical ventilation?**

About 75%

❍ **What is the differential diagnosis of acute pancreatitis include?**

Cholecystitis, perforated viscous, penetrating ulcer, hepatitis, intestinal obstruction, mesenteric ischemia, vasculitis, myocardial infarction, pneumonia, renal colic, DKA and appendicitis.

❍ **What is a pancreatic pseudocyst?**

Collections of necrotic tissue, fluid and blood that develop near the pancreas over a period of 1-4 weeks without a true capsule.

❍ **When should surgical drainage be considered?**

Larger cysts (larger than 5 cm), those not resolving or decreasing after 6 weeks of onset.

❍ **What are the complications of pseudocyst?**

Infection, perforation, hemorrhage.

❍ **What are the clinical features of chronic pancreatitis?**

Abdominal pain, pancreatic calcifications, malabsorption, and diabetes mellitus.

❍ **What is the commonest cause?**

Chronic alcoholism

❍ **What does chronic pancreatitis result from?**

Progressive damage and permanent destruction of exocrine and endocrine functions.

❍ **What is the treatment of chronic pancreatitis?**

Supportive. Pain management, malabsorption management with enzyme supplements, nutritional support and management of diabetes.

❍ **T/F: Once cirrhosis develops as a result of hepatitis C virus (HCV) infection, the risk of hepatocellular carcinoma is approximately 1-4% per year.**

True. Severe progression of hepatitis C to cirrhosis occurs in approximately 20% of persons with chronic infection. HCV infection is largely responsible for the recent increase in the incidence of hepatocellular carcinoma in the United States.

❍ **Which extraintestinal manifestations of Crohn's disease does not improve with improvement in bowel pathology?**

Ankylosing spondylitis and sacroiliitis, which cause hip and back pain, may antedate bowel disease by several years and may persist after surgical or medical remission of the disease.

❍ **Which common manifestation of ulcerative colitis is an uncommon manifestation of Crohn's disease?**

Gastrointestinal bleeding.

❍ **A 38-year-old man with severe acute necrotizing pancreatitis, following several weeks of binge alcohol drinking, is in his second week of hospitalization in the intensive care unit. He continues to have intermittent spiking fevers and leukocytosis, despite appropriate antibiotic therapy. What is the best immediate next step in his treatment?**

CT-guided needle aspiration of pancreatic necrosis for Gram stain and culture The key question is whether this patient has infected or sterile pancreatic necrosis. Infected pancreatic necrosis requires surgical debridement for a successful clinical outcome. Surgery does not clearly benefit patients with sterile pancreatic necrosis, and these patients should continue their treatment in the intensive care unit.

❍ **During a routine blood evaluation, a 39-year-old asymptomatic woman was found to have an alkaline phosphatase level of 437 IU. The antimitochondrial antibody titer was 1:320. A liver ultrasound was performed, with normal findings. Results of a liver biopsy demonstrated ductopenia, lymphocytic aggregates, and cholestasis. The histological picture is compatible with primary biliary cirrhosis (PBC) stage II. What type of treatment is recommended at this point?**

Ursodeoxycholic acid (UDCA). UDCA has been found to improve the survival rate in patients without cirrhosis and is recommended as the first-line treatment at a dose of 12-15 mg/kg/d.

METABOLIC AND ENDOCRINE

We are here on earth to do good for others. What the others are here for, I don't know.
W.H. Auden

❍ **Which types of nodules are more likely to be malignant on a thyroid scan, hot or cold?**

Cold. This procedure should not be considered confirmatory. Cysts and benign adenomas can also read as cold. Some types of thyroid cancers will read as "warm" and thus be dismissed. Use caution when interpreting results.

❍ **What test should be performed to distinguish a benign cystic nodule from a malignant nodule?**

Fine needle aspiration biopsy and cytological evaluation.

❍ **What is a solitary thyroid nodule most likely to be?**

A nodular goiter (50%). Other possibilities to consider include cancer (20%), adenoma (20%), cyst (5%), or thyroiditis (5%).

❍ **What are some causes of factitious hyponatremia?**

Hyperglycemia, hyperlipidemia, and hyperproteinemia.

❍ **How does hyperglycemia lead to hyponatremia?**

Because glucose stays in the extracellular fluid, hyperglycemia draws water out of the cell into the extracellular fluid. Each 100 mg/dl increase in plasma glucose decreases the serum sodium by 1.6 to 1.8 mEq/L.

❍ **What are the signs and symptoms of hyponatremia?**

Weakness, nausea, anorexia, vomiting, confusion, lethargy, seizures, and coma.

❍ **What is central pontine myelinolysis (osmotic demyelination syndrome)?**

The complication of brain dehydration following the rapid correction of severe hyponatremia. Correct hyponatremia slowly, i.e., < 12 mEq/day for chronic hyponatremia.

❍ **What are the signs and symptoms of hypernatremia?**

Confusion, muscle irritability, seizures, respiratory paralysis, and coma.

❍ **What are the most common causes of hypotonic fluid loss leading to hypernatremia?**

Diarrhea, vomiting, hyperpyrexia, and excessive sweating.

❍ **What are the ECG findings of a patient with hypokalemia?**

Flattened T waves, depressed ST segments, prominent P and U waves, and prolonged QT and PR intervals.

❍ **What are the ECG findings of a patient with hyperkalemia?**

Peaked T waves, prolonged QT and PR intervals, diminished P waves, depressed T waves, QRS widening, and with levels near 10 mEq/L, a classic sine wave.

❍ **What is the quickest way to treat hyperkalemia?**

Calcium gluconate (10%), 10 to 20 ml IV (onset of action of 1 to 3 minutes).

❍ **What are the causes of hyperkalemia?**

Acidosis, tissue necrosis, hemolysis, blood transfusions, GI bleed, renal failure, Addison's disease, primary hypoaldosteronism, excess oral K^+ intake, RTA Type IV, and medication, such as succinylcholine, beta-blockers, captopril, spironolactone, triamterene, amiloride, and high-dose penicillin.

❍ **What are the causes of hypocalcemia?**

Shock, sepsis, multiple blood transfusions, hypoparathyroidism, vitamin D deficiency, pancreatitis, hypomagnesemia, alkalosis, fat embolism syndrome, phosphate overload, chronic renal failure, loop diuretics, hypoalbuminemia, tumor lysis syndrome, and medication, such as Dilantin, phenobarbital, heparin, theophylline, cimetidine, and gentamicin.

❍ **What is the most common cause of hyperkalemia?**

Lab error. Chronic renal failure is the most common cause of "true" hyperkalemia.

❍ **In order of prevalence, what are the three most common causes of hypercalcemia?**

Malignancy, primary hyperparathyroidism, and thiazide diuretics.

❍ **What are the signs and symptoms of hypercalcemia?**

The most common gastrointestinal symptoms are anorexia and constipation. Remember:

Stones:Renal calculi

Bones:Osteolysis

Abdominal groans:Peptic ulcer disease and pancreatitis

Psychic overtones:Psychiatric disorders

❍ **What is the initial treatment for hypercalcemia?**

Restoration of the extracellular fluid with 5 to 10 L of normal saline within 24 hours. After the patient is rehydrated, administer furosemide in doses of 1 to 3 mg/kg. Patients with hypercalcemia are dehydrated because high calcium levels interfere with ADH and the ability of the kidney to concentrate urine.

❍ **A patient with a history of alcohol abuse presents after a recent tonic-clonic seizure. What particular electrolyte abnormality should be considered and treated during evaluation?**

Hypomagnesemia. Treat the patient with $MgSO_4$, 2 g IV over 1 hour. Total deficit is often 5-10 grams.

❍ **What is the most common cause of hyperphosphatemia?**

Acute and chronic renal failure.

❍ **What are the two primary causes of primary adrenal insufficiency?**

Tuberculosis and autoimmune destruction. Together, they account for 90% of cases.

❍ **What are the signs and symptoms of primary adrenal insufficiency?**

Fatigue, weakness, weight loss, anorexia, hyperpigmentation, nausea, vomiting, abdominal pain, diarrhea, and orthostatic hypotension.

❍ **What characteristic lab findings are associated with primary adrenal insufficiency?**

Hyperkalemia, hyponatremia, hypoglycemia, azotemia (if volume depletion is present), and a mild metabolic acidosis.

❍ **How should acute adrenal insufficiency be treated?**

Administration of hydrocortisone, 100 mg IV, and crystalloid fluids containing dextrose.

❍ **What are the main causes of death during an adrenal crisis?**

Circulatory collapse and hyperkalemia-induced arrhythmias.

❍ **What are the causes of acute adrenal crisis?**

Major stress, such as surgery, severe injury, myocardial infarction, or any other acute illness in a patient with primary or secondary adrenal insufficiency.

❍ **What is thyrotoxicosis? What causes it?**

A hypermetabolic state occurring secondary to excess circulating thyroid hormone. Thyrotoxicosis is caused by thyroid hormone overdose, thyroid hyperfunction, or thyroid inflammation.

❍ **What are the hallmark clinical features of myxedema coma?**

Hypothermia (75%) and coma.

❍ **What is the most important initial step in treating DKA?**

Volume replacement, with the first liter administered over about 60 minutes.

❍ **What principle hormone protects the human body from hypoglycemia?**

Glucagon.

❍ **What drugs potentiate the hypoglycemic effects of sulfonylurea?**

Salicylates, alcohol, sulfonamides, phenylbutazone, and bis-hydroxycoumarin. Chlorpropamide is the sulfonylurea compound most likely to induce hypoglycemic events. It also causes the most prolonged hypoglycemia.

❍ **How is sulfonylurea-induced hypoglycemia treated?**

IV glucose alone may be insufficient. It may require diazoxide, 300 mg slow IV over 30 minutes, repeated every 4 hours.

❍ **What are the neurologic signs and symptoms associated with hypoglycemia?**

Hypoglycemia may produce mental and neurologic dysfunction. Neurologic manifestations can include paresthesias, cranial nerve palsies, transient hemiplegia, diplopia, decerebrate posturing, and clonus.

❍ **What lab findings are expected with diabetic ketoacidosis?**

Elevated beta-hydroxybutyrate, acetoacetate, acetone, and glucose. Ketonuria and glucosuria are present. Serum bicarbonate levels, pCO_2, and pH are decreased. Potassium levels may be elevated but will fall when the acidosis is corrected.

❍ **What is the basic treatment for DKA?**

Administer fluids. Start with normal saline (the total deficit may be 5 to 10 L), followed by potassium, 100 to 200 mEq in the first 12 to 24 hours. Prescribe insulin, 20 units bolus followed by 5 to 10 units/hour. (Editors' note: Many physicians no longer give bolus). Add glucose to the IV fluid when the glucose level falls below 250 mg/dl and give the patient a phosphate supplement when the levels drop below 1.0 mg/dl.

❍ **A 42 year-old female presents with a history of palpitations, sweating, diplopia, blurred vision, and weakness. The husband states she has been confused, most notably before breakfast. What is the probable diagnosis?**

Islet cell tumor of the pancreas, which can result in fasting hypoglycemia.

❍ **What are the key features of non-ketotic hyperosmolar coma?**

Hyperosmolality, hyperglycemia, and dehydration. Blood sugar levels should be > 800 mg/dl, serum osmolality should be > 350 mOsm/kg, and serum ketones should be negative.

❍ **What is the treatment for non-ketotic hyperosmolar coma?**

Normal saline and potassium, 10 to 20 mEq/hour, and insulin, 5 to 10 units/hour. Glucose should be added to the IV if the blood sugar level drops below 250 mg/dl.

❍ **Distinguish between lactic acidosis type A and B.**

Type A is associated with inadequate tissue perfusion, the resultant anoxia, and subsequent lactate and hydrogen ion accumulation. This condition usually occurs because of shock and is often seen in the ED. Type B includes all forms of acidosis in which there is no evidence of tissue anoxia.

❍ **What pathognomonic findings and confirmatory lab tests are diagnostic of thyroid storm?**

None. Diagnosis and thyroid storm is based on a clinical impression.

❍ **What is the most common precipitant of thyroid storm?**

Pulmonary infections.

❍ **What signs and symptoms are helpful for diagnosing thyroid storm?**

Eye signs of Graves' disease, a history of hyperthyroidism, widened pulse pressure, hypertension, a palpable goiter, tachycardia, fever, diaphoresis, increased CNS activity, emotional lability, heart failure, and coma.

❍ **What are some diagnostic findings of thyroid storm?**

Tachycardia, CNS dysfunction, cardiovascular dysfunction, GI system dysfunction, and a temperature > 37.8° C (100° F).

❍ **What are the complications of bicarbonate therapy in DKA?**

Paradoxical CSF acidosis, cardiac arrhythmias, decreased oxygen delivery to tissue, and fluid and sodium overload.

❍ **What is the overall mortality rate of non-ketotic hyperosmolar coma?**

Approximately 50%.

❍ **What is the most common cause of hypothyroidism?**

Primary thyroid failure (as opposed to secondary or pituitary etiology). The primary etiology of hypothyroidism in adults is the use of radioactive iodine or subtotal thyroidectomy in the treatment for Graves' disease. The second most common cause is autoimmune thyroid disorders.

❍ **What is the most common cause of secondary adrenal insufficiency and adrenal crisis?**

Iatrogenic adrenal suppression from prolonged steroid use. Rapid withdrawal of steroids may lead to collapse and death.

❍ **What pH decrease is expected with an increase of pCO_2 of 10 mm Hg?**

0.08.

❍ **What pH increase is expected with a decrease of pCO_2 of 10 mm Hg?**

0.13.

❍ **What pH increase is expected with a rise in HCO_3 of 5.0 mEq/L?**

0.08.

❍ **What decrease in pH is expected with a decrease in HCO_3 of 5.0 mEq/L?**

0.10.

❍ **How is the anion gap calculated from electrolyte values?**

Anion gap = $Na - Cl - CO_2$. The normal gap is 12 ± 4 mEq/L.

❍ **Acidosis is closely related to anion gap measurement. What are the causes of increased anion gap acidosis?**

A MUD PILE CAT

Alcohol	Methanol	Paraldehyde	Carbon monoxide
	Uremia	Iron and isoniazid	Aspirin
	DKA	Lactic acidosis	Toluene
		Ethylene glycol	

❍ **How can the magnitude of the anion gap be useful in narrowing the differential of an anion gap acidosis?**

An anion gap > 35 mEq/L is usually caused by ethylene glycol, methanol, or lactic acidosis. An anion gap 23 to 30 mEq/L may be due to an increase in organic acids, and an anion gap 16 to 22 mEq/L may be a result of advanced uremia.

❍ **How is the osmolar gap determined?**

Osmolality is a measure of the concentration of particles in a solution with units of osmoles per kg water. Osmolarity is a measure of osmoles per liter of solution. For dilute solutions, like body fluids, these two measures are roughly equivalent. An osmolar gap is the difference between the measured osmolality and the calculated osmolarity.

(Normally 275 to 285 mOsm/L.)

❍ **How much do different substances contribute to the osmolar gap?**

	mg/dl to increase serum osmol 1 mOsm/L	mOsm/L increase per mg/dl
Methanol	2.6	0.38
Ethanol	4.3	0.23
Ethylene glycol	5.0	0.20
Acetone	5.5	0.18
Isopropyl alcohol	5.9	0.17
Salicylate	14.0	0.07

Small amounts of methanol cause greater increases in osmolality. Large amounts of salicylate will eventually increase the osmolar gap. Note also that the contribution to an osmolar gap due to ethanol may be calculated; this can be useful when a mixed alcohol ingestion is suspected.

❍ **What else can narrow the differential of an anion gap acidosis?**

Methanol:Visual disturbances and headache are common; can produce wide gaps

Uremia:Must be advanced to contribute to gap

Diabetic ketoacidosis:Usually occurs with both hyperglycemia and glucosuria

Alcoholic ketoacidosis:Often has lower blood sugar and mild or absent glucosuria

Salicylates:High levels required to contribute to gap

Lactic acidosis:Can check serum level and has a broad differential

Ethylene glycol:Causes calcium oxalate or hippurate crystals in urine

❍ **What causes an oxygen saturation curve to shift to the right?**

A shift to the right delivers more O_2 to the tissue. Remember:

CADET! Right face!

Hyper	Carbia
	Acidemia
2,3	DPG
	Exercise
Increased	Temperature
	Release to tissues

❍ **When body waste materials, urine, and stool are internally recycled, they can cause a normal anion gap metabolic acidosis. What are the causes of normal anion gap metabolic acidosis?**

USED CRAP

Ureteroenterostomy
Small bowel fistula
Extra chloride (NH_4Cl or amino acid chlorides)
Diarrhea

Carbonic anhydrase inhibitors
Renal tubular acidosis
Adrenal insufficiency
Pancreatic fistula

❍ **What are the two primary causes of metabolic alkalosis?**

Loss of hydrogen and chloride from the stomach and overzealous diuresis with loss of hydrogen, potassium, and chloride.

❍ **What should one suspect in a patient with DKA, fever and necrotic eschar on the palate?**

Rhinocerebral mucor.

❍ **What are the key treatments used in DKA?**

Vigorous intravenous hydration and intravenous regular insulin.

❍ **What is the usual pathogen in a diabetic patient with septic arthritis?**

Staphylococcus aureus.

❍ **What are the key predisposing factors to hypoglycemia in diabetic patients on insulin?**

Exercise, poor oral intake, worsening renal function, medications are the key predisposing factors to consider.

❍ **What are the key therapies used to treat non ketotic hyperosmolar coma?**

Intravenous fluids. Usually, only small doses of insulin are required.

❍ **What is the major mechanism of hyponatremia in DKA patients?**

Dilution of sodium due to shifting of water out of the cells into the vascular space.

❍ **What will orthostatic drops in blood pressure in a diabetic patient will usually reflect?**

Autonomic dysfunction.

❍ **What major insults are likely to lead to DKA in an otherwise controlled diabetic?**

Always look for infection (even a minor one), cardiac ischemia, medications, lack of compliance with insulin and diet.

❍ **Which medications are likely to worsen glucose control in a diabetic patient?**

The list is long but includes thiazide diuretics, beta-blockers, steroids, estrogens, Dilantin, cyclosporin, diazoxide.

❍ **What is the most common time for hypoglycemia to occur in a diabetic patient?**

50% of all episodes occur at night or before breakfast.

❍ **What is the agent that may cause lactic acidosis in a diabetic patient?**

Metformin.

❍ **What are the key factors leading to hypernatremia in a patient with non-ketogenic hyperosmolar coma?**

Profound dehydration with greater losses of water than salt as well as impaired thirst.

❍ **Severe cellulitis with high fever, marked leukocytosis and rapid clinical demise should suggest what severe illness?**

Necrotizing fasciitis.

❍ **What are some complications of hypophosphatemia seen in treated DKA?**

Rhabdomyolysis, cardiac dysfunction, arrhythmias, hemolysis, poor neutrophil function.

❍ **What are the key factors predisposing to diabetic soft tissue infections?**

Microvascular disease, poor wound healing and trauma often masked by neuropathy.

❍ **What are usual glucose levels seen in patients with non-ketogenic coma?**

Glucose usually between 800-1000 mg/dl.

❍ **What are some agents used to treat severe diabetic gastroparesis?**

Cisapride and metochlorpromide are the key agents. Erythromycin has also been tried in very severe cases.

❍ **What are some life threatening abdominal infections in a diabetic?**

Emphysematous cholecystitis, ischemic bowel, diverticular abscess, emphysematous pyelonephritis or pyonephrosis.

❍ **Antibiotic regimen used to treat an elderly diabetic patient admitted to the hospital with a bilobar pneumonia?**

Regimen should include a third generation cephalosporin with erythromycin.

❍ **Diffuse abdominal pain with bloody stools and a high serum lactate in a diabetic might suggest what gastrointestinal disease?**

One should strongly consider ischemic or necrotic bowel.

❍ **What clues suggest osteomyelitis in a diabetic patient with a soft tissue infection?**

A draining sinus tract in a patient with persistent fever and anon healing ulcer. Radiographic studies will show devitalized bone and periostial elevation.

❍ **What medications are likely to lead to acute hyperkalemia in a diabetic patient?**

NSAID's, ACE inhibitors, beta-blockers, potassium sparing diuretics and salt substitutes (these are usually potassium salts).

❍ **Common causes of sudden visual loss in a diabetic patient might suggest what eye disorder?**

Vitreous hemorrhage or retinal detachment.

❍ **What key complication is seen in diabetic patient on CAPD?**

Peritonitis.

❍ **What are the major causes of sudden mortality in diabetic patients on dialysis?**

Usually due to vascular events including cardiac ischemia, CVA's, and ischemia leading to ventricular arrhythmias.

❍ **What are the common causes of abdominal pain, nausea and vomiting in a diabetic patient?**

Diabetic gastoparesis, gallbladder disease, pancreatitis, and perhaps, ischemia bowel.

❍ **Severe hyperkalemia in a diabetic patient are usually due to what causes?**

Usually a Type IV renal tubular acidosis with a lack of insulin.

❍ **What refeeding phenomenon is seen in DKA patients undergoing treatment?**

Shifting of potassium, magnesium and phosphorous into cells.

❍ **Atypical chest pain in elderly diabetic individual should always suggest what syndrome?**

Diabetic patients have high a high risk of cardiac ischemia and this must always be strongly considered even if the pain is somewhat atypical.

❍ **What is a necrotizing perineal infection in a diabetic male?**

Fournier's gangrene which can spread very rapidly with a high mortality.

❍ **What necrotizing ear infection is seen in patient with DKA?**

Malignant otitis externa.

❍ **What is the most desirable agent used to treat severe hyperglycemia in pregnancy?**

These patients must have tight control achieved by multiple injections of insulin.

❍ **What is not a usual adverse effect of Metformin if taken in an overdose in a diabetic?**

Metformin does not cause hypoglycemia.

❍ **What common factors predispose diabetics to severe foot infections?**

Poor foot care, micotrauma with poor wound healing and microvascular disease. Trauma may be prevalent as these patients often have sensory neuropathy.

❍ **What is the mortality rate in a patient with non ketogenic hyperosmolar coma?**

Mortality rate is very high, especially in the elderly. It may exceed 60-70%.

❍ **Increasing quantities of acetone seen during treatment of DKA are due to what phenomenon?**

The conversion of beta-hydroxybutyrate into acetone.

❍ **What do profound polyuria and dehydration in DKA reflect?**

Severe osmotic diuresis caused by glycosuria.

❍ **What are the usual causes of metabolic acidosis on patients with diabetes?**

In addition to ketoacidosis, diabetic patients are at risk for renal tubular acidosis as well as lactic acidosis.

❍ **What is the possible adverse effect seen during very rapid correction of severe hyperglycemia?**

Cerebral edema.

❍ **What are the major risks of cholecystitis in patients with diabetes?**

Precipitation of DKA, necrotizing or emphysematous cholecystitis and pancreatitis as a result of biliary disease.

❍ **What are the major adverse effects of intravenous radiocontrast given to diabetic patients?**

Acute tubular necrosis is well known. One should also watch for worsening of CHF, precipitation of angina pectoris and hemodynamic compromise.

❍ **Primary adrenal insufficiency refers to destruction of which component of the hypothalamic-pituitary-adrenal axis?**

Adrenal gland.

❍ **If autoimmune adrenal disease is the underlying disorder, which zone of the adrenal is spared?**

Medulla.

❍ **Secretion of which adrenal hormone is not impaired by secondary adrenal insufficiency?**

Aldosterone. Aldosterone secretion is more dependent upon angiotensin II than corticotropin, and aldosterone deficiency is not a problem in hypopituitarism. Selective aldosterone hypersecretion can manifest as a result of increased renin and angiotensin II formation.

❍ **What is the most common cause of chronic primary adrenal insufficiency (Addison's disease)?**

Autoimmune disease, although iatrogenic through the use of glucocorticoids could be considered as a common use.

❍ **What are the causes of acute abrupt primary adrenal insufficiency?**

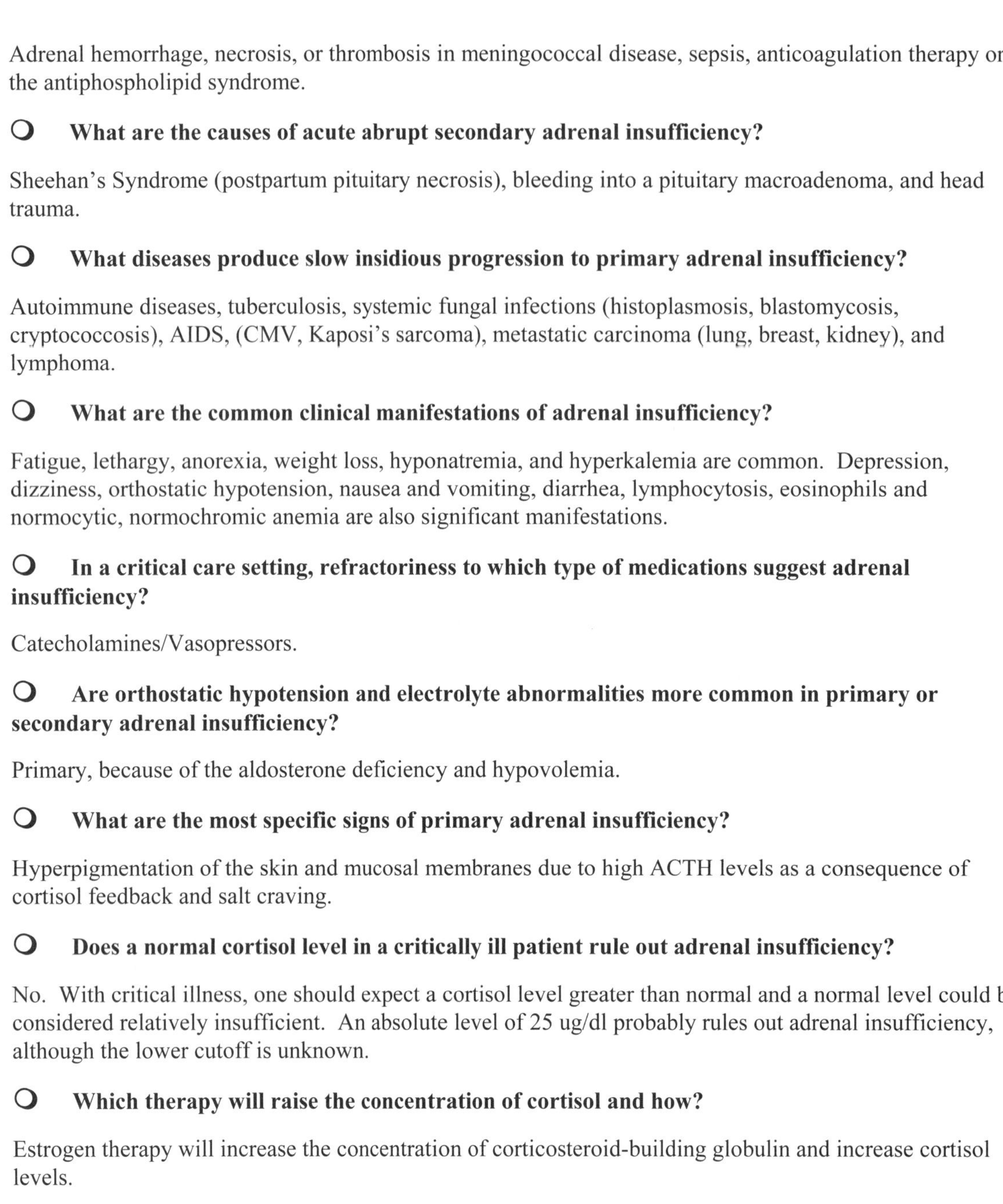

Adrenal hemorrhage, necrosis, or thrombosis in meningococcal disease, sepsis, anticoagulation therapy or the antiphospholipid syndrome.

❍ **What are the causes of acute abrupt secondary adrenal insufficiency?**

Sheehan's Syndrome (postpartum pituitary necrosis), bleeding into a pituitary macroadenoma, and head trauma.

❍ **What diseases produce slow insidious progression to primary adrenal insufficiency?**

Autoimmune diseases, tuberculosis, systemic fungal infections (histoplasmosis, blastomycosis, cryptococcosis), AIDS, (CMV, Kaposi's sarcoma), metastatic carcinoma (lung, breast, kidney), and lymphoma.

❍ **What are the common clinical manifestations of adrenal insufficiency?**

Fatigue, lethargy, anorexia, weight loss, hyponatremia, and hyperkalemia are common. Depression, dizziness, orthostatic hypotension, nausea and vomiting, diarrhea, lymphocytosis, eosinophils and normocytic, normochromic anemia are also significant manifestations.

❍ **In a critical care setting, refractoriness to which type of medications suggest adrenal insufficiency?**

Catecholamines/Vasopressors.

❍ **Are orthostatic hypotension and electrolyte abnormalities more common in primary or secondary adrenal insufficiency?**

Primary, because of the aldosterone deficiency and hypovolemia.

❍ **What are the most specific signs of primary adrenal insufficiency?**

Hyperpigmentation of the skin and mucosal membranes due to high ACTH levels as a consequence of cortisol feedback and salt craving.

❍ **Does a normal cortisol level in a critically ill patient rule out adrenal insufficiency?**

No. With critical illness, one should expect a cortisol level greater than normal and a normal level could be considered relatively insufficient. An absolute level of 25 ug/dl probably rules out adrenal insufficiency, although the lower cutoff is unknown.

❍ **Which therapy will raise the concentration of cortisol and how?**

Estrogen therapy will increase the concentration of corticosteroid-building globulin and increase cortisol levels.

❍ **How is a corticotropin (ACTH) stimulation test performed to rule out adrenal insufficiency?**

After a baseline cortisol level is obtained (time0), 250 ug of Cosyntropin is given IV (or IM), and cortisol levels are obtained at 30 and 60 minutes post-injection. Adrenal function is thought to be normal if the cortisol level drawn at the time 30 minutes or 60 minutes is $\geq$ 20 ug/dl.

❍ **How can the ACTH stimulation test be normal in secondary adrenal insufficiency of recent origin?**

The results of an ACTH stimulation test can show a normal cortisol production response as the gland has not yet atrophied and retains the ability to be stimulated. The 250 ug dose of ACTH is also far in excess of the 5 or 10 ug that maximally stimulates a normal adrenal cortex. A low dose of 1 ug ACTH stimulation test may allow for assessment of mild insufficiency.

❍ **What are the three tests used to evaluate secondary adrenal insufficiency?**

Insulin induced hypoglycemia, short-term Metyrapone tests, and the corticotropin releasing hormone test.

❍ **What is the basis of the insulin induced hypoglycemia test for secondary adrenal insufficiency?**

Hypoglycemia induced by 0.1 unit insulin/kg stimulates the entire HPA, sympathetic nervous system and plasma cortisol levels should exceed 20 ug/dl. This test is contraindicated in patients with cardiac disease and a history of seizures, as well as unnecessarily in patients with low basal cortisol levels.

❍ **What is the short-term Metyrapone test?**

Metyrapone (30mg/kg given with snack at midnight) inhibits adrenal 11-hydroxylase. Normally, the cortisol precursor 11-deoxycortisol increases to at least 7 ug/dl. This is in response to the decreased production of cortisol and loss of negative feedback of cortisol to the HPA axis; hence stimulation of corticotropin (ACTH). This is indicative of secondary adrenal insufficiency only in the setting of a previously measured cortisol level of $\leq$ 8 ug/dl.

❍ **After an endocrinologic diagnosis has been established by hormonal studies, the radiologic study of choice to assess for pituitary or hypothalamic tumor would be?**

MRI with analysis of the sagittal and coronal sections. A CT scan can be helpful if bony invasion is suspected.

❍ **Are imaging studies of the adrenal glands necessary in primary adrenal insufficiency?**

Yes. In cases other than autoimmune or adrenal myeloneuropathy, a CT scan of the adrenal should be performed to aid in the differential diagnosis. Enlarged glands with/without calcifications in patients with TB are a sign of active disease and warrant anti-infective therapy. Enlargement also occurs in other fungal infections, lymphoma, cancer and AIDS. A biopsy by CT guidance may also be helpful.

❍ **What is the emergent steroid replacement in adrenal insufficiency?**

Hydrocortisone 50-100 mg IV every eight hours initially.

❍ **What is the daily replacement of hydrocortisone once the patient is stabilized?**

Hydrocortisone 15 mg in the a.m. and 10 mg in the p.m. The dose should be the smallest possible to alleviate clinical symptoms yet prevent weight gain and osteoporosis. Measurements of urinary cortisol may help determine the appropriate dosing.

❍ **Which patients should receive fludrocortisone?**

Patients with primary adrenal insufficiency should receive 50-200 ug/day of fludrocortisone as a substitute for aldosterone, guided by measurements of blood pressure, potassium and plasma renin activity.

❍ **What added precautions should be taken by all patients with adrenal insufficiency?**

They should wear a medic alert bracelet, carry a card detailing their medications and the recommendations for treatment in emergencies, and to double or triple their dose of hydrocortisone when they sustain injury or illness. They should secure ampules of glucocorticoids for self injection or suppositories when vomiting or unable to take oral steroids.

❍ **What accounts for the almost immediate effect of cortisol on blood pressure in patients with adrenal insufficiency?**

Cortisol exerts a permissive effect on catecholamine vascular responsitivity and a vital role in the maintenance of vascular tone, vascular permeability and distribution of body water within the vascular compartment.

❍ **What is the characteristic hemodynamic pattern of adrenal insufficiency?**

Predominantly, decreased systemic vascular resistance to a lesser degree, decreased cardiac contractility depending upon the volume status.

❍ **How long after routine surgery do the serum corticotropin and cortisol concentrations return to normal?**

24-28 hours.

❍ **What is the amount of increased cortisol production that accompanies surgery?**

It depends upon the surgery; 85% above baseline for up to two days post laparotomy and 35% above baseline for more minor procedures involving joints, breasts or neck.

❍ **What is the relationship between the serum cortisol level and the illness severity score?**

The higher the score, the higher the level and the higher the mortality.

❍ **What drugs can impair cortisol synthesis in the critically ill patient?**

Ketoconazole, etomidate, and aminoglutethimide.

❍ **Which drugs can increase the metabolism of cortisol?**

Phenytoin, phenobarbital. and Rifampin.

❍ **The use of which sedating agent has been shown to increase mortality in critically ill patients by inducing primary adrenal insufficiency?**

Etomidate. This sedating agent is a selective inhibitor of adrenal 11-hydroxylase, the enzyme that converts deoxycortisol to cortisol. Mortality reportedly increased in a trauma unit that began using etomidate by continuous infusion for sedation and for this reason, etomidate is not used for continuous sedation in the critically ill.

❍ **Is there any evidence to support the use of corticosteroids in septic shock?**

No beneficial effects of corticosteroids have been shown in sepsis or septic shock. In fact, they may be harmful, according to several studies.

❍ **Randomized propspective trials have shown benefit from corticosteroids in which disease states?**

Bacterial meningitis, acute spinal injury, typhoid fever, Pneumocystis carinii pneumonia, and possibly treatment of the fibroproliferative phase of acute respiratory distress syndrome.

❍ **What symptoms should increase the suspicion of adrenal insufficiency in the critically ill?**

Unexplained circulatory instability, high fever without cause, unresponsive to antibiotics, hypoglycemia, hyponatremia, hyperkalemia, neutropenia, eosinophilia, unexplained mental status changes, disparate anticipated severity of disease and the actual state of the patient.

❍ **What is the best correlation between the degree/duration of hypothalamic-pituitary-adrenal suppression in patients previously on exogenous steroid therapy?**

Previously, it was thought that the highest dose, the duration and total cumulative dose were important predictors of HPA suppression, but recent data suggests that high dose and prolonged treatment do not necessarily correlate with the degree and duration of HPA suppression.

❍ **Which study is probably the best predictor of adrenal adequacy in patients previously receiving steroids who are scheduled for surgery?**

Although the insulin induced hypoglycemia test and Metyrapone tests can be useful, the best indicator of maximal serum cortisol concentration during surgery was the peak cortisol level after administration of corticotropin.

❍ **What is the daily normal production of cortisol?**

Previously thought to be 12-15 mg/m2, but current estimates are 5 mg/m2. This correlates to about 10-12 mg of oral hydrocortisone replacement per m2 because of decreased bioavailability secondary to first pass hepatic metabolism.

❍ **How much cortisol is produced per 24 hours in patients undergoing minor and major surgery?**

50 mg and 75-100 mg respectively; production rates seldom exceed 200-300 mg/day hence the recent recommendations to decrease the stress from the traditional 300 mg/day.

❍ **What are the adverse effects of using excessive dosing when covering for stress?**

Catabolic effects on muscle, impaired wound healing, antagonizing insulin and the effects on glucose metabolism and the anti-inflammatory effect on active infection.

❍ **What are the current dosing recommendations for stress doses in patients with suspected adrenal insufficiency?**

Minor stress25 mg/day

Moderate stress50-75 mg/day

Major stress100-150 mg/day

❍ **Are stress dose steroids necessary in patients receiving topical or intranasal steroids?**

HPA axis suppression is rare in these patients and withholding additional corticosteroids during minor or moderate surgical procedures is reasonable as long as the clinical course is unremarkable.

❍ **How is the etiology of type-1 DM different from type-II DM?**

Type-I DM is associated with Human Leukocyte Antigens (HLA), autoimmunity, and or islet cell antibodies. Type-II DM usually involves a genetic mutation resulting in inactive pancreatic and liver enzymes as well as insulin receptor defects.

❍ **What etiologies are responsible for secondary DM?**

Exocrine pancreatic diseases like cystic fibrosis, pancreatic cancer and Cushing's disease.

❍ **What condition should be suspected in a patient with a serum glucose of 942 mg/dl, mild ketonuria, depressed sensorium and positive Babinski sign?**

Non-ketotic hyperosmolar coma (NKHC).

❍ **What is the appropriate mixture of regular and intermediate-acting insulin in a daily insulin injection regimen?**

2/3 of the total dose should be intermediate acting with 1/3 being regular insulin. The single injection should be given 30 minutes prior to breakfast.

❍ **What is the appropriate mixture or regular and intermediate acting insulin in a twice daily insulin injection regimen?**

2/3 of the dose should be given 30 minutes prior to breakfast; the remaining 1/3 given 30 minutes prior to dinner. Both injections should be 2/3 intermediate acting and 1/3 short acting insulin.

❍ **What is the significance of the Hgb-A1C?**

It represents the fraction of hemoglobin that has been non-enzymatically glycosylated. It provides an accurate estimation of the relative BGL over the preceding 6-8 weeks.

❍ **What is the Somogyi phenomenon?**

A hyperglycemic event that results from an over zealous response by counter regulatory hormones during a period of hypoglycemia.

❍ **What happens to a patient with hyperthyroidism when exogenous TRH is administered?**

The TRH receptors are blocked thus preventing a rise in TSH levels. In a patient with a normal thyroid a concomitant rise in TSH would occur.

❍ **What are the causes for elevated TBG levels?**

Pregnancy, newborn state, estrogens, and heroin.

❍ **What is the most common cause of a acquired hypothyroidism?**

Lymphocytic thyroiditis.

❍ **What are the clinical manifestations of acquired hypothyroidism?**

Myxedema of the skin, cold intolerance, constipation, low pitched voice, menorrhagia, mental and physical slowing, dry skin, coarse brittle hair, and decreased energy level with increased need for sleep.

❍ **What is the most common clinical manifestation of Lymphocytic thyroiditis?**

The appearance of a goiter.

❍ **Patients with lymphocytic thyroiditis are usually hypothyroid, euthyroid, or hyperthyroid?**

The majority will be euthyroid. However , many will eventually become hypothyroid, while only a few will manifest the symptoms of hyperthyroidism.

❍ **What is Schmidt's syndrome?**

A type II polyglandular autoimmune disease involving Addison's disease and IDDM, with or without lymphocytic thyroiditis.

❍ **What is deQuervain's disease?**

A subacute, nonsupparative thyroiditis. Clinical manifestations involve a tender thyroid, fever and chills usually remitting within several months.

❍ **What is the etiology of DeQuervain's thyroiditis?**

Most likely due to a viral infection such as mumps or Coxsackie virus.

❍ **Which medications are commonly found to result in sporadic goiters?**

Lithium, amiodarone and iodide containing asthma inhalers.

❍ **What is a thyrotropin receptor-stimulating antibody?**

An antibody commonly found in Grave's disease, which binds to the TSH receptor leading to thyroid stimulation and goiter production.

❍ **Which HLA is associated with Grave's disease?**

HLA-DR3. The association of this HLA type represents a seven fold relative risk for Grave's disease.

❍ **Is Grave's disease more common in boys or girls?**

Girls are affected five times more than boys.

❍ **What are the classical signs and symptoms of Grave's disease?**

Emotional liability, autonomic hyperactivity, exophthalmos, tremor, increased appetite with no weight gain or weight loss, diarrhea, and a goiter in nearly all affected individuals.

❍ **How is Grave's disease confirmed by laboratory testing?**

Increased bound and free T3 and T4 with decreased TSH. Frequently, the presence of thyroid peroxidase and TSH receptor stimulating antibodies are present.

❍ **What treatment options exist for patients with Grave's disease? What treatment is recommended?**

Patients can be managed medically with propylthiouracil (PTU) or methimazole, surgically with a subtotal thyroidectomy or with radioiodine therapy. Medical management is the treatment of choice.

❍ **What are the differences between PTU and methimazole?**

Methimazole is ten times more potent on a weight basis, allowing it to be a once a day medication. PTU is predominately protein bound making it a better choice in pregnant and nursing mothers as its ability to cross the placental membrane is limited.

❍ **What are the respective doses of PTU and methimazole?**

PTU is given at 5 - 10 mg/kg/d given T.I.D. Methimizole is .5 - 1.0 mg/kg/d given either Q.D. or B.I.D.

❍ **How much time must pass before noticing a clinical response when using medical treatment for Grave's disease?**

2 - 3 weeks.

❍ **What medication is available to treat the autonomic hyperactivity associated with Grave's disease?**

Propranolol, a beta-blocker dosed at .5 - 2.0 mg/kg/d given T.I.D.

❍ **What are the three largest concerns with surgical management of Grave's disease?**

Hyper or hypothyroidism depending on the amount of tissue removed, vocal cord paralysis and hypoparathyroidism.

❍ **If fine needle aspiration of a thyroid nodule reveals parafollicular cells, what type of carcinoma should be suspected?**

Medullary carcinoma of the thyroid.

❍ **What combination of disorders account for multiple endocrine neoplasia type-IIA?**

Medullary carcinoma of the thyroid, adrenal medullary hyperplasia or pheochromocytoma, and parathyroid hyperplasia.

❍ **What is the mode of inheritance of MEN Type-IIA?**

Autosomal dominant.

❍ **How is MEN Type-IIA different from MEN Type-IIB?**

Men Type-IIB is associated with multiple neuromas. It, too, is autosomal dominant.

❍ **What are the hallmarks of polyglandular autoimmune disease type-I?**

Autoimmune hypoparathyroidism, Addison's disease, and chronic mucocutaneous candidiasis.

❍ **What are the symptoms of a thyroid storm?**

Tachycardia, systolic hypertension, tremulousness, delirium and hyperthermia.

❍ **How do you manage acute thyrotoxicosis?**

Propranolol at 10 mg/kg IV over 10-15 minutes for hypertension and increased metabolic rate. Lugol's iodide, 5 drops PO every eight hours or sodium iodide 125-250 mg/dl IV over 24 hours will stop thyroxine production.

❍ **What measures can be taken to further reduce peripheral conversion of T4 to T3?**

Oral dexamethasone at .2 mg/kg or oral hydrocortisone 5 mg/kg.

❍ **What is the differential diagnosis of acute primary adrenal insufficiency?**

Congenital adrenal hypoplasia, autoimmunity, TB, infection, trauma, and adrenal hemorrhage.

❍ **What are the clinical manifestations of adrenocortical insufficiency?**

Low blood pressure, muscular weakness, weight loss, anorexia and salt craving.

❍ **What emergency should be suspected in patients who present with cyanosis, cold skin, thready pulse, hypotension and tachypnea?**

Addison's crisis.

❍ **What conditions have been implicated in precipitating adrenal crisis?**

Infection, trauma, fatigue, and various medications.

❍ **How is adrenal insufficiency diagnosed?**

Plasma levels of cortisol are measured before and after administration of ACTH.

❍ **What is the Waterhouse-Fredrickson Syndrome?**

Primary adrenal insufficiency due to adrenal hemorrhage. It is often secondary to meningococcemia-induced shock.

❍ **What are the causes of secondary adrenal insufficiency?**

Diminished ACTH levels secondary to long term glucocorticoid treatment.

❍ **Does the clinical presentation of adrenal insufficiency differ between primary and secondary causes?**

Yes. Primary causes involve the adrenals directly, while secondary causes involve the hypothalamic-pituitary axis. Also, primary insufficiency involves both glucocorticoids and mineral corticoids, while secondary insufficiency will only involve glucocorticoids.

❍ **Is hyperpigmentation a common finding with acute adrenal insufficiency?**

No. It is usually seen with chronic primary adrenal insufficiency.

❍ **How do you manage a patient in acute adrenal insufficiency?**

Therapy includes fluid replacement and exogenous glucocorticoids.

❍ **Name four conditions that can be attributed to hyperadrenocortical stimulation.**

Cushing's syndrome, hyperaldosteronism, adrenogenital syndrome, and feminization.

❍ **What is the most common cause of primary adrenal insufficiency?**

Autoimmune destruction of the adrenal glands.

❍ **What is a pheochromocytoma?**

An uncommon tumor derived from neural crest cells found in the adrenal medulla.

❍ **What two autosomal dominant diseases have a high prevalence of pheochromocytomas?**

Neurofibromatosis and Von Hippel-Lindau disease.

❍ **What laboratory tests will help to make the diagnosis of pheochromocytoma?**

Look for increased total 24 hour urinary catecholamines and their metabolites (i.e., epinephrine, norepinephrine, metanephrine and VMA).

❍ **What are the classic signs and symptoms of pheochromocytomas?**

Paroxysmal hypertension, autonomic hyperactivity, headache, visual changes and weight loss.

❍ **Which class of antihypertensive drugs are recommended for the temporary treatment of pheochromocytoma associated hypertension?**

Alpha-adrenergic blocking agents like phenoxybenzamine and prazosin.

❍ **How do you manage a hypertensive crisis in a patient with a pheochromocytoma?**

1 mg of IV phentolamine or .5-.8mg/kg/min of sodium nitroprusside.

❍ **What is central diabetes insipidus?**

A lack of ADH secretion which results in an inability to concentrate the urine despite functioning kidneys.

❍ **What specific disease process should be considered in a child who presents with dehydration, hypernatremia, decreased urine osmolarity and a high level of circulating ADH?**

Nephrogenic diabetes insipidus.

❍ **How is the diagnosis of diabetes insipidus made?**

A presumptive diagnosis can be made by finding hypernatremia, increased serum osmolarity and decreased urine osmolarity.

❍ **What is the danger of rigorously hydrating a patient who has hypernatremia due to diabetes insipidus?**

Cerebral edema, seizures and death.

❍ **A serum sodium of _____ mEq/L without obvious signs of pathology still requires admission?**

160 mEq/L.

❍ **What additional adjuncts can be used in addition to volume replacement in a patient with diabetes insipidus?**

Intranasal administration of DDAVP at 0.4 mg/kg.

❍ **What should the physician do if the patient fails to respond to the initial dose of DDAVP?**

The patient should be given a second dose from a different bottle. DDAVP may fail due to inappropriate administration or outdated preparations that have lost their potency.

❍ **What should the physician consider if the patient with diabetes insipidus continues to diurese despite repeated doses of DDAVP?**

The patient most probably has nephrogenic diabetes insipidus, due to unresponsive kidney receptors for ADH, whether the ADH is endogenous or exogenous.

❍ **If nephrogenic diabetes insipidus is assumed, what further pharmacological treatment may be helpful?**

Thiazide diuretics have a paradoxical effect and may work in decreasing fluid losses.

❍ **How frequently should the physician monitor the serum sodium and urine osmolarity when correcting a hypernatremic state in a patient with diabetes insipidus?**

At least every four hours.

❍ **What is acromegaly?**

A condition resulting from overproduction of growth hormone individuals with closed epiphyses.

❍ **What are the clinical manifestations of acromegaly?**

Coarse facial features, enlarged tongue, enlargement of the distal extremities and hypogonadism.

❍ **What medical modality can be used to suppress exogenous growth hormone production?**

Octreotide, an analogue of somatostatin.

❍ **What pituitary tumor is the most common?**

Prolactinomas.

❍ **What are the common presenting signs of a prolactinoma?**

Headache, amenorrhea and galactorrhea.

❍ **What two options exist for the treatment of prolactinomas?**

Bromocriptine and surgery via a transphenoidal approach.

❍ **What is Cushing's disease?**

Pituitary adenomas leading to increased ACTH secretion with resultant bilateral adrenal hyperplasia and elevated cortisol levels.

❍ **Is Cushing's disease different than Cushing's syndrome?**

Cushing's disease results from pituitary adenomas, while Cushing's syndrome is elevated cortisol levels from various causes, including paraneoplastic syndromes, primary adrenal tumors, and exogenous use of cortisol.

❍ **What clinical manifestations are common to all patients with Cushing's syndrome?**

Moon faces, buffalo hump, obesity, hypertrichosis, hypertension, growth retardation, easy bruising, purple striae on the hips and abdomen, and amenorrhea in girls.

❍ **How is Cushing's syndrome diagnosed?**

Using the dexamethasone suppression test. Patients with ACTH dependent Cushing's demonstrate suppression with the larger doses of dexamethasone while those with ectopic tumors cannot be suppressed at any level.

❍ **What is Conn's syndrome?**

Primary, hyperproduction of adrenal mineralcorticoids usually resulting from an aldosteronoma.

❍ **What are the clinical manifestations of primary aldosteronism?**

Hyperplasia of the zona glomerulosa leading to hypertension, sodium and water retention, hypokalemia and decreased serum renin levels.

❍ **What is hypergonadotropic hypogonadism in males?**

Primary hypogonadism resulting from a defect in androgen production often leading to pseudohermaphrodism.

❍ **What are the clinical manifestations of primary hypogonadism?**

Failure of development of the secondary sexual characteristics with abnormally small penis and testes.

❍ **What is hypogonadotropic hypogonadism?**

A delayed onset of puberty, due to decreased levels of FSH and LH, with functioning ovaries or testes.

❍ **How is the diagnosis of primary hypogonadism made?**

The levels of FSH and LH are abnormally elevated for the corresponding age. Testosterone levels remain low and show little response to the administration of hCG.

❍ **What is the deficient hormone in secondary hypogonadism?**

FSH or LH. The defect is in the pituitary rather than in the testes or ovaries.

❍ **What is Kallmann's syndrome?**

Hypogonadotropic hypogonadism with anosmia.

❍ **Is the pituitary gland responsible for parathyroid regulation?**

No. Unlike the thyroid gland, the parathyroids are not regulated by the pituitary gland, but rather, by circulating calcium levels.

❍ **What is the difference between primary and secondary hyperparathyroidism?**

In primary hyperparathyroidism, the defect is in the parathyroid gland, (i.e., an adenoma or hyperplasia), while in secondary hyperparathyroidism, the elevated PTH is a physiologic response to a low calcium level, usually a result of renal disease.

❍ **What are the diagnostic laboratory findings seen in hyperparathyroidism?**

Elevated serum calcium and PTH with concomitant decreased phosphorous levels.

❍ **What is Von Recklinghausen's disease?**

Hyperparathyroidism, leading to cystic changes in bone, due to osteoclastic resorption with fibrous replacement, forming non-neoplastic "brown tumors".

❍ **What is Pseudohypoparathyroidism?**

An autosomal recessive disorder characterized by kidney unresponsiveness to PTH, shortened fourth and fifth metacarpals and metatarsals, and short stature, all occurring without evidence of parathyroid dysfunction.

❍ **What other mineral must be considered in the patient who appears hypocalcemic?**

Magnesium. Giving calcium will not correct the problem; however the administration of magnesium will correct both the calcium level and the magnesium level.

❍ **What renal manifestation may occur in patients with hyperparathyroidism?**

Nephrocalcinosis due to the high calcium load delivered to the kidneys.

❍ **What are the clinical manifestations of polycystic ovarian disease (PCO)?**

Obesity, hirsuitism, secondary amenorrhea and bilaterally enlarged polycystic ovaries.

❍ **How are patients with PCO treated?**

Contraceptive pills for menstrual regulation and ovarian suppression.

❍ **What laboratory findings are seen in PCO?**

Most patients have increased ratio of LH to FSH and an increased amount of LH due to an exaggerated response to GnRH.

❍ **What is Klinefelter's syndrome?**

Males with 47, XXY. These individuals usually display mental retardation, small testes, long body habitus, gynecomastia and infertility.

❍ **What is Turner's syndrome?**

A chromosomal defect 45, XO. This manifests in girls as short stature, cubitus valgus, webbed neck, streaked ovary, widely spaced nipples and pigmented nevi.

❍ **What are the sodium concentrations of the most common commercially available IV fluids?**

0.9 normal saline = 154 mEq/l
0.45 normal saline = 77 mEq/l
0.3 normal saline = 54 mEq/l
0.2 normal saline = 33 mEq/l

❍ **What disorder has autosomal dominant inheritance and is associated with episodic weakness or paralysis along with transient alterations in serum potassium?**

Periodic paralysis, most commonly associated with episodes of hypokalemia, but may occur with hyperkalemia as well. Patients are normal between attacks . The condition becomes progressively worse in adulthood.

❍ **What is the definition of malnutrition?**

A nutritional deficit associated with increase risk of adverse clinical events, and decreased risk of such events when corrected.

❍ **What is the primary goal of nutritional support in critically ill patients?**

To provide usable substrates to meet energy needs, conserve lean body mass, and restore physiologic homeostasis.

❍ **What proportion of critically ill and injured patients are catabolic or hypermetabolic?**

Nearly all.

❍ **Are immunocompetence and vital organ function dependent upon nutritional support?**

Absolutely. Both are secondary goals of nutritional support.

❍ **What is the predominant energy source used during starvation by a healthy subject?**

Lipids.

❍ **How long does the body's reserve of carbohydrates last during starvation?**

Glycogen stores are consumed within 24 hours.

❍ **Does the metabolic rate increase or decrease during starvation in a healthy subject?**

Decrease.

❍ **Are adaptation mechanisms seen with starvation similar to those seen in critically ill patients?**

No. There is impaired protein conservation and a persistent hypermetabolic response in the critically ill patient.

❍ **With the onset of critical illness, what factors are thought to raise resting energy expenditure and protein turnover?**

Catecholamines and cortisol.

❍ **How does the insulin resistance associated with critical illness affect substrate use?**

Insulin resistance decreases the peripheral use of glucose and increases proteolysis.

❍ **Is there any rationale for overfeeding or underfeeding critically ill patients?**

No. Both have been shown to be detrimental. The goal is to meet the metabolic needs of the patient.

❍ **What is the utility of anthropometric (e.g., weight change), biochemical (e.g., serum albumin level), or immunologic (e.g., absolute lymphocyte count) indices as a measures of nutritional status in the critical care setting?**

Low. Too many other factors such as fluid retention, changes in protein synthesis priorities, and underlying infections make these indices less reliable than in otherwise healthy patients.

❍ **What are the serum half-lives of albumin and prealbumin?**

18 days and 2 to 3 days, respectfully.

❍ **What two methods are frequently used to assess nutritional status in critically ill patients?**

Indirect calorimetry and nitrogen balance.

❍ **As a patient's FIO_2 requirements increases, is indirect calorimetry more or less accurate in measuring energy expenditure?**

Less.

❍ **What other factors are sources of errors with indirect calorimetry?**

Air leak from endotracheal tubes and the need for extrapolation of measurements to 24 hours.

❍ **What is the equation for nitrogen balance?**

Nitrogen Balance = Nitrogen intake - (Nitrogen loss)

= (Protein (g) / 6.25) - ((Urine Urea Nitrogen / 0.8) + 3)

❍ **How much protein is required for balance in a healthy stable adult?**

Approximately 0.6 g/kg ideal body weight/day.

❍ **What is the recommended starting point for protein needs in hypermetabolic critically ill patients?**

Approximately 1.5 to 2.5 g/kg ideal body weight/day.

❍ **What is the goal of protein delivery?**

To achieve a positive nitrogen balance.

❍ **What is the optimal calorie-to-nitrogen ratio for critically ill patients?**

100 : 1 to 200 : 1.

❍ **What is the recommended starting point for non-protein calories needs for hypermetabolic critically ill patients?**

25 kcal/kg ideal body weight/day.

❍ **What is the most common manifestation of excessive carbohydrate administration?**

Hyperglycemia.

❍ **Can lipid emulsions be useful in patients needing volume restriction or demonstrating carbohydrate intolerance?**

Yes. Lipids are calorie dense compared to dextrose solutions.

❍ **What minimum percent of total calories should be supplied as lipid to prevent fatty acid deficiency?**

Five percent of total calories at minimum.

❍ **How long does it take non-stressed patients receiving lipid-free total parenteral nutrition (TPN) to demonstrate evidence of essential fatty acid deficiency?**

Within four weeks. Hypermetabolic patients within ten days.

❍ **What is the optimal amount of lipids that should be given during critical illness?**

There is no consensus.

❍ **Can lipids administered parenterally hurt cellular immunity?**

There is data to suggest lipids cause reticuloendothelial dysfunction and immune suppression.

❍ **What clinical symptoms are seen with hypophosphatemia brought on by refeeding a malnourished patient?**

Weakness and congestive heart failure.

❍ **Which form of protein, peptides or amino acids, is more uniformly and efficiently absorbed from the gut?**

Peptides.

❍ **How much glutamine has been included in standard amino acid solutions used with total parenteral nutrition (TPN)?**

None, due to its instability in parenteral solutions.

❍ **Is glutamine an essential amino acid?**

No. However, during times of metabolic stress, intracellular glutamine stores are markedly depleted indicating supplementation may be beneficial.

❍ **Arginine, a semi-essential amino acid, is considered to be vital to what body system?**

The immune system.

❍ **Can branched-chain amino acids improve the outcome in critically ill patients?**

No. Some suggest it may be helpful in patients with hepatic encephalopathy.

❍ **Have immunoenriched diets, containing substrates such as omega-3 fish oils, arginine, and RNA nucleotides, been found to improve outcome?**

Yes, a number of recent studies suggest improvement using enteral immunoenriched formulas.

❍ **Which is the preferred route for the delivery of nutrition, enteral or parenteral?**

The enteral route, although there is still some debate.

❍ **When should nutritional support be started?**

As soon as a hypermetabolic state (e.g., trauma or sepsis), underlying malnutrition, or an expected delay in resuming an oral diet of > 5-10 days is recognized.

❍ **Has early initiation of enteral feedings been shown to decrease septic complications in trauma patients compared to early parenteral nutrition?**

Yes. It appears those most severely injured gain the greatest benefit.

❍ **What complications are associated with enteral nutrition?**

Complications involving routes of access to the GI tract (e.g., feeding tube displacement or obstruction), the GI tract itself (e.g., nausea, vomiting, diarrhea), or metabolic (e.g., hyperglycemia, hypophosphatemia).

❍ **T/F: Bowel sounds are a good index of small bowel motility.**

False.

❍ **Has preoperative nutritional support for malnourished patients been shown to reduce postoperative morbidity?**

Yes, for those with severe malnutrition.

❍ **In which patients is parenteral nutritional support indicated?**

When enteral access is unobtainable, enteral feeding contraindicated, or when level of enteral nutrition fails to meet requirements.

❍ **In which patients is intravenous nutritional support unlikely to be of benefit?**

Those expected to start oral intake in 5 to 7 days or with mild injuries.

❍ **Typically, which feeding route requires a greater length of time to reach full support?**

Enteral.

❍ **Can lipids be given through a peripheral vein?**

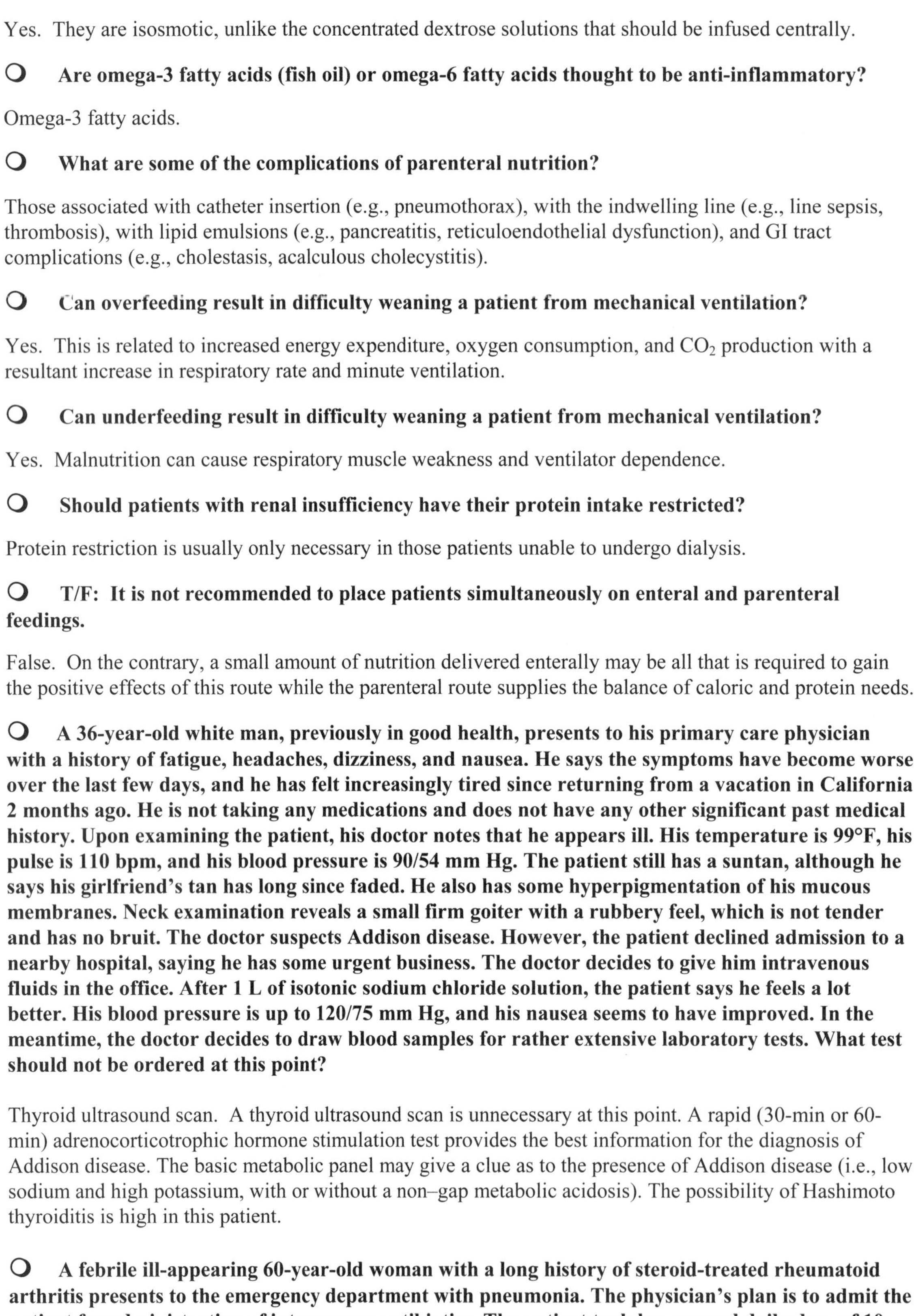

Yes. They are isosmotic, unlike the concentrated dextrose solutions that should be infused centrally.

❍ **Are omega-3 fatty acids (fish oil) or omega-6 fatty acids thought to be anti-inflammatory?**

Omega-3 fatty acids.

❍ **What are some of the complications of parenteral nutrition?**

Those associated with catheter insertion (e.g., pneumothorax), with the indwelling line (e.g., line sepsis, thrombosis), with lipid emulsions (e.g., pancreatitis, reticuloendothelial dysfunction), and GI tract complications (e.g., cholestasis, acalculous cholecystitis).

❍ **Can overfeeding result in difficulty weaning a patient from mechanical ventilation?**

Yes. This is related to increased energy expenditure, oxygen consumption, and CO_2 production with a resultant increase in respiratory rate and minute ventilation.

❍ **Can underfeeding result in difficulty weaning a patient from mechanical ventilation?**

Yes. Malnutrition can cause respiratory muscle weakness and ventilator dependence.

❍ **Should patients with renal insufficiency have their protein intake restricted?**

Protein restriction is usually only necessary in those patients unable to undergo dialysis.

❍ **T/F: It is not recommended to place patients simultaneously on enteral and parenteral feedings.**

False. On the contrary, a small amount of nutrition delivered enterally may be all that is required to gain the positive effects of this route while the parenteral route supplies the balance of caloric and protein needs.

❍ **A 36-year-old white man, previously in good health, presents to his primary care physician with a history of fatigue, headaches, dizziness, and nausea. He says the symptoms have become worse over the last few days, and he has felt increasingly tired since returning from a vacation in California 2 months ago. He is not taking any medications and does not have any other significant past medical history. Upon examining the patient, his doctor notes that he appears ill. His temperature is 99°F, his pulse is 110 bpm, and his blood pressure is 90/54 mm Hg. The patient still has a suntan, although he says his girlfriend's tan has long since faded. He also has some hyperpigmentation of his mucous membranes. Neck examination reveals a small firm goiter with a rubbery feel, which is not tender and has no bruit. The doctor suspects Addison disease. However, the patient declined admission to a nearby hospital, saying he has some urgent business. The doctor decides to give him intravenous fluids in the office. After 1 L of isotonic sodium chloride solution, the patient says he feels a lot better. His blood pressure is up to 120/75 mm Hg, and his nausea seems to have improved. In the meantime, the doctor decides to draw blood samples for rather extensive laboratory tests. What test should not be ordered at this point?**

Thyroid ultrasound scan. A thyroid ultrasound scan is unnecessary at this point. A rapid (30-min or 60-min) adrenocorticotrophic hormone stimulation test provides the best information for the diagnosis of Addison disease. The basic metabolic panel may give a clue as to the presence of Addison disease (i.e., low sodium and high potassium, with or without a non–gap metabolic acidosis). The possibility of Hashimoto thyroiditis is high in this patient.

❍ **A febrile ill-appearing 60-year-old woman with a long history of steroid-treated rheumatoid arthritis presents to the emergency department with pneumonia. The physician's plan is to admit the patient for administration of intravenous antibiotics. The patient took her normal daily dose of 10 mg of prednisone 5 hours earlier, but she vomited 3 hours later. How should the physician manage this patient's steroids?**

Administer 80 mg hydrocortisone intravenously immediately. This scenario should raise a clinical suspicion for a risk of adrenal crisis. During acute illnesses, stress doses of glucocorticoids are appropriate when this suspicion arises.

❍ **A 27-year-old woman, a nurse, presents with complaints of dry cough, low-grade fevers, sore throat, palpitations, fatigue, muscle aches, and increased sweating. She admits to taking medicine samples from her workplace to treat her pain. Examination reveals a blood pressure of 148/80 mm Hg, pulse of 88 beats/min, and temperature of 98°F. She has a visible goiter but declines further neck examination, stating her neck is sore. She has minimally noticeable tremor of the hands, with slightly diaphoretic palms. Her thyroid-stimulating hormone (TSH) level is <0.001 mIU/L (0.5-5). The following studies are pending CBC, TSH, total thyroxine (T4), total triiodothyronine (T3), and T3 uptake. In addition to beta-blockers, what should the next step be?**

Order sedimentation rate, thyroid uptake, and initiate nonsteroidal anti-inflammatory agents. This patient has a painful subacute thyroiditis that probably has viral origins. The symptoms of a viral illness followed by hyperthyroidism and tender thyroid are typical. Sedimentation rate and thyroglobulin are elevated. Treatment is with salicylates, bedrest, and beta-blockers if hyperthyroid symptoms are prominent. The patient is a healthcare worker. Malingering and factitious thyroid hormone ingestion is a legitimate consideration. An ultrasound will not change management at this time. Iodine uptake by the thyroid is minimal or absent in both subacute thyroiditis and thyroid hormone ingestion, whereas it is increased in most other hyperthyroid states. Fine-needle aspiration biopsy is not appropriate at this time, nor is radioactive iodine ablation without complete thyroid studies.

❍ **Regarding hyperparathyroidism, medullary thyroid carcinoma, Hirschsprung disease, gastrinoma, or pheochromocytoma, which of the following is not a known complication in multiple endocrine neoplasia, type 2 (MEN 2)?**

Gastrinoma is a feature of MEN, type 1. All of the others are features of MEN, Type II.

NEUROLOGY

Logic is the art of going wrong with confidence.
Joseph Wood Krutch

❍ **A 50 year-old female with hearing loss over the last six months presents at 2 a.m. with vertigo that has progressively become worse over the last two months. Upon examination, she is mildly ataxic. What is the diagnosis?**

Eighth nerve lesion, possibly an acoustic schwannoma or meningioma.

❍ **What is a vestibular schwannoma?**

An acoustic neuroma or a tumor of the eighth cranial nerve. In addition to hearing loss and vertigo, patients also present with tinnitus. Surgical removal is the treatment of choice because this tumor may spread to the cerebellum and the brainstem.

❍ **Where are congenital berry aneurysms located?**

In the circle of Willis.

❍ **What is the prognosis for a patient recently diagnosed with amyotrophic lateral sclerosis (ALS)?**

Death 3 to 10 years after the onset of symptoms. ALS, also known as Lou Gehrig's disease, involves a progressive loss of the anterior horn cell function of the motor neurons. No sensory abnormalities are involved, just gradual weakness and atrophy of the muscles.

❍ **Which type of bacteria are most commonly cultured from brain abscesses, aerobic or anaerobic?**

Anaerobic.

❍ **What is an Argyll-Robertson pupil?**

A small and irregular pupil that can narrow to focus but not in response to light. This can be a sign of neurosyphilis. Other symptoms include headache, dizziness, diplopia, nuchal rigidity, weakness, paralysis, tabes dorsalis, memory loss, dementia, lethargy, and delusions.

❍ **A patient presents with facial droop on the left and weakness of the right leg. Where is the most likely site of the lesion?**

The brainstem, specifically the left pons.

❍ **What area of the brain is dysfunctional when a patient has Cheyne-Stokes respirations?**

The cortex. The nervous system is relying on diencephalic control.

❍ **What are the most common origins of metastatic brain lesions in adults?**

Breast adenocarcinoma, bronchogenic carcinoma, and malignant melanoma. Twenty percent of adult brain tumors are metastatic.

❍ **A 25 year-old was knocked unconscious for ten seconds while playing touch football one week ago. Since then, he has had intermittent vertigo, nausea, vomiting, blurred vision, a headache, and malaise. His neurological examination and CT are normal. What is the diagnosis?**

Post-concussive syndrome. Most individuals recover fully over a 2 to 6 week time span. A small percentage of patients with post-concussive syndrome will have persistent deficits.

❍ **Differentiate between decerebrate and decorticate posturing.**

Decerebrate posturing: elbows and legs extended (indicative of a midbrain lesion).

Decorticate posturing: elbows flexed and legs extended (suggesting a thalamic lesion).

Remember: DeCORticate = hands by the heart.

❍ **When does the onset of epilepsy usually occur?**

Before age 20.

❍ **How long must a generalized tonic-clonic seizure last without a period of consciousness to be considered status epilepticus?**

30 minutes. Status epilepticus may result from grand mal seizures or anticonvulsant therapy withdrawal.

❍ **What is the most common malignant brain tumor in adults?**

Glioblastoma.

❍ **What is the most common benign brain tumor in adults?**

Meningioma.

❍ **What happens if light is directed into the eyes of a patient who is in a diabetic coma?**

The pupils will constrict.

❍ **Distinguish between the gait of a patient with a cerebellar lesion and that of a patient with an extrapyramidal lesion.**

A patient with a cerebellar lesion will have truncal ataxia, an unsteady, irregular gait with broad steps. A patient with an extrapyramidal lesion will have a festinating gait, several small, shuffling steps taken without swinging the arms.

❍ **Weber's test is performed on a patient complaining of hearing loss. The patient hears sounds more loudly in his right ear. Which types of hearing loss may this patient have?**

Conductive hearing loss on the right or sensory hearing loss on the left.

❍ **Describe Rinne's test and expected normal findings.**

Rinne's test is performed by placing the tip of the tuning fork on the mastoid process until the patient can no longer hear the tone. The fork is relocated to just in front of the pinna until the patient can no longer hear the tone. In normal patients, the ratio is 1:2 of the duration of time the patient can hear the fork.

❍ **What is the most common cause of subarachnoid hemorrhage?**

Saccular aneurysm.

❍ **What are other common causes of a subarachnoid hemorrhage?**

Rupture of cerebral artery aneurysm and arteriovenous malformation. These patients present with an abrupt, severe headache that can progress to syncope, nausea, vomiting, nuchal rigidity, and non-focal neurological changes.

❍ **Damage to the middle meningeal artery results in what kind of hematoma?**

Epidural.

❍ **A 29 year-old drunken male presents after having his head pounded into the concrete. The patient had a brief episode of LOC, but was then ambulatory and alert. Now he appears drowsy and just threw up on you. What is the diagnosis?**

Epidural hematoma.

❍ **Which is more common, subdural or epidural hemorrhaging?**

Subdural. Subdural hemorrhaging can result from the tearing of the bridging veins. Bleeding occurs less rapidly because the veins, not arteries, are damaged.

❍ **A 26 year-old woman complains of a throbbing, dull, unilateral headache that lasts for hours then goes away with sleep. She also has been nauseated and has vomited twice. She reports small areas of visual loss plus strange zig-zag lines in her vision. What is the diagnosis?**

Classic migraine headache. Classic migraine accounts for only 1% of migraines. It can be differentiated from the common migraine because it involves visual disturbances of scotomata and fortification spectra, in addition to all the other migraine symptoms.

❍ **What factors may precipitate migraine headaches?**

Bright lights, cheese, hot dogs and other foods containing tyramine or nitrates, menstruation, monosodium glutamate, and stress.

❍ **A 36 year-old man with severe orbital and temporal pain on the right side has tearing out of the right eye but not the left. The patient's pain tends to occur when he arrives home from work. Also, he knows he will get a headache if he comes home and grabs a beer. The headaches last only about an hour. What syndrome can be associated with this man's headache?**

Horner's syndrome (anhidrosis, miosis, and ptosis). This man has a cluster headache, which typically occurs in men ranging from ages 20 to 50. A cluster headache can recur at the same time and location each day, and is exacerbated by alcohol and vasodilators. Relief is achieved with 100% O_2, ergots, lithium, or prednisone. Intranasal viscous lidocaine can also be effective

❍ **Which type of headache usually afflicts adults?**

Tension headaches. This is a bilateral "band-like" fronto-occipital headache accompanied by constant pain. Tension headaches are generally muscular in nature; therefore, a patient may also have tense neck and scalp muscles.

❍ **Describe the key signs and symptoms of classic, common, ophthalmoplegic, and hemiplegic migraine headaches.**

Common: This headache is indeed the most common. It is a slowly evolving headache that lasts for hours to days. A positive family history as well as two of the following are prevalent: nausea or vomiting, throbbing quality, photophobia, unilateral pain, and increase with menses. A lack of visual symptoms distinguishes common migraine from classic migraine.

Classic: Prodrome lasts up to 60 minutes. The most common symptom is visual disturbance (homonymous hemianopsia, scintillating scotoma, fortification spectra, and photophobia). Lip, face, and hand tingling, aphasia and extremity weakness. Nausea and vomiting may occur.

Ophthalmoplegic: Most frequently manifests in young adults. The patient has an outwardly deviated, dilated eye with ptosis. The third, fourth, and sixth nerves are usually involved.

Hemiplegic: Unilateral motor and sensory symptoms and mild hemiparesis to hemiplegia are exhibited.

❍ **How can you tell if a headache is caused by an intracranial tumor?**

Through a CT or MRI. However, everyone who walks into the office complaining of a headache cannot be subjected to these procedures. Patients complaining of the "worst headache of their life" have written a ticket for a scan and LP. Other signs that may suggest a serious underlying disease are headaches that (1) wake patients from their sleep (although cluster headaches may do this), (2) are worse in the morning, (3) increase in severity with postural changes or Valsalva maneuvers, (4) are associated with nausea and vomiting (though migraines have similar symptoms), (5) are associated with focal defects or mental status changes, and (6) occur with a new onset of seizures.

❍ **A man developed Huntington's chorea at the age of 44. What are the chances of his daughter developing the same disease?**

50%. Huntington's chorea is an autosomal dominant disorder that first manifests itself between ages 30 to 50. Symptoms include dementia, amnesia, delusions, emotional instability, depression, paranoia, antisocial behavior, and irritability. If the daughter inherits the disease, she will also develop chorea, bradykinesia, hypertonia, hyperkinesia, clonus, schizophrenia, intellectual impairment, and bowel incontinence. She will eventually die a premature death about 15 years after the onset of her symptoms.

❍ **What chromosome carries the genetic defect for Huntington's chorea?**

The short arm of chromosome 4.

❍ **Differentiate between Korsakoff's psychosis and Wernicke's encephalopathy.**

Korsakoff's psychosis: Inability to process new information, i.e., to form new memories. This is a reversible condition resulting from brain damage induced by a thiamine deficiency that is generally secondary to chronic alcoholism.

Wernicke's encephalopathy: Also due to an alcohol-induced thiamine deficiency. This is an irreversible disease in which the brain tissues break down, become inflamed, and bleed. Patients experience decreased muscle coordination, ophthalmoplegia, and confusion.

❍ **A 35 year-old woman with a history of flu-like symptoms (URI) one week ago presents with vertigo, nausea, and vomiting. No auditory impairment or focal deficits are noted. What is the likely diagnosis?**

Labyrinthitis or vestibular neuronitis.

❍ **A 50 year-old female with acute vertigo, nausea, and vomiting reports similar episodes over the last 20 years that are sometimes associated with hearing change, hearing loss, and tinnitus. She has permanent right > left sensorineural hearing loss. What is the diagnosis?**

Meniere's disease.

❍ **What organism is frequently responsible for bacterial meningitis in adults?**

Neisseria meningitides.

❍ **How does bacterial meningitis differ from viral meningitis in terms of the corresponding CSF lab values?**

Bacterial meningitis is associated with low glucose and high protein levels, while viral meningitis will have normal glucose and normal protein levels.

❍ **On LP, opening pressure is markedly elevated. What should be done?**

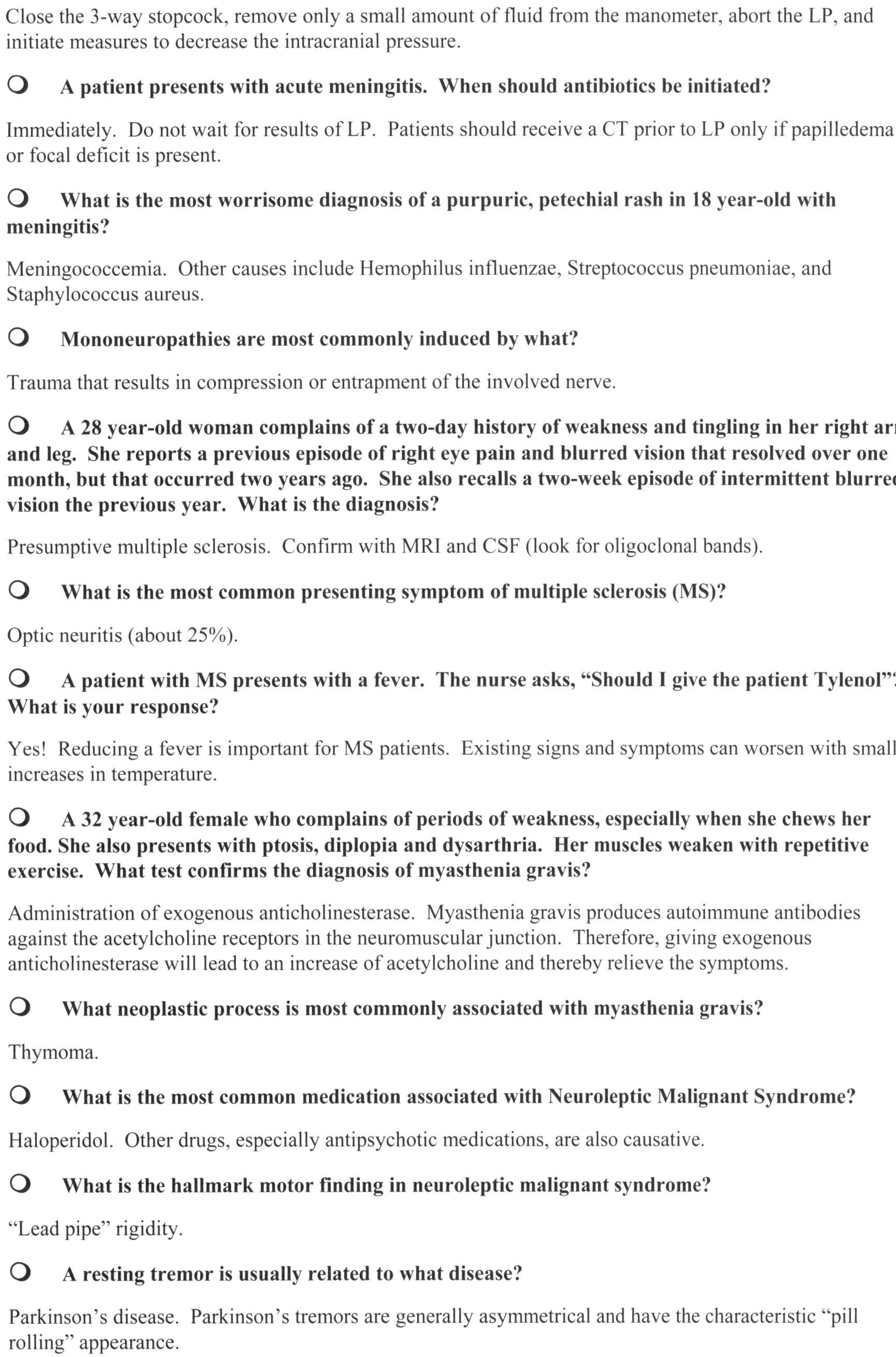

Close the 3-way stopcock, remove only a small amount of fluid from the manometer, abort the LP, and initiate measures to decrease the intracranial pressure.

❍ **A patient presents with acute meningitis. When should antibiotics be initiated?**

Immediately. Do not wait for results of LP. Patients should receive a CT prior to LP only if papilledema or focal deficit is present.

❍ **What is the most worrisome diagnosis of a purpuric, petechial rash in 18 year-old with meningitis?**

Meningococcemia. Other causes include Hemophilus influenzae, Streptococcus pneumoniae, and Staphylococcus aureus.

❍ **Mononeuropathies are most commonly induced by what?**

Trauma that results in compression or entrapment of the involved nerve.

❍ **A 28 year-old woman complains of a two-day history of weakness and tingling in her right arm and leg. She reports a previous episode of right eye pain and blurred vision that resolved over one month, but that occurred two years ago. She also recalls a two-week episode of intermittent blurred vision the previous year. What is the diagnosis?**

Presumptive multiple sclerosis. Confirm with MRI and CSF (look for oligoclonal bands).

❍ **What is the most common presenting symptom of multiple sclerosis (MS)?**

Optic neuritis (about 25%).

❍ **A patient with MS presents with a fever. The nurse asks, "Should I give the patient Tylenol"? What is your response?**

Yes! Reducing a fever is important for MS patients. Existing signs and symptoms can worsen with small increases in temperature.

❍ **A 32 year-old female who complains of periods of weakness, especially when she chews her food. She also presents with ptosis, diplopia and dysarthria. Her muscles weaken with repetitive exercise. What test confirms the diagnosis of myasthenia gravis?**

Administration of exogenous anticholinesterase. Myasthenia gravis produces autoimmune antibodies against the acetylcholine receptors in the neuromuscular junction. Therefore, giving exogenous anticholinesterase will lead to an increase of acetylcholine and thereby relieve the symptoms.

❍ **What neoplastic process is most commonly associated with myasthenia gravis?**

Thymoma.

❍ **What is the most common medication associated with Neuroleptic Malignant Syndrome?**

Haloperidol. Other drugs, especially antipsychotic medications, are also causative.

❍ **What is the hallmark motor finding in neuroleptic malignant syndrome?**

"Lead pipe" rigidity.

❍ **A resting tremor is usually related to what disease?**

Parkinson's disease. Parkinson's tremors are generally asymmetrical and have the characteristic "pill rolling" appearance.

❍ **A patient with a stooped posture, festinating gait (small shuffling steps), mask-like facies, poor balance, slow starting speech, decreased movement, muscular rigidity, and a "pill rolling" tremor should be treated with what?**

Dopaminergic agonists, such as amantadine, bromocriptine, and levodopa; and cholinergic antagonists such as benztropine. Parkinson's syndrome is caused by a loss of dopaminergic cells in the substantia nigra. Most people lose these neurons at a rate of 0.5% a year. Individuals with Parkinson's disease lose them at a rate of 1% per year.

❍ **What ECG finding makes phenytoin relatively contraindicated?**

Second or third degree heart block. If the patient is in status epilepticus, there may be no other choice. Phenytoin is relatively ineffective for seizures due to cyclic antidepressant overdose.

❍ **What is the classic EEG finding associated with petite mal seizures?**

A three second spike and wave pattern.

❍ **What is Shy-Drager syndrome?**

A rare, gradually progressive nerve disorder characterized by very low blood pressure, lack of coordination, muscle wasting, stiffness, and lack of bladder and/or bowel control. This syndrome occurs most often in young people.

❍ **What artery is most commonly involved in stroke?**

Middle cerebral artery.

❍ **Unilateral occlusion of the vertebral-basilar arterial distribution results in what kind of symptoms?**

Ipsilateral cranial nerve abnormalities and contralateral motor and sensory deficits.

❍ **A patient with aphasia most likely had a stroke involving which hemisphere?**

The dominant hemisphere. Patients who stroke in the non-dominant hemisphere have apraxia and sensory neglect.

❍ **What is the most common cause of syncope?**

Vasovagal or simple fainting (50%).

❍ **In order for a patient to faint from cardiac causes, to what level must the cardiac output fall?**

50% the normal capacity. Cardiac syncope can occur because of mechanical causes, such as aortic or pulmonic obstruction and arrhythmias, or because of ischemic causes, such as MI or aortic dissection.

❍ **What is tabes dorsalis?**

Progressive loss of all or part of the body's reflexes. The large joints of affected limbs are destroyed. Patients experience severe, stabbing pains in their legs, sensory deficits, and difficulty walking. Forty percent of patients with neurosyphilis are afflicted with tabes dorsalis.

❍ **What body parts are most commonly affected in an essential tremor?**

Head and upper extremities. Essential tremors are sporadic and slowly progressive. These tremors are rare at rest but become worse when the limbs are used.

❍ **If a patient with a tremor drinks alcohol and the tremor temporarily subsides a bit, what kind of tremor is it?**

An essential tremor or a familial tremor. Botulinum toxin injections, beta-blockers, and primidone are the conventional treatments.

❍ **A 74 year-old male presents with a unilateral burning headache that is worse around his temples and his eye. He also complains of visual disturbances and pain in his jaw after heavy use. Upon examination, you palpate a prominent temporal artery that is very tender. What tests should be run to make a diagnosis?**

Biopsy of the temporal artery. This patient most likely has temporal arteritis or giant cell arteritis. A sedimentation rate of over 50 mm/hr suggests this diagnosis.

❍ **Why is the above case a medical emergency?**

Giant cell arteritis affects the large blood vessels. It usually involves the arteries branching off of the carotids. Therefore, involvement of the temporal artery may also indicate involvement of the central retinal artery. Twenty-five percent of patients with temporal arteritis have thromboses in the central retinal artery, which leads to blindness. An immediate course of high dose prednisone should be started to decrease the inflammation in all patients.

❍ **A 67 year-old woman complains of severe episodes of pain in her nose, cheek, and upper lip. She says it feels like a "lightening bolt hitting my face". What is the diagnosis?**

Trigeminal neuralgia. This is a nerve condition of unknown etiology, possibly a microvascular compression causing a neuronal breakdown. It involves the trigeminal nerve and is most common in the V1 and V2 branches, although it may affect all three.

❍ **How is the above patient treated?**

Perform an MRI to rule out a brainstem process, such as a tumor. Carbamazepine treats trigeminal neuralgia.

❍ **For the following clinical presentations, identify which are associated with peripheral vertigo or with central vertigo.**

1) Intense spinning, nausea, hearing loss, diaphoresis
2) Swaying or impulsion, worse with movement, tinnitus, acute onset
3) Unidirectional nystagmus inhibited by ocular fixation, fatigable
4) Mild vertigo, diplopia, and ataxia
5) Multidirectional nystagmus not inhibited by ocular fixation, non-fatigable
Answers: peripheral vertigo: (1), (2), and (3); central vertigo: (4) and (5).

❍ **A patient has an irritative lesion in the left hemisphere. What way do the eyes deviate?**

To the right.

❍ **What motor deficit occurs with an anterior cerebral artery infarct?**

Leg weakness greater than arm weakness on the contralateral side.

❍ **What two signs are displayed in a middle cerebral artery stroke?**

1) Contralateral sensory/motor deficits

2) Arm/face weakness greater than leg weakness

❍ **What is the significance of bilateral nystagmus with cold caloric testing?**

It signifies that an intact cortex, midbrain, and brainstem are present.

❍ **How are upper motor neuron (UMN) lesions of CN VII (facial nerve) distinguished from peripheral lesions?**

UMN: A unilateral weakness of the lower half of the face

Peripheral: Involves the entire half of the face

❍ **What symptoms form the classic tetrad seen in kernicterus?**

Choreoathetosis, supranuclear ophthalmoplegia, sensorineural hearing loss, and enamel hypoplasia.

❍ **What are the two main forms of neurofibromatosis?**

Type 1 (NF1), Von Recklinghausen's disease or peripheral neurofibromatosis, consists of cafe-au-lait spots, neurofibromas, plexiform neuromas, iris hamartomas (Lisch nodules), optic gliomas, and osseous lesions. It is caused by a mutation in the gene on chromosome 17, and accounts for 85% of all neurofibromatosis. Type 2 (NF2), central neurofibromatosis, involves tumors of cranial nerve VIII and the gene is linked to chromosome 18.

❍ **What is the immunological abnormalities associated with ataxia-telangiectasia?**

These include increased susceptibility to sinopulmonary infections and increased risk of malignancy, such as lymphoma. Often absent or low levels of IgA, normal or low levels of IgG and increased or normal levels of IgM can be utilized to help make the diagnosis.

❍ **Heterozygotes for homocystinuria can present with what problem in adulthood?**

Deficiency of cystathionine beta-synthetase is the most common cause of homocystinuria. Homozygotes present early in life with ectopia lentis, mental retardation and early strokes. Adults who are heterozygotes for homocystinuria can present with a history of stroke at a younger age than expected.

❍ **What are the two disorders involving copper metabolism?**

Wilson's disease (hepatolenticular degeneration), with diminished ceruloplasmin and copper accumulation and Menkes disease (Kinky hair disease), with maldistribution of copper leading to decreased synthesis of copper-containing enzymes.

❍ **What is the enzyme defect in Lesch-Nyhan disease?**

Hypoxanthine-guanine phosphoribosyltransferase (HGPRT).

❍ **Which neurons are spared in Huntington's disease?**

Cholinergic interneurons whose axons terminate in the striatum and interneurons expressing somatostatin and neuropeptide Y.

❍ **Which are the two most common organisms to cause meningitis in patients with a ventriculo-peritoneal (VP) shunt?**

Staphylococcus epidermidis and Staphylococcus aureus.

❍ **Which vitamin should be given routinely during the treatment of tuberculous meningitis?**

Isoniazid can induce a peripheral neuropathy, which can be prevented by the co-administration of vitamin B6.

❍ **What are the three most common predisposing factors in the formation of a brain abscess?**

Cyanotic heart disease, otitis and sinusitis.

❍ **What is the most common cranial neuropathy seen in Borreliosis (Lyme disease)?**

Unilateral or bilateral facial palsy. Less frequently, the VIII cranial nerve can also be affected.

❍ **Which is the cranial nerve most affected in pseudotumor cerebri?**

Cranial nerve IV can be involved with clinical signs of diplopia. Other findings include decreased visual acuity and restricted peripheral fields with enlargement of the blind spot.

❍ **When should steroids be used in the treatment of increased intracranial pressure (ICP)?**

Steroids are beneficial in the treatment of vasogenic edema, so they should be used to treat increased ICP associated with tumors, abscesses and brain trauma.

❍ **What cutaneous manifestation is seen in patients with Sturge-Weber disease?**

A Port-wine stain, or angiomatous naevus, is seen in the distribution of cranial nerve V. This may be associated with pial angiomas. Seizures are the main clinical manifestation, but hemiparesis can also be seen.

❍ **Why is a family history of deafness important in evaluating a patient with episodes of sudden loss of consciousness?**

Jervell-Lange-Nielson syndrome is associated with prolonged Q-T and neurosensory hearing loss. Prolonged Q-T syndromes must be identified because they can lead to sudden death.

❍ **The 'Alice in Wonderland' sensory changes are seen most often in what neurologic condition?**

Migraines

❍ **What percent of migraine patients have their onset of headaches prior to age 5 years of age?**

20%

❍ **Ophthalmoplegic migraine affects which cranial nerve?**

Cranial nerve III.

❍ **What are the clinical findings of Klein-Levin syndrome?**

This syndrome occurs in adolescent males and presents with episodes of hypersomnia, hyperphagia and frontal lobe-type personality changes.

❍ **Which metabolic peripheral neuropathy can be clinically misdiagnosed as Friedreich's ataxia?**

Vitamin E deficiency.

❍ **What is the time window for treatment of acute ischemic stroke with t-PA?**

The maximum allowed time from onset of symptoms to treatment is 3 hours.

❍ **A 63 year-old previously healthy man awakens at 6 AM with weakness of the left arm and leg and difficulty walking. He arrives at the hospital at 7 AM and a CT scan is immediately performed, the results of which are normal. What dose of t-PA should he receive?**

It must be assumed that the stroke onset was the time the patient was last known to be normal, i.e., when he went to sleep. Thrombolysis is contraindicated beyond 3 hours.

❍ **What blood pressure parameters must be met for an acute stroke patient to receive thrombolytic treatment?**

The SBP must be no greater than 185 mmHg and the DBP no greater than 110 mmHg.

❍ **What was the risk of symptomatic intracranial hemorrhage in patients who receive t-PA?**

Six percent. The risk of fatal intracranial hemorrhage is 3 percent.

❍ **What effect does t-PA have on 3-month mortality?**

The 3-month mortality of patients receiving t-PA was 17%, compared to 21% for conventional treatment.

❍ **Carotid endarterectomy is indicated for symptomatic patients with what degree of stenosis?**

70% or greater.

❍ **The benefit of carotid endarterectomy assumes a reasonably low rate of perioperative complications. What is the incidence of perioperative death or stroke in patients undergoing carotid endarterectomy?**

Approximately 6%.

❍ **What is the single most important modifiable risk factor for stroke?**

Hypertension.

❍ **Which region of the United States has the highest incidence of stroke?**

The southeastern United States, also known as "the Stroke Belt".

❍ **What are three vitamin deficiencies that lead to elevated levels of plasma homocysteine, a risk factor for peripheral vascular disease?**

Folate, Vitamin B6 and Vitamin B12.

❍ **According to recent observational studies, what effect does postmenopausal replacement estrogen therapy have on the risk of stroke?**

Estrogen replacement treatment has been associated with a decreased incidence of stroke.

❍ **What is the prevalence of patent foramen ovale in the general population?**

Approximately 15%. The prevalence of patent foramen ovale in patients with cryptogenic ischemic stroke is about 50%.

❍ **Aortic arch atheroma are an independent risk factor for stroke. What characteristic denotes an especially increased risk?**

Plaque thickness greater than or equal to 4 mm.

❍ **When is maximum cerebrospinal fluid xanthochromia observed after subarachnoid hemorrhage?**

48 hours.

❍ **Which of the following signs is not part of the classic Wallenberg syndrome: nystagmus, Horner's syndrome, contralateral hemiparesis, ipsilateral ataxia, contralateral loss of pain and temperature sense.**

Hemiparesis.

❍ **What is the usual localization of the pure sensory stroke?**

Thalamus.

❍ **Does hypothermia increase or decrease ischemic injury in experimental models of stroke?**

Hypothermia decreases ischemic injury.

❍ **Nitric oxide plays both a beneficial and a deleterious role in the ischemic cascade. The toxicity of nitric oxide is mediated largely through free radical damage. By what mechanism does nitric oxide have a protective effect?**

Nitric oxide induces vasodilation.

❍ **Rank the following vascular malformations in order of risk of hemorrhage: arteriovenous malformation, capillary telangiectasia, cavernous malformation, and venous angioma.**

1) arteriovenous malformation, 2) cavernous malformation, 3) capillary telangiectasia, 4) venous angioma.

❍ **What stroke type is increased most in the postpartum period?**

Cerebral venous thrombosis.

❍ **What disorder presents with ischemic and hemorrhagic stroke associated with progressive occlusion of arteries at the Circle of Willis?**

Moyamoya disease.

❍ **What arterial disorder is characterized by the pathological findings of smooth muscle hyperplasia or thinning, elastic fiber destruction, fibrous tissue proliferation, and arterial wall disorganization?**

Fibromuscular dysplasia.

❍ **Which of the following laboratory findings are not seen in antiphospholipid antibody syndrome: positive ANA, false-positive VDRL, decreased PTT, lupus anticoagulant, anti-cardiolipin antibody?**

Decreased PTT.

❍ **What recently discovered condition causes activated protein C resistance and a hypercoagulable state?**

The factor V Leiden mutation.

❍ **Which viral infection classically causes a delayed stroke syndrome?**

Herpes zoster.

❍ **Bilateral cortical hemorrhagic infarcts associated with increased intracranial pressure are observed in what stroke syndrome?**

Superior sagittal sinus syndrome.

❍ **What disorder presents with chemosis, proptosis, and an ocular bruit?**

Carotid-cavernous fistula.

❍ **What are the antiplatelet mechanisms of action of aspirin and ticlopidine?**

Aspirin interferes with platelet function by inhibiting the enzyme cyclooxygenase. Ticlodipine inhibits ADP-induced platelet aggregation.

❍ **What potential adverse effect requires monitoring in patients treated with ticlopidine?**

Neutropenia.

❍ **What recently described disease of autosomal dominant inheritance causes a cerebral vasculopathy and subcortical infarcts?**

Cerebral autosomal dominant angiopathy with subcortical infarcts and leukoencephalopathy (CADASIL).

❍ **What is the CSF volume in a typical adult?**

150 ml.

❍ **A head trauma patient develops hyponatremia. What criteria would diagnose SIADH?**

The criteria are: 1) Hyponatremia, a normal or increased extracellular fluid volume, 2) elevated urinary osmolarity (>100 mOsm), 3) elevated urine sodium (>25 mEq/L), 4) no adrenal, thyroid, or renal disease.

❍ **How is SIADH distinguished from cerebral salt wasting syndrome?**

In cerebral salt wasting syndrome, urinary sodium loss persists, despite fluid restriction, and there is a normal or reduced extracellular fluid volume.

❍ **Rapid correction of chronic hyponatremia will cause which neurologic disorder?**

Central pontine myelinolysis may be caused by rapid correction of serum sodium level (> 0.5 mEq/L).

❍ **What are the clinical features of myxedema coma?**

Non-pitting edema, hypothermia, bradycardia, dry skin, and brittle hair.

❍ **What are the neurological causes of diabetes insipidus?**

Lesions of the hypothalamus or pituitary such as post-operative state, head trauma, sarcoid, lymphoma, craniopharyngioma, pituitary adenoma and metastatic tumors.

❍ **What are the clinical features of epidural abscess?**

Spinal tenderness, fever, radicular pain, myelopathy, elevated CSF protein and CSF pleocytosis.

❍ **What is the treatment of epidural abscess?**

Immediate laminectomy, drainage of the abscess, and antibiotic therapy. A delay may result in permanent myelopathy.

❍ **What are the causes of subdural empyema?**

Sinusitis, meningitis, head trauma, otitis, and osteomyelitis.

❍ **What are the clinical features of H. simplex encephalitis?**

Personality changes, fever, headache, delerium followed by coma, focal or generalized seizures, aphasia, and focal motor symptoms.

❍ **What are the CSF, EEG and MRI findings in H. simplex encephalitis?**

CSF shows elevated protein, mononuclear pleocytosis, normal glucose and often red cells. H. simplex DNA may be detected in CSF by PCR testing. EEG may show periodic temporal lobe sharp wave complexes. MRI may show lesions in the medial temporal lobe, insula, inferior-medial frontal lobes and cingulate gyrus.

❍ **What drug is used to treat H. simplex encephalitis?**

Acyclovir.

❍ **What is the drug treatment for acute traumatic spinal cord injury?**

The treatment for acute (<8 hours) spinal cord injury is Methylprednisolone 30 mg/kg bolus followed by 5.4 mg/kg-hour for the next 23 hours.

❍ **What are the complications that occur following subarachnoid hemorrhage?**

Vasospasm, recurrent hemorrhage, hydrocephalus, seizures, cardiac arrhythmias, hypertension, neurogenic pulmonary edema, stress ulcers and SIADH.

❍ **What drug will reduce the risk of vasospasm following subarachnoid hemorrhage?**

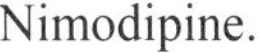

Nimodipine.

❍ **What are the causes of cerebral hemorrhage?**

Trauma, hypertension, ruptured aneurysms, cerebral amyloid angiopathy, vascular malformations, hemorrhage into a tumor (e.g. melanoma, choriocarcinoma, renal cell carcinoma), anticoagulant use, hemophilia, thrombocytopenia, stimulant drugs (amphetamines, cocaine, phenylpropanolamine) and vasculitis (e.g. Wegener's granulomatosis).

❍ **What drug is used to treat acute ischemic stroke?**

TPA, within 3 hours, 0.9 mg/kg not to exceed 90 mg. The initial 10% is given over 1 minute and the remaining dose is given over the remaining 1 hour.

❍ **What is the drug treatment for convulsive status epilepticus?**

Lorazepam (0.1 mg/kg) administered at 2 mg/minute, followed by intravenous fosphenytoin (18 mg of phenytoin equivalent/kg).

❍ **What are the clinical features of spinal cord compression from metastatic cancer?**

Localized spinal tenderness, radicular pain, sensory level, paraparesis or quadriparesis, bowel-bladder incontinence, brisk deep tendon reflexes, upgoing plantar reflexes, and spasticity.

❍ **What is the treatment for acute spinal cord compression from metastatic cancer?**

Usually with high dose corticosteroids and radiation therapy. Surgical therapy is used instead of radiation therapy if the primary cancer type is unknown, the tumor is radioresistant, spinal instability makes surgery necessary or the patient has received the maximum radiation dose.

❍ **What are the medical complications in Guillain-Barré syndrome?**

Respiratory failure, dysautonomia, deep vein thrombosis, pulmonary embolus, SIADH, and respiratory and urinary tract infections.

❍ **What is myasthenic crisis?**

A myasthenia gravis patient with significant impairment in respiratory function. Myasthenic crisis may require emergency intubation and assisted ventilation.

❍ **What are the features of neuroleptic malignant syndrome?**

The features are altered mental status, fever, rigidity, irregular pulse, irregular blood pressure, tachycardia, diaphoresis and elevated CPK.

❍ **What is the treatment for neuroleptic malignant syndrome?**

Immediate withdrawal of the neuroleptic drug. Sinemet, bromocriptine or dantrolene may be used as needed.

❍ **What is the treatment for hepatic coma?**

Treat the precipitating causes such as GI bleeding, alkalosis, hypokalemia, narcotics, sedatives, and infection. Treatment may include reduced dietary protein, lactulose, oral neomycin and flumazenil.

❍ **What are the features of botulism infection?**

The features are a history of recent ingestion of home canned or prepared foods, followed by sudden onset of diplopia, dysphagia, muscle weakness, dry mouth, fixed dilated pupils and respiratory paralysis.

❍ **What is the medical treatment of confirmed botulism?**

Botulism antitoxin.

❍ **What are the features of hypertensive encephalopathy?**

The features are diastolic blood pressure usually over 130 Torr, papilledema, and impaired mental status.

❍ **What are the features of giant cell arteritis?**

The features may include: age > 50 years, visual loss, unilateral headache, tender nodular temporal artery, pain and stiffness of shoulders and pelvic girdle area, malaise, fever, weight loss, jaw claudication, anemia, elevated sedimentation rate and a temporal artery biopsy showing giant cell arteritis.

❍ **What is the treatment for giant cell arteritis?**

Prednisone (60 mg/day) is started immediately prior to biopsy to prevent blindness.

❍ **What are the earliest clinical features of uncal herniation?**

Uncal herniation begins with a unilateral enlarged pupil and a sluggish pupillary light reaction.

❍ **How is a subarachnoid hemorrhage diagnosed?**

CT scan may show blood in the suprasellar cistern, interhemispheric fissure, sylvian fissure, or surface of the brain. If the CT scan is normal, a spinal tap may show xanthochromia.

❍ **What is the Cushing reflex?**

Elevation in blood pressure and reduction in pulse that follows a increase in intracranial pressure. It is a brainstem mediated reflex.

❍ **What are the criteria for diagnosis of brain death?**

The criteria are: (1) coma is present from a known cause, (2) reversible causes of coma such as hypothermia (temperature < 32° C) or drug intoxication have been excluded, (3) there is no clinical evidence of brain or brainstem function.

❍ **What is the apnea test?**

Determines spontaneous ventilatory activity.

❍ **What is the treatment for cerebral metastatic brain tumors?**

High dose corticosteroids to reduce the mass effect from cerebral edema, and usually radiation therapy. Surgery replaces radiation if biopsy for diagnosis of a metastatic lesion is needed, or if a single metastatic lesion is present.

❍ **What age group and sex is affected more by multiple sclerosis?**

25-30 (average 29) years with women to men ratio of 1.4 - 2.2 to 1.

❍ **Does MS have any racial, geographical distribution?**

Yes; whites are more susceptible than blacks and Asians. People living between latitudes 40 degrees North and 40 degrees South are less susceptible.

❍ **Are there any psychiatric symptoms seen in MS?**

In about 50% of cases, depression, irritability, low mood, anxiety, and poor concentration occur. Less common is confusion and psychosis.

❍ **Does multiple sclerosis affect cognition?**

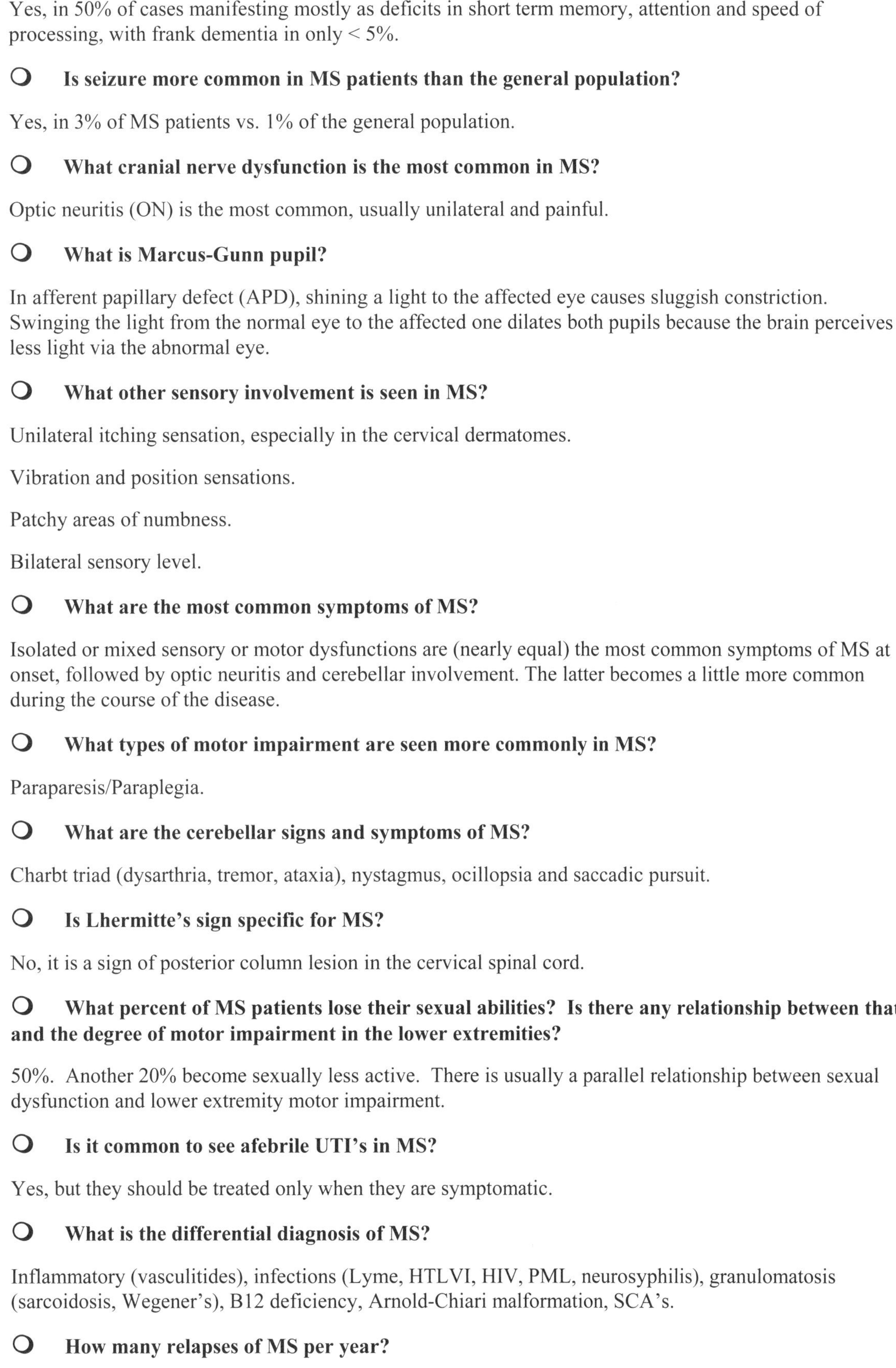

Yes, in 50% of cases manifesting mostly as deficits in short term memory, attention and speed of processing, with frank dementia in only < 5%.

❍ **Is seizure more common in MS patients than the general population?**

Yes, in 3% of MS patients vs. 1% of the general population.

❍ **What cranial nerve dysfunction is the most common in MS?**

Optic neuritis (ON) is the most common, usually unilateral and painful.

❍ **What is Marcus-Gunn pupil?**

In afferent papillary defect (APD), shining a light to the affected eye causes sluggish constriction. Swinging the light from the normal eye to the affected one dilates both pupils because the brain perceives less light via the abnormal eye.

❍ **What other sensory involvement is seen in MS?**

Unilateral itching sensation, especially in the cervical dermatomes.

Vibration and position sensations.

Patchy areas of numbness.

Bilateral sensory level.

❍ **What are the most common symptoms of MS?**

Isolated or mixed sensory or motor dysfunctions are (nearly equal) the most common symptoms of MS at onset, followed by optic neuritis and cerebellar involvement. The latter becomes a little more common during the course of the disease.

❍ **What types of motor impairment are seen more commonly in MS?**

Paraparesis/Paraplegia.

❍ **What are the cerebellar signs and symptoms of MS?**

Charbt triad (dysarthria, tremor, ataxia), nystagmus, ocillopsia and saccadic pursuit.

❍ **Is Lhermitte's sign specific for MS?**

No, it is a sign of posterior column lesion in the cervical spinal cord.

❍ **What percent of MS patients lose their sexual abilities? Is there any relationship between that and the degree of motor impairment in the lower extremities?**

50%. Another 20% become sexually less active. There is usually a parallel relationship between sexual dysfunction and lower extremity motor impairment.

❍ **Is it common to see afebrile UTI's in MS?**

Yes, but they should be treated only when they are symptomatic.

❍ **What is the differential diagnosis of MS?**

Inflammatory (vasculitides), infections (Lyme, HTLVI, HIV, PML, neurosyphilis), granulomatosis (sarcoidosis, Wegener's), B12 deficiency, Arnold-Chiari malformation, SCA's.

❍ **How many relapses of MS per year?**

0.4 - 0.6 per year. Relapses are more frequent during the early years of the disease.

❍ What percent of MS patients will never experience a relapse?

15%.

❍ What is primary progressive MS?

The illness is progressive from the onset, without attacks (19%).

❍ What is secondary progressive MS?

Initial course being relapsing-remitting then evolved to a progressive phase (15%).

❍ What exogenous factors may exacerbate MS?

Gamma-interferon and TNF-alpha, produced by the immune cells during viral infections.

❍ What is the pathology of MS?

Demyelination of CNS (white matter) with relative axonal preservation, although there are evidences of a moderate degree of axonal loss as well as some plaques encroaching upon the cortex with sparing of neuronal cell bodies and axis cylinders.

❍ What type of immunity is suggested to be causing MS?

T-cell mediated immunity.

❍ What is the etiology of MS?

Unknown, but probably due to predisposition, immune or viral mediated and triggered by environmental factors.

❍ What are the good prognostic indicators?

Female sex, younger age at onset, relapsing-remitting form, less rate of relapses early in the course, long first inter-attack interval, and initial symptom is sensory or cranial nerve dysfunction (especially ON).

❍ What form of MS course do younger patients develop?

Relapsing-remitting, progressive form being more common in older age group.

❍ Does MS increase mortality?

There is a progressive increase in the 25-year survival of MS patients of 69% versus 87% in the control population. MS patients live six years (women) and eleven years (men) less than age-matched controls.

❍ Are MS patients at higher risk for suicide? What age group?

Yes, seven times more common. Suicide is a significant cause of death in MS particularly in the younger, less disabled patients.

❍ Does a patient with two clinically evident attacks, but no CSF evidence or paraclinical (neuroimaging, electrophysiological or urological) support, have MS?

Yes. According to the Poser Committee diagnostic criteria for multiple sclerosis, this patient has "clinically definite" MS.

❍ Do most of the MS patients have normal WBC count in CSF?

Two-thirds of them have a normal CSF WBC count. Less than 5% have more than 15 cells (and only rarely above 50). T-cells are the predominant cells.

❍ Is CSF protein level normal in the majority of MS patients?

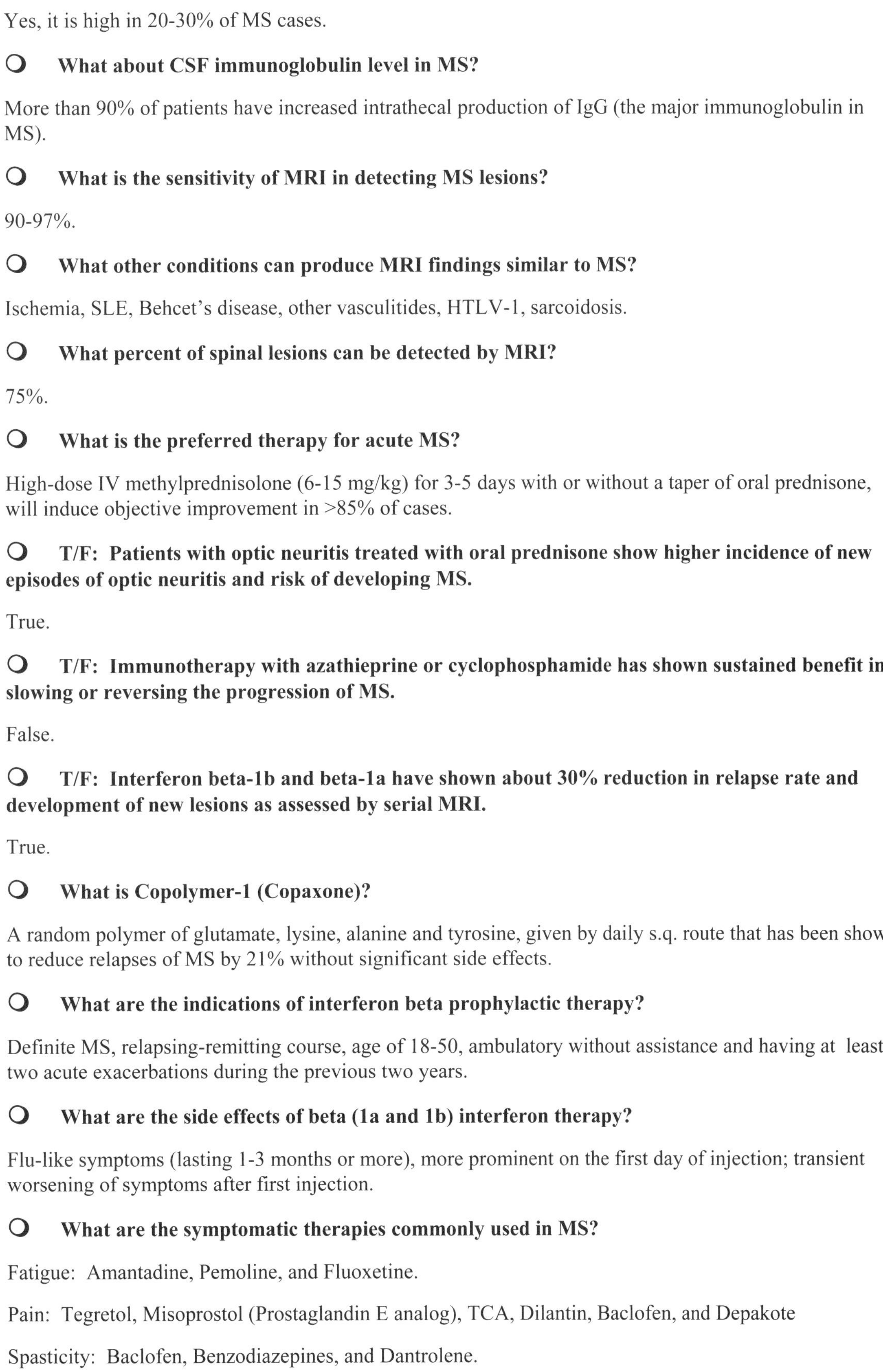

Yes, it is high in 20-30% of MS cases.

❍ **What about CSF immunoglobulin level in MS?**

More than 90% of patients have increased intrathecal production of IgG (the major immunoglobulin in MS).

❍ **What is the sensitivity of MRI in detecting MS lesions?**

90-97%.

❍ **What other conditions can produce MRI findings similar to MS?**

Ischemia, SLE, Behcet's disease, other vasculitides, HTLV-1, sarcoidosis.

❍ **What percent of spinal lesions can be detected by MRI?**

75%.

❍ **What is the preferred therapy for acute MS?**

High-dose IV methylprednisolone (6-15 mg/kg) for 3-5 days with or without a taper of oral prednisone, will induce objective improvement in >85% of cases.

❍ **T/F: Patients with optic neuritis treated with oral prednisone show higher incidence of new episodes of optic neuritis and risk of developing MS.**

True.

❍ **T/F: Immunotherapy with azathieprine or cyclophosphamide has shown sustained benefit in slowing or reversing the progression of MS.**

False.

❍ **T/F: Interferon beta-1b and beta-1a have shown about 30% reduction in relapse rate and development of new lesions as assessed by serial MRI.**

True.

❍ **What is Copolymer-1 (Copaxone)?**

A random polymer of glutamate, lysine, alanine and tyrosine, given by daily s.q. route that has been shown to reduce relapses of MS by 21% without significant side effects.

❍ **What are the indications of interferon beta prophylactic therapy?**

Definite MS, relapsing-remitting course, age of 18-50, ambulatory without assistance and having at least two acute exacerbations during the previous two years.

❍ **What are the side effects of beta (1a and 1b) interferon therapy?**

Flu-like symptoms (lasting 1-3 months or more), more prominent on the first day of injection; transient worsening of symptoms after first injection.

❍ **What are the symptomatic therapies commonly used in MS?**

Fatigue: Amantadine, Pemoline, and Fluoxetine.

Pain: Tegretol, Misoprostol (Prostaglandin E analog), TCA, Dilantin, Baclofen, and Depakote

Spasticity: Baclofen, Benzodiazepines, and Dantrolene.

Intention tremor: Clonazepam, Inderal, and Artane.

❍ **What about treating urgency? What is the cause?**

Oxybutinin or propantheline (anticholinergics). Detrusor hyperreflexias are the cause of urinary urgency.

❍ **Is there any predisposing factor to Guillain-Barré syndrome (GBS)?**

Viral infection, gastrointestinal infection, immunization or surgery often precede the neurological symptoms by 5 days to 3 weeks.

❍ **Can Guillain-Barré syndrome (GBS) involve respiratory muscles quickly?**

Yes. It can start as rapidly progressing symmetric weakness, facial diplegia, oropharyngeal and respiratory paresis, loss of DTRs, and impaired sensation in the hands and feet.

❍ **When do GBS symptoms "level off"?**

After several days to three weeks.

❍ **Does early treatment with IVIG or plasmapheresis accelerate recovery?**

Yes. It also diminishes the incidence of long-term neurologic disability.

❍ **Does activity of the disease correlate with the appearance of serum antibodies to peripheral nerve myelin?**

Yes.

❍ **What is the incidence of GBS?**

With 0.6 to 1.9 per 100,000, GBS is the most common acquired demyelinating neuropathy.

❍ **What age group is more prone to the disease?**

The incidence increases with age (men as equally as women).

❍ **What factor triggers axonal variant of GBS?**

Campylobacter jejuni or parenteral injection of Gangliosides.

❍ **Is there any increase in CSF cells in GBS?**

Usually not. Occasionally 10-100 monocytes. Protein is usually increased.

❍ **Can GBS be fatal?**

Yes. Especially with autonomic dysfunction, but very uncommonly.

❍ **What percent of patients will develop permanent residual weakness, atrophy or hyperreflexia?**

35%, if untreated.

❍ **Does relapse occur in GBS?**

Yes, in 10% but after full recovery it drops to 2%.

❍ **How would you differentiate acute anterior poliomyelitis from GBS?**

The former shows asymmetry of paralysis, signs of meningeal irritation, fever and CSF pleocytosis.

❍ **What are the other differential diagnoses of GBS?**

1- porphyria (normal CSF protein, mental symptoms, recurrent abdominal crisis, onset after exposure to drugs like barbiturates).

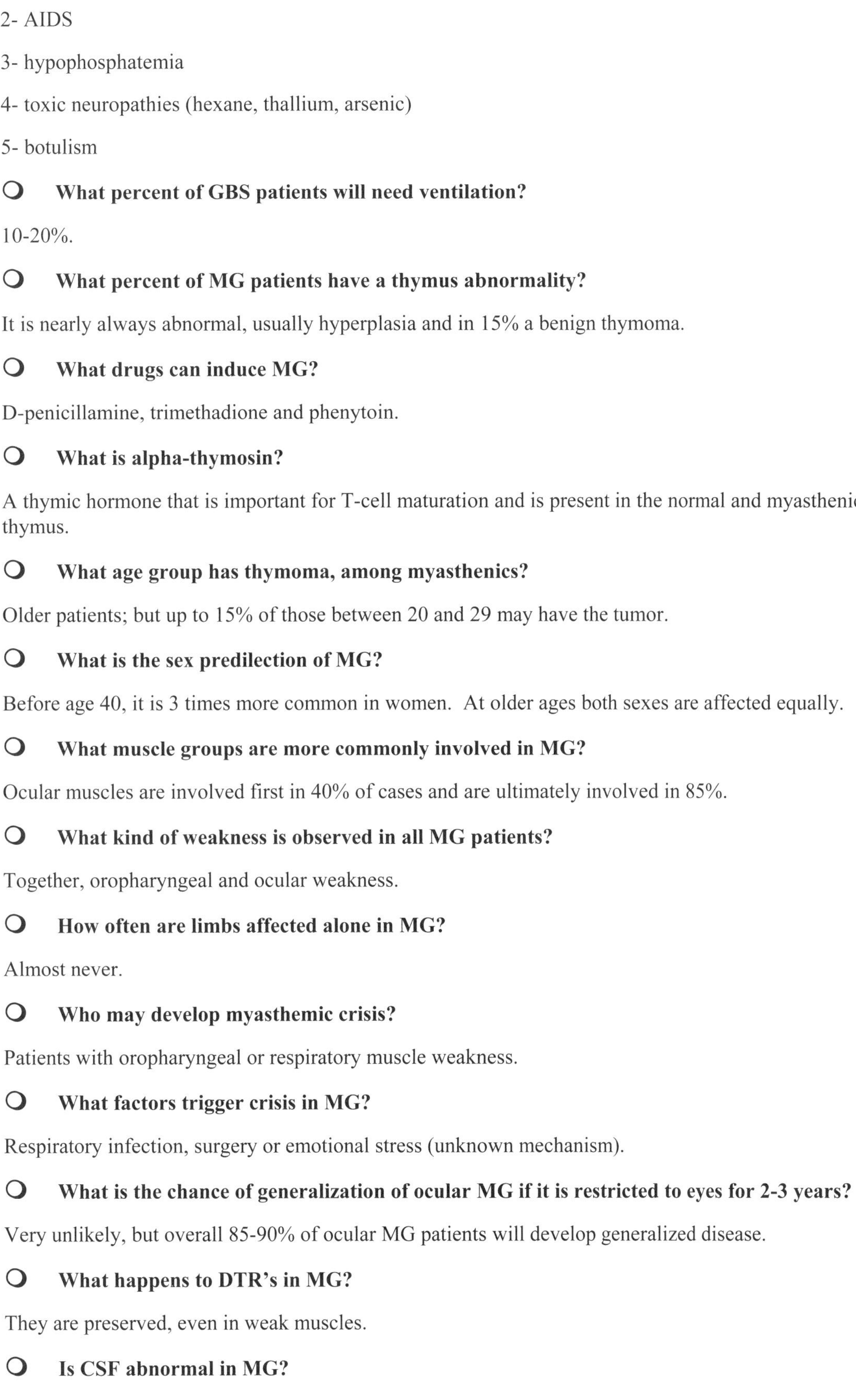

2- AIDS

3- hypophosphatemia

4- toxic neuropathies (hexane, thallium, arsenic)

5- botulism

❍ **What percent of GBS patients will need ventilation?**

10-20%.

❍ **What percent of MG patients have a thymus abnormality?**

It is nearly always abnormal, usually hyperplasia and in 15% a benign thymoma.

❍ **What drugs can induce MG?**

D-penicillamine, trimethadione and phenytoin.

❍ **What is alpha-thymosin?**

A thymic hormone that is important for T-cell maturation and is present in the normal and myasthenic thymus.

❍ **What age group has thymoma, among myasthenics?**

Older patients; but up to 15% of those between 20 and 29 may have the tumor.

❍ **What is the sex predilection of MG?**

Before age 40, it is 3 times more common in women. At older ages both sexes are affected equally.

❍ **What muscle groups are more commonly involved in MG?**

Ocular muscles are involved first in 40% of cases and are ultimately involved in 85%.

❍ **What kind of weakness is observed in all MG patients?**

Together, oropharyngeal and ocular weakness.

❍ **How often are limbs affected alone in MG?**

Almost never.

❍ **Who may develop myasthemic crisis?**

Patients with oropharyngeal or respiratory muscle weakness.

❍ **What factors trigger crisis in MG?**

Respiratory infection, surgery or emotional stress (unknown mechanism).

❍ **What is the chance of generalization of ocular MG if it is restricted to eyes for 2-3 years?**

Very unlikely, but overall 85-90% of ocular MG patients will develop generalized disease.

❍ **What happens to DTR's in MG?**

They are preserved, even in weak muscles.

❍ **Is CSF abnormal in MG?**

No.

❍ **What is the remission rate after thymectomy in MG patients without thymoma?**

80%.

❍ **Is thymectomy recommended for most MG patients with generalized thymoma?**

Yes. It must be considered in disabling ocular myasthenia as well.

❍ **Do MG patients with thymoma have more severe disease?**

Yes. They benefit less from thymectomy.

❍ **What percent of MG patients experiences crisis?**

10%.

❍ **What types of memory are impaired earliest in Alzheimer's disease?**

Episodic, explicit, declarative, and short-term memory.

❍ **What is the difference between dysarthria and aphasia?**

Dysarthria is a disorder of speech, a motor function. Aphasia is a disorder of language, a higher cortical function.

❍ **What is the most common psychiatric diagnosis among patients with neurologic disorders?**

Depression. It occurs in up to 50% of patients with Alzheimer's disease, Parkinson's disease, Huntington's disease, stroke, epilepsy, multiple sclerosis, and traumatic brain injury.

❍ **What are the typical features of transient global amnesia?**

Abrupt onset of amnesia that spares personal identity, resolves within 24 hours, has no other neurologic deficits, and occurs typically between ages 50 and 70.

❍ **How is delirium distinguished from dementia?**

Delirium is characterized by rapid onset, fluctuations in alertness and level of consciousness, and reversibility over hours to days with correction of the underlying toxic or metabolic disturbance. Delirium may also be accompanied by asterixis, tremulousness, and a diffusely slow EEG.

❍ **How is depression distinguished from dementia?**

In depression, onset of symptoms is usually more acute, progression more rapid and self-report of mental impairment more common affect is depressed. Memory impairment is more inconsistent over time, and psychometric testing produces variable and effort-related results. There may be a history of psychiatric illness, recent life stress, and somatic disturbances (anorexia and insomnia).

❍ **Are all dementias progressive?**

No. For example, a single closed head injury may cause a non-progressive dementia.

❍ **What symptoms and signs suggest a diagnosis of multi-infarct (vascular) dementia?**

An abrupt onset with stepwise progression and evidence of two or more strokes by history, examination, or imaging studies.

❍ **What functions are preserved in fronto-temporal dementias, e.g., Pick's disease, as compared to Alzheimer's disease?**

Memory, calculations, and visuospatial abilities. (Both are associated with language disturbances and personality alterations are prominent in fronto-temporal dementias).

❍ **Headache, altered mentation, seizures, and an EEG showing periodic lateralized epileptiform discharges suggest what diagnosis?**

Herpes simplex encephalitis.

❍ **What is the characteristic triad of normal pressure hydrocephalus?**

Dementia, incontinence, and a gait Ataxia (often described as a "magnetic" gait due to difficulty picking up the feet).

❍ **The post-concussive syndrome includes what symptoms?**

Headaches, dizziness, impaired memory and concentration, irritability, and depression.

❍ **What is the Wernicke-Korsakoff syndrome?**

Chronic, severe impairment in anterograde memory (Korsakoff's syndrome) with acute confusion, ataxia, ophthalmoplegia, and nystagmus (Wernicke's encephalopathy). This syndrome results from lesions of the dorsomedial nuclei of the thalamus and mamillary bodies.

❍ **How should Wernicke's encephalopathy be treated?**

Immediate intravenous thiamine replacement.

❍ **Alzheimer's disease is associated with what pattern on single photon emission computed tomography (SPECT) imaging?**

Bilateral hypoperfusion in inferior parietal and posterior temporal association cortices.

❍ **What are the major risk factors for Alzheimer's disease?**

Age, Down's syndrome (Trisomy-21), and family history/genetics.

❍ **How do donepezil (Aricept) and tacrine (Cognex) treat Alzheimer's disease?**

Both are acetylcholinesterase inhibitors and help compensate for the cholinergic deficits in Alzheimer's disease.

❍ **What is Tourette's syndrome?**

A tic disorder with motor and vocal tics developing before age 18. Vocal tics may be unformed or formed (words). Coprolalia (cursing) and echolalia may occur.

❍ **What other disorders may co-exist with Tourette's syndrome?**

Tourette's syndrome may be accompanied by Attention Deficit Disorder and Obsessive Compulsive Disorder.

❍ **What are the clinical characteristics of Klein-Levin syndrome?**

Periodic hypersomnolence and hyperphagia in a young man.

❍ **What are symptoms of Attention Deficit Disorder?**

Impulsivity, distractibility, and often hyperactivity.

❍ **What are some disorders of myelination in the CNS?**

Multiple sclerosis is an autoimmune disorder of central myelin.

Pelizaeus-Merzbacher is a hereditary CNS demyelinating disorder caused by a mutation in myelin proteolipid protein.

Metabolic demyelinating diseases include metachromatic leukodystrophy (deficiency of arylsulfatase A), adrenoleukodystrophy (faulty metabolism of very long chain fatty acids) and Krabbe's globoid cell leukodystrophy.

Central pontine myelinolysis, a catastrophic disruption of corticospinal pathways in the brainstem resulting in a "locked-in" syndrome, occurs with overrapid correction of hypo- or hypernatremia.

Progressive multifocal leukoencephalopathy (PML) is a viral patchy white matter encephalopathy (due to JC virus, but associated with HIV infection).

❍ **What are some disorders of peripheral nervous system myelin.**

Guillain-Barré Syndrome (GBS, a.k.a. acute inflammatory demyelinating polyradiculoneuropathy, AIDP) is an autoimmune attack on peripheral myelin, often after a viral or bacterial illness, resulting in sudden rapidly progressive weakness and areflexia. EMG shows slowing of nerve conduction and conduction block. Prognosis is worse if Campylobacter jejuni is involved. Treatment options include plasma exchanges or intravenous IgG.

CIDP (chronic immune demyelinating polyradiculoneuropathy) is a chronic or relapsing form of GBS. CIDP responds to steroids; GBS doesn't.

Charcot-Marie-Tooth is an autosomal recessive (usually) or X-linked (rarely) distal peripheral neuropathy; mutations in myelin membrane binding proteins (P_o) or connexin gap junction proteins result in progressive demyelination, distal weakness and atrophy with foot drop and a "stork-like" gait. There is also an axonal form (HSMN2).

❍ **What drugs act at the neuromuscular junction?**

d-Tubocurarine (curare) is a nicotinic AChR antagonist that binds to the receptor and prevents channel opening. It is used as a non-depolarizing neuromuscular blocker in general anesthesia. Succinylcholine binds to and persistently activates nAChRs, resulting in depolarization blockade and paralysis; it is also used for induction of general anesthesia. Neither agent depresses mental status! Anticholinesterases (neostigmine, pyridostigmine) prolong the duration of ACh in the synaptic cleft, and are used in treatment of MG. The tensilon (edrophonium) test is an anticholinesterase challenge that usually improves strength (or ptosis) rapidly but briefly in untreated patients. Alpha-bungarotoxin, a snake venom, binds to and blocks nAChRs.

❍ **What is the main excitatory neurotransmitter in brain?**

Glutamate.

❍ **What is the role of glutamate receptors in disease?**

Glutamate receptors, particularly kainate and NMDA receptors, have been implicated in excitotoxicity, a form of neuronal cell death induced by overstimulation by excitatory inputs resulting in accumulation of intracellular calcium ions. Excitotoxicity may be a mechanism involved in neurodegenerative diseases including Huntington's chorea and Alzheimer's disease.

❍ **What is the main inhibitory neurotransmitter in the brain?**

Gamma-aminobutyric acid

❍ **What drugs act at GABA receptors?**

Benzodiazepines (e.g. diazepam), barbiturates (phenobarbital), neurosteroids, and the novel anticonvulsant loreclezole enhance GABA receptors. They are inhibited by convulsants including bicuculline, picrotoxin, penicillin, and Zn^{++}.

❍ **What is the role of GABA receptors in disease?**

Loss of GABAnergic neurons may contribute to the development of epilepsy. GABA receptors are the site of action of many anticonvulsants and anxiolytics.

❍ What is the main inhibitory neurotransmitter in the spinal cord?

Glycine, an essential amino acid, is the major inhibitory transmitter in the spinal cord. Glycine receptors are blocked by strychnine and picrotoxin.

❍ What are the major monoamine neurotransmitters in the CNS?

Acetylcholine, epinephrine, norepinephrine, serotonin, dopamine, and histamine.

❍ What drugs act at CNS muscarinic acetylcholine receptors?

Antimuscarinic agents (atropine, scopolamine, etc.) and antimuscarinic side effects of other agents (e.g. tricyclic antidepressants) result in initial CNS excitation, irritability, hallucinations or delirium, progressing to coma and respiratory paralysis. Clinical uses include decreasing secretions or GI motility, paralyzing the iris, reversing bradycardia or bronchospasm, preventing motion sickness, and inducing sleep. Anticholinergics are sometimes helpful in treating early Parkinson's disease, especially for tremor, but can cause confusion, dry mouth, and urinary retention.

Anticholinesterases (physostigmine, neostigmine) are used to treat hypotonic bladder, glaucoma, and myasthenia gravis (see above). Tacrine (Cognex) and donepezil (Aricept) cause modest symptomatic improvement of Alzheimer's disease.

Organophosphate insecticides irreversibly inhibit AChE resulting in sweating, salivation, lacrimation, urination, defecation (SLUD), bradycardia, hypotension and death.

❍ What is the role of acetylcholine in CNS disease?

Loss of cholinergic neurons may be responsible for some of the symptoms of Alzheimer's Disease, and has led to use of AChE inhibitors in treatment (see above). A mutation in the membrane spanning region of the a4 subunit of the nicotinic AChR is likely responsible for autosomal dominant frontal lobe epilepsy; the disease mechanism is unknown.

❍ What pathologies are associated with dopamine?

Parkinson's disease (PD) results from loss of SNc dopaminergic neurons. Schizophrenia is undoubtedly related to dopamine receptor function, but the etiology remains elusive. Long-term treatment with neuroleptics can result in dopamine receptor upregulation and tardive dyskinesia/dystonia.

❍ What drugs act at CNS dopamine receptors?

Sinemet is a preparation of L-DOPA and carbidopa, which prevents peripheral metabolism of L-DOPA and reduces side effects (nausea). Bromocriptine is a direct dopamine agonist, used occasionally in PD, for suppression of pituitary prolactinomas, and formerly used to stop lactation (parlodel), but is now restricted due to incidence of hypertension, seizure and stroke. Antidopaminergics (neuroleptics) are used to treat psychosis/schizophrenia and other problems. Clozapine is an antipsychotic D4 receptor antagonist that does not exacerbate Parkinson's disease. Deprenyl, an MAO-type B inhibitor, provides minimal symptomatic benefit in early PD; latest analyses of the DATATOP study data no longer support a protective effect on SNc neurons.

❍ What drugs act as adrenergic receptors?

Alpha-2 agonist agents (clonidine) suppress sympathetic outflow in hypertension. Beta-1 receptors are found in the cerebral cortex and beta-2 in the cerebellum. Isoproterenol is a relatively pure beta-agonist. Deprenyl and pargyline are antidepressants that inhibit catabolism of epinephrine and NE by blocking MAO. Desipramine and other tricyclic antidepressants (TCA's) block NE reuptake. Amphetamine blocks reuptake and facilitates increased release of NE. Beta-blockers (propranolol, nadolol, atenolol, etc.) are used in hypertension, to prevent arrhythmias, and in migraine prophylaxis.

❍ **What drugs act on the serotonin system?**

Selective serotonin reuptake inhibitors (SSRIs, e.g. fluoxetine) are useful in major depression, obsessive-compulsive disorder and migraine. TCAs are less selective and also block reuptake of other monoamines. Reserpine and tetrabenazine block reuptake and storage of serotonin in granules, depleting serotonin stores. Sumatriptan is a $5HT_{1C}$ receptor agonist, used in migraine. Ondansetron, a $5HT_3$ antagonist, is a potent nonsedating antiemetic. The hallucinogen LSD is a $5HT_6$ or $5HT_7$ agonist. Clozapine is a $5HT_{6/7}$ antagonist. P-chlorophenylalanine blocks tryptophan hydroxylase.

❍ **What disease states have been linked to the serotonin system?**

You name it. Disturbances of 5HT systems are implicated in depression, obsessive-compulsive disorder, sleep disturbances, anxiety disorders, headache, chronic pain, schizophrenia, eating disorders, substance abuse, post-traumatic stress disorder, etc., etc.

❍ **What drugs act on histamine receptors?**

Antihistamines, of course, and the antihistamine side effects of drugs used for other problems. Doxepin, chlorpheniramine, pyrilamine and cyproheptadine are H1 antagonists; newer non-sedating agents include terfenadine (Seldane, don't give with erythromycin or ketoconazole). Meclizine (Antivert) is useful in Meniere's disease for temporary symptomatic relief. The sedative and weight gain side effects of TCA's (doxepin, amitriptyline) and antipsychotics (clozapine, thioridazine) may be due to anti-H1 effects. H2 antagonists are used in GI ulcer prophylaxis: cimetidine, ranitidine, etc.

❍ **What are the major peptide neurotransmitters in the CNS?**

Opioid peptides, substances P and Y, and "gut peptides" including somatostatin, colecystokinin, neurotensin, VIP, calcitonin gene-related peptide, corticotropin releasing factor, etc., are present in neurons, and may act as neurotransmitters or neuromodulators. Substance P is one of several tachykinin peptides, which is present in dorsal root ganglion neurons that project to the substantia gelatinosa of dorsal spinal cord (pain modulation), also in projection neurons from striatum back to substantia nigra.

❍ **What drugs act at opioid receptors?**

Narcotics (morphine, oxycodone, codeine, meperidine, heroin, etc.) act at mu receptors; naloxone is a mu receptor antagonist.

❍ **What is the diagnostic yield of lumbar puncture for organisms causing brain abscess?**

About 20%. Proximity to the ventricles or cortical edge (in contact with CSF) may affect results.

❍ **What is considered a safe time interval for acutely re-opening an internal carotid artery occlusion?**

About six hours. In the acute and subacute phases, the risk of reperfusion injury increases with time.

❍ **What percentage of the available cardiac output, glucose, and oxygen does the brain use?**

15 - 20% of that consumed by the entire body per unit time.

❍ **Below what value of cerebral perfusion pressure (CPP) is autoregulation of cerebral blood flow impaired?**

40 - 50 mm Hg: CPP = MAP - ICP, where MAP is mean arterial pressure and ICP is intracranial pressure.

❍ **How long should seizure prophylaxis be offered to a patient after severe traumatic brain injury?**

Seven days: After that, the risk/benefit ratio of prophylaxis increases. Effective agents include phenytoin and carbamazepine.

❍ **What is the recommended duration of antibiotic therapy for brain abscess?**

Six to eight weeks of intravenous antibiotics.

❍ **What are the CSF findings in a patient with subdural empyema?**

Normal glucose, mild pleiocytosis and protein elevation, and negative cultures. While CSF examination is rarely helpful, completely normal CSF makes the diagnosis unlikely.

❍ **What is appropriate empirical antibiotic therapy for spinal epidural abscess?**

A penicillinase-resistant anti-Staphylococcal penicillin, such as nafcillin or oxacillin: The majority of cases are caused by methicillin-sensitive Staphylococcus aureus.

❍ **What are the three most-common forms of disturbed water balance after traumatic brain injury?**

Diabetes insipidus, the syndrome of inappropriate antidiuretic hormone secretion, and cerebral salt-wasting.

❍ **What are the features of neurogenic pulmonary edema?**

1- Onset within 24 hours after brain injury of decreased lung compliance without elevation of the pulmonary capillary wedge (pulmonary artery occlusion) pressure
2- Diffuse roentgenographic infiltrates
3- Hypoxemia

This syndrome usually occurs after severe injuries as a result of alveolar flooding by protein rich, blood tinged fluid.

❍ **What are common electrocardiographic changes seen with brain injuries?**

Sinus tachycardia, QT-interval prolongation, and pan-precordial T-wave inversion. More severe findings include QRS-widening and ventricular tachycardia.

❍ **What cerebral artery is commonly injured in the setting of lateral transtentorial herniation?**

The posterior cerebral artery, most commonly, the calcarine branch.

❍ **Why is shock after spinal cord injury called "warm shock"?**

Disruption of the descending sympathetic tracts impairs vasoconstriction caudal to the injury.

❍ **Are fixed and dilated pupils only found with structural dysfunction?**

No. Metabolic dysfunction (e.g., hepatic encephalopathy) or toxins (e.g., atropinics) can give enlarged unreactive pupils.

❍ **What are "pontine pupils"?**

"Pinpoint," but reactive, pupils secondary to injury of the sympathetic fibers descending through the tegmentum. It results from intrinsic pontine tegmental injury or from cerebellar or other posterior fossa mass effect causing compression of the tegmentum: Narcotic administration causes similar pupillary findings.

❍ **What is meant by the term "communicating" (or "non-obstructive") hydrocephalus?**

All of the ventricles are dilated, including the cerebral aqueduct and basal cisterns: Obstructive hydrocephalus is either secondary to aqueductal stenosis or CSF outflow blocked by a mass.

❍ **Lesions containing what substances are of high attenuation on unenhanced CT scan?**

Blood, calcium, or melanin. High attenuation with blood results from the protein fraction of hemoglobin (92 - 93%), rather than the iron, which only contributes 7 - 8% to the brightness.

❍ **What are the two most common locations for cerebral contusions?**

The frontal and temporal poles.

❍ **Do anterior cord syndrome patients usually regain the ability to walk without assistance?**

Fewer than 50% do. Patients with central cervical cord injury usually do, but only about half of these patients regain useful hand function.

❍ **What diagnosis must be investigated in the patient presenting with pulsating exophthalmos?**

Carotid-cavernous fistula. Patients without a history of trauma, usually women, over forty years of age, often present with orbito-fronto-temporal headache, dilated conjunctival veins, and may have a sixth nerve palsy.

❍ **What are the two most common tumor types to develop after radiation therapy to the brain?**

Meningioma and fibrosarcoma.

❍ **What is the most common symptom of a glioblastoma multiforme?**

Headache, in 3/4 of patients.

❍ **What is the median postoperative survival for patients with glioblastoma multiforme who do not receive radiation therapy following surgery?**

Four months: Radiation therapy increases the median survival to 9 months.

❍ **Carotid bifurcation aneurysms may cause intracerebral hemorrhage into what areas of the brain?**

Frontal lobe, temporal lobe, and basal ganglia.

❍ **What is the risk of cerebral infarction in the first 5 years following posterior circulation transient ischemic attacks?**

35%.

❍ **What are the common presenting symptoms of a glomus jugulare tumor?**

Hearing loss and pulsatile tinnitus.

❍ **How long after spinal radiation does transverse myelitis occur?**

6 months to 5 years.

❍ **What is the most common tumor of the third ventricle?**

Colloid cyst.

❍ **What is the most common tumor of the sellar and parasellar region?**

Pituitary adenoma.

❍ **What is the most common primary posterior fossa tumor in adults?**

Hemangioblastoma, a histologically benign tumor found only in the neuraxis often associated with Von Hippel-Lindau disease.

❍ **Which tumor markers are secreted by certain pineal tumors?**

Alpha-fetoprotein is secreted by yolk sac tumors, endodermal sinus tumors, and embryonal carcinomas. Human chorionic gonadotropin is secreted by choriocarcinoma and embryonal cell carcinomas.

❍ **What is the most common endocrine disorder associated with suprasellar extension of pineal tumors?**

Diabetes insipidus.

❍ **What is the best treatment for symptomatic epidermoid and dermoid tumors?**

Complete surgical resection: Chemotherapy and radiation therapy play no role.

❍ **What is the most common initial symptoms of an acoustic neuroma?**

Tinnitus, hearing loss, and unsteadiness.

❍ **What is the 5-year survival of patients with intracranial ependymomas who undergo surgery and radiation therapy?**

Infratentorial 90%. Supratentorial 80%.

❍ **What condition sometimes requires emergency transphenoidal surgery?**

Pituitary apoplexy, fulminant expansion of a pituitary tumor due to infarction and hemorrhage. Need for surgery depends on status of and impending threat to the visual apparatus.

❍ **What symptoms related to lumbar disc herniation are indications for emergency surgery?**

Urinary retention, perineal numbness, and motor weakness of more than a single nerve root. These are findings suggestive of cauda equina compression.

❍ **An extreme lateral lumbar disc herniation at L4-5 typically compresses which nerve root?**

L4. Unlike more common medial disc herniations which compress the root exiting a level below, extreme lateral disc herniations compress the root exiting at that level.

❍ **What are potential causes of delayed neurological deterioration in patients following intracranial aneurysm rupture?**

Re-bleeding, vasospasm, hydrocephalus and seizures.

❍ **What is the most common location of a posterior fossa aneurysm?**

Basilar bifurcation. 15% of intracranial aneurysms are in the posterior fossa.

❍ **What species of bacteria is most commonly associated with mycotic aneurysms?**

Streptococcus. The next most common is Staphylococcus.

❍ **What are the most common clinical problems seen at the initial presentation of an intracranial arteriovenous malformation?**

Seizures and hemorrhage.

❍ **What is the management of an incidental venous angioma of the brain?**

No treatment is necessary.

❍ **A patient presenting with symptoms of neurogenic claudication would have what spinal condition?**

Lumbar spinal stenosis.

❍ **Do a normal EMG and nerve conduction studies rule out carpal tunnel syndrome?**

No. Studies may be normal in 25% of patients with carpal tunnel syndrome.

❍ **What spinal abnormality is commonly seen in rheumatoid arthritis?**

Atlanto-axial subluxation, present in 25% of patients.

❍ **What is the prevalence of obstructive sleep apnea in the United States?**

3%. Among persons aged 30 to 60, approximately 4% of men and 2% of women have obstructive sleep apnea syndrome.

❍ **What are the symptoms of narcolepsy?**

1- Cataplexy, a brief loss of strength following a display of emotion such as laughter, surprise, or anger; 2- Hypnagogic hallucinations; 3- Sleep paralysis; and 4-Sleep attacks. Recent reports suggest that all these symptoms except cataplexy may also occur in obstructive sleep apnea and other disorders of excessive daytime sleepiness.

❍ **What measures besides medication can be taken to help a patient with narcolepsy?**

Narcoleptics benefit from highly regular sleep schedules, one or several brief, scheduled naps during the day, and narcolepsy support groups.

❍ **What medications are useful in the treatment of cataplexy?**

Noradrenergic reuptake inhibitors and specifically tricyclic antidepressants are the agents most commonly used. Imipramine, clomipramine, desipramine, and protriptyline are effective. Fluoxetine can also help but may not be as effective.

❍ **A 47 year-old man cannot stay awake at work and is in danger of losing his job He falls asleep even at meetings with his supervisors. He had several near-miss accidents because of drowsiness while driving. He obtains 7 to 8 hours of sleep each night but is unrefreshed on awakening, even when he sleeps more. His wife states that he snores loudly at night, but she has never witnessed him stop breathing during his sleep. Could this patient still have obstructive sleep apnea?**

Yes. Although a bedpartner's observation of apneas during sleep can certainly increase the suspicion that sleep apnea is present, the absence of observed apneas in patients who have the disorder is common and may relate to the soundness of the bedpartner's sleep or other factors.

❍ **What other symptoms should you ask about?**

Nocturnal reflux, excessive sweating at night, nocturia, dry mouths or sore throats on awakening, morning headaches, difficulty with memory or concentration, or episodes of automatic behavior.

❍ **If this patient is confirmed to have obstructive sleep apnea, without any underlying neurological condition, what treatments might he be offered?**

Nasal continuous positive airway pressure (CPAP) is the most common treatment. Others include surgical procedures, oral appliances, medication (tricyclic antidepressants), and behavioral techniques.

❍ **In what sleeping position is obstructive sleep apnea usually worst?**

Supine. The tongue may be more likely to fall back into the throat.

❍ **A patient with a history and physical exam strongly suggestive of obstructive sleep apnea is given a portable sleep study at home, and has a normal result. What should you do next?**

Complete diagnostic polysomnography in a sleep laboratory. Portable sleep studies usually record several cardiorespiratory variables and can confirm a diagnosis of obstructive sleep apnea. However, a negative study does not have sufficient negative predictive value to rule out the possibility that obstructive sleep apnea would be demonstrated on a laboratory study.

❍ **A patient had a stroke within the last 2 weeks. Why might his or her risk for obstructive sleep apnea be high?**

Patients with transient ischemic attacks and no residual weakness, or with strokes have a high (about 70%) risk for obstructive sleep apnea. Strokes that affect the musculature of the upper airway might allow closure of the airway during sleep. Increasing evidence suggests sleep apnea may precede or contribute to stroke in many cases, but prospective studies are lacking.

❍ **What surgical techniques are used to treat obstructive sleep apnea?**

Uvulopalatopharyngoplasty (UPPP), tonsillectomy, genioglossal advancement, hyoid suspension, maxillary and mandibular advancement, and tracheostomy.

❍ **What disorders should be considered in the differential diagnosis of nocturnal paroxysmal dystonia?**

Other parasomnias (sleep terrors, sleep walking, confusional arousals, REM sleep behavior disorder) and epilepsy, especially frontal lobe epilepsy.

❍ **What are the current indications for treatment with melatonin?**

None. Melatonin is not classified as a drug in the USA Preparations of uncertain quality and dose are widely available but use should not be recommended until more information is gathered and reliable preparations are available.

❍ **What are typical sleep complaints of patients with Parkinson's disease?**

Insomnia, difficulty getting out of bed without help, getting to the bathroom, or turning over in bed. Patients may experience leg cramps, pain related to prolonged time in one position, limb jerking, nightmares, or hallucinations. Tremor usually disappears with sleep but may occur briefly during arousals, stage 2 sleep, or changes in sleep state.

❍ **How is melatonin secretion by the pineal gland regulated?**

Light information, relayed by the suprachiasmatic nucleus

❍ **What sleep problems are common in patients with Tourette's Syndrome?**

About half of these patients complain of insomnia and sleep walking is common.

❍ **A patient has complex partial seizures. During which stage of sleep are seizures least likely to occur?**

REM sleep. Interictal epileptiform activity is also least likely to appear in REM sleep.

❍ **In what stage of sleep do nightmares occur?**

REM sleep.

❍ **What are some symptoms commonly associated with repeated episodes of central sleep apnea?**

Insomnia, disrupted sleep due to frequent awakenings, and gasping for breath are described. Excessive daytime sleepiness is less common in patients with central sleep apnea than in those with obstructive sleep apnea.

❍ **With what neurological disorders is this condition often associated?**

Autonomic neuropathies (diabetes mellitus, Shy-Drager, familial dysautonomia), medullary dysfunction (post-polio syndrome, tumor, infarct, hemorrhage, or encephalitis), and neuromuscular diseases (muscular dystropy, myasthenia gravis).

❍ **What are some characteristics of sleep during acute alcohol withdrawal in alcoholics?**

Short total sleep time, sleep fragmentation, and decreased stages 3 and 4 sleep are seen. Sometimes increased REM sleep (REM rebound) occurs, since alcohol suppresses REM sleep.

❍ **What is the effect of most tricyclic medications on sleep architecture?**

REM sleep suppression. A "REM rebound" effect may be seen after withdrawal of tricyclics.

❍ **How long does it take to recover from jet lag?**

Generally, one day per hour of time zone changed.

❍ **What three types of headaches can be triggered by sleep.**

Migraine, cluster, and chronic paroxysmal hemicrania.

❍ **Which of these is more commonly reported to be relieved by sleep rather than triggered by it?**

Migraine.

❍ **A 21-year-old fell from a horse. The patient is unconscious and has decerebrate posturing. What is the diagnosis?**

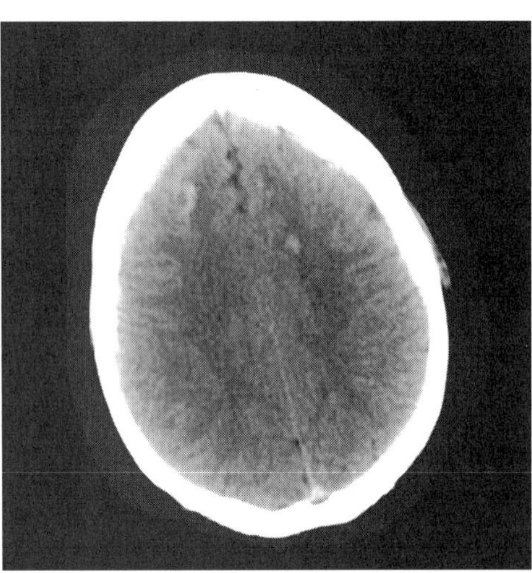

Petechial acute hemorrhages at the gray/white junction in a patient with diffuse axonal injury caused by shearing at the junction of axons and cell bodies from rotational forces.

❍ **A 66-year-old presents with new onset left ptosis. What is the diagnosis?**

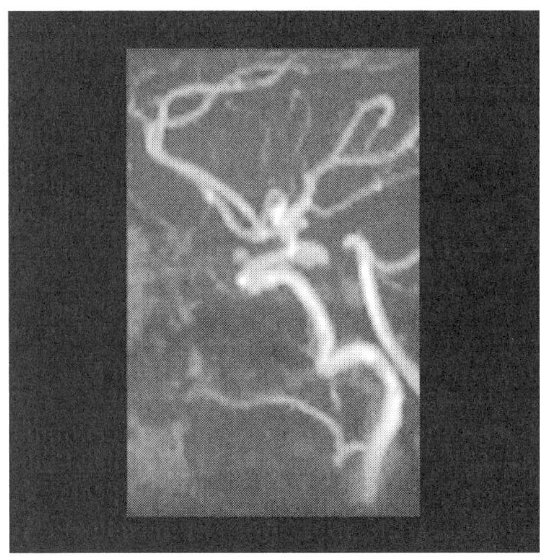

MR angiography demonstrates a large left posterior communicating artery aneurysm. Did you also note the left ophthlmic artery origin aneurysm? Not shown is a right posterior communicating artery aneurysm incidentally noted.

❍ **A 62-year-old patient presents with right shoulder pain. What is the diagnosis?**

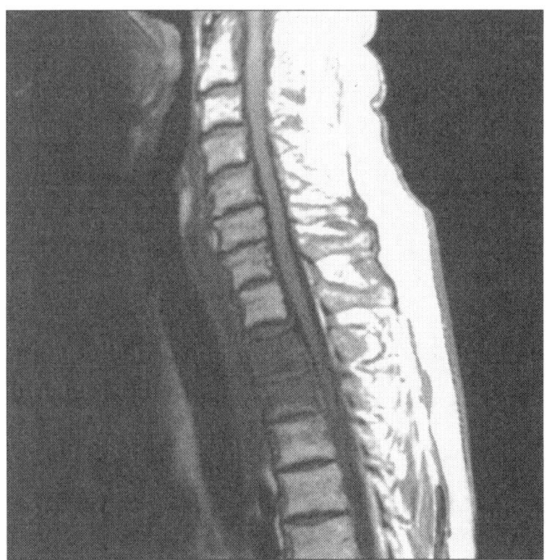

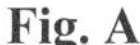

Fig. A

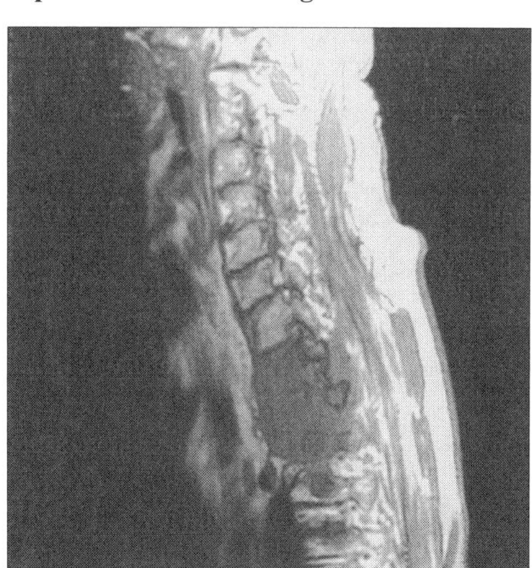

Fig. B

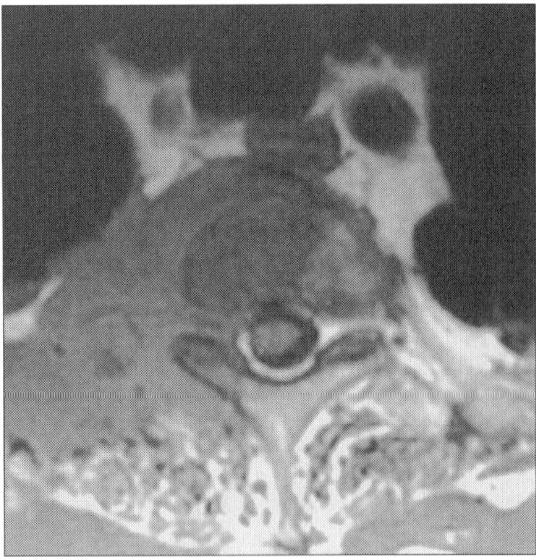

Fig. C

Sagittal (Fig. A and B) and axial T1 (Fig. C) noncontrast sections through the upper thoracic spine demonstrate a mass lesion involving both vertebral bodies and the nearby lung pleura with some extension into the epidural space on the right. This patient was subsequently shown to have a Pancoast tumor at biopsy.

❍ **A 36-year-old presents with altered mental status and history of a fall with severe headache. What is the diagnosis after viewing only the CT? (Fig. A)**

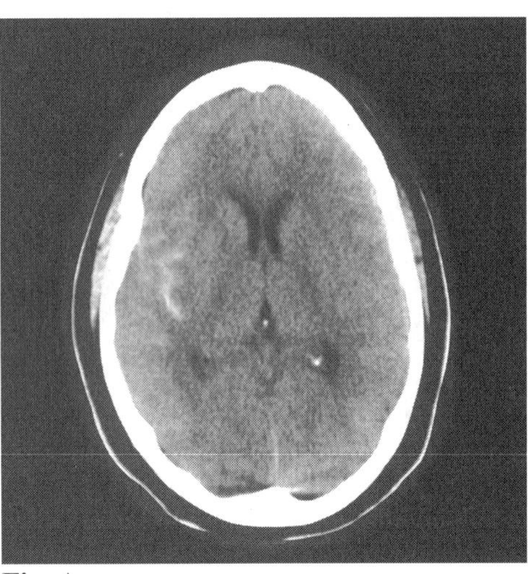

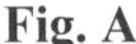

Fig. A

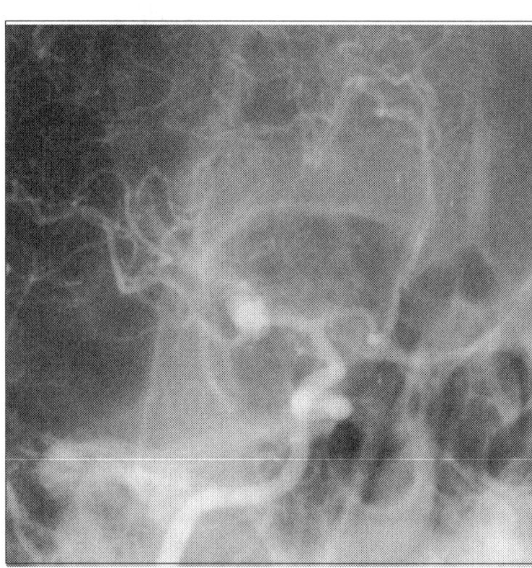

Fig. B

Acute right-sided subarachnoid hemorrhage confined mostly to the sylvian fissure. The differential diagnosis is between trauma and ruptured intracerebral aneurysm. In this patient, a large right middle cerebral artery trifurcation aneurysm is confirmed by contrast angiography. (Fig. B)

❍ **A 35-year-old presents with new onset inability to close the right eye. There are two separate findings.**

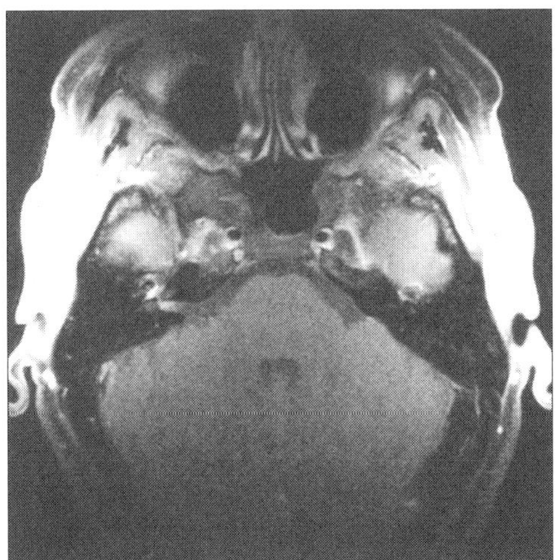
Fig. A

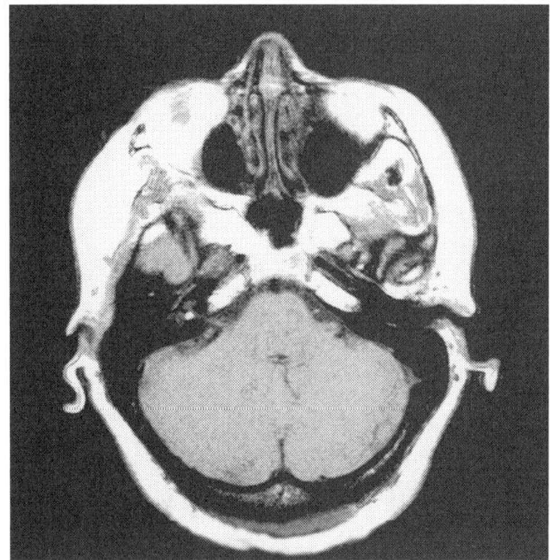
Fig. B

Enhancement along the course of the right 7th nerve in the internal auditory canal extending into the genu consistent with Bell's palsy (Fig. A). This should be followed to assure that it resolves as occasionally a small 7th nerve Schwannoma can have this appearance. Incidental note is also made on precontrast axial T1 sections of a small lipoma in the right IAC (Fig. B). Note that precontrast images are essential so as not to mistake a lipoma for an enhancing lesion and fat saturation is utilized on the post contrast images to suppress signal from the lipoma.

❍ **This is a 68-year-old with new onset right homonomous hemianopsia. Based on the images shown, what is the diagnosis? (Fig. A)**

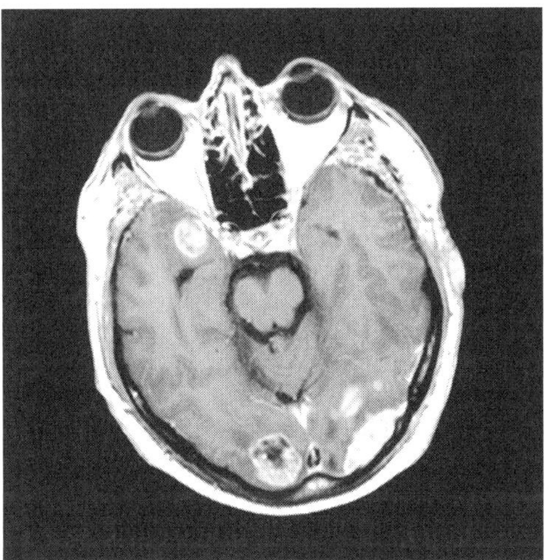
Fig. A

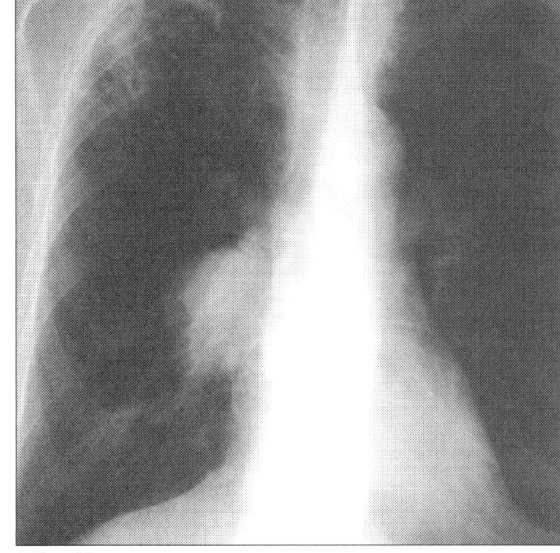
Fig. B

Multiple inhomogeneously enhancing lesions are present throughout the brain, several of which are shown here. The left occipital lesion would explain the patient's visual symptoms. The chest x-ray demonstrates a large mass in the right hilum (Fig. B) in this patient with lung carcinoma and multiple brain metastases.

❍ A 69-year-old presents with confusion of new onset. What is the diagnosis?

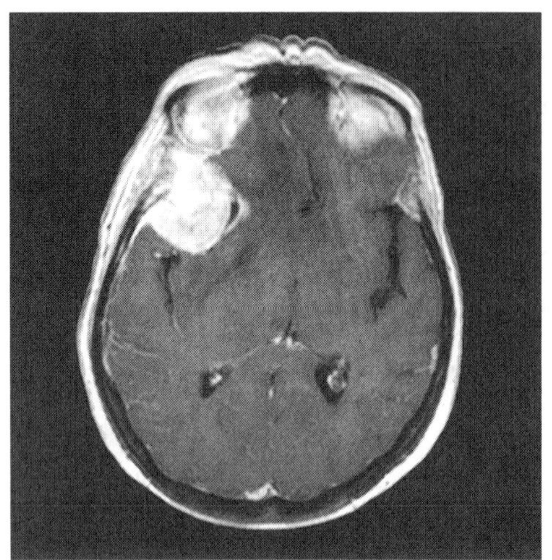

A large dural based enahncing mass with a dural tail arises near the greater wing of the sphenoid at the junction of the right frontal and temporal lobes. The mass has characteristics of an extra-axial lesion and is consistent with a meningioma. Note that the finding of a small dural tail of enhancement along the edge of the mass is quite characteristic of meningioma along with its broad-based dural attachment.

CLINICAL PHARMACOLOGY AND TOXICOLOGY

The young physician starts life with twenty drugs for each disease.
The old physician ends life with one drug for twenty diseases.
William Osler

❍ **Name 6 primary actions of cyclic antidepressant overdose.**

1) Inhibition of amine reuptake
2) Sodium channel blockade, which causes negative inotropy
3) Anticholinergic effects, primarily antimuscarinic
4) CNS depression
5) α-Adrenergic antagonism, which contributes further to hypotension
6) GABA antagonism

❍ **What is the appropriate treatment for QRS widening in tricyclic antidepressant (TCA) poisoning?**

$NaHCO_3$ is administered intravenously for patients with a QRS > 100 ms. One to two mEq/kg are initially administered and repeated until the blood pH is between 7.50 and 7.55 A continuous infusion of $NaHCO_3$, 3 amps in 1 L of D_5W, may then be initiated and titrated in over 4 to 6 hours to maintain an appropriate pH. Potassium levels must be closely monitored as supplementation may be required to prevent hypokalemia.

❍ **What is the appropriate treatment for TCA-induced seizures?**

Benzodiazepines and barbiturates are the agents of choice. Phenytoin is not generally effective. Bicarbonate and alkalosis are the main stays of treatment.

❍ **What TCA may induce seizures without concomitant cardiac toxicity?**

Amoxapine.

❍ **What is the treatment for TCA-induced hypotension?**

Isotonic saline and pepid alkalinization. If the patient is resistant to fluid resuscitation, a directly acting α-agonist, such as norepinephrine, should be started. Dopamine acts in part by releasing norepinephrine. This agent may already be depleted by the reuptake inhibition of the cyclic antidepressant and by stress.

❍ **What is the clinical presentation of anticholinergic poisoning?**

Mydriasis, tachycardia, hypoactive bowel sounds, urinary retention, dry axilla, hyperthermia, and mental status changes. Remember:

Dry as a bone,
Red as a beet,
Mad as a hatter,
Hot as hades,
Blind as a bat.

❍ **What period of observation is required prior to medically clearing a TCA overdose?**

6 hours.

❍ **A 32 year-old female is prescribed meperidine (Demerol) for an open fracture. The patient is chronically on fluoxetine (Prozac). What is a potential complication?**

The serotonin syndrome.

❍ **What signs and symptoms are typical of the serotonin syndrome?**

Agitation, anxiety, sinus tachycardia, hyperthermia shivering, tremor, hyperreflexia, myoclonus, muscular rigidity, and diarrhea.

❍ **What are potential pharmacological treatments for the serotonin syndrome?**

Serotonin antagonists, such as methysergide and cyproheptadine. Benzodiazepines and propranolol have also been successfully employed.

❍ **A patient chronically on Nardil, an MAO inhibitor, drinks a glass of red wine. What potential toxicity may result?**

The tyramine reaction.

❍ **A patient, who ingests a toxic quantity of an MAOI inhibitor, is in a hyperadrenergic state with a blood pressure of 240/160. What is the appropriate treatment?**

Short-acting antihypertensives, such as phentolamine and nitroprusside, should be employed because the patient may soon develop refractory hypotension.

❍ **What are the major pharmacological effects of neuroleptics?**

Blockade of dopamine, α-adrenergic, muscarinic, and histamine receptors.

❍ **What level of lithium is generally considered toxic?**

2.0 mEq/L.

❍ **Will charcoal bind lithium?**

No.

❍ **What are the signs and symptoms of lithium toxicity?**

Neurological signs and symptoms include tremor, hyperreflexia, clonus, fasciculations, seizures, and coma. GI signs and symptoms consist of nausea, vomiting, and diarrhea. Finally, signs and symptoms associated with CV are ST-T wave changes, bradycardia, conduction defects, and arrhythmias.

❍ **What is the treatment for lithium toxicity?**

Supportive care, normal saline diuresis, hemodialysis for patients with clinical signs of severe poisoning, i.e., seizures and arrhythmias, renal failure, or decreasing urine output.

❍ **What is the pharmacological effect of barbiturates and benzodiazepines?**

Both enhance chloride influx through the GABA receptor-associated chloride channel. Benzodiazepines increase the frequency of channel opening, whereas barbiturates increase the duration of channel opening.

❍ **Alkalization of the urine is beneficial in the management of what barbiturates?**

Long-acting barbiturates, such as phenobarbital.

❍ **What syndrome is atypical for sedative hypnotics but unique to glutethimide?**

Anticholinergic poisoning syndrome.

❍ **What is the mixture of alcohol and chloral hydrate commonly called?**

A "Mickey Finn."

❍ **At what rate is alcohol metabolized in an acutely intoxicated person?**

About 20 mg/dl/hour.

❍ **What is the pharmacological treatment for alcohol withdrawal?**

Benzodiazepines or barbiturates.

❍ **Isopropanol is metabolized by what enzyme to what metabolite?**

Isopropanol is metabolized by alcohol dehydrogenase to acetone in the liver.

❍ **What is a normal osmolar gap?**

< 10 mOsm.

❍ **What is the toxic metabolic end product in methanol poisoning?**

Formic acid.

❍ **What cofactor is required to convert formic acid to carbon dioxide and water?**

Folate. Leucovorin, folinic acid, the active form of folate, is preferentially administered at 1 mg/kg. Folate may be substituted at the same dose if leucovorin is not available.

❍ **Is $NaHCO_3$ beneficial in the management of methanol poisoning?**

Yes. In animal models, maintenance of a normal pH through bicarbonate administration decreased toxicity, including visual impairment.

❍ **What methanol level mandates dialysis?**

50 mg/dl. Other indications include visual impairment, severe metabolic acidosis, and ingestion of greater than 30 cc.

❍ **What cofactors are administered to a patient with ethylene glycol poisoning?**

Thiamine and pyridoxine. These cofactors will aid in transforming glyoxylic acid to nontoxic metabolites. Both are administered intravenously in 100 mg increments.

❍ **Name the three clinical phases of ethylene glycol poisoning?**

Stage I: Neurological symptomatology (i.e., inebriation)
Stage II: Metabolic acidosis and cardiovascular instability
Stage III: Renal failure

❍ **When should dialysis be initiated for an ethylene glycol poisoning case?**

When the serum level is > 25 mg/dl, or when renal insufficiency or severe metabolic acidosis occurs.

❍ **Which valve is most commonly infected in an IV drug-abuser?**

The tricuspid valve, usually by Staphylococcus aureus.

❍ **What is the toxic dose of naloxone?**

None. Narcan is a safe drug and may be given in large quantities. The usual adult dosage is 2 mg IV; the usual pediatric dose is 0.01 mg/kg. Narcan may precipitate acute withdrawal and may therefore be titrated to effect.

❍ **What is the etiology of non-cardiogenic pulmonary edema after heroin injection?**

Unknown. May be delayed 24 to 48 hour after injection, although most patients present immediately after injection. Treatment is the same as with any patient with ARDS.

❍ **How does treatment for a cocaine-induced MI differ from a typical MI?**

Both are treated the same except that beta-blockers must be used in concert with nitrates and calcium channel blockers to reverse the intense coronary vasospasm that occurs with cocaine. The tachycardia of a cocaine associated MI is first treated with benzodiazepine sedation.

❍ **What is the mechanism of salicylate toxicity?**

Salicylates uncouple oxidative phosphorylation and thereby halt cellular ATP production.

❍ **Which acid-base disturbance is typical for salicylate poisoning?**

Mixed respiratory alkalosis, secondary to central respiratory center stimulation, and metabolic acidosis, secondary to uncoupling of oxidative phosphorylation.

❍ **T/F: A patient who ingests a large amount of enteric-coated aspirin, but is asymptomatic for six hours in the emergency department, may be safely discharged home.**

False. The enteric coating delays absorption. Any patient who has ingested 150 mg/kg of enteric coated aspirin should be admitted to the hospital to determine serial salicylate levels and for observation.

❍ **A patient has an arterial pH of 7.5 through alkalization, but her urine pH is still low. What electrolyte is probably responsible?**

Potassium. When reabsorbing sodium, the renal tubules will preferentially excrete hydrogen ions into the tubular lumen rather than potassium ions. Thus, potassium should be maintained at 4.0 mmol/L.

❍ **What is the treatment for a prolonged prothrombin time in salicylate poisoning?**

Parenteral vitamin K_1 administration. Salicylates inhibit vitamin K_1 epoxide reductase in poisoning, resulting in an ability for the inactive vitamin K_1 epoxide to be regenerated into the active vitamin K_1.

❍ **What are the indications for dialysis in salicylate poisoning?**

Persistent CNS involvement, ARDS, renal failure, severe acid-base disturbance despite appropriate care, acute salicylate level > 100 mg/dl.

❍ **Can a patient present with salicylate poisoning and a therapeutic level?**

Yes. Patients with chronic salicylate poisoning have a large Vd and thus may present with mental status changes and a therapeutic level.

❍ **What are the 4 stages of acetaminophen (APAP) poisoning?**

Stage I:30 minutes to 24 hours, nausea and vomiting
Stage II:24 to 48 hours, abdominal pain and elevated LFT's
Stage III:72 to 96 hours, LFT's peak, nausea and vomiting
Stage IV: 4 days to 2 weeks, resolution or fulminant hepatic failure

❍ **APAP poisoning produces which type of hepatic necrosis?**

Centrilobular necrosis. The toxic metabolite of APAP is generated in the liver via the P-450 system, which is located in the centrilobular region.

❍ **What is the toxic metabolite of APAP?**

NAPQI. When the glucuronidation and sulfation pathways are saturated, APAP is metabolized by the

P-450 system to the toxic metabolite N-acetyl-para-benzoquinoneimine (NAPQI).

❍ **What hepatic laboratory parameter is the first to become abnormal in APAP poisoning?**

The prothrombin time (PT).

❍ **An acutely intoxicated, nonalcoholic, otherwise healthy patient ingests APAP. Is this patient more or less likely to develop hepatotoxicity?**

Less likely. An acute ingestion of alcohol will tie up the P-450 system thereby inhibiting the formation of NAPQI. A chronic alcoholic has an induced P-450 system and will suffer greater APAP hepatic toxicity through increased NAPQI formation.

❍ **According to the Rumack-Matthew nomogram, at what four hour APAP level should treatment be initiated?**

150 mg/ml.

❍ **How is the nomogram utilized in a patient who ingests an Extended Relief formulation of APAP?**

4 hour and 8 hour levels are obtained. If either level is in the "possible" hepatotoxic range, the patient should be treated.

❍ **What is the proposed mechanism of theophylline-induced seizures?**

Adenosine antagonism. Adenosine is released into the synaptic cleft from presynaptic terminals along with excitatory neurotransmitters. Adenosine binds to presynaptic adenosine receptors, inhibiting the release of more excitatory neurotransmitters.

❍ **What is the appropriate initial treatment of theophylline-induced seizures?**

Benzodiazepines and barbiturates. Theophylline-induced seizures warrant hemodialysis or hemoperfusion.

❍ **What is the treatment of theophylline-induced hypotension?**

Fluid administration and beta-blockers. Theophylline-induced cardiovascular instability is secondary to beta-agonist effects. Therefore, beta-blockers can be beneficial in the treatment of arrhythmias and hypotension.

❍ **What are absolute indications for hemodialysis or hemoperfusion in theophylline toxicity?**

Seizures or arrhythmias that are unresponsive to conventional therapy.

❍ **Why is multidose activated charcoal administration advocated for theophylline poisoning?**

Theophylline undergoes enterohepatic circulation.

❍ **What abnormal laboratory parameters are typical in a patient with acute theophylline poisoning?**

Hypokalemia, hyperglycemia, and leukocytosis. The beta-agonist properties of theophylline produce these abnormalities.

❍ **What are the absolute indications for Digibind administration in digoxin poisoning?**

Ventricular arrhythmias, hemodynamically significant bradyarrhythmias that are unresponsive to standard therapy, and a potassium level greater than 5.0 mEq/L.

❍ **Why is calcium chloride administration contraindicated in digoxin poisoning?**

Digoxin inhibits the Na^+-K^+-ATPase. This mechanism increases the intracellular concentration of sodium. The sodium-calcium exchange pump is then activated, which leads to high intracellular concentrations of calcium. Calcium chloride administration would further increase intracellular calcium, which would cause myocardial irritability.

❍ **Can the digoxin level be followed after the administration of Digibind?**

No. Extremely elevated digoxin levels are measured after Digibind administration.

❍ **A patient on Digoxin is bradycardic and hypotensive with significantly peaked T waves. What is the initial line of treatment?**

Administer 10 vials of Digibind intravenously while simultaneously treating the presumed hyperkalemia with insulin and glucose, sodium bicarbonate, and Kayexalate. After the Digibind is administered, hyperkalemic-induced arrhythmias may safely be treated with calcium chloride.

❍ **What is the antidote for beta-blocker poisoning?**

Glucagon.

❍ **What is the biochemical rational for treatment with glucagon?**

Glucagon receptors, located on myocardial cells, are G protein-coupled receptors that activate adenylate cyclase, leading to increased levels of intracellular c-AMP. Thus, glucagon administration causes the same intracellular effect as beta-agonist.

❍ **A 25 year-old female presents status post ingestion of a sustained release calcium channel blocker. What is the disposition?**

Hospital admission to a monitored setting. Sustained release preparations have the capability of producing delayed toxicity.

❍ **What are potential treatment modalities for a calcium channel blocker poisoning?**

Admit symptomatic patients to an intensive care unit; treatment can be guided by pulmonary artery catheter hemodynamic measurements. Therapeutic interventions include IV calcium, isoproterenol, glucagon, transvenous pacer, atropine, and vasopressors, such as norepinephrine, epinephrine, or dopamine.

❍ **What is the mechanism and treatment for clonidine-induced hypotension?**

Mechanism: Decreased cardiac output secondary to a decreased sympathetic outflow from the CNS.

Treatment: Includes IV fluid administration and dopamine.

❍ **What typical eye response is related to clonidine poisoning?**

Pinpoint pupils.

❍ **At what adrenergic receptor is clonidine active?**

Clonidine is an α-2 agonist.

❍ **Does oral phenytoin poisoning require cardiac monitoring in an otherwise healthy patient?**

No. Oral phenytoin poisoning has resulted in arrhythmias in only two case reports. These two individuals had previous underlying cardiac abnormalities.

❍ **What is the pharmacological basis of the anticonvulsant effect of phenytoin?**

Sodium channel blockade.

❍ **Why does IV phenytoin administration lead to cardiovascular toxicity?**

The propylene glycol diluent is a myocardial depressant and vasodilator.

❍ **What are the four stages of iron poisoning?**

Stage I: Initial hour; gastrointestinal symptomatology, which is abdominal pain, vomiting, and diarrhea secondary to the corrosive effects of iron
Stage II: 6 to 24 hours; quiescent period during which iron is absorbed
Stage III: > 12 hours; shock, metabolic acidosis, hepatic dysfunction, heart failure, cerebral dysfunction, and renal failure
Stage IV: 1 day to 1 week; gastric outlet or small bowel obstruction secondary to scarring

❍ **What dose of iron is expected to produce clinical toxicity?**

20 mg/kg of elemental iron.

❍ **What 4 hour iron level is generally considered toxic?**

300 to 350 mg/dl.

❍ **What are indications for deferoxamine therapy?**

1) All symptomatic patients exhibiting more than merely transient symptomatology
2) Patients with lethargy, significant abdominal pain, hypotension, or metabolic acidosis
3) Patients with a positive KUB
4) Any symptomatic patient with a level greater than 300 mg/dl

❍ **What is the standard dose of deferoxamine?**

15 mg/kg/hour continuous IV infusion.

❍ **What are the criteria for stopping deferoxamine therapy?**

1) The patient must be asymptomatic.
2) A KUB must be negative.
3) The serum iron concentration must be normal or low. Most laboratories cannot accurately measure serum iron in the presence of deferoxamine. Therefore, the iron level should be less than 100 mg/dl in these facilities.
4) The vin rose urine should clear.

❍ **Chronic solvent abusers develop what metabolic complication?**

Renal tubular acidosis.

❍ **Carbon tetrachloride poisoning produces which type of liver damage?**

Centrilobular necrosis.

❍ **Methylene chloride is metabolized to which toxin?**

Carbon monoxide.

❍ **Oral hydrofluoric acid exposure may result in what life-threatening electrolyte abnormalities?**

Hyperkalemia and hypocalcemia.

❍ **What is the antidote for cutaneous hydrofluoric acid exposures?**

Intradermal injection or intra-arterial infusion of calcium gluconate.

❍ **What enzyme is inhibited by organophosphates?**

Cholinesterase.

❍ **What are the two principle antidotes used for organophosphate poisoning?**

Atropine and pralidoxime.

❍ **What is the mechanism of cyanide toxicity?**

Electron transport inhibition. Cyanide binds to the ferric ion in cytochrome oxidase.

❍ **What antihypertensive agent may induce cyanide poisoning?**

Nitroprusside. One molecule of sodium nitroprusside contains five molecules of cyanide. To prevent toxicity with long duration infusions, sodium thiosulfate should be infused with sodium nitroprusside at a ratio of 10:1, thiosulfate to nitroprusside. Beware of thiocyanate toxicity!

❍ **What is "arterialization" of venous blood?**

High partial pressure of oxygen in venous blood. In cyanide poisoning, electron transport is inhibited that leads to an inability to utilize oxygen as an electron acceptor. Therefore, venous blood will contain a high partial pressure of oxygen.

❍ **A patient who is chronically on an oral hypoglycemic agent presents with a depressed mental status. Bedside glucose level is 20 mg/dl. After an amp of D_{50} is administered, the patient returns to a normal mental status rapidly. What is the disposition of this patient?**

Hospital admission with serial glucose level determination. Oral hypoglycemic agents are long acting thus, patients must be admitted and observed for recurrent hypoglycemia.

❍ **What is the antidote for isoniazid-induced seizures?**

Pyridoxine. Dose intravenously gram for gram. For unknown overdoses, administer 5 grams.

❍ **A patient is administered a topical Cetacaine spray prior to an endoscopy. The patient then complains of shortness of breath and is noted to be cyanotic. What is the antidote?**

Methylene blue, 1 mg/kg intravenously. Methemoglobinemia developed secondary to the local anesthetic.

❍ **A 32 year-old female complains of vomiting and diarrhea which developed eight hours after ingesting an unknown type of mushroom. Is the mushroom potentially a hepatotoxin?**

Yes. Hepatotoxic cyclopeptide-containing mushrooms induce a delayed onset of gastrointestinal symptomatology, generally occurring 6 hours after ingestion. The benign mushrooms with gastrointestinal toxins induce symptomatology within 0.5 to 3 hours.

❍ **A patient presents with seizures 6 hours status post mushroom ingestion. What is the antidote?**

Atropine.

❍ **What is the treatment for cyanide overdose?**

1) Place on oxygen, CPR P.R.N.
2) Provide amyl nitrite pearle inhaled.
3) Administer sodium nitrite: 10 ml of 3% solution in an adult, which is 300 mg, or 0.2 to 0.33 ml/kg in a child.
4) Administer sodium thiosulfate at five times the volume of sodium nitrite, 12.5 mg in an adult, which is 50 ml of a 25% solution, or 1.0 to 1.5 ml/kg in a child.

❍ **The mechanism of action for nitrates in the above response is not completely understood, although the formation of methemoglobin is presumably important. Methemoglobin rapidly combines with cyanide to form cyanomethemoglobin. Now that cyanide has been stripped off its binding site to cytochrome A_3, how is the cyanomethemoglobin handled?**

The intrinsic enzyme, rhodanese, catalyzes the transport of cyanide from cyanomethemoglobin to sulfur forming thiocyanate. This reaction is limited by sulfur availability. Sodium thiosulfate is administered to act as a sulfur donor. Thiocyanate is excreted by the kidney.

❍ **What order are the kinetics of elimination for an ASA overdose?**

Zero-order elimination with hepatic enzymatic clearance saturated and renal clearance becoming important.

❍ **Remember to think of ASA poisoning when a patient presents with mental status changes associated with respiratory alkalosis and metabolic acidosis. Recall that salicylate toxicity can be associated with elevated, normal, or decreased glucose levels. What mechanisms induce hyperglycemia and hypoglycemia?**

Hyperglycemia is caused by salicylate-induced mobilization of glycogen, whereas hypoglycemia is caused by the salicylate inhibition of gluconeogenesis.

❍ **Is ARDS more likely to be a complication of acute ASA poisoning or chronic ASA poisoning?**

Chronic.

❍ **What is the "magic number" for the dose of a non-enteric-coated ASA that must be exceeded to cause toxicity (mg/kg)?**

150 mg/kg.

❍ **What is the 'magic number" for the dose of an enteric-coated ASA that must be exceeded to require admission for observation and for the determination of serial salicylate levels?**

150 mg/kg.

❍ **Metabolic acidosis favors the formation of which form of salicylate, ionized or un-ionized?**

Un-ionized. This is crucial in two respects:

1) It is the reason to therapeutically produce an alkaline urine. More of the free salicylate is thereby converted to the ionized form that cannot be reabsorbed by tubules and is instead excreted.
2) It is the reason for the large changes in amount of free drug that diffuses into the tissue. Small decreases in pH result in decreased protein binding. Therefore, more salicylate in the un-ionized form diffuses into tissue increasing its volume of distribution. Remember to always treat the patient and not the level-serum levels can decrease as salicylate moves into tissue!

❍ **Under what circumstance is the use of A.D. Done's nomogram appropriate?**

Only when the patient has an acute single ingestion of a non-enteric-coated ASA without recent prior use.

❍ **Is hemodialysis used to treat salicylate toxicity?**

Yes. For severely poisoned patients, i.e., coma, ARDS, cardiac toxicity, serum levels > 100 mg/dl, and for patients who are unresponsive to maximal therapy.

❍ **What minimum ingestion level of acetaminophen (N-acetyl-para-aminophenol, APAP) is necessary to cause hepatic toxicity in an adult? In a child?**

7.5 g.

❍ **How is APAP usually metabolized in non-overdose conditions?**

Most APAP is metabolized is by glucuronidation. However, some APAP metabolism occurs in conjugation with sulfate. This percentage increases with decreasing age. Four percent or less APAP is transformed into an extremely toxic intermediary compound by P-450 MFO's. It is theorized that this toxic intermediary immediately conjugates with glutathione and is harmlessly excreted in the urine.

❍ **How does N-acetylcysteine (NAC, Mucomyst) work?**

The precise mechanism is still not well understood. However, it is known that NAC enters cells and is metabolized to cysteine, which serves as a glutathione precursor.

❍ **Which measure of hepatic function is a better prognostic indicator in APAP overdose: liver enzyme levels or bilirubin level and prothrombin time?**

Bilirubin level and prothrombin time.

❍ **Clonidine is a centrally acting presynaptic α-2 adrenergic agonist that decreases the central sympathetic outflow. Although its primary use is to treat hypertension, clonidine has additional emergency value in blunting withdrawal symptoms from opiates and ethanol. A clonidine overdose closely resembles an overdose with which other class of drugs?**

Opiates.

❍ **Toxicity from clonidine (Catapress) usually occurs within what time period?**

Within 4 hours.

❍ **Which agent is a useful "antidote" for clonidine overdose?**

Naloxone.

❍ **What are a few substances that have anticholinergic properties?**

Antihistamines, cyclic antidepressants, phenothiazine, atropine, amanita sp., Jimson weed.

❍ **What ECG abnormality is most common in patients who suffer from anticholinergic toxicity?**

Sinus tachycardia. Other dangerous arrhythmias include conduction problems and ventricular tachycardia.

❍ **Digitalis increases myocardial inotropy by inhibiting Na^+-K^+-ATPase, thereby allowing intracellular Na^+ to increase. More substrate thus is provided for the Na^+-Ca^{2+} membrane exchange which leads to elevated intracellular (sarcoplasmic) Ca^{2+} concentrations. Does it also increase vagal tone and slow conduction through the AV node?**

Yes.

❍ **Serum potassium can soar to very high levels with acute digitalis toxicity. Is this also true for chronic digitalis poisoning?**

No, not really.

❍ **T/F: A patient with acute digitalis overdose presents with frequent multifocal PVC's, peaked T waves, and a K^+ of 6.2 mEq/L. The correct treatment is to first administer $CaCl_2$, as this is the fastest acting agent for reducing hyperkalemia.**

False! Although $CaCl_2$ is the fastest acting agent for decreasing hyperkalemia, you don't want to give any more Ca^+ to a patient with digitalis-induced cardiac toxicity.

❍ **What are the signs and symptoms of phenytoin toxicity?**

Seizure, heart blocks, bradyarrhythmias, hypotension, and coma. All dangerous cardiovascular complications of phenytoin overdose result from parenteral administration. High levels after oral doses do not cause such signs in a stable patient.

❍ **What is the treatment for a phenytoin overdose?**

Systemic support, charcoal, atropine for bradyarrhythmias, and phenobarbital, 20 mg/kg IV, for seizures.

❍ **Nystagmus, ataxia, and lethargy generally occur at what serum level of phenytoin?**

Nystagmus: 20 mg/ml
Ataxia: 30 mg/ml
Lethargy: 40 mg/ml

❍ **What rhythm and ECG findings are expected with phenytoin toxicity?**

Bradycardia, AV block, ventricular tachycardia, VF, and asystole. ECG findings might also include increased PR interval and a wide QRS.

❍ **Beta-adrenergic antagonists have what three main effects on the heart?**

Negative chronotropy
Negative inotropy
Decrease AV nodal conduction velocity

❍ **T/F: Beta-adrenergic antagonists can cause mental status changes and seizures.**

True.

❍ **A patient with a history of cyclic antidepressant overdose is found awake and alert by paramedics. What is the prognosis?**

25 to 50% of patients who die from cyclic overdose are awake and alert at the scene.

❍ **In cyclic antidepressant overdose, is the degree of toxicity closely related to QRS duration?**

QRS > 100 ms has a specificity of 75% and a sensitivity of 60% for serious complications. A normal ECG will not rule out a serious overdose! Of those with QRS > 100 ms, 30% will seize; of those with QRS > 160 ms, 50% will develop arrhythmias.

❍ **How is pulmonary edema associated with heroin use treated?**

Naloxone and ventilatory support. Diuretics, digitalis, and rotating tourniquets are not effective.

❍ **What is the treatment for narcotic overdose?**

Naloxone, 0.4 to 2.0 mg in an adult. Naloxone's duration of action is about 1 hour. Higher doses and continuous infusion may be required.

❍ **A cocaine addict presents with chest pain but his ECG is normal. What are the odds that he will have abnormal CPK and CPK-MB isoenzymes?**

6 to 19%.

❍ **What is the most common cause of chronic heavy metal poisoning?**

Lead.

❍ **Organophosphates are found in what kinds of compounds?**

Pesticides, flame retardants and plasticizers.

❍ **What is an iatrogenic source of cyanide?**

Nitroprusside.

❍ **What are the constituent gases of hydrogen cyanide?**

Ammonia (NH_3) and methane (CH_4).

❍ **What is the rate limiting step in the metabolism of ethanol?**

The conversion of ethanol to acetaldehyde by alcohol dehydrogenase.

❍ **T/F: In a lethargic or unresponsive, ethanol intoxicated patient, there is little need to search for further pathology.**

False. Before attributing a change in mental status simply to alcohol intoxication other etiologies such as hypoglycemia, subdural hematoma, hypothermia, subarachnoid bleed, or ingestion of other drugs must be considered.

❍ **What is the most common arrhythmia induced by chronic, heavy ethanol binge ?**

Atrial fibrillation.

❍ **In a non-drinker what blood ethanol level will cause confusion or stupor?**

180mg/dl to 300mg/dl.

❍ **In a nondrinker, what is the minimum blood alcohol level that can cause coma?**

300mg/dl.

❍ **In chronic alcohol users, alcohol withdrawal seizures occur approximately how many hours after cessation of heavy alcohol consumption?**

6-48 hours from the time of the last drink.

❍ **T/F: In chronic heavy alcohol users a normal serum magnesium generally reflects normal total body magnesium levels.**

False. Heavy or chronic alcohol users are very likely to have total body magnesium deficits and generally require magnesium supplementation.

❍ **Delirium tremens occur how long after the cessation of alcohol consumption?**

On average 3-5 days.

❍ **What is the only proven means to enhance ethanol elimination?**

Hemodialysis.

❍ **Is there a role for phenytoin in the prevention or treatment of pure alcohol withdrawal seizures?**

No. Careful titration of benzodiazepines or Phenobarbital should be used if necessary.

❍ **What is the class of drugs currently felt to best treat Delirium Tremens?**

Benzodiazepines. Other drugs have been suggested such as clonidine, Phenobarbital and beta blockers. However, current literature favors benzodiazepines, such as Valium or Ativan along with hydration and supportive therapy.

❍ **T/F: Status epilepticus is commonly seen in alcohol withdrawal seizures.**

False. Status epilepticus is rare in alcohol withdrawal seizures and should suggest the need to find other causative pathology.

❍ **Chronic alcohol abusers who are poorly nourished may develop Wernicke's encephalopathy as a result of what deficiency?**

Thiamine.

❍ **What is the classic triad of Wernicke's encephalopathy?**

Global confusion, oculomotor disturbances and ataxia.

❍ **Alcoholic patients are at greater risk for what type of pneumonia?**

Aspiration pneumonia. They are also at increased risk for Klebsiella pneumonia when compared to the general population.

❍ **What is the likely diagnosis in a chronic heavy alcohol abuser with the following history: little or no alcohol ingested for the past 1-2 days, abdominal pain, recurrent nausea and vomiting, decreased food intake, dehydration, a high anion gap acidosis and positive serum and urine ketones?**

Alcoholic ketoacidosis.

Methanol.

❍ **Which of the following alcohol intoxications may present with calcium oxalate crystals in the urine: methanol, isopropyl alcohol or ethylene glycol?**

Ethylene glycol.

❍ **Are ethylene glycol levels necessary to determine toxicity or institute therapy?**

No. The diagnosis of ethylene glycol toxicity can be based on history , clinical exam and examination of the urine. Urine may show calcium oxalate crystals. Labs should reveal metabolic acidosis. Ethylene glycol levels should be sent. If there will be a delay until the results are available, therapy can be started.

❍ **What is the treatment for ethylene glycol toxicity?**

Ethanol, usually by IV infusion, and sodium bicarbonate by IV infusion. Hemodialysis may be required. A new medication, IV fomepizole, has recently been released to replace the use of ethanol.

❍ **T/F: Ethylene glycol is found most commonly in antifreeze/coolant fluids.**

True.

❍ **What is the approximate lethal dose ingestion of ethylene glycol?**

0.5-1.0 ml/kg or about 100 ml. However, ingestions of as little as 0.1ml/kg of pure ethylene glycol may result in potentially toxic levels.

❍ **Peak levels of ethylene glycol occur how many hours after ingestion?**

1 - 4 hours.

❍ **What constellation of findings should prompt consideration of ethylene glycol toxicity?**

Ethanol-like intoxication (with no odor), large anion gap acidosis, increased osmolal gap, altered mental status leading to coma, and calcium oxalate crystals in the urine

❍ **In a methanol overdose, what is the serum level of methanol at which hemodialysis is generally recommended?**

50mg/dl .

❍ **What is the accepted antidote for methanol poisoning?**

Ethanol administration. It is usually administered intravenously to maintain ethanol level between 100 - 150 mg/dl. Patients with high serum levels or who are very ill may also require hemodialysis. If dialysis is performed the dose of alcohol must be increased.

❍ **What are 4 indications for the use of ethanol in methanol overdose?**

1- Peak methanol level over 20mg/dl.
2- History of ingestion of 0.4 ml/kg of methanol or more. Even smaller ingestions can be toxic.
3- Acidosis
4- Consideration for hemodialysis

❍ **Hypocalcemia is most common in which alcohol ingestion: ethylene glycol, methanol, ethanol or isopropyl alcohol?**

Ethylene glycol.

❍ **In which type of alcohol ingestion may the urine appear to fluoresce under a Woods lamp?**

Ethylene glycol.

❍ **Is activated charcoal of any value in ethylene glycol or methanol ingestions?**

Yes. According to recent literature activated charcoal has been advocated. Although it is not considered definitive therapy, it is considered a part of supportive therapy.

❍ **T/F: In significant theophylline toxicity activated charcoal should be given every six hours.**

False. In theophylline toxicity , charcoal should be administered every 2 - 4 hours (.5 - 1g/kg). Repeated doses of charcoal significantly decrease the half-life of theophylline and increases total body clearance.

❍ **T/F: In a patient with a significant theophylline poisoning and recurrent vomiting, activated charcoal should be discontinued.**

False. For a patient with recurrent vomiting metoclopramide or ondansetron can be given to decrease vomiting and a slow continuous infusion through a nasogastric tube may be tried.

❍ **T/F: Syrup of ipecac is helpful in theophylline overdoses.**

False. It often leads to recurrent vomiting and makes the administration of repeat doses of activated charcoal more difficult.

❍ **In a suspected or known theophylline overdose, how often should a theophylline level be checked?**

Levels should be drawn as frequently as every 2 hours until the levels begin to decline, then every 4 - 6 hours.

❍ **Why is a distinction made between an acute theophylline overdose and an acute on chronic overdose?**

Patients with acute overdoses can generally tolerate higher levels with better outcomes.

❍ **In life threatening theophylline overdose, what is definitive management?**

Charcoal hemoperfusion.

❍ **What are two clear indicators for charcoal hemoperfusion in theophylline overdose?**

Theophylline level > 90mcg/ml in an acute ingestion, or theophylline level > 40mcg/ml in an acute on chronic ingestion. Other indications include a level > 40mcg/ml and any of the following: protracted vomiting (unable to tolerate charcoal), seizures, hypotension, ventricular arrhythmias.

❍ **Which of the following is not a common manifestations of significant theophylline toxicity: seizures, dysrhythmias, hypotension, or visual disturbances?**

Visual disturbances.

❍ **T/F: Chronic exposure to theophylline leads to toxicity at lower levels than acute exposures.**

True.

❍ **What drugs should be used as initial therapy for seizures in theophylline toxicity?**

Intravenous diazepam, lorazepam or phenobarbital.

❍ **What is the initial therapy for hypotension in the theophylline toxicity?**

Fluid administration.

❍ **Will serious theophylline toxicity likely result in hypertension or hypotension?**

Hypotension.

❍ **After ingestion of standard theophylline tablets, when does the maximum plasma concentration occur?**

Usually peak plasma levels occur 4 hours after ingestion.

❍ **When will sustained released theophylline tablets produce peak plasma concentrations?**

12-24 hours after ingestion.

❍ **Lithium is the drug of choice for the treatment of what disorder?**

Bipolar affective disorder.

❍ **T/F: Lithium has a narrow therapeutic-toxic range.**

True. Therapeutic lithium levels are between .5 - 1.5 mEq/L, and must be monitored closely.

❍ **How is lithium eliminated after metabolism?**

By renal excretion.

❍ **Which electrolyte abnormality may enhance lithium toxicity?**

Hyponatremia. Reabsorption of lithium will be enhanced.

❍ **Does activated charcoal bind lithium?**

No.

❍ **What are the typical CNS findings in mild lithium toxicity?**

Rigidity, tremor, hyperreflexia.

❍ **What are the typical CNS findings in severe lithium toxicity?**

Seizures, coma, myoclonic jerking.

❍ **When comparing potential lithium toxicity following an acute ingestion, which patient is at greater risk: a patient who has not previously received lithium, or a patient on chronic maintenance lithium therapy?**

The patient on chronic therapy.

❍ **What is the primary system affected by lithium toxicity?**

Central nervous system.

❍ **T/F: Hydration status has little effect on lithium toxicity.**

False. Patients with lithium toxicity and dehydration require aggressive rehydration to establish euvolemia and normal urine output, while avoiding fluid overload.

❍ **What constitutes definitive therapy for moderate to severe lithium toxicity?**

Hemodialysis.

❍ **What are the indications for hemodialysis in lithium toxicity?**

Serum lithium level above 4.0 mEq/l, renal failure and severe clinical symptoms (stupor, seizures etc.).

❍ **Is there a need to draw serial lithium levels?**

Yes. This is necessary to determine if delayed absorption is occurring, allowance for more accurate assessment in terms of current therapy, and potential need for intensive care monitoring or dialysis.

❍ **T/F: Permanent neurologic sequelae (encephalopathy) can develop from lithium toxicity.**

True.

❍ **A 30 year-old man presents to the ED 20 minutes after ingesting 30 tablets of Amitripyline. What is the preferred method of gastric emptying?**

Immediate gastric lavage using a large (34-36 French) orogastric tube. Ipecac should not be used due to the potential for a rapid deterioration in mental status and seizures.

❍ **What is the treatment of seizures secondary to cyclic antidepressant poisoning?**

Benzodiazepines. Phenytoin should be avoided because of its potential cardiotoxicity.

❍ **What are the ECG findings in cyclic antidepressant overdoses?**

Sinus tachycardia, QRS prolongation, and rightward terminal 40 msec of the frontal plane QRS complex (an R wave in lead aVR)

❍ **What level correlates with toxicity in cyclic antidepressant overdoses?**

There is no correlation between serum levels and symptoms of serious toxicity.

❍ **A 22 year-old female presents to the ED lethargic, flushed with a temperature of 100.9° F. Her mother states she's been very upset recently after a break up with her boyfriend. The patient has no past medical history but the mother has a history of manic depression. The patient's ECG show sinus tachycardia, QRS interval of .12 and a short run of ventricular tachycardia. What is the initial treatment for the ventricular tachycardia?**

Bolus the patient with $NaHCO_3$ 1-2 mEq/kg and continue a bicarbonate infusion to maintain pH between 7.45 to 7.55. Alkalinization of the serum to prevent ventricular dysrhythmia can either be done by hyperventilation or bicarbonate infusion. In this case, bicarbonate is used because the patient is not intubated.

❍ **If this patient continues to have ventricular arrythmias despite serum alkalinization what antidysrhythmic medication would you use?**

Lidocaine

❍ **What class of antidysrhythmics are contraindicated in cyclic antidepressant overdoses?**

The type 1A and 1C antidysrhythmics. They have quinidine-like effects on the sodium channels and will enhance the cardiotoxcity of the cyclic antidepressants.

❍ **A 40 year-old female with a history of depression presents to the ED after taking a handful of her Doxepin. She is awake and alert, vital signs are normal and the ECG show normal sinus**

rhythm, with a QRS interval of .8 msec. If there is no change in her condition after what time interval can you safely discharge the patient for further psychiatric evaluation.

Six hours. Most patients will manifest toxicity within the first 2 hours after ingestion and virtually everyone within 6 hours.

❍ **Along with continuous ECG monitoring and observation in the ED, what other treatment should this patient receive?**

Gastric lavage may be performed. The patient should definitely receive activated charcoal 1 g/kg with cathartic. The activated charcoal, without cathartic can be repeated every 2-4 hours in a patient with intact gut motility.

❍ **What is the initial treatment for hypotension in antidepressant overdose?**

Intravenous fluids - normal saline or Ringer's lactate

❍ **What vasopressor should be used to treat hypotension not responsive to IV fluids in antidepressant overdose?**

Norepinephrine should be used because it is a direct acting alpha-adrenergic agonist.

❍ **The onset of toxicity of monoamine oxidase inhibitors (MAOI) can occur up to what period of time after ingestion?**

12 to 24 hours.

❍ **What over the counter cold medications should not be used by people taking MAOIs?**

Decongestants, antihistamines and products containing dextromethorphan

INFECTIOUS DISEASES

No man really becomes a fool until he stops asking questions.
Charles Steinmetz

❍ **Describe the pathophysiologic features of HIV.**

HIV attacks the T4 helper cells. The genetic material of HIV consists of single-stranded RNA. HIV has been found in semen, vaginal secretions, blood and blood products, saliva, urine, cerebrospinal fluid, tears, alveolar fluid, synovial fluid, breast milk, transplanted tissue, and amniotic fluid. There has been no documentation of infection from casual contact.

❍ **How quickly do patients infected with HIV become symptomatic?**

5-10% develop symptoms within three years of seroconversion. Predictive characteristics include a low T4 count and a hematocrit less than 40. The mean incubation time is about 8.23 years for adults and 1.97 years for children less than 5 years old. When AIDS develops, the survival duration is about 9 months. However, new treatments may prolong this time period.

❍ **Name the most common causes of fever in HIV-infected patients.**

Mycobacterium avium-intracellularae, CMV, non-Hodgkin's and Hodgkin's lymphoma.

❍ **An HIV-positive patient presents with a history of weight loss, diarrhea, fever, anorexia, and malaise. She is also dyspneic. Lab studies reveal abnormal LFT's and anemia. What is the diagnosis?**

Mycobacterium avium-intracellularae. Lab confirmation is made by an acid-fast stain of body fluids or by a blood culture.

❍ **What is the most common complication of AIDS?**

Pneumocystis carinii pneumonia (PCP). Kaposi's sarcoma is the second most common.

❍ **What is the most common cause of focal encephalitis in AIDS patients?**

Toxoplasmosis. Symptoms include focal neurologic deficits, headache, fever, altered mental status, and seizures. Ring enhancing-lesions are evident on CT.

❍ **Which drugs are used to treat CNS toxoplasmosis in AIDS patients?**

Pyrimethamine plus sulfadiazine.

❍ **The differential diagnosis of ring-enhancing lesions in AIDS patients is:**

Lymphoma, cerebral tuberculosis, fungal infection, CMV, Kaposi's sarcoma, toxoplasmosis, and hemorrhage.

❍ **What are the signs and symptoms of CNS cryptococcal infection in an AIDS patient?**

Headache, depression, lightheadedness, seizures, and cranial nerve palsies. A diagnosis is confirmed by an India ink prep, a fungal culture, or by a testing for the presence of cryptococcal antigens in the CSF.

❍ **What is the presentation of an AIDS patient with tuberculous meningitis?**

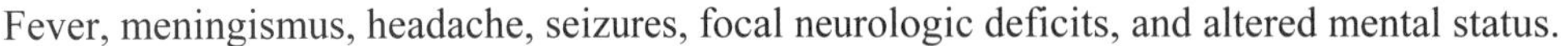

Fever, meningismus, headache, seizures, focal neurologic deficits, and altered mental status.

❍ **What is the most common eye finding in AIDS patients?**

Cotton wool spots. It has been proposed that the cotton-wool spots are associated with PCP. These finding may be hard to differentiate from the fluffy, white, often perivascular retinal lesions that are associated with CMV.

❍ **An AIDS patient has decreased visual acuity, photophobia, redness, and eye pain. What is the diagnosis?**

Retinitis or malignant invasion of the periorbital tissue or eye.

❍ **What is the most common cause of retinitis in AIDS patients?**

Cytomegalovirus. Findings include photophobia, redness, scotoma, pain, or a change in visual acuity. On examination, fluffy white retinal lesions may be evident.

❍ **What is the most common opportunistic infection in AIDS patients?**

PCP. Symptoms may include a non-productive cough and dyspnea. A chest x-ray may reveal diffuse interstitial infiltrates, or it may be negative. Although Gallium scanning is more sensitive, false positives occur. Initial treatment includes TMP-SMX. Pentamidine is an alternative.

❍ **How is Candida of the esophagus diagnosed?**

An air-contrast barium swallow shows ulceration with plaques. In contrast, herpes esophagitis produces punched-out ulcerations with no plaques.

❍ **What is the most common gastrointestinal complaint in AIDS patients?**

Diarrhea. Hepatomegaly and hepatitis are also typical. Conversely, jaundice is an uncommon finding. Cryptosporidium and Isospora are the common causes of prolonged watery diarrhea.

❍ **What is the risk of contracting HIV after occupational exposure?**

0.32%. 80% of the occupational exposure-related infections are from needle sticks.

❍ **A patient is infected with Treptonema pallidum. What is the treatment?**

The type of treatment depends upon the stage of the infection. Primary and secondary syphilis are treated with benzathine penicillin G (2.4 million units IM X 1 dose) or doxycycline (100 mg bid po for 14 day). Tertiary syphilis is treated with benzathine penicillin G, 2.4 million units IM X 3 doses 3 weeks apart.

❍ **Describe the lesions associated with lymphogranuloma venereum (LV).**

LV caused by Chlamydia presents as painless skin lesions with lymphadenopathy. Lesions may be papular, nodular, or herpetiform vesicles. Sinus formation, involving the vagina and rectum, are common in women.

❍ **What is the cause of chancroid?**

Hemophilus ducreyi. Patients with this condition present with 1 or more painful necrotic lesions. Suppurating inguinal lymphadenopathy may also be present.

❍ **What is the cause of granuloma inguinale?**

Calymmatobacterium granulomatis. Onset occurs with small papular, nodular, or vesicular lesions that develop slowly into ulcerative or granulomatous lesions. Lesions are painless and are located on mucous membranes of the genital, inguinal, and anal areas.

❍ **What causes tetanus?**

Clostridium tetani. This organism is a Gram-positive rod; it is vegetative and a spore former. It produces tetanospasmin, an endotoxin, which induces the disinhibition of the motor and autonomic nervous systems and thus the exhibition of tetanus clinical symptoms.

❍ **What is the incubation period of tetanus?**

Hours to over 1 month. The shorter the incubation period, the more severe the disease. Most patients who contract tetanus in the US are over 50 years old.

❍ **What is the most common presentation of tetanus?**

"Generalized tetanus" with pain and stiffness in the trunk and jaw muscles. Trismus develops and results in risus sardonicus, i.e., a sardonic smile.

❍ **Which cranial nerve is most commonly involved in cephalic tetanus?**

Cephalic tetanus usually occurs after injuries to the head and typically involves the seventh cranial nerve.

❍ **Outline the treatment for tetanus.**

Respiratory: Administer succinylcholine for immediate intubation if required.

Immunotherapy: Human tetanus immune globulin will neutralize circulating tetanospasmin and the toxin in the wound. However, it will not neutralize toxin fixed in the nervous system. Dose TIG 3000 to 5000 units. Prescribe tetanus toxoid, 0.6 ml IM, at 1 week and 6 weeks and 6 months.

Antibiotics: Clostridium tetani is sensitive to cephalosporins, tetracycline, erythromycin, and penicillin, but penicillin G is the drug of choice.

Muscle relaxants: Administer diazepam or dantrolene.

Neuromuscular block: Prescribe pancuronium bromide, 2 mg plus sedation.

Autonomic dysfunction: Prescribe labetalol, 0.25 to 1.0 mg/minute IV, or magnesium sulfate, 70 mg/kg IV load, then 1 to 4 g/hour continuous infusion is used to treat autonomic dysfunction. Administer MS, 5 to 30 mg IV infusion every 2 to 8 hours, and clonidine, 3 mg po every 8 hours per NG.

Note: Fatal cardiovascular complications have occurred in patients treated with beta-adrenergic blocking agents alone. Adrenergic blocking agents used to treat autonomic dysfunction may precipitate myocardial depression.

❍ **Which is the most common tapeworm in the US?**

Hymenolepis nana. Infections occur in institutionalized patients.

❍ **A patient presents with fever, dyspnea, cough, hemoptysis, and eosinophilia. What is the likely diagnosis?**

Ascaris lumbricoides. This helminth is a roundworm. Serologic tests include an ELISA, a bentonite flocculation, and an indirect hemagglutination. Treat with pyrantel pamoate (pyrimidine pamoate) or mebendazole. An obstruction of the intestine may require surgery.

❍ **Where is the hookworm Necator americanus infection acquired?**

In areas where human fertilizer is used and people don't wear shoes. Patients present with chronic anemia, cough, low-grade fever, diarrhea, abdominal pain, weakness, weight loss, eosinophilia, and guiac positive stools. A diagnosis is confirmed if ova is present in the stool. Treatment includes mebendazole or pyrantel pamoate.

Editor's note: This is not a zebra. (MEZ)

❍ **What are the signs and symptoms of Trichuris trichiura?**

This hookworm lives in the cecum. Complaints include anorexia, abdominal pain (especially RUQ), insomnia, fever, diarrhea, flatulence, weight loss, pruritus, eosinophilia, and microcytic, hypochromic anemia. The diagnosis is made by examining for ova in the stool. Mebendazole is the treatment of choice.

❍ A patient attended a walrus, bear and pork roast. He now has N/V/D/F, urticaria, myalgia, splinter hemorrhages, muscle spasm, headache, and a stiff neck. What physical finding will clinch the diagnosis?

Periorbital edema is pathognomonic for infection with Trichinella spiralis. Patients may have acute myocarditis, nonsuppurative meningitis, and catarrhal enteritis bronchopneumonia. Lab studies may reveal leukocytosis, eosinophilia, ECG changes, and elevated CPK. Diagnosis is confirmed with a latex agglutination, skin test, complement fixation, or bentonite flocculation test. A stool examination is not helpful after the initial GI phase for confirming the diagnosis.

❍ What are three common protozoa that can cause diarrhea?

Entamoeba histolytica. Found worldwide. Although half of the infected patients are asymptomatic, the usual symptoms consist of N/V/D/F, anorexia, abdominal pain, and leukocytosis. Determine the presence of this organism by ordering stool tests and performing an ELISA for extraintestinal infections. Treatment is with metronidazole or tinidazole followed by chloroquine phosphate.

Giardia lamblia. Found worldwide. This organism is one of the most common intestinal parasites in the US. Symptoms include explosive watery diarrhea, flatus, abdominal distention, fatigue, and fever. The diagnosis is confirmed via a stool examination. Treatment is with metronidazole.

Cryptosporidium parvum. Found worldwide. Symptoms are profuse watery diarrhea, cramps, N/V/F, and weight loss. Treatment is supportive care. Medications may be needed for immunocompromised patients.

❍ What is the pathophysiology of rabies?

Infection occurs within the myocytes for the first 48 to 96 hours. It then spreads across the motor endplate and ascends and replicates along the peripheral nervous sysytem, axoplasm, and into the dorsal root ganglia, spinal cord, and CNS. From the gray matter, the virus spreads by peripheral nerves to tissues and organ systems.

❍ What is the characteristic histologic finding associated with rabies?

Eosinophilic intracellular lesions within the cerebral neurons, called Negri bodies, are the sites of CNS viral replication. Although these lesions occur in 75% of rabies cases and are pathognomonic for rabies, their absence does not eliminate the possibility of rabies.

❍ What are the signs and symptoms of rabies?

Incubation period of 12 to 700 days with an average of 20 to 90 days. Initial signs and systems are fever, headache, malaise, anorexia, sore throat, nausea, cough, and pain or paresthesias at the bite site.

In the CNS stage, agitation, restlessness, altered mental status, painful bulbar and peripheral muscular spasms, bulbar or focal motor paresis, and opisthotonos are exhibited. As in the Landry-Guillain-Barré syndrome, 20% develop ascending, symmetric flaccid and areflexic paralysis. In addition, hypersensitivity to water and sensory stimuli to light, touch, and noise may occur.

The progressive stage includes lucid and confused intervals with hyperpyrexia, lacrimation, salivation, and mydriasis, along with brainstem dysfunction, hyperreflexia, and extensor planter response.

Final stages include coma, convulsions, and apnea, followed by death between the fourth and seventh day for the untreated patient.

❍ What is the diagnostic procedure of choice in rabies?

Fluorescent antibody testing (FAT).

❍ **How is rabies treated?**

Wound care includes debridement and irrigation. The wound must not be sutured; it should remain open. This will decrease the rabies infection by 90%.

RIG 20 IU/kg, half at wound site and half in the deltoid muscle, should be administered along with HDCV, 1 ml doses IM on days 0, 3, 7, 14, and 28, also in the deltoid muscle.

❍ **A patient presents has a 40° C fever and an erythematous, macular, and blanching rash, which becomes deep red, dusky, papular, and petechial. The patient is vomiting and has a headache, myalgias, and cough. Where did the rash begin?**

Rocky Mountain Spotted Fever (RMSF) rash typically begins on the flexor surfaces of the ankles and wrists and spreads in a centripetal and centrifugal manner.

❍ **Which test confirms RMSF?**

Immunofluorescent antibody staining of a skin biopsy or serologic fluorescent antibody titer. The Weil-Felix reaction and complement fixation tests are no longer recommended.

❍ **Which antibiotics are prescribed for the treatment of RMSF?**

Tetracycline or chloramphenicol. Antibiotic therapy should not be withheld pending serologic confirmation.

❍ **What is the most deadly form of malaria?**

Plasmodium falciparum.

❍ **What is the vector for malaria?**

The female Anopheline mosquito.

❍ **What lab findings are expected for a patient with malaria?**

Normochromic normocytic anemia, a normal or depressed leukocyte count, thrombocytopenia, an elevated sedimentation rate, abnormal kidney and LFT's, hyponatremia, hypoglycemia, and a false-positive VDRL.

❍ **How is malaria diagnosed?**

Visualization of parasites on Giemsa-stained blood smears. In early infection, especially with

P. falciparum, parasitized erythrocytes may be sequestered and undetectable.

❍ **How is P. falciparum diagnosed on blood smear?**

1) Small ring forms with double chromatin knobs within the erythrocyte.
2) Multiple rings infected within red blood cells.
3) Rare trophozoites and schizonts on smear.
4) Pathognomonic crescent-shaped gametocytes.
5) Parasitemia exceeding 4%.

❍ **What is the drug of choice for treating P. vivax, ovale, and malariae?**

Chloroquine.

❍ **How is uncomplicated chloroquine-resistant P. falciparum treated?**

Quinine plus pyrimethamine-sulfadoxine plus doxycycline or mefloquine.

❍ **How is complicated chloroquine-resistant P. falciparum treated?**

Quinidine gluconate IV plus doxycycline IV.

❍ **Which complication of quinine and quinidine therapy should be considered?**

Insulin release, which may result in hypoglycemia.

❍ **What are the adverse effects of chloroquine?**

N/V/D/F, pruritus, headache, dizziness, rash, and hypotension.

❍ **Which type of parasitic infection commonly occurs with a papular pruritic rash?**

Schistosomiasis.

❍ **Which type of parasite infections do not typically result in eosinophilia?**

Protozoa infections, such as amebas, Giardia, Trypanosomiasis, and Babesia.

❍ **Name the most common intestinal parasite in the US.**

Giardia. Cysts are obtained from contaminated water or by hand-to-mouth transmission. Symptoms include explosive foul-smelling diarrhea, abdominal distention, fever, fatigue, and weight loss. Cysts reside in the duodenum and upper jejunum.

❍ **How is Chagas' disease transmitted?**

The blood-sucking Reduviid "kissing" bug, blood transfusion, or breast-feeding. A nodule or chagoma develops at the site. Symptoms include fever, headache, conjunctivitis, anorexia, and myocarditis. CHF and ventricular aneurysms can occur. The myenteric plexus is involved and may result in megacolon. Lab findings include anemia, leukocytosis, elevated sedimentation rate, and ECG changes, such as PR interval, heart block, T wave changes, and arrhythmias.

❍ **Which two diseases are transmitted by the deer tick, Ixodes dammini?**

Lyme disease and Babesia.

❍ **How do patients present with Babesia infection?**

Intermittent fever, splenomegaly, jaundice, and hemolysis. The disease may be fatal in patients without spleens. Treatment is with clindamycin and quinine.

❍ **What is the most frequently transmitted tick-borne disease?**

Lyme disease. The causative agent is spirochete, Borrelia burgdorferi; the vectors are Ixodes dammini, I. pacificus, Amblyomma americanum, and Dermacentor variabilis.

❍ **When are patients most likely to acquire Lyme disease?**

Late spring to late summer with the highest incidence in July.

❍ **How is Lyme disease diagnosed?**

Immunofluorescent and immunoabsorbent assays identify the antibodies to the spirochete. Treatment includes doxycycline or tetracycline, amoxicillin, IV penicillin (V in pregnant patients), or erythromycin.

❍ **Which type of paralysis does tick paralysis cause?**

Ascending paralysis. The venom that causes the paralysis is probably a neurotoxin. A conduction block is induced at the peripheral motor nerve branches and thereby prevents the release of acetylcholine at the neuromuscular junction. Forty-three species of ticks have been implicated as causative agents.

❍ **What is the most common sign of tularemia?**

Lymphadenopathy, usually cervical in children and inguinal in adults. It is caused by Francisella tularensis and is transmitted by the vectors Dermacentor variabilis and Amblyomma americanum.

❍ **A patient presents with sudden onset of fever, lethargy, a retro-orbital headache, myalgias, anorexia, nausea, and vomiting. She is extremely photophobic. The patient has been on a camping trip in Wyoming. What tick-borne disease might cause these symptoms?**

Colorado tick fever. This is caused by a virus of the genus Orbivirus and the family Reoviridae. The vector is the tick D. andersoni. The disease is self-limited; treatment is supportive.

❍ **What is the most common cause of cellulitis?**

Streptococcus pyogenes. Staphylococcus aureus can also cause cellulitis, though it is generally less severe and more often associated with an open wound.

❍ **What is the most common cause of cutaneous abscesses?**

Staphylococcus aureus.

❍ **What percentage of dog and cat bites become infected?**

About 10% of dog bites and 50% of cat bites become infected. Pasteurella multocida are the causative agents for 30% of dog bites and 70% of cat bites.

❍ **A 26 year-old female presents with headache, fever, malaise, and tender regional lymphadenopathy about a week after a cat bite. A tender papule develops at the site. What is the diagnosis?**

Cat-scratch disease. This condition usually develops 3 days to 6 weeks following a cat bite or scratch. The papule typically blisters and heals with eschar formation. A transient macular or vesicular rash may also develop.

❍ **What is the probable cause of an animal bite infection arising that develops in less than 24 hours? More than 48 hours?**

Less than 24 hours: Pasteurella multocida or streptococci. More than 48 hours: Staphylococcus aureus.

❍ **A patient involved yesterday in a work-related crush injury to his foot is now in shock. He has a fever, severe pain, and a horrible smell coming from his foot. On palpation you feel crepitus. What is the diagnosis?**

Gas gangrene. Gas from the infection quickly invades the fascial planes, which accounts for the crepitus. Treat with wound debridement and systemic antibiotics. The drug of choice is penicillin G; an alternative is chloramphenicol.

❍ **What is the most common cause of gas gangrene?**

Clostridium perfringens.

❍ **What is the most common site of a herpes simplex I infection?**

The lower lip. These lesions are painful and can frequently recur since the virus remains in the sensory ganglia. Stress, sun, and illness generally trigger recurrences.

❍ **Among patients with cystic fibrosis, what bacteria are seen with increased frequency as causes of pneumonia?**

Pseudomonas aeruginosa and Staphylococcus aureus.

40%.

❍ **What are the four indications for drainage of a pleural effusion associated with pneumonia?**

Positive gram stain or culture, the presence of gross pus, pleural fluid glucose less than 40 mg/dl or fluid pH less than 7.0.

❍ **An air-fluid level in the pleural space suggests what pathologic process?**

Bronchopleural fistula.

❍ **Is the vasculitis that is seen in syphilis, a large or a small vessel disease?**

Both. Large vessel (Heubner arteritis) is caused by adventitial lymphocytic proliferation of large vessels, and is commonly seen in the late meningovascular syphilis. The small vessel (Nissl-Alzheimer) vasculitis is the dominant vasculitic pattern in the paretic neurosyphilis.

❍ **What is the recommended treatment for neurosyphilis?**

Intravenous penicillin G. Follow up CSF examinations are mandatory.

❍ **What complication may arise from aggressive treatment of neurosyphilis with penicillin?**

Jarisch-Herxheimer reaction. It is due to a release of endotoxin when large numbers of spirochete are lysed during the penicillin treatment, and consists of mild fever, malaise, headache, arthralgia, and may produce a temporary worsening of the neurological status.

❍ **At which stage of Lyme disease does neurological involvement occur?**

The second and third stages. 2nd stage-cranial neuropathies, meningitis and radiculoneuritis. 3rd stage-encephalitis, and a variety of CNS manifestations including stroke like syndromes, extrapyramidal and cerebellar involvement.

❍ **Which is the vector responsible for the transmission of Lyme disease?**

Deer tick. Ixodus damnii.

❍ **What important feature in history should be sought in a patient in whom a neurological involvement from Lyme disease is being considered?**

History of Erythema Chronicum Migrans (ECM), which is present in nearly 60-80% of patients early in the disease.

❍ **What are the main differences between the European and the American patterns of Lyme disease?**

The European variety has been seen to have more of peripheral nervous system involvement, with relatively fewer joint and cardiac complications.

❍ **What is the currently recommended treatment for Lyme disease?**

Amoxicillin or doxycycline.

❍ **What is Weil's disease?**

Weil's syndrome is the less common variety of leptospirosis, with icterus, marked hepatic and renal involvement along with a bleeding diasthesis being the main features, and hence the name leptospirosis-ictero-hemorrhagica.

❍ **What is the commonest neurological feature of leptospirosis?**

Aseptic meningitis (present in over 50%).

❍ **What clinical feature of leptospirosis sets it apart from other infections of the nervous system and hints at the diagnosis?**

Hemorrhagic complications. These are not uncommon, and intraparenchymal and subarachnoid hemorrhages have been reported.

❍ **Which organism causes Weil's disease?**

Leptospirosis interrogans.

❍ **What are the neurological features of brucellosis?**

Mainly a chronic meningitis and the vascular complications thereof. However, cranial neuropathies, demyelination and mycotic aneurysms have all been described.

❍ **How is brucellosis spread?**

By ingestion of contaminated milk and milk products. It may also be spread by contact with an infected animal (usually cattle).

❍ **Which organism is responsible for brucellosis?**

Brucella Melitensis.

❍ **Which infectious disease characteristically causes dementia and a supranuclear palsy?**

Whipple's disease, which is caused by a gram positive argyrophillic bacillus.

❍ **What neurological findings are almost exclusively found in Whipple's disease?**

Oculo-facial-skeletal-myoarrythmia. In this condition, there is a convergence of the eyes or a pendular nystagmus that is synchronous with movements of the jaw or other parts of the body.

❍ **What is the neuropathological characteristic of Whipple's disease?**

A nodular ependymitis, mainly of the third and fourth ventricles, and the cerebral aqueduct. There is also a microgranulomatous polioencephalitis that may involve inferior frontal, temporal cortex and cerebellar nuclei. Spinal cord grey matter may be involved.

❍ **What is the diagnostic test for Whipple's disease?**

Examination of the jejunal mucosa, where PAS positive macrophages are seen in the lamina propria. These PAS positive structures are within the macrophages, are the remnants of the bacilli, and seen under the electron microscope.

❍ **What are the characteristic features of cerebral amebiasis, and what is the pathogenic organism?**

Cerebral amebiasis is usually a secondary infection, and patients often have intestinal or hepatic amebiasis. The causative organism is Entamoeba Histolytica. The clinical features are that of intracerebral abscesses causing focal neurological signs. Frontal lobes and basal nuclei are common sites of abscess formation.

❍ **What are the differences between cerebral amebiasis and primary amebic meningoencephalitis?**

The former is caused by E. Histolytica, and is usually a secondary infection. The latter is caused by the free-living Naegleria species. This organism causes an acute meningoencephalitis.

❍ **What is the treatment for amebiasis with neurological involvement?**

E. Histolytica is treated with metronidazole, emetine and chloroquine. Naegleria species is treated with amphotericin and rifampicin.

❍ **What is the nature of the myopathy in AIDS?**

HIV disease is directly related to development of a myopathy. Polymyositis that is clinically indistinguishable from the idiopathic variety has been seen. Prolonged use of high dose AZT has also been associated with development of a myopathy.

❍ **What are the typical features of Zidovudine associated myopathy?**

AZT is known to cause myopathy when used in high doses over prolonged periods. There is typically severe myalgia, and striking atrophy of the gluteal muscles.

❍ **What are the pathological features of AZT myopathy?**

AZT causes a mitochondrial cytopathy, and ragged red fibres are characteristically seen.

❍ **What is the nature of peripheral neuropathy in AIDS?**

Peripheral neuropathy in AIDS is divided into three main groups. A distal sensorimotor neuropathy, an acute inflammatory demyelinating neuropathy (AIDP), and a mononeuropathy multiplex.

❍ **Which organism is mainly responsible for causing polyradiculopathy in AIDS?**

Cytomegalovirus is notorious for causing polyradiculopathies and occasionally polyradiculomyelopathy. It is a late complication of AIDS, and usually occurs with CD4 counts less than 100 cells/ul.

❍ **What is the commonest cause of intracranial mass lesion in HIV disease?**

Intracranial toxoplasmosis. About 20-30% of AIDS patients with positive serology for toxoplasmosis will develop toxoplasma encephalitis. The second most common intracranial mass lesion is lymphoma.

❍ **What pathological findings are seen in the brain biopsy of toxoplasma encephalitis?**

Presence of tachyzoites around the necrotic lesion.

❍ **What are some important radiological differences between intracranial toxoplasmosis and lymphoma?**

1. Intracranial toxoplasmosis is usually multiple, whereas lymphomas are usually solitary, at least in the beginning. Rarely one may see a solitary toxoplasma lesion and multiple lymphoma lesions
2. Enhancement. Both may enhance with gadolinium on the MRI scan, however, toxoplasma lesions are usually round and discrete in comparison to the lymphoma.
3. Thallium 201 SPECT scan. Lymphomas usually show increased activity in the Thallium scans compared to toxoplasmosis, which has poor uptake.
4. Location. Toxoplasmosis is usually in the deeper structures such as basal ganglia, or the grey white junction, whereas the lymphomas usually present themselves in the periventricular areas. However, biopsy is still necessary to make the diagnosis since imaging studies may overlap.

❍ **What is the current recommended treatment for intracranial toxoplasmosis in HIV disease?**

This is usually a combination therapy with sulfadiazine, pyrimethamine, and folinic acid.

❍ **What is the rational for using folinic acid in the treatment of intracranial toxoplasmosis with pyrimethamine, and sulfadiazine combination?**

Folinic acid is thought to decrease the incidence of bone marrow suppression.

❍ **What percentage of patients with HIV disease develop CNS lymphoma?**

Approximately 2% of AIDS patients will develop primary CNS lymphoma. Up to 0.6% will present with primary CNS lymphoma concurrent with a diagnosis of AIDS.

❍ **What is the nature of CNS lymphoma in AIDS?**

They are almost all tumors of B cell origin. They may be large cell immunoblastic, or small non-cleaved cell lymphoma.

❍ **Which virus is considered responsible for AIDS associated CNS lymphoma?**

Epstein-Barr virus

❍ **What is the usual treatment modality for AIDS associated primary CNS lymphoma (PCNSL)?**

PCNSL is very radiosensitive, and responds well to about 4000 rads over 3 weeks.

❍ **What is the typical clinical presentation of progressive multifocal leucoencephalopathy (PML)?**

PML commonly presents with focal neurological signs such as hemisensory or motor signs, and visual field deficits.

❍ **Which virus is responsible for causing PML?**

JC virus, which is a Papovavirus that infects oligodendrocytes.

❍ **PML is seen in which other immune disorders?**

Cell mediated immunedeficiency. It is thus seen in HIV disease, chronic myeloid leukemia, Hodgkin's disease, chemotherapy patients and rarely sarcoidosis.

❍ **What are the common radiological features of PML?**

Hypodensities in the subcortical white matter on the CT scan. T1 images on the brain MRI are hypointense, and T2 images hyperintense. They are nonenhancing and usually start in the parietooccipital region of the subcortical white matter.

❍ **What is the commonest cause of meningitis in HIV disease?**

Cryptococcal followed by HIV.

❍ **What are some common causes of myelopathy associated with HIV disease?**

Vacuolar myelopathy is probably the commonest cause of myelopathy in AIDS patients. Other infectious and non-infectious causes are cytomegalovirus (CMV), herpes simplex virus (HSV), varicella zoster virus (VZV), human T cell lymphotrophic virus 1 (HTLV1), and mass lesions such as lymphoma and toxoplasmosis.

❍ **Which amongst the following is responsible for subacute sclerosing panencephalitis (SSPE). Paramyxoviruses, enteroviruses or polyomaviruses?**

It is caused by the measles virus, which belongs to the morbillivirus subgroup of the paramyxoviruses.

❍ **What are characteristic findings in the cerebrospinal fluid in SSPE?**

Normal cells and glucose. Normal to raised protein content, positive oligoclonal bands, and a raised titer of measles antibody. The measles-specific antibody index is greater than 10.

❍ **Which virus is considered responsible for Tropical Spastic Paraparesis (TSP)?**

Human T cell Lymphotrophic Virus type 1.

❍ **What are the modes of transmission of HTLV 1?**

Vertical: Mother to Child. Horizontal: Through sexual contact, and blood transfusion.

❍ **Which is the commonly ascribed pathogen for endemic TSP?**

This is caused by HTLV1 and this virus can also be associated with Adult T cell Leukemia/Lymphoma (ATLL).

❍ **What are some common features of HTLV1 associated myelopathy?**

Aside from the upper motor neuron signs, dysaesthesias are common. Absent ankle jerks and bladder symptoms are commonly seen.

❍ **What are four other infectious causes of paraparesis?**

Syphilis, Tuberculosis with Pott's disease of the spine, Leptospirosis, VZV.

❍ **What is the single most helpful antemortem test for supportive diagnosis of Creutzfeldt-Jakob disease (CJD)?**

EEG. 1-2 cycles per second triphasic sharp waves superimposed on a depressed background. They are usually asymmetrical and slow with advancing disease.

❍ **How is botulism contracted, and what are the principle clinical features?**

It is contracted by consumption of contaminated foods, by injury from non-sterile objects (wound botulism) and in infants from intestinal colonization by Clostridium botulinum (lack of normal intestinal flora permit this colonization). The clinical features are that of a descending paralysis with complete ophthalmoplegia, bulbar and somatic palsy.

❍ **Is the motor paralysis induced by botulinum toxin reversible?**

It's an irreversible paralysis, and recovery is from axonal sprouting from old sarcolemmal area to a new locus.

❍ **Which condition resembles Guillain-Barré syndrome, the appropriate treatment of which results in miraculous complete improvement often within a day?**

Tick paralysis, which results in an ascending paralysis within a few days of attack by the tick Dermacentor (hard tick). This releases a toxin in its saliva, which is responsible for the neuromuscular blockade. Removal of the tick results in resolution of the weakness that begins within hours.

❍ **What is the cause of Sydenham's chorea, and what are the principal clinical features?**

This is caused by an immunological cross-reaction after group A streptococcus infections. The development often occurs several months after the acute infection. It is characterized by development of involuntary choreiform movements that may be unilateral, and remits spontaneously after a while. There are also associated behavioral changes that may reach the severity of obsessive compulsive disorder.

❍ **What are the long-term sequelae of Sydenham's chorea?**

There may be no further problems, but these patients are at higher risk for drug induced chorea or chorea gravidarum.

❍ **What is epidemic pleurodynia (Bornholm's disease)?**

An upper respiratory tract infection followed by pleuritic chest pain and tender muscles.

❍ **Which is the organism responsible for causing Bornholm's disease?**

Coxsackie viruses are a group of enteroviruses responsible for the epidemic myalgia (Bornholm's disease) where pleurodynia is also a common feature. Specifically, the disease is thought to occur due to a Coxsackie group B virus.

❍ **What are the neurological manifestations of Poliomyelitis?**

Spinal poliomyelitis, bulbar poliomyelitis, and the encephalitic form, in descending order of frequency.

❍ **What is the CSF characteristic of Polio?**

In the acute stages, it is associated with a lymphocytic pleocytosis, elevated protein and normal glucose. There may be a neutrophilic response very early in the disease. Chronic residual polio has normal CSF.

❍ **What are three paralytic diseases caused by infectious agents other than Polio?**

Paralytic rabies, Botulism and Tick paralysis.

❍ **To which group of viruses does the Poliovirus belong?**

Poliovirus is an enterovirus that belongs to the picornavirus group.

❍ **What is the meaning of the term reverse transcriptase in the description of HIV?**

Under normal circumstances, the transcription of a protein in a human cell occurs in a forward direction going from DNA to RNA. In reverse transcriptase, the transcription proceeds from RNA to DNA. HIV is a reverse transcriptase or a 'retrovirus' that needs to be incorporated into the human genome by the reverse transcription before replicating.

❍ **Where is the location of the P24 antigen?**

P24 antigen is the principle core protein of the virus, and measures 24,000 Daltons in molecular weight.

❍ **Name the three principle genes of the HIV.**

GAG. Group associated antigen, which codes amongst other things for the P24 antigen. POL Polymerase or the reverse transcriptase gene (P51), ENV. Envelop glycoprotein genes that code for two proteins, P41 of 41,000 Daltons molecular weight, and P120 of 120,000 Daltons molecular weight.

❍ **Is the immune deficiency in HIV disease principally a cell mediated or a humoral deficiency?**

Cell mediated immunity is slowly eroded in HIV disease.

❍ **Name some common causes of myelopathy associated with HIV disease.**

Vacuolar myelopathy is probably the commonest cause of myelopathy in AIDS patients. Other infectious and non-infectious causes are CMV, HSV, VZV, HTLV1 and lymphomas.

❍ **Is AIDS dementia a cortical or subcortical dementia?**

Cortical. There is no evidence of myelin breakdown in AIDS dementia. The white matter pallor is probably secondary to blood brain barrier breakdown

❍ **What are the most common causes of otitis media?**

S. pneumoniae, H. influenzae, and M. catarrhalis.

❍ **What are the best agents to use against cytomegalovirus?**

Ganciclovir, and foscarnet.

❍ **A 31 year-old stepped on a nail at his job. The nail pierced through his sneaker and into his foot. His tetanus status is up to date. What is you main concern?**

Infection with Pseudomonas that can lead to osteomyelitis. Pseudomonal infection is soon most commonly in association with hot, moist environments, such as sneakers.

❍ **What is the most common cause of infectious arthritis in patients with sickle cell disease? What joint is most commonly affected?**

Staph. aureus remains the most common cause, as in otherwise healthy children. However, Salmonella is more commonly seen in septic arthritis in children with hemoglobinopathies. The hip is most commonly affected.

❍ **What is necessary for the diagnosis of fever of unknown origin?**

1) History of fever over 1 week, 2) documentation of fever by health provider, 3) lack of a diagnosis after one week of investigation.

❍ **What specific substance in the body is the cause of fever?**

PGE_2.

❍ **Why should a patient with suspected idiopathic thrombocytopenic purpura (ITP) be tested for HIV?**

Because thrombocytopenia may be the presenting sign for HIV infection.

❍ **How do viral meningitis and bacterial meningitis differ with regards to CSF pressure? CSF leukocytes? CSF glucose?**

The pressure in bacterial infection is increased, whereas it is normal or slightly increased in viral. The leukocytosis is greater than 1000 (up to 60K) in bacterial, and rarely over 1000 in viral meningitis. The glucose concentration is decreased in bacterial meningitis and is generally normal in viral.

❍ **Why do so many patients with meningitis become hyponatremic?**

Because a majority of patients with this disease develop some degree of SIADH.

❍ **What is the sine-quo-non of botulism poisoning presentation?**

Bulbar palsy.

❍ **Which cephalosporins cover Listeria monocytogenes?**

None. That is why ampicillin is usually added to the antibiotic regimen when infection with this organism is a possibility.

❍ **Where does the rash of Rocky Mountain Spotted Fever usually start?**

On the wrists and ankles. It then spreads to the trunk and extremities within hours.

❍ **What should you suspect in a patient that presents with tender and swollen pectoral nodes?**

Cat-scratch disease.

❍ **What is the causative agent of cat-scratch disease?**

Bartonella henselae.

❍ **What is thought to be the mode of inoculation in cat-scratch disease?**

Rubbing the eye after contact with a cat.

❍ **Cat-scratch disease is the most common cause of what type of conductivities?**

Parinaud oculoglandular syndrome.

❍ **A patient is diagnosed with impetigo from group A streptococcus. What sequelae do you have to keep an eye out for?**

Acute post-streptococcal glomerulonephritis. It will not lead to rheumatic fever, however, for reasons that are not fully understood (possibly the strains for pharyngitis and impetigo are different).

❍ **What is the usual ideological agent of a hordeolum (stye)?**

Staph. aureus.

❍ **What are the major Jones criteria used to diagnose rheumatic fever?**

Carditis, chorea (Sydenham's), erythema marginatum, migratory polyarthritis, and subcutaneous nodules. The diagnosis requires either 2 major or 1 major and 2 minor with evidence of previous strep. infection.

❍ **What Jones criteria alone is sufficient for the diagnosis of rheumatic fever?**

Sydenham's chorea. Deterioration in handwriting and increased clumsiness are commonly seen.

❍ **What is the drug of choice for meningococcal disease?**

Aqueous penicillin G (250k-300k units/kg/day IV in 6 doses) is the ideal, though patients can be started effectively on empiric cefotaxime or ceftriaxone for suspected cases and in patients with penicillin allergy.

❍ **Should people who have had contact with patients with meningococcal meningitis be given prophylactic antibiotics?**

Yes. Rifampin or ceftriaxone are recommended.

❍ **What is, overall, the most common cause of aseptic meningitis?**

Enteroviruses.

❍ **Generally speaking, how do exudates of viral conjunctivitis differ from bacterial conjunctivitis?**

Viral is serous, and bacterial is mucopurulent or purulent.

❍ **What is the recommended initial treatment for cases of gonorrhea?**

Third generation cephalosporins (especially ceftriaxone) plus either doxycycline (100 mg BID for seven days) or azithromycin (1 gram PO x 1 dose) for presumptive coinfection with chlamydia.

❍ **What is the cause of epidemic keratoconjunctivitis?**

Adenovirus.

❍ **Clinically, how can you distinguish orbital cellulitis from periorbital cellulitis?**

Extra-ocular muscle dysfunction, decreased pupillary reflexes, decreased visual acuity and changes in globe position are seen only in orbital cellulitis.

❍ **What is the drug of choice for streptococcal pharyngitis?**

Penicillin V.

❍ **After initiation of therapy for streptococcal pharyngitis, when should a patient be allowed back to work?**

At least 24 hours should elapse.

❍ **After finishing the prescribed dosage of penicillin for pharyngitis, your patient's repeat culture still grows streptococcus. What do you do?**

Nothing. Most people are asymptomatic carriers and in most cases it is inconsequential.

❍ **What are the most common causes Herpangina?**

Coxsackie A and B viruses, and Echovirus.

❍ **Does trismus more commonly occur with a peritonsillar abscess or peritonsillar cellulitis?**

Peritonsillar abscess.

❍ **Why does therapy for TB take several months, when other infections usually clear in a matter of days?**

Because the mycobacterium divide very slowly and have a long dormant phase, during which time they are not responsive to medications.

❍ **What is the most common side effect of rifampin?**

Orange discoloration of urine and tears.

❍ **What negative outcome can be avoided by supplementing pyridoxine in patients receiving isoniazid?**

Peripheral neuritis and convulsions.

❍ **What are five infectious diseases that give false positive treponemal tests (FTA, MHA-TP, TPI) for syphilis?**

Yaws, pinta, leptospirosis, rat-bite fever (Spirillum minus) and Lyme disease.

❍ **What are five diseases that give false positive non-treponema (VDRL, RPR) tests for syphilis?**

Infectious mononucleosis, connective tissue diseases, tuberculosis, endocarditis, and intravenous drug abuse.

❍ **What are the organisms most commonly thought to be associated with Guillain-Barré Disease?**

CMV, EBV, Coxsackie virus, Campylobacter jejuni, and Mycoplasma pneumoniae.

❍ **In what disease is cerebrospinal fluid albuminocytologic dissociation seen and what does it mean?**

Guillain-Barré Disease. An increase in cerebrospinal fluid protein without a corresponding increase in cerebrospinal fluid white cells is referred to as albuminocytologic dissociation.

❍ **Patients with HIV infections who go on to develop AIDS are most commonly infected with what organisms?**

Pneumocystis carinii, cytomegalovirus, candida, aspergillus, nocardia, cryptococcus, and mycobacteria.

❍ **Adults with sickle cell disease most commonly are affected with what organisms?**

Streptococcus pneumoniae, Haemophilus influenzae B, and particularly severe Mycoplasma pneumoniae infections.

❍ **How is the diagnosis of histoplasmosis made?**

By culture or staining from sputum, bronchoalveolar lavage or tissue, and by a positive serology.

❍ **How is the diagnosis of coccidiomycosis made?**

By culture or staining of sputum, bronchoalveolar lavage or tissue, and by a positive serology.

❍ **How is the diagnosis of pulmonary blastomycosis made?**

By culture from sputum, bronchial washing or tissue.

❍ **How does one make the diagnosis of pulmonary sporotrichosis?**

This condition is diagnosed by culture from the sputum or tissue and also from skin test or positive serology.

❍ **How is the diagnosis of pulmonary zygomycosis made?**

By biopsy.

❍ **How is the diagnosis of pulmonary cryptococcosis made?**

By culture or biopsy.

❍ **How does one diagnose invasive aspergillosis?**

By biopsy.

❍ **How is an aspergilloma diagnosed?**

By chest x-ray.

❍ **How does one go about making the diagnosis of allergic Bronchopulmonary aspergillosis?**

Patients will have eosinophilia, Aspergillus fumigatus in the sputum and serum lgE to aspergillus.

❍ **What is the evaluation of foreign body in the lung?**

Chest x-ray and bronchoscopy.

❍ **What is the evaluation for candida of the lung?**

Fresh sputum or transtracheal aspirate should reveal yeast and pseudohyphae. Mycelia and blastospores will be seen in established colonization, so a tissue exam is needed for definitive proof.

❍ **What are some of the most convenient ways to make the diagnosis of Mycoplasma pneumonia?**

Cold agglutinin levels of > or = to 1:32 with consistent clinical findings will make presumptive diagnosis. A complement fixation level to Mycoplasma pneumoniae may be seen of > or = to 1:256, or Mycoplasma pneumoniae specific lgA or lgM will be elevated.

❍ **What are the most common causes of non-infectious stomatitis?**

Behcet's syndrome, Stevens-Johnson syndrome, cancer chemotherapy, and Kawasaki syndrome.

❍ **What organisms are known to cause renal and perinephric abscesses?**

The most common organisms are Staphylococcus aureus, Escherichia coli, Proteus spp., Pseudomonas spp., and enterococcus.

❍ **If a patient with underlying heart disease that has a tendency towards the development of endocarditis is undergoing a genitourinary or gastrointestinal procedure, what prophylactic antibiotic should be administered?**

Intravenous or intramuscular ampicillin and gentamicin thirty minutes prior to the procedure followed by the same, or amoxicillin eight hours after the procedure. Alternatively, intravenous vancomycin and gentamicin just prior to the procedure and repeated eight hours later is also acceptable. For a low risk procedure where the patient remains conscious, amoxicillin may be given one hour before and repeated six hours later.

❍ **What are five infectious agents associated with erythema nodosum?**

Erythema nodosum has been associated with many infectious and some non-infectious processes. Some of its better known associates are Group A streptococcus, meningococcus, syphilis, Mycobacterium tuberculosis, and Mycobacterium leprae, as well as histoplasmosis, coccidiomycosis, blastomycosis and herpes simplex virus. Some of the less common associates of erythema nodosum include Chlamydia trachomatis, Chlamydia psitacci, Corynebacterium diphtheriae, Campylobacter, Haemophilus ducreyi, Yersinia, Rochalimea henselae, trichophyton, filariasis, sarcoidosis, and various drugs.

❍ **What is the most common infectious disease problem in patients with lupus that are not on steroid therapy?**

Urinary tract infections and urosepsis.

❍ **What infectious disease problem is both characteristic of and potentially devastating in patients with lupus, whether on steroids or not on steroids?**

Meningitis.

❍ **How often is herpes simplex virus cultured from the cerebrospinal fluid of an adult with HSV encephalitis?**

Herpes simplex virus may be cultured from the cerebrospinal fluid of an adult with herpes encephalitis only 5% of the time.

❍ **What rapid diagnostic test is now available to diagnose herpes simplex virus encephalitis in patients of all ages and how reliable is it considered to be?**

HSV polymerase chain reaction (PCR) on cerebrospinal fluid is considered to be highly sensitive and specific in the diagnosis of HSV encephalitis.

❍ **What are the three questions that every victim of a dog bite should be asked?**

1) Was the attack provoked or unprovoked? 2) Was the dog known or unknown? 3) Has the dog had its rabies shots?

❍ **Do bite wounds caused by humans usually become infected with one or with multiple organisms?**

The average human bite wound contains 5.4 organisms per wound.

❍ **What are the most common organisms found in human bite wounds?**

Staphylococcus aureus, Streptococcus species, and Eikenella corrodens. Anaerobes are also commonly seen.

❍ **What is the risk of transmission of HIV from and HIV-infected person following a needle stick exposure?**

0.3%-0.5%.

❍ **Is it necessary to treat the male sexual partner of women with vaginal bacterial vaginosis?**

No. Affected women should be treated with oral or intra-vaginal metranidozole or clindamycin.

❍ **In the United States, are cats or are dogs more likely to be the most commonly infected domestic animal with rabies?**

Cats. Among wild animals, rabies is most commonly found among raccoons, skunks, foxes and coyotes.

❍ **Pasteurella multocida infection from an animal bite is best treated with which antibiotic?**

Penicillin is the drug of choice.

❍ **What is the intervention most likely to be successful in the treatment of onychomycosis of the toenail: a) removal of the toenail or b) antifungal therapy for four to eighteen months?**

231B) Drug therapy with Itraconazole (Sporonox) is the easiest and shortest term of the various antifungal drug regimens. Treatment can be given for one week each month for three to four months. Other medications that are useful include terbinafine, ketoconazole, and griseofulvin. Therapy with griseofulvin can take as long as eighteen months.

❍ **A patient who develops encephalitis following a near drowning episode is most likely to be infected with what organism?**

Acanthamoeba. Granulomatous amebic encephalitis may also be seen to occur in patients with systemic lupus erythematosus, AIDS, steroids or lymphoreticular malignancies.

❍ **What two common urinary pathogens do not give a positive urine nitrate test?**

Enterococcus and Staphylococcus saprophyticus. Acinobacter also fails to give a positive urine nitrate test.

❍ **What are the features of typhoid fever?**

Bradycardia, Insiduous onset, Rose spots, Dicrotic pulse, Splenomegaly, Fever, Leukopenia, Epidemic, Widal reaction. (BIRDS FLEW).

❍ **In a patient who presents with diarrhea, high fever, headache, lethargy, confusion, a normal lumbar puncture, 45% band forms on the differential of his white blood count, and a blood culture that is positive for Escherichia coli, what is the most likely cause of the diarrhea?**

Shigella. Blood cultures in shigella diarrhea are virtually never positive for shigella. When they are positive, they are more likely to be positive for Escherichia coli. Perhaps this is due to the fact that while Shigella is locally quite invasive at the mucosal level, it is very poorly invasive at the systemic level. Resident Escherichia coli in the gut, however, take advantage of the disrupted mucosa and invade the blood stream.

❍ **What percent of dog and cat bites result in cellulitis?**

Approximately 30% of cat bites and 6% of dog bites.

❍ **While on the farm, Coxiella burnetii is most commonly associated with sheep. In the city a parturient cat can aerosolize enough organisms n a closed space to be infective to people for days. What illness does Coxiella burnetii cause?**

Q Fever. This usually presents as an atypical pneumonia.

❍ **What are the two most common organisms known to be transmitted by unpasteurized Mexican cheese?**

Brucella and Listeria.

❍ **What is the most productive source of positive cultures for patients with Brucellosis?**

While blood, abscess and tissue cultures may be useful, bone marrow is the most productive source of positive cultures.

❍ **Which hemoglobin provides the greatest innate resistance to falciparum malaria?**

Erythrocytes of patients that are heterozygous for sickle cell hemoglobin (sickle cell trait) are resistant to malaria.

❍ **What is the most common infectious disease complication of both measles and influenza?**

Pneumococcal pneumonia.

❍ **Which rickettsial infection is most common in the United States?**

Rocky Mountain Spotted Fever, caused by Rickettsia rickettsia.

❍ **What prophylactic antibiotic should be given systemically to burn victims?**

None. Prophylactic agents with antibacterial activity should be given topically. Chief among these is Silvadene.

❍ **On Tuesday you are driving home from work in rural California and pass a dead squirrel. On Wednesday, taking a different route, you pass two more dead squirrels. The following morning you see a twenty-six year old male with enlarged tender lymphadenitis and a 105° F fever. What illness do you suspect?**

Cases of human plague (Yersinia pestis) are sometimes heralded by squirrel die-offs. A squirrelly die-off occurs when the organism is introduced into a highly susceptible mammalian population, causing a high mortality rate among infected animals. This is referred to as epizootic plague.

❍ **One day after a previously healthy adult has been admitted to the hospital after an accidental overdose of oral iron, she appears to become septic. What is the most likely organism causing her sepsis?**

Yersinia enterocolitica. The growth of Y. enterocolitica appears to be enhanced after exposure to excess iron. This combined with intestinal damage to the mucosa by the iron may play a role in pathogenesis.

❍ **Helicobacter pylori have been isolated from the gastric antrum in what percentage of patients with duodenal ulcer?**

Up to 100%. While a casual role for H. pylori in the development of duodenal ulcers has not been proven conclusively, when the organism is treated with an antibiotic effective against H. pylori, the relapse rate is approximately 20%. If the organism is not effectively eradicated, approximately 80% of these patients relapse.

❍ **T/F: Care must be taken in interpreting the results of a PPD in a patient who has been tested multiple times (more than ten times) because 30-50% of these patients will become positive from the PPD itself.**

False. It is believed that no amount of PPD testing will make a patient PPD positive.

❍ **If the result of a patient's PPD is read as 3 mm of induration and then 15 mm of induration following the placement of the second PPD two weeks later, which study should be considered the more reliable?**

The second study with an induration of 15 mm. With time, the body's memory of the tuberculosis infection may want. The placement of a PPD may stimulate that memory. This is what is referred to as the "booster phenomenon". The boosted result is considered to be the reliable result.

❍ **In a patient with a chest x-ray typical of tuberculosis, the PPD is negative. A repeat PPD two weeks is still negative. A panel of skin tests is placed and all of them prove to be positive. Does this rule out tuberculosis as a cause of the chest x-ray abnormality?**

No. Patients with tuberculosis can be selectively anergic. If one suspects tuberculosis, one must continue to maintain a high index of suspicion for that disease. Other more aggressive approaches will need to be taken to prove the diagnosis such as gastric washings, or if the patient's condition warrants, bronchoscopy or lung biopsy.

❍ **A patient from the Philippines has a hypo-pigmented patch that is lacking in sensation. What is the most likely cause of his problem?**

Leprosy (Mycobacterium leprae).

❍ **Which intestinal parasites are known to cause anemia as their major manifestation?**

Hookworms. Three species of hookworms affect humans. These include Ancylostoma duodenale, Necator americanus, and Ancylostoma ceylanicum.

❍ **What are the three most common causes of bacterial meningitis beyond the neonatal period?**

Pneumococcus, meningococcus and hemophilus influenzae.

RHEUMATOLOGY, IMMUNOLOGY AND ALLERGY

I don't want to achieve immortality through my work.
I want to achieve it through not dying.
Woody Allen

❍ **Which class of immunoglobulins is responsible for urticaria (hives) and angioedema?**

IgE.

❍ **Which class of immunoglobulins is responsible for food allergies?**

IgE.

❍ **What are the most common food allergies?**

Dairy products, eggs, and nuts.

❍ **When do the clinical manifestations of a new drug allergy usually become apparent?**

One to 2 weeks after starting the drug.

❍ **Which class of drugs is commonly associated with angioedema?**

Angiotensin-converting-enzyme (ACE) inhibitors. A patient who has suffered angioedema from one ACE inhibitor should not be prescribed another one. Complication can result from any member of this class of antihypertensive agents. ACE-triggered angioedema can occur at any time during the course of therapy.

❍ **What drug is the most common pharmaceutical cause of true allergic reactions?**

Penicillin. It accounts for approximately 90% of true allergic drug reactions and more than 95% of fatal anaphylactic drug reactions. Parenterally administered penicillin is more than twice as likely to cause a fatal anaphylactic reaction as compared to orally administered penicillin.

❍ **How long after exposure to an allergen does anaphylaxis occur?**

Seconds to 1 hour.

❍ **After penicillin, what is the most common cause of anaphylaxis-related deaths?**

Insect stings. Approximately 100 deaths occur in the US annually because of anaphylaxis induced by insect stings.

❍ **A patient on beta-blockers who develops anaphylactic cardiovascular collapse may not respond to epinephrine or dopamine infusions. What drug can be used in this setting?**

Glucagon, 5 to 15 mg/minute IV.

❍ **Are the nodules of erythema nodosum more often symmetrical or asymmetrical in distribution?**

Symmetrical. These nodules are distinctive, bilateral, tender nodules with underlying red or purple shiny patches of skin that develop in a symmetric distribution along the shins, arms, thighs, calves, and buttocks.

❍ **Is there an effective treatment for erythema nodosum?**

No. The disease usually lasts several weeks, but the pain associated with the tender lesions can be relieved with non-steroidal anti-inflammatory agents.

❍ **A patient presents with fever and acute polyarthritis or migratory arthritis a few weeks after a bout of streptococcal pharyngitis. What disease should be suspected?**

Acute rheumatic fever. Although the early symptoms may be nonspecific, a physical examination eventually reveals signs of arthritis (60 to 75%), carditis (30%), choreiform movements (10%), erythema marginatum, or subcutaneous nodules.

❍ **What treatment should be started when acute rheumatic fever has been diagnosed?**

Penicillin or erythromycin. This treatment should be started even if cultures for group A streptococci are negative. High-dose aspirin therapy is used at an initial dose of 75 to 100 mg/kg/day. Carditis is treated with prednisone, 1 to 2 mg/kg/day. Congestive heart failure is best treated with ACE inhibitors and/or diuretics.

❍ **What is Lhermitte's sign in ankylosing spondylitis?**

A sensation of electric shock that radiates down the back when the neck is flexed. This is a sign that atlanto-axial subluxation and C-spine instability may be present.

❍ **What other diseases may produce Lhermitte's sign?**

Rheumatoid arthritis and multiple sclerosis.

❍ **What rheumatic syndrome may lead to corneal irritation, ulceration, and infection?**

Sjogren's syndrome. This syndrome involves the lymphocytic infiltration of the lacrimal and salivary glands and may occur as an independent entity or as an accompaniment to other rheumatologic diseases. Patients with Sjorgren's syndrome present with a dry mouth and eyes.

❍ **What organisms are typically responsible for septic arthritis and osteomyelitis of the foot in an immunocompetent adult?**

Staphylococcus and Pseudomonas.

❍ **How is gout distinguished from pseudogout, using a microscope with a polarizing filter?**

When the plane of polarization is perpendicular to the crystal, pseudogout (calcium pyrophosphate) crystals appear yellow and rhomboidal, while gout (uric acid) crystals appear blue and needle-shaped. The mnemonic CUB, or "crossed urate blue" is a reminder.

❍ **Is the onset of pain more rapid in gout or in pseudogout?**

Gout. The onset of pain in acute gouty arthritis occurs over a few hours, whereas the pain associated with pseudogout usually evolves over a day or more.

❍ **Cite an example for each of the four major types of allergic reactions: Type I (immediate hypersensitivity); type II (cytotoxic); type III (Arthus reaction); and type IV (delayed hypersensitivity).**

Type I: Asthma, food allergies (IgE).
Type II: Transfusion reaction (IgG and IgM).
Type III: Serum sickness, post streptococcal glomerulonephritis (complex activates complement).
Type IV: Skin testing (activated T-lymphocytes).

❍ **Which of the four types of allergic reactions can be caused by a drug allergy?**

All of them.

❍ **What is the normal atlantodental distance on lateral flexion views of the C-spine?**

3.5 mm in adults.

❍ **Myocardial infarction can occur with which two rheumatic diseases?**

Kawasaki disease and polyarteritis nodosa (PAN).

❍ **What diagnostic procedure is indicated for a patient with rheumatoid arthritis who presents with dysphagia, hoarseness, and stridor?**

Urgent laryngoscopy to assess the paired cricoarytenoid joints. These joints can cause airway compromise if they become fixed in a closed position.

❍ **What is the most common cause of anaphylactoid reactions?**

Radiographic contrast media.

❍ **A bacterial infection and an allergic phenomenon can both cause a generalized confluent exfoliation of the skin. What are the two diseases and what test should be performed to distinguish between them?**

Bacterial infection: Ritter's disease. This disorder is caused by Staphylococcus and is also known as staphylococcal scalded skin syndrome. Ritter's disease causes exfoliation at the superficial granular layer of the epidermis.

Allergic phenomenon: Toxic epidermal necrolysis (TEN).

A skin biopsy distinguishes between the two conditions because the exfoliative cleavage plane is deeper at the dermal-epidermal junction or lower with TEN.

❍ **How is mucocutaneous lymph node syndrome (Kawasaki disease) diagnosed in a young patient with prolonged fever?**

Diagnosis requires four of the following findings:

1) Conjunctival inflammation
2) Rash
3) Adenopathy
4) Strawberry tongue and injection of the lips and pharynx
5) Erythema and edema of extremities

Desquamation of the fingers and the toes may be striking, but it is a late finding and is not one of the key clinical features of the disease.

❍ **What is the treatment of choice for a patient in anaphylactic shock?**

Epinephrine, 0.3 to 0.5 mg intravenously. If there is no IV access, inject the medication into the venous plexus at the base of the tongue.

❍ **How long should a patient with a generalized anaphylactic reaction be observed?**

24 hours. Recurrence of hemodynamic collapse and airway compromise is common within this period of time. Treat with antihistamines and steroids for 72 hours.

❍ **How does relapsing polychondritis affect the airway?**

Approximately 50% of patients with relapsing polychondritis have airway involvement and may present with pain and tenderness over the cartilaginous structures of the larynx. Dyspnea, stridor, cough, hoarseness, and erythema and edema of the oropharynx and nose may also be exhibited.

❍ **How should patients with airway involvement from relapsing polychondritis be managed?**

Admit these patients for high-dose steroids and for close observation. Repeated exacerbations may lead to severe airway compromise and asphyxiation.

❍ **How common is pleurisy in patients with systemic lupus erythematosus (SLE)?**

Approximately half of the patients with SLE will develop symptoms of pleurisy at some time.

❍ **What is the diagnostic approach for SLE with pleurisy?**

All pleural effusions in patients with rheumatic disease require thoracentesis to distinguish inflammatory effusions from infectious effusions. Pulmonary embolisms are common in patients with SLE; thus, a nuclear ventilation-perfusion (V/Q) scan is also indicated.

❍ **What percentage of patients with Kawasaki disease will develop coronary artery aneurysms because of improper therapy?**

Approximately 20%. 1 to 2% of these patients will die from acute myocardial infarction during the resolution phase of the illness.

❍ **A patient on chronic steroids presents with weakness, depression, fatigue, and postural dizziness. What pathological process should be suspected? What is the treatment?**

Adrenal insufficiency. The treatment is to administer large "stress doses" of steroids.

❍ **If adrenal insufficiency is suspected, what test should be performed? What drug should be prescribed?**

A serum cortisol level should be drawn before administering a large dose of steroids. Dexamethasone is the preferred agent because it will not interfere with subsequent tests if they are needed.

❍ **What cardiac complication commonly occurs with SLE, juvenile rheumatoid arthritis, and rheumatoid arthritis?**

Pericarditis.

❍ **What is the normal atlantodental distance on lateral flexion views of the C-spine? What rheumatologic diseases commonly alter this?**

Up to 3.5 mm in adults. Ankylosing spondylitis and rheumatoid arthritis can destroy ligamentous supporting structures and produce atlanto-axial subluxation with widening of this space.

❍ **What are the symptoms of atlanto-axial subluxation?**

Changes in bowel or bladder function, limb paresthesias, or new weakness.

❍ **What vascular disease is accompanied by polymyalgia rheumatica in 10 to 30% of the cases?**

Temporal arteritis.

❍ **A patient is suspected of having a new onset of acute gouty arthritis. What must be determined?**

The exclusion of a septic arthritis must assume top priority because the signs and symptoms of the two diseases may be indistinguishable.

❍ **What complication of rheumatoid arthritis may produce signs and symptoms that mimic those of deep vein thrombosis (DVT)?**

A Baker's cyst. This cyst can occasionally be distinguished clinically from DVT when deep hemorrhage from the ruptured cyst produces bruising or staining in a purple crescent below the malleoli, or when localized swelling at the site of the ruptured popliteal cyst spares the more distal parts of the leg and the foot.

❍ **Arthritis of the elbow joint causes limitation of all motion at the joint. In what way does olecranon bursitis differ?**

Pain from olecranon bursitis may limit flexion and extension at the elbow, but it usually does not affect pronation and supination.

❍ **How should a potentially septic olecranon bursitis be treated?**

Aspirate as much fluid as possible from the bursa via a large-bore needle. Antibiotics should be started immediately.

❍ **How does the white blood cell count in fluid aspirated from septic bursitis differ from that detected with septic arthritis?**

The white blood cell count in the fluid from a septic joint is usually 10 times higher than the white blood cell count in the fluid from a septic bursitis.

❍ **What are the articular symptoms of disseminated, Stage II Lyme disease?**

Migratory arthritis, bursitis, and tendonitis. The attacks associated with migratory arthritis are usually brief.

❍ **What are the articular symptoms of late, Stage III Lyme disease?**

Chronic arthritis, especially in the knee, periostitis, and tendonitis.

❍ **How should a new monoarthritis be approached in a patient with rheumatoid arthritis?**

Assume it is septic until proven otherwise. The risk for infection is higher in a joint that has been previously injured or affected by arthritis.

❍ **What painful bone abnormality often complicates steroid therapy in patients with rheumatoid arthritis or systemic lupus erythematosus?**

Avascular necrosis of the femoral head, femoral condyles, or bones of the feet.

❍ **What is the diagnosis for a preadolescent child with activity-related knee pain and a thickened and tender patellar tendon?**

Osgood-Schlatter. This disease is an inflammatory repetitive-injury process in which cartilaginous fragments are pulled loose from the tibial tuberosity by the ligamentum patellae of the quadriceps tendon. Treatment involves several months of restriction from excessive physical activity.

❍ **What disease is suspected in an adolescent with a tender, purpuric dependent rash on the lower extremities, colicky abdominal pain, migratory polyarthritis, and microscopic hematuria?**

Henoch-Schonlein purpura, a leukoblastic vasculitis. Intestinal or pulmonary hemorrhage may occur, and 7 to 9% of the cases will develop chronic renal sequelae. Salicylates are effective for the arthritis. Other treatments are directed at the symptoms. However, steroids are not particularly effective.

❍ **A 17 year-old female has painful swollen joints along with a spiking high fever, shaking chills, signs of pericarditis, and a pale erythematous coalescing rash on the trunk, palms, and soles. Hepatosplenomegaly is found. What is your diagnosis?**

Systemic juvenile rheumatoid arthritis. Arthrocentesis is necessary to eliminate the possibility of septic arthritis. The rheumatoid factor and the antinuclear antibody usually are negative; one-fourth of patients will proceed to have joint destruction. This is the least common of the three types of JRA.

❍ **What treatment, besides aspirin, prevents the complications of Kawasaki disease?**

IV immunoglobulins can reduce the incidence of coronary artery aneurysms to less than 5%.

❍ **What joint is typically involved in the most common form of juvenile rheumatoid arthritis?**

The knee; it does not lead to joint destruction. Reiter's syndrome, iridocyclitis, and inflammatory bowel disease may all be associated with this "pauciarticular" form of the disease.

❍ **A patient presents with pain along the radial aspect of the wrist extending into the forearm. What is the diagnostic test of choice?**

Finkelstein's test. This test confirms the diagnosis of de Quervain's tenosynovitis, an overuse inflammation of the extensor pollicis brevis and the abductor pollicis where they pass along the groove of the radial styloid. Finkelstein's test is performed by instructing the patient to make a fist with his thumb tucked inside the other fingers. The test is positive if pain is reproduced when the examiner gently deviates the fist in the ulnar direction.

❍ **In carpal tunnel syndrome, Tinel's sign is produced by tapping the volar wrist over the median nerve. If the test is positive, what does the patient experience?**

Paresthesias extending into the index and long fingers.

❍ **A patient with shoulder pain radiating to the medial forearm also has a reduction in the radial pulse upon passive abduction of the shoulder. What is your diagnosis?**

Thoracic outlet syndrome. Compression of the brachial plexus can produce pain and paresthesias that sometimes radiate all the way down to the ring and small fingers.

❍ **What condition is suspected when a patient with shoulder pain has palpable fullness in the supraclavicular fossa?**

A Pancoast's tumor in the superior sulcus of the lung.

❍ **What are the three most common cervical problems that produce pain radiating to the shoulder?**

Degenerative disease of the C-spine, degenerative disc disease, and herniated nucleus pulposus.

❍ **What herniated cervical disc causes pain that mimics the pain of a rotator cuff injury?**

C5-C6.

❍ **A 70 year-old patient has had progressive pain and motion restriction of the shoulder for several months. There is minimal tenderness to palpation, but active and passive range of motion is limited in abduction and rotation. What is the probable diagnosis?**

Adhesive capsulitis. The pain is usually a poorly localized diffuse ache that is often worse at night. The etiology is unclear but the condition commonly follows injury or chronic inflammation, particularly after immobilization.

❍ **A 40 year-old patient complains of sudden-onset shoulder pain while at rest. Any shoulder movement reproduces the pain. There is crepitus with motion, and the point of maximum tenderness is over the proximal humerus at the insertion of the rotator cuff. What will an x-ray reveal? What is the diagnosis?**

The x-ray will reveal calcified deposits in the rotator cuff, typical of calcific tendonitis. The cause is unknown, but the calcific deposits are painless until they begin to undergo spontaneous resorption. The symptoms are self-limited.

❍ **What disease produces erythematous plaques with dusky centers and red borders resembling bull's eye targets?**

Erythema multiforme. This disease can also produce non-pruritic urticarial lesions, petechiae, vesicles, and bullae.

❍ **What is the appropriate management for toxic epidermal necrolysis (TEN)?**

Admit the patient for management similar to that required for extensive second-degree burns. The mortality rate of TEN can be as high as 50% because of fluid loss and secondary infections.

❍ **What drugs are most commonly implicated in toxic epidermal necrolysis?**

Sulfonamides and sulfones, phenylbutazone and related drugs, barbiturates, other antiepileptic drugs, and antibiotics.

❍ **What can cause erythema multiforme?**

Viral or bacterial infections, drugs of nearly all classes, and malignancy.

❍ **What is the most common cause of allergic contact dermatitis?**

Toxicodendron species, such as poison oak, poison ivy, and poison sumac. These allergens are responsible for more cases than all the other allergens combined.

❍ **Why does scratching spread poison oak and poison ivy?**

The antigenic resin contaminates hands and fingernails. A single contaminated finger can produce more than 500 reactive groups of lesions.

❍ **How is the antigen of poison oak or poison ivy inactivated?**

Careful washing with soap and water destroys the antigen. Special attention must be paid to the fingernails, as the antigenic resin can be carried for weeks.

❍ **What underlying illnesses should be considered in a patient with nontraumatic uveitis?**

Collagen vascular diseases, sarcoid, ankylosing spondylitis, Reiter's syndrome, tuberculosis, syphilis, toxoplasmosis, juvenile rheumatoid arthritis, and Lyme disease.

❍ **What is the difference between episcleritis and scleritis?**

Both are associated with collagen vascular disorders however, episcleritis is a benign superficial inflammation of the tissues between the sclera and the conjunctive. Conversely, scleritis is a more severe and more painful inflammation of the deep sclera and it can result in vision loss.

❍ **What cervical radiculopathy produces pain that mimics cardiac ischemia?**

C6-C7.

❍ **What anatomic fact makes cervical radiculopathies confusing?**

Motor and sensory roots are separate at the neural foramina; therefore, severe sensory complaints and findings often lack a motor component.

❍ **Neck pain and upper extremity hyperreflexia suggest a cervical lesion at which level?**

Above C5.

❍ **What cervical root is usually involved when radiculopathy causes bilateral shoulder pain?**

C6. This myotome encompasses most of the proximal shoulder muscles. The C6 nerve root is the earliest and most commonly affected root by cervical disc syndromes.

❍ **What bony abnormality can produce Horner's syndrome, radicular symptoms without neck pain, vertebral-basilar insufficiency, and painless weakness in an upper-extremity myotome?**

Osteophytes encroaching on cervical neural foramina.

❍ **A patient presents with acute lower back pain. What are the criteria for admission?**

Paralysis, paraparesis, loss of bowel or bladder function, inability to stand or sit, the need to sleep in an upright position, intractable pain and spasticity, or metastatic cancer.

❍ **Which type of spinal lesion should be suspected when back pain forces a patient to sleep in an upright position?**

Thoracic root lesions.

❍ **In what way does trochanteric bursitis mimic lumbar radiculopathy?**

Both conditions produce pain that involves the hip and radiates along the iliotibial band to the lateral knee.

❍ **A patient with sudden, symmetric, multilevel areflexia, lower extremity muscle weakness, and bowel or bladder incontinence may have what neurologic problem?**

A midline herniation of a lumbar disk with compromise of the distal cauda equina. Emergency decompression may restore function and prevent permanent paraparesis.

❍ **What spinal lesion can produce shin splints?**

Compromise of the L5 and S1 nerve roots. This lesion may also produce calf pain that mimics the symptoms of deep vein thrombosis.

❍ **A patient with back pain who cannot walk on his/her toes has a lesion at which level?**

S1.

❍ **A patient with back pain who cannot walk on his/her heels has a lesion at which level?**

L5.

❍ **A patient has back pain when his hip and knee are flexed and the sciatic nerve is instrumented in the popliteal fossa. What is your diagnosis?**

A disc herniation with nerve root impingement.

❍ **A patient has myalgias, arthralgias, headache, and an annular erythematous lesion accompanied by central clearing. What is your diagnosis?**

Stage I Lyme disease with the classic lesion of erythema chronicum migrans (ECM). The primary lesion occurs at the site of the tick bite.

❍ **What rheumatologic ailments produce pulmonary hemorrhage?**

Goodpasture's disease, systemic lupus erythematosus, Wegener's granulomatosis, and non-specific vasculitides.

❍ **What rheumatologic ailments can produce pulmonary fibrosis?**

Ankylosing spondylitis, scleroderma, and rheumatoid arthritis (less common).

❍ **What rheumatologic ailments can produce respiratory muscle failure?**

Dermatomyositis and polymyositis.

❍ **What rheumatologic ailments can produce acute airway obstruction?**

Relapsing polychondritis and rheumatoid arthritis.

❍ **What infectious agents can produce a chronic smoldering arthritis with sterile aspiration cultures?**

Tuberculosis and fungal infections. A synovial biopsy may be required to confirm the diagnosis.

❍ **How is septic bursitis contracted?**

A puncture wound or an overlying cellulitis are the typical sources for septic bursitis.

❍ **The T cell receptor is co-expressed with what clusters of differentiation molecule (CD)?**

CD3.

❍ **What lymphocyte surface molecule is responsible for activating the alternate T cell activation pathway?**

CD2.

❍ **What lymphocyte surface molecule is responsible for HLA class II antigens?**

CD4.

❍ **What lymphocyte surface molecule is responsible for HLA class I antigens?**

CD8.

❍ **Which are the only complement fixing immunoglobulins?**

IgG and IgM.

❍ **Which is the major immunoglobulin protective of external secretions?**

IgA.

❍ **Which immunoglobulin is the major host defense against parasites?**

IgE.

❍ **What are the two main functions of T cells?**

To signal B cells to make antibody, and to kill virally infected or tumor cells.

❍ **T/F: CD4 to CD8 ratio in infants is 1.5 : 2.1.**

False. T cells are actually present in a higher numbers in infants due to the higher absolute lymphocyte counts; therefore the ratio is 3.5 : 4.1, rather than 1.5 : 2.1 ratio seen in children.

❍ **What are the <u>most reliable</u> and <u>cost effective</u> tests for assessing T, B, and, NK cell function?**

CBC and sedimentation rate. If the sedimentation rate is normal, a chronic bacterial infection is unlikely. If the absolute lymphocyte count is normal, the patient is not likely to have a severe T cell defect. If the RBCs are without Howell-Jolly bodies, congenital splenism is excluded. If the platelet count is normal, then Wiscott-Aldrich syndrome is excluded.

❍ **Blood products given to an individual with selective IgA deficiency must be prepared in what way?**

Washed normal donor erythrocytes or blood products. 44% of IgA deficient patients have auto-IgA antibody. When present, it may precipitate anaphylaxis and result in death from transfusion of unprepared donor cells.

❍ **Is immune serum globulin (IVIG) therapy indicated for Selective IgA deficiency?**

No.

❍ **What complex syndrome exhibits clinical features which include progressive cerebellar ataxia, oculocutaneous telangiectasia, chronic sinopulmonary infections, high incidence of malignancy (lymphoreticular being the most common), and variable cellular and humoral immunodeficiency?**

Ataxia-telangiectasia.

❍ **Which X-linked recessive syndrome is characterized by atopic dermatitis, thrombocytopenic purpura, small defective platelets, and undue susceptibility to infection?**

Wiskott-Aldrich syndrome.

❍ **Which rare primary immunodeficiency presents with recurrent severe staphylococcal abscesses, sinopulmonary tract infections, allergic rhinitis, asthma, keraconjuntivitis, and markedly elevated levels of serum IgE and IgD?**

Hyper IgE or Job's syndrome.

❍ **In patients with Hyper IgE syndrome and history of recurrent staphylococcal abscesses, what long-term management should you employ?**

Prophylactic penicillinase.

❍ **A patient presents with classic malar rash, fever, fatigue, myalgia, and arthalgia. A kidney biopsy demonstrated a membranoproliferative glomerulonephritis. However, all SLE serologic tests are negative. What disease etiology is most likely?**

Deficiency of the complement component C1q.

❍ **For those patients with C5, C6, C7 or C8 deficiency, which types of infections are they most susceptible to?**

Recurrent Neisseria.

❍ **Why are patients with C2 deficiency not unusually susceptible to infection?**

Protective function of alternative pathway is still intact.

❍ **X-linked agammaglobulinemia (Bruton's) and C3 complement deficiency share what common clinical feature?**

Susceptibility to pyogenic infections.

❍ **Why do patients with C1 esterase inhibitor deficiency suffer from hereditary angioedema?**

Episodic localized, nonpitting edema results from vasodilatory effects of kinins on the post-capillary venule, due to uncontrolled C1 activity, and hence, C4 and C2 breakdown with kinin release.

❍ **What causes fatality in hereditary angioedema?**

Edema of the larynx.

❍ **What is the functional defect of paroxysmal nocturnal hemogloinuria (PNH)?**

A hemolytic anemia disorder that occurs as a result of DAF, CD59, C8bp not being expressed on the erythrocyte surface, resulting in inappropriate anchoring of cell membrane proteins.

❍ **Patients with systemic lupus erythematosis (SLE) and their asymptomatic family members often have a partial deficiency of which complement component?**

Deficiency of CR1, which increases the risk of developing immune complex disease.

❍ **Patients suffering from Familial Mediterranean Fever (FMF) have a genetic deficiency in a protease whose function is to inactivate chemotactic factor C5a and IL-8. How does the disease manifest clinically?**

Patients with this rare disorder suffer from recurrent episodes of fever with associated painful inflammation of joints, pleural, and peritoneal cavities.

❍ **Acute neutrophilia occurs during what physiologic events?**

Physical exercise.

Epinephrine induced reaction, such as a panic response.

❍ **Reactive leukocytosis, resembling a leukemia-like picture, can occur in what clinical scenarios?**

Sepsis
Systemic mycotic or protozoan
Hepatic failure
Diabetic acidosis
Azotemia

❍ **What is the definition of neutropenia?**

Absolute Neutrophil Count (ANC) < 1500 cell/ml.

❍ **Aside from chemotherapeutics, which suppress bone marrow, what other agents are most commonly implicated?**

Phenothiazines
Semisynthetic penicillin
NSAID's
Aminopyrine derivatives
Antithyroid medications

❍ **What is the most common cause of transient neutropenia?**

Viral infections which most commonly include Hepatitis A, Hepatitis B, Influenza A and B, measles, rubella, and varicella.

❍ **How long would you expect the neutropenia to persist?**

It may persist for the first three to six days of the acute viral syndrome.

❍ **What nutritional deficiencies may precipitate neutropenia?**

Vitamin B12, folic acid, and copper.

❍ **Neutropenia and bacterial infection may herald the onset of?**

Overwhelming sepsis.

❍ **What is the likely symptomtology of individuals with hereditary myeloperoxidase deficiency?**

A majority of individuals remain asymptomatic. Remarkably, the incidence of disease is high, with 1 in 2,000 individuals affected in the United States.

❍ **Briefly explain the cellular basis for the Type I hypersensitivity reaction (wheal and flare). Give a clinical example.**

This immediate type or anaphylactic hypersensitivity is mediated by circulating basophils and mast cells, which become activated by crosslinking of IgE on their membrane surface. The prototypic IgE mediated disease is ragweed hay fever. Other, sometimes fatal, anaphylactic reactions are the classic insect venom or food induced allergies.

❍ **Briefly explain the cellular basis for the Type II hypersensitivity reaction (cytotoxic). Give a clinical example.**

These immune interactions involve integral cellular antigen components and IgG and IgM antibody formation to these foreign antigen determinants. The classic example is immune mediated hemolysis such as that seen in transfusion reaction, or hemolytic disease of the newborn.

❍ **Briefly explain the cellular basis for the Type III hypersensitivity reaction (Arthus or immune complex). Give a clinical example.**

Tissue injury is caused by immune complex deposition in various tissues, which are toxic to that tissue, by mechanisms, such as complement activation or proteolytic enzyme release. Examples include immune complex pericarditis, and arthritis following meningococcal, or H. influenzae infection.

❍ **In Type IV hypersensitivity reaction (cell-mediated or delayed type), pathologic changes follow interaction of antigen with what cellular component of the immune system?**

Antigen specific sensitized T cells.

❍ **Which hypersensitivity reaction is responsible for a majority of the glomerulopathies?**

90% of glomerulonephritis is Type III or immune complex disease.

❍ **What is a prototypic DTH type IV reaction?**

Contact allergy, such as chemical induced contact dermatitis or poison ivy.

❍ **In taking a history, when one suspects allergy, what are some of the most important components to include?**

History of exposure to potential allergens
Frequency, duration, location, and progression of symptoms
Seasonal symptoms
Onset of symptoms
Relieving factors (medication, diurnal variation, and change in location)
Nature of symptoms (dry vs. productive cough, clear vs. purulent sputum)

❍ **What features of the physical exam which should be highlighted when examining an atopic individual?**

Height and weight
Pulsus paradoxus
Alae nasi flaring
Mouth breathing
Allergic ‘shiner’
Allergic ‘salute’ (transverse nasal creasing from habitual nose wiping)
Dennie lines (wrinkles beneath lower eyelids)

❍ **What test is most cost effective, sensitive, and specific in the diagnosis of allergy?**

In vivo skin testing.

❍ **What in vitro tests may be useful in the diagnosis of allergic conditions?**

WBC with differential
Immunoglobulin serum content
RAST
Leukocyte histamine release test

❍ **What other conditions would you see eosinophilia?**

Neoplasm (Hodgkin’s lymphoma)
Immunodeficiency
Parasitic infestation

Addison's disease
Collagen vascular disease
Cystic fibrosis
Infections (CMV, EBV, Leprosy, systemic Candidiasis, Coccidioidmycosis)
Guillain-Barré
Hemosiderosis
Interstitial nephritis
Kawasaki disease

❍ **A patient has a 5-mm "wheal and flare" reaction to ragweed, but denies seasonal allergic symptoms. What does this indicate?**

The patient has been exposed to the allergen, but may not be allergic.

❍ **What percent of patients with mild allergic or extrinsic asthma benefit from inhaled cromolyn sodium inhalation?**

70%.

❍ **What mast cell stabilizer is most effective for treatment of vernal keratoconjunctivitis, vernal conjunctivitis, or vernal keratitis?**

Lodoxamide tromethamine.

❍ **What effects of corticosteroids are likely after two hours?**

A fall in peripheral eosinophils and lymphocytes.

❍ **What effects of corticosteroids are likely after six to eight hours?**

An improvement in pulmonary function in asthmatics and hyperglycemia.

❍ **What are the clinical effects of phenobarbital and phenytoin on corticosteroids?**

Increased steroid clearance and hence decreased plasma concentration.

❍ **What is the most common adverse effect on chronic systemic corticosteroid use?**

Suppression of linear growth.

❍ **What are some other possible adverse effects of chronic steroid use?**

Posterior subcapsular cataract
Osteoporosis
Hypertension
Diabetes mellitus
Cushingoid body habitus
Infections
Pancreatitis
Gastritis
Myopathy.

❍ **What is the preferred dosing regimen of prednisone or prednisolone to lessen the hypothalmic-pituitary-adrenal axis suppressive effect?**

It is recommended that alternate day regimen given as a single dose between 6:00 and 8:00 am. If daily dosing is required, administer a single dose between 6:00 and 8:00 am.

❍ **What is the basis of antigen desensitization?**

Injection of antigenic extract into patients blunts the anamnestic rise of IgE via production of IgG, which effectively sequesters antigen by binding it.

❍ **What patients are not good candidates for immunotherapy desensitization?**

Patients with atopic dermatitis or food allergy.

❍ **When should immunotherapy be discontinued?**

If significant improvement is seen after three years, discontinue injections and observe for symptom recurrence. If no substantial improvement is seen after two years, therapy is unlikely to be of benefit.

❍ **What precaution should be taken each time immunotherapy is administered?**

Observe the patient in the office for at least twenty minutes, as potentially fatal reactions are more likely to occur within this time.

❍ **What are the likely causative agents implicated in perennial allergic rhinitis?**

Components of house dust, feathers, allergens, dander of household pets, and mold spores are the most common inciting agents.

❍ **What constitutes triad asthma?**

The syndrome of nasal polyps, asthma, and aspirin intolerance comprise triad asthma.

❍ **What is the most effective treatment of allergic rhinitis?**

Topical use of corticosteroids, such as beclomethasone nasal spray.

❍ **What are the major risk factors of asthma?**

Poverty
Black race
Maternal age <20 year old
Birth weight < 2,500 grams
Maternal smoking
Small home size
Intense allergic exposure (dust mite)
Large family size
Frequent respiratory infection

❍ **Is cor pulmonale, resulting from sustained pulmonary hypertension, a common complication of asthma?**

No.

❍ **What is extrinsic asthma?**

Asthmatic exacerbation following environmental exposure to allergens such as dust, pollens, and dander.

❍ **What is intrinsic asthma?**

Asthmatic exacerbation not associated with an increase in IgE or a positive skin.

❍ **Is clubbing a feature of severe asthma?**

Rarely observed in either mild or severe asthma.

❍ **Why are acute asthmatic exacerbations more common at night?**

Patency of the airway decreases at night, which precipitate an acute attack.

❍ **A 20 year-old obese, African-American, who appears pale and alert, comes to the ER with shortness of breath. He can only speak in short phrases, his respiratory rate is 28/min, he has audible inspiratory and expiratory wheezing, and obvious intercostal retractions and chest hyperinflation are noted on exam. A blood gas demonstrates oxygen saturation of 90-95% and carbon dioxide of 39. What is the estimated asthma severity?**

Moderate.

❍ **When administering epinephrine in the treatment of asthma, how might the side effects of epinephrine be minimized?**

Side effects, such as pallor, tremor, anxiety, palpitations, and headache, can be minimized if doses of no more than 0.3 ml are given.

❍ **If the response to epinephrine and bronchodilator are unsatisfactory what might be administered next and at what dose?**

Aminophylline may be given IV at a dose of 5mg/kg for 5-15 minutes at rate no greater than 25 mg/min.

❍ **What are the historical risk factors for status asthmaticus?**

Chronic steroid-dependent asthma
Prior ICU admission
Prior intubation
Recurrent ER visits in past 48 hours
Sudden onset of severe respiratory
Poor therapy compliance
Poor clinical recognition of attack severity
Hypoxic seizures

❍ **What should be reserved for refractory status asthmaticus after the patient has been intubated?**

Halothane anesthesia produces prompt bronchodilation, but is difficult to administer and is therefore reserved for the most severe cases.

❍ **The same 20 year-old asthmatic, in the previous question, has had a poor response to treatment in the ER. His PEFR is still 40% below baseline, his oxygen desaturation is at 91%, and he now exhibits pulsus paradoxus on physical exam. What is your next step in management?**

Hospitalize.

❍ **What are the criteria for ICU admission in a severe asthma case?**

PEFR <30% baseline

PCO_2 >40 mm Hg

O_2 saturation <90%

Severe wheezing on auscultation with evidence of decreased air movement

Pulsus paradoxus >15 mmHg.

❍ **What is the mortality rate of asthma?**

In the United States, the mortality rate is 2.0/100,000.

❍ **What is atopic dermatitis?**

An inflammatory skin disorder characterized by erythema, edema, pruritus, exudation, crusting, and scaling.

❍ **What percent of patients with atopic dermatitis have elevated serum IgE levels above normal?**

80%.

❍ **What is the clinical manifestation of urticaria?**

Well-circumscribed, erythematous raised skin lesions.

❍ **What is the most common form of urticaria caused by physical factors?**

Cold urticaria.

❍ **What is the most effective treatment for control of urticaria?**

0.5 mg/kg Hydroxyzine (Atarax) is the most effective therapy, but diphenhydramine (Benadryl) is also useful.

❍ **What are the 9 major causes of anaphylaxis?**

Drugs
Foods
Insect bites
Biological agents (i.e., blood products)
Food additives
Latex
Exercise induced
Idiopathic pseudoallergic.

❍ **What is pseudoallergic anaphylaxis?**

Anaphylactoid reactions may occur which is not necessarily IgE mediated. Some substances can, by themselves, induce mast cell degranulation.

❍ **What substances can induce pseudoallergic anaphylaxis?**

Iodinated radiocontrast media, opiates, D-tubocurarine, thiamine, aspirin, and captopril.

❍ **When do most anaphylactic reactions occur following exposure?**

30 minutes.

❍ **What are typical initial symptoms of an anaphylactic reaction?**

Initially patients usually report a tingling sensation around the mouth followed by a warm feeling and tightness in chest or throat.

❍ **What is standard treatment of an anaphylactic reaction?**

Aqueous epinephrine 1: 1000 at 0.1 ml/kg.

❍ **Patients with severe allergic reaction to eggs should avoid receipt of which vaccines?**

Influenza and yellow fever vaccines.

❍ **Which antitoxoids are still prepared with horse serum and such may precipitate serum sickness?**

Crotalid envenomation and clostridia antitoxin.

❍ **What is the most serious complication of serum sickness?**

The most serious complications are Guillain-Barré syndrome, and peripheral neuritis, most commonly of the brachial plexus.

❍ **What is the major cause of serum sickness?**

Drug allergy, particularly penicillin.

❍ **Are atopic individuals at an increased risk for developing adverse drug reactions?**

No. They may, however, suffer a more severe reaction if they do aquire a drug allergy.

❍ **What is the most common manifestation of an adverse drug reaction?**

Cutaneous eruption with urticarial, exanthematous, and eczematoid reaction

❍ **What cell wall inhibitor does not cross react with penicillin allergic patients?**

Aztreonam.

❍ **When treatment with penicillin is absolutely necessary, which route of desensitization is safest?**

Oral.

❍ **What infectious agent is implicated in chronic blepharitis infection?**

Staphylococcal.

❍ **In idiopathic aplastic anemia, the curative treatment of choice is?**

Bone marrow transplantation (BMT) with an HLA matched donor.

❍ **What should be avoided in patients with aplastic anemia if BMT is an option?**

Transfusions should be avoided as it increases the likelihood of blood product sensitization and hence increases the risk for graft rejection.

❍ **What may be administered as part of the preparative regime to lessen the likelihood of rejection in patients with aplastic anemia who have received transfusions?**

Anti-thymocyte globulin (ATG) with cyclophosphamide.

❍ **What are the indications for BMT in patients with acute myelogenous leukemia (AML)?**

For all those who do <u>not</u> enter remission.
Children with acute megakaryocytic (M7) leukemia.
For all who have entered their first remission, as disease-free survival ranges from 55-83% after BMT.
BMT is indicated if an HLA-matched donor exists.

❍ **Which AML is treated by pharmacological means only, with BMT usually <u>not</u> being considered unless a relapse occurs?**

M3 or promyelocytic leukemia is usually quite responsive to all trans-retinoic acid and consolidation chemotherapy.

❍ **What percent of children with acute lymphoblastic leukemia (ALL) are cured by conventional chemotherapy?**

70%.

❍ **Patients with ALL, considered at high risk for relapse following conventional chemotherapy, are considered for BMT. What patients are included in this group?**

Congenital or infant (<1 year) ALL
Chromosomal translocation t (4,11), t (9,22)-Philadelphia, t (8,14)
FAB L-3 morphology (Burkitt's)
WBC > 100,000

More than I month to achieve remission
Relapse while on chemotherapy
More than one extramedullary site of relapse without a marrow relapse
Second and subsequent remissions.

❍ **What is the disease free survival of patients with ALL after BMT?**

15% to 65% with relapse rates of 30%-70%.

❍ **In general, which patients have the best prognosis, after BMT, for disease-free survival?**

Those which have been transplanted in remission or those that went into an earlier remission.

❍ **What is the incidence of infection with autologous BMT?**

5-10%.

❍ **When is BMT recommended for those with chronic myelogenous leukemia?**

Within one year of diagnosis.

❍ **When is BMT recommended for patients with either non-Hodgkin's or Hodgkin's lymphoma?**

Early after relapse when there is little bulky disease and a greater chance to tolerate the BMT regimen.

❍ **What blood dyscrasias are currently being considered for treatment through BMT?**

Fanconi's anemia, thalassemia major, sickle cell disease, Diamond-Blackfan syndrome, and congenital sideroblastic anemia.

❍ **What is graft versus host disease (GVHD)?**

Engraftment of immunocompetent donor cells into an immunocompromised host, resulting in cell-mediated cytotoxic destruction of host cells if an immunologic incompatibility exists.

❍ **What are the common factors which influence engraftment and graft rejection?**

HLA disparity - most important
Pretransplant alloimmunization by transfusions
Conditioning regimen
Transplanted marrow cell dose
Marrow stroma/microenviroment
Post-transplant immunosupression
Donor T cells
Drug toxicity
Viral infections

❍ **When does acute GVHD present and what are the typical manifestations?**

Acute GVHD typically occurs around day 19 (median), just as the patient begins to engraft, and is characterized by erythroderma, cholestatic hepatitis, and enteritis.

❍ **A 30 year-old female is 21 days status-post BMT and presents with a fever, maculopapular rash over 30% of her body, >1,000 ml diarrhea/ day, and rising LFT's, with a total bilirubin of 4 mg/100ml. What is the clinical stage of GVHD?**

Stage 2.

❍ **The patient, in the previous question, 4 days later, has evidence of generalized erythroderma with desquamation, severe abdominal pain with no bowel movements, and a total bilirubin of 16mg/100ml. What is the clinical stage of GVHD?**

The patient has progressed to a worse clinical stage or stage 4.

❍ **What is the clinical definition of chronic GVHD (cGVHD)?**

As early as 60-70 days status-post engraftment, the patient exhibits signs of a systemic autoimmune process, manifesting as Sjogren's syndrome, systemic lupus erythrematosus, scleroderma, primary bililary cirrhosis, and commonly experiences recurrent infection with encapsulated bacteria, fungus, or viruses.

❍ **What are the risk factors for development of cGVHD?**

Advanced age
Prior acute GVHD
Buffy coat transfusions
Parity of female donor.

❍ **How long is immunosuppressive treatment required for BMT recipients?**

Usually 6-12 months or until a state of tolerance is attained.

❍ **What agent may be a treatment alternative for patients with high risk GVHD, or with refractory chronic GVHD?**

Thalidomide has been shown to have a 59% response rate with a 76% survival for those with refractory GVHD and a 48% survival for those with high-risk cGVHD.

❍ **What are the potential risks for treatment of GVHD with T cell depletion techniques?**

By depleting the T cell population, the success of engraftment decreases, as well as the ability to defend against potential malignancies.

❍ **What is the typical dosing regimen of methotrexate given to prevent GVHD?**

Given on post-transplant days 1,3,6 and 11 and weekly thereafter.

❍ **Treatment with methotrexate may result in what complications and how is it treated?**

Methotrexate may worsen renal impairment, resulting in fluid retention and may aggravate existing mucositis. In these situations, rescue of the dihydrofolate reductase system with leucovorin is indicated.

❍ **What is the mechanism of action of cyclosporine?**

It selectively inhibits the translation of IL-2 m-RNA by helper T cells, thus attenuating the T cell activation pathways.

❍ **What drugs <u>increase</u> blood levels of cyclosporine?**

Ketoconazole
Erythromycin
Methylprednisone
Warfarin
Verapamil
Ethanol
Imipenem-cilastatin
Metaclopramide
Fluconazole

❍ **What drugs <u>decrease</u> blood levels of cyclosporine?**

Phenytoin
Phenobarbital
Carbamazepine

Valproate
Nafcillin
Rifampin

❍ **What are significant toxic side effects of cyclosporine therapy?**

Neurotoxic - Tremors, paraesthesia, headache, confusion, somnolence, seizures, coma.
Hepatotoxic - Cholestasis, cholelithiasis, hemorrhagic necrosis.
Endocrine - Ketosis, hyperprolatinemia, hypertestosteronemia, gynecomastia, impaired spermatogenesis.
Metabolic - Hypomagnesemia, hyperuricemia, hyperglycemia, hyperkalemia, hypocholestrolemia.
Vascular - Hypertension, vasculitic hemolytic-uremic syndrome, atherogenesis.
Nephrotoxic - Oliguria, acute tubular damage, fluid retention, interstitial fibrosis, tubular atrophy.

❍ **What drugs may exacerbate the nephrotoxicity of cyclosporine?**

Aminogylcosides, amphotercin B, acyclovir, digoxin, furosemide, indomethacin, and trimethoprim.

❍ **What is the incidence of cataracts in patients who have received single dose total body irradiation (TBI), fractionated TBI, and chemotherapeutics alone?**

The incidence of cataracts with single dose TBI is 80%, with fractionated TBI 20%-50%, and 20% after chemotherapy alone.

❍ **What are the long-term effects of corticosteroid treatment?**

Growth failure, Cushingoid appearance, hypertension, cataracts, GI bleeding, pancreatitis, psychosis, hyperglycemia, osteoporosis, aseptic necrosis of the femoral head, and suppression of the pituitary-adrenal axis.

❍ **What is the overall risk for developing a secondary malignancy, as compared to the general population?**

The risk is 6.7 times that of the general population.

❍ **What solid tumor malignancy is most common in patients who have received radiation?**

Thyroid carcinoma.

❍ **How long does recovery of immune cell function take in post transplant patients?**

B cells- response to mitogenic stimulation in 2 to 3 months. However, adequate serum IgG levels may take as long as 7 to 9 months and IgA levels may lag up to two years. CD8 T cells- 4 months

CD4 T cells- 6 to 9 months.

❍ **What are the most common types of infections seen pre-transplant after bone marrow ablation (day 0-14)?**

Mucositis, cellulitis, sepsis, pneumonia, and urinary tract infections.

❍ **What are the most common types of infections seen post-transplant engraftment (day 0-30)?**

Oral thrush, bacterial sepsis, catheter infections, fungal infections, pneumonia, and sinusitis.

❍ **What are the most common types of infections seen in post-transplant postengraftment (day 30-100)?**

CMV and EBV infection, viral hepatitis, toxoplasmosis, diffuse interstitial pneumonia, and cystitis.

❍ **What are the most common types of infections seen post-transplant postengraftment (day 100-365)?**

Varicella, herpes, CMV, toxoplasmosis, Pnuemocystis carnii pneumonia, viral hepatitis, and common bacterial infections.

❍ **With BMT recipients 30 to 100 days post-transplant, what percentage of patients will be infected with cytomegalovirus if prophylaxis is not used?**

50 to 60 %.

❍ **When should re-immunization be instituted in patients with no evidence of chronic GVHD?**

Diphtheria and tetanus toxoid-3 to 6 months status post transplant
Inactivated (Salk) polio-6 to 12 months
Measles, mumps, and rubella (MMR)-1 to 2 years.

❍ **How are cardiac allografts matched for transplant recipients?**

ABO blood group
Body weight
HLA matching is not currently used

❍ **Immediately postoperative immunosuppression of cardiac transplant patients consists of?**

Cyclosporine 10 mg/kg/24 hr
Azathioprine 2 mg/kg/24 hr
Prednisone 0.6 mg/kg/24 hour
Antilymphocyte preparation within the first 1-2 weeks

❍ **In what post-operative time period is acute rejection the greatest?**

3 months status post transplantation.

❍ **T/F: Most clinical cardiac transplant rejections occur without detectable clinical symptoms.**

True. Cyclosporine has significantly modified the clinical course of rejection and the most reliable method of monitoring patients for rejection is myocardial biopsy.

❍ **What is the five-year survival of a heart transplant recipient?**

72%.

❍ **What neoplastic disease is most commonly associated with post transplantation patients?**

Lymphoproliferative disease (LPD), which is associated with Epstein-Barr virus infection.

❍ **What infectious agent accounts for 25% of all infectious episodes of allograft heart recipients?**

Cytomegalovirus.

❍ **What is the most common site of bacterial infection in all types of transplant patients?**

Lung (35%).

❍ **What is the most commonly seen side effect of cyclosporine therapy?**

Hypertension, as a result of plasma volume expansion and defective renal sodium excretion.

❍ **What are the three most frequent causes of mortality in heart transplant patients.**

Infection
Rejection
Coronary artery disease

❍ **Fever, sternal tenderness, erythema, and purulent drainage suggest what diagnosis 48 hours postoperative heart transplantation?**

Mediastinitis, caused by S. aureus, S. epidermidis, or gram negative bacilli.

❍ **What commonly used immunosuppressive agent would be contraindicated in heart-lung transplant patients?**

Steroids. Their use may affect airway healing.

❍ **What is the leading cause of death for these patients?**

Infection.

❍ **What tests should be performed for rejection surveillance in a heart-lung transplant recipient?**

Pulmonary function tests
Systemic arterial oxygen tension
Chest roentgenogram
Transbronchial biopsy

❍ **What is the most sensitive and specific sign of an infectious disease in an immunocompromised host?**

Fever.

❍ **At what absolute neutrophil count (ANC) are neutropenic patients at risk for serious infection and what two types of infectious agents are most responsible?**

At an of ANC $<0.5 \times 10^9$ cells/liter, the risk for infection is inversely proportional to the cell count with the most common infectious agents being bacterial or fungal.

❍ **At what CD4 cell count is prophylaxis indicated in these patients and what antimicrobial is used?**

Just as with immunodeficiency virus, a CD4 count of <200cells/mm^3 is indication for prophylaxis with TMP-SMX (Bactrim) being used.

❍ **What is the most important pre-liver transplantation management for a patient?**

Ensure adequate nutritional status with regard to caloric intake, vitamins, and mineral supplementation.

❍ **Which immunosuppressive agent is associated with a lower rate of acute rejection and reduced use of corticosteroids, but has a higher incidence of renal impairment, perturbed glucose metabolism, and neurologic complications?**

FK 506 (Tacrolimus)

❍ **What percent of liver transplant patients will become infected with cytomegalovirus if prophylaxis is not given?**

50%.

❍ **Common types of early infections of liver transplant patients include?**

Gram negative enteric pneumonia
Cholangitis
Soft tissue wound infections,
Intraabdominal abscess
Peritonitis
Disseminated candidiasis

❍ **During the first six months post-liver transplant, patients have a 15% chance of developing what type of hepatitis?**

CMV Hepatitis.

❍ **What tissue typing studies are necessary prior to renal transplantation?**

HLA-A, B, C, D/DR, and ABO.

❍ **What viral antibody titers must be tested in both the donor and recipient prior to renal transplantation?**

Hepatitis A, B, and C; Epstein-Barr; Cytomegalovirus; Herpes; and Varicella.

❍ **In patients requiring renal transplantation, which type of transplant is associated with the most favorable prognosis, live or cadaver?**

39 months after transplantation, 80% of live donor kidneys and 58% cadaver kidneys are functional.

❍ **One month after renal transplant, what infectious agent most commonly causes a urinary tract infection?**

Psuedomonas aeruiginosa.

❍ **What percent of patients have recurrence of original disease?**

7%.

❍ **What type of glomerulopathy is most likely to recur?**

Focal segmental glomerulosclerosis.

❍ **A renal transplant patient, 30 days post-transplant, presents with fever, oliguria, hypertension, elevated serum creatinine. What two diagnostic tests would you perform next?**

Renal ultrasound and renal scan to evaluate renal blood flow.

❍ **What diagnostic study is necessary to differentiate between rejection reaction, acute tubular necrosis, cyclosporine toxicity, or recurrence of renal disease?**

Renal biopsy.

❍ **What percent of renal transplant patients will have at least one episode of rejection reaction?**

100%.

❍ **Of patients experiencing rejection reaction, what percent are successfully treated during the first episode?**

62%.

❍ **Sequential immunsupression post transplantation commonly employs which drugs?**

Azathioprine, cyclosporine, and prednisone.

❍ **What is the major cause of death in renal transplant recipients one year following transplant?**

Infection.

❍ **What is the most common infection seen in renal transplant patients?**

CMV.

O What are the most common post-transplantation complications in renal patients?

Acute tubular necrosis
Rejection reaction
Vascular or urological block
Recurrence of original disease
Drug toxicity
Infection
Bleeding
Pancreatitis
Lymphocele
Uroma
Bowel obstruction.

O A transplant patient presents with nausea, vomiting, and mild dehydration. What is your next step?

ADMIT. Any condition, which impairs the ability to take or absorb medication, requires hospital admission and parenteral administration of immunosuppressive agents.

O In transplant patients receiving immunosuppressive therapy, how does one evaluate abdominal pain?

Chronic steroid use often masks abdominal catastrophes. Therefore, abdominal pain in a transplant patient is a surgical EMERGENCY until otherwise proven.

O When is Pneumocystis carinii pneumonitis most likely to be seen in a transplant patient?

Most commonly 2 to 6 months post transplantation.

O In what three patterns might CMV infection occur?

As a primary infection with recipient having no prior exposure

Reactivation infection

Superinfection with seropositivity

O What immunosuppressive agents have the highest risk of reactivating CMV infection?

Azathioprine and OKT3/antilymphocyte globulin.

O Of those with clinically diagnosed CMV, 33% will develop what complication?

Pulmonary involvement, which may rapidly progress to respiratory failure and death.

O Following an acute episode of CMV, patients with renal or liver transplants are at an increased risk for?

GRAFT REJECTION. CMV has been shown to upregulate MHC II D/DR in allografts, which may precipitate rejection reaction.

O EBV infection is linked with what late complication (years)?

Post transplant lymphoproliferative disorder.

O A transplant patient on chronic immunosuppressive agents presents with two-week history of persistent, severe headache without fever. Your diagnostic management?

Neurological exam, CT scan, MRI, and a lumbar puncture, unless contraindicated by evidence of increased intracranial pressure (DO a fundiscopic exam).

❍ **A liver transplant patient presents with increased liver aminotransferase and direct bilirubin without pain or fever. Which diagnostic test would be most useful?**

Doppler flow study to rule out arterial thrombosis.

❍ **What would you suspect if liver transplant patient presented with rapidly increasing ascites and liver dysfunction?**

Portal vein thrombosis.

❍ **What is the mechanism of immunosuppression with treatment modalities intravenous immunoglobulin (IVIG) or colloidal gold?**

Inhibition of phagocytosis.

❍ **What is the mechanism of immunosuppression with hydroxychloroquine?**

Alkalinization of proteolytic vesicles.

❍ **Anti-dsDNA antibodies are most indicative for what disease?**

Systemic lupus erythematosus.

❍ **The presence of antineutrophil cytoplasmic antibodies (c-ANCA) with a diffuse staining pattern in serum immunofluorescence is most commonly associated with what disease?**

Wegener's granulomatosus.

❍ **The above-described staining pattern may be associated with what other diseases?**

Kawasaki disease and HIV.

❍ **Patients with the presence of anti phospholipdid antibodies in either primary or secondary antiphopholipid syndromes are at increased risk for what diseases?**

Risk of thrombotic events
Thrombocytopenia
Hemolytic anemia
Stroke
Chorea
Transverse myelitis
Vascular heart disease

❍ **What are the HLA allele associations for the following types of Juvenile Rheumatoid Arthritis (JRA); Pauciarticular Type I and Type II, and polyarticular rheumatoid factor positive?**

JRA Pauciarticular Type I: HLA-DR5, -DR6, and -DR8
JRA Pauciarticular Type II: HLA-B27
Polyarticular RA positive: HLA-DR4

❍ **Which two subgroups of JRA is joint destruction more likely?**

RA factor positive polyarticular and systemic-onset JRA.

❍ **What is the percent of above that develop severe arthritis?**

> 50%.

❍ **What forms of JRA are ANA negative?**

Pauciarticular Type II and JRA systemic onset.

❍ **Regardless of joint disease activity, what should all children with pauciarticular onset disease be screened for and how?**

Children with this form of JRA are at increased risk of chronic ocular inflammation regardless of systemic activity and hence serious sequelae such as cataracts, glaucoma, ocular globe degeneration, and permanent blindness can result. It is therefore mandatory to perform slit lamp examinations every 3 to 4 years on these children.

❍ **The most common form of JRA is at risk for what chronic disease manifestation?**

The most common form, Pauciarticular onset disease type I, which primarily affects young girls, are at increased risk of developing chronic iridocyclitis.

❍ **In Pauciarticular JRA Type I, would one expect a positive rheumatoid factor?**

No. Over 90% of patients however will be ANA positive.

❍ **Which of the JRA predominantly affects young boys older than 8 years old?**

Pauciarticular disease type II.

❍ **What are the most common manifestations of Juvenile Rheumatoid Arthritis (JRA)?**

High intermittent fever, rheumatoid rash, arthralgia or myalgia during febrile episodes, and persistent arthritis of greater than six weeks duration.

❍ **What is the overall prognosis of JRA patients?**

At least 75% of patients with JRA will have long term remissions without significant residual deformity or loss of function.

❍ **A 16 year-old girl presents with intermittent fever, arthralgia, and complaint of bilateral knee stiffness and pain. What tests would be most helpful in your diagnosis?**

Roentgenogram of affected joints
Joint fluid analysis and culture
PPD with anergy panel
B. burgdorferi antibody titer
CBC with differential

❍ **What pharmacological treatment is NOT indicated in the treatment of JRA?**

Corticosteroids.

❍ **How does ankylosing spondylitis differ from rheumatoid arthritis?**

Involvement of the sacroiliac joints and lumbodorsal spine, predilection for males, occurrence of aortitis, familial incidence, a negative RF, and lack of rheumatoid nodules or incidence of acute iridocyclitis characterize ankylosing spondilitis.

❍ **Reiter's disease may occur following infection with which microbial agents?**

Shiella, Yersinia, Enterocolitica, Camphylobacter, and Chlamydia.

❍ **What percent of patients with inflammatory bowel disease have articular manifestations if the disease?**

10%.

❍ **What are the most frequent early symptoms of SLE?**

The most frequent early symptoms in children are fever, malaise, arthritis or arthralgia, and rash.

❍ **What is the best screening test for SLE?**

ANA should be demonstrable in all patients with active SLE.

❍ **What hematologic conditions are seen in patients with SLE?**

Anemia, thrombocytopenia, and leukopenia occur frequently.

❍ **What neurologic disorders, if present, serve as diagnostic criteria for SLE?**

Seizures and psychosis.

❍ **What pharmacologic agents are most commonly associated with drug-induced lupus?**

Anticonvulsants, hydralazine and isoniazid.

❍ **What are the major causes of SLE mortality?**

Nephritis, with resultant renal failure
Central nervous system complications
Infection
Pulmonary lupus
Myocardial infarction

❍ **When is anticoagulation therapy indicated in SLE?**

Patients with the persistent presence of antiphospholipid antibodies (because of the risk of venous or arterial thrombosis), migraine, recurrent fetal loss, TIA, stroke, avascular necrosis, transverse myelitis, pulmonary hypertension or embolus, livedo reticularis, leg ulcers, or thrombocytopenia.

❍ **What are the possible complications of Kawasaki disease during the acute phase of the illness?**

Arthritis
Myocarditis
Pericarditis
Mitral insufficiency
CHF
Iridocyclitis
Meningitis
Sterile pyuria

❍ **What are the diagnostic criteria for Kawasaki disease?**

Fever lasting at least 5 days
Presence of four of the following five conditions:
Bilateral nonpurulent conjunctival injection.
Changes in the mucosa of the oropharynx, including infected pharynx, dry fissured lips, strawberry tongue.
Changes in peripheral extremities, such as edema and/or erythema of the hands or feet desquamation.
Primarily truncal rash.
Cervical lymphadenopathy.
Illness not explained by any other known disease process

❍ **Which form of vasculitis may be seen after infection with Hepatitis B?**

Polyarteritis nodosa.

❍ **What side effects might one rarely see with administration of IV gamma globulin?**

Anaphylaxis
Chills
Fever

Headache
Myalgia.

❍ **Which tissue biopsy is most helpful for diagnosis of Polyarteritis nodosa, but seldomly employed?**

Testicular biopsy.

❍ **A 30 year-old patient presents with progressive destruction and ulcerations of upper respiratory tract and associated arthritis and acute glomerulitis. The presumptive diagnosis of Wegener's granulomatosis is made. What are the therapeutic options?**

Corticosteroids, cyclosporine, or trimethoprim-sulfmethoxazole (Bactrim)

❍ **What rare vasculitis should be considered in an 18 year-old African-American girl with obscure hypertension, increased ESR, and fever?**

Takayasu's arteritis.

❍ **Patient with slowly progressive course of dermatomyositis is most susceptible to what disease complication.**

Calcinosis, which is deposition of calcium in subcutaneous tissue.

❍ **What is the mortality of untreated dermatomyositis?**

40%.

❍ **What are two late complications of dermatomyositis?**

Lipodystrophy with insulin resistance and hyperandrogenism.

❍ **The clinical histologic biopsy of a patient with scleroderma will demonstrate?**

Fibrosis with minimal inflammation and occlusive vasculitis affecting the capillaries and small blood vessels.

❍ **What clinical manifestations differentiate SYSTEMIC from FOCAL scleroderma?**

In focal one sees cutaneous fibrosis and does not see systemic involvement, such as diffuse fibrosis or Raynaud's phenomenon, both of which are components of systemic scleroderma.

❍ **What characteristic features would serve to differentiate EOSINOPHILIC FASCIITIS from SYSTEMIC SCLERODERMA?**

In Eosinophilic fasciitis, one sees isolated inflammation of the fascial layers, particularly the limbs, with sparing of the skin, prominent eosinophilia, and absence of Raynaud's phenomenon. Joint contractures of the hand are characteristic of both diseases.

❍ **An 18 year-old female presents with complains of fever and malaise one week prior to the development of 1-3 cm painful, red, ovoid nodules on her shins bilaterally. The patient's mom states she had an episode of severe sore throat the previous week also. Hilar lymphadenopathy is demonstrated on chest x-ray. What is the diagnosis?**

Erythema nodosum.

❍ **Erythema nodosum is most common in which age group?**

This disease progressively increases in frequency up to the third decade in life.

❍ **Behcet syndrome is characterized by recurrent oral and genital ulcers and ocular inflammation. What additional symptoms are associated with a particularly poor prognosis?**

CNS abnormalities, such as cranial nerve palsies and psychosis.

❍ **The combination of pain, tenderness, and swelling of the costosternal junction is referred to as what syndrome?**

Tietze's syndrome or costochondritis.

❍ **What is the clinical scenario of Familial Mediterranean Fever and what is the attributed cause?**

Amyloid deposition is the cause of this condition, which manifests with proteinuria that progresses to nephrotic syndrome and renal failure.

❍ **What is the treatment?**

Colchicine, which may greatly lessen the occurrence of the amyloid deposition.

❍ **What inflammatory conditions might one expect in secondary amyloidosis?**

JRA, cystic fibrosis, inflammatory bowel disease, and chronic infections, such as tuberculosis.

❍ **What diseases are not associated with secondary amyloidosis?**

SLE and dermatomyositis.

❍ **What is the mortality of untreated dermatomyositis?**

40%.

❍ **What connective tissue disease is characterized by sicca complex and anti-SSA and SSB autoantibodies?**

Sjogren's syndrome.

❍ **Which vasculitis affects predominantly the extracranial vessels?**

Takayasu's arteritis.

❍ **What complement deficiency is associated with the greatest mortality and morbidity?**

C3 deficiencies. Patients with C3 deficiencies have an especially poor clinical course. The key location of C3 in the complement cascade leaves patients with a C3 deficiency with decreased abilities in both opsonization and the formation of the membrane attack complex. As a result, these patients are highly susceptible to severe, overwhelming infection, especially with encapsulated organisms.

❍ **T/F: Treatment of possible meningitis in a patient with a known complement deficiency should include coverage of *Streptococcus pneumoniae, Haemophilus influenzae, and Neisseria meningitides.***

True. Patients with complement deficiencies (in particular C3 deficiency) are especially susceptible to infections with encapsulated organisms, such as S pneumoniae, H influenzae, and N meningitidis. Treatment of infection should provide empiric coverage for these organisms.

❍ **What medications would be the best choice for single-agent, first-line therapy in an otherwise healthy 36-year-old woman with a 4-month history of daily hives that occur without apparent reason?**

The first-line treatment for chronic urticaria is use of an H1 antihistamine, such as cetirizine (Zyrtec), desloratadine (Clarinex), fexofenadine. The second-generation H1 blockers have a much better safety profile than do the first-generation H1 blockers. Cetirizine causes sedation of 10% of patients.

Desloratadine, fexofenadine and loratadine cause sedation at a rate similar to placebo (approximately ≤5%). Long-term therapy with corticosteroids, such as prednisone, should be avoided unless absolutely necessary because of adverse systemic effects. Cyclosporin is a potentially toxic drug that should be reserved for use when all conventional therapies have failed, and it should be used only by a specialist skilled in its use. H2 blockers, such as ranitidine, can be helpful as adjuncts to H1 antihistamines but are not effective when used alone. Aspirin is not known to be of benefit in urticaria, and it can exacerbate the condition in some patients.

❍ **T/F: Laryngeal edema is the most feared complication of hereditary angioedema (HAE).**

True. Laryngeal edema is the most feared complication of HAE and can cause an immediate life threatening emergency. Dental work and surgery involving the head and neck are common precipitants, but laryngeal edema can be spontaneous. Patients describe a choking sensation, as if something is caught in the throat. They may rapidly progress to stridor and airway obstruction and require emergency intubation or tracheostomy to ensure adequate airways.

GENITOURINARY

Trust only movement. Life happens at the level of events not of words. Trust movement.
Alfred Adler

❍ **What is the most common cause of acute renal failure?**

Acute tubular necrosis. This occurs after toxic or ischemic renal injuries caused by shock, surgery, or rhabdomyolysis.

❍ **What percentage of men with BPH are afflicted with occult prostate cancer?**

10 to 30%.

❍ **How well does the size of the prostate in BPH correlate with the symptoms?**

Not well. Symptoms can arise because of a small fibrous prostate as well as a large one. Additional symptoms can also develop as a result of median bar hypertrophy of the posterior vesicle neck, detrusor muscle decompensation, or instability.

❍ **Which is the most common type of bladder cancer?**

Transitional cell carcinoma. Schistosomiasis infection, aniline dyes, smoking, and the male gender are all risk factors.

❍ **Why is surgical correction of cryptorchidism important?**

Surgical correction is required to inhibit infertility, but the procedure has no bearing on the future development of testicular cancer. Surgery must be performed before age 5 to preserve fertility.

❍ **How is testicular torsion distinguished from epididymitis?**

By the rate of the onset of the pain. Torsional pain begins instantaneously at maximum intensity, whereas epididymal pain grows steadily over hours or days. Clinically, elevation of the scrotum will relieve pain related to epididymitis but is not effective with torsional pain.

❍ **What is the most common cause of epididymitis?**

Prepubertal boys:Coliform bacteria
Men younger than 35:Chlamydia or Neisseria gonorrhea
Men older than 35:Coliform bacteria
Epididymitis is also frequently caused by urinary reflux, prostatitis, or urethral instrumentation.

❍ **What does epididymitis in childhood suggest?**

Obstructive or fistulous urinary defects. Epididymitis is rare in children.

❍ **What does a blue dot sign suggest?**

Torsion of the epididymis or appendix testis. With transillumination of the testis, a blue reflection occurs. When detected early, a patient with torsion of the appendix testis will experience intense pain near the head of the epididymis or testis, which is frequently associated with a palpable tender nodule. If normal flow to the affected testis can be confirmed by a testicular ultrasound, immediate surgery can be avoided. Most appendages will calcify or degenerate within 10 to 14 days without harm to the patient.

❍ **How does the pain associated with epididymitis differ from that produced by prostatitis?**

Epididymitis: Pain begins in the scrotum or groin and radiates along the spermatic cord. It intensifies rapidly, is associated with dysuria, and is relieved with scrotal elevation (Prehn's sign).

Prostatitis: Patients have frequency, dysuria, urgency, bladder outlet obstruction, and retention. They may have low back pain and perineal pain, associated with fever, chills, arthralgias, and myalgias.

❍ **What percentage of patients with epididymitis will also have pyuria?**

25%.

❍ **What is the eponym for idiopathic scrotal edema? How is this disease treated?**

Fournier's gangrene is a polymicrobial infection of the subcutaneous tissue that is characterized by widespread tissue necrosis. Treatment consists of broad-spectrum parenteral antibiotics and immediate surgical debridement.

❍ **What four clinical findings are indicative of acute glomerulonephritis (GN)?**

1) Oliguria
2) Hypertension
3) Pulmonary edema
4) Urine sediment containing RBCs, WBC's, protein, and RBC casts.

❍ **What is the most common cause of post-infectious GN?**

Post streptococcal Group A beta-hemolytic glomerulonephritis. However, other infections may also produce GN-related infections. GN is caused by an immune-complex deposition in glomeruli. Most patients completely recover normal renal function, spontaneously, within a few weeks.

❍ **What syndrome is characterized by a rapidly progressive, anti-glomerular basement membrane antibody-induced GN that is preceded by pulmonary hemorrhage and hemoptysis?**

Goodpasture's syndrome.

❍ **What is the most common cause of hematuria?**

Lesions of the bladder or lower urinary tract. When hematuria originates in a kidney, the probable causes are polycystic kidney disease and nephropathy.

❍ **What are some causes of false-positive hematuria?**

Food coloring, beets, paprika, rifampin, phenothiazine, Dilantin, myoglobin, or menstruation.

❍ **A urinalysis reveals RBC casts and dysmorphic RBCs. What is the probable origin of hematuria?**

Glomerulus.

❍ **A 17 year-old male presents with a painless mass in his scrotum that fluctuates in size with palpation. The mass transilluminates. What is the probable diagnosis?**

A communicating hydrocele. An inguinal-scrotal ultrasound should distinguish hydrocele from bowel, and a testicular nuclear scan should rule out testicular torsion.

❍ **What percentage of urinary calculi are radiopaque?**

90%.

❍ **What are the admission criteria for patients with renal calculi?**

Infection with concurrent obstruction, a solitary kidney and complete obstruction, uncontrolled pain, intractable emesis, or large stones. Only 10% of stones > 6 mm pass spontaneously. Other indications include renal insufficiency and complete obstruction or urinary extravasation, as demonstrated by the IVP.

❍ **What percentage of patients with urinary calculi do not have hematuria?**

10%.

❍ **A urinary pH of 7.3 is conducive to the formation of what kind of stones?**

Struvite and phosphate stones. Alkaline urine actually inhibits the formation of uric acid and cystine stones. Conversely, struvite and phosphate stones are inhibited by a more acidic urine.

❍ **Which type of stone formation is caused by a genetic error?**

Cysteine stones. These stones are produced because there is an error in the transport of amino acids, resulting in cystinuria.

❍ **Where is kidney stone formation most likely to occur?**

In the proximal portion of the collecting system.

❍ **What is the 5-year recurrence rate for kidney stones?**

50%. The 10-year recurrence rate is 70%.

❍ **What percentage of patients spontaneously pass kidney stones?**

80%. This is largely dependent on size. Seventy-five percent of stones less than 4 mm pass spontaneously, while only 10% of those larger than 6 mm pass spontaneously. Analgesics and increased fluid intake aid in outpatient management of kidney stones.

❍ **What is the most common systemic cause of impotence?**

Diabetes.

❍ **What is the most common form of incontinence?**

Detrusor instability.

❍ **What is the post-void residual volume that suggests urinary retention?**

A volume greater than 60 cc.

❍ **What is the most common cause of nephrotic syndrome in children? In adults?**

Children: Minimal change disease. Adults: Idiopathic glomerulonephritis.

❍ **What are some common nephrotoxic agents?**

Aminoglycoside, NSAID's, contrast dye, and myoglobin.

❍ **What is the definition of oliguria? Of anuria?**

Oliguria:Urine output < 500 ml/day

Anuria:Urine output < 100 ml/day

❍ **When is a retrograde urethrogram necessary to evaluate a patient with a penile fracture?**

Patients with hematuria, blood at the urethral meatus, or the inability to void should undergo this procedure to rule out a urethral injury. A penile fracture is rupture of the corpus cavernosum with tearing of the

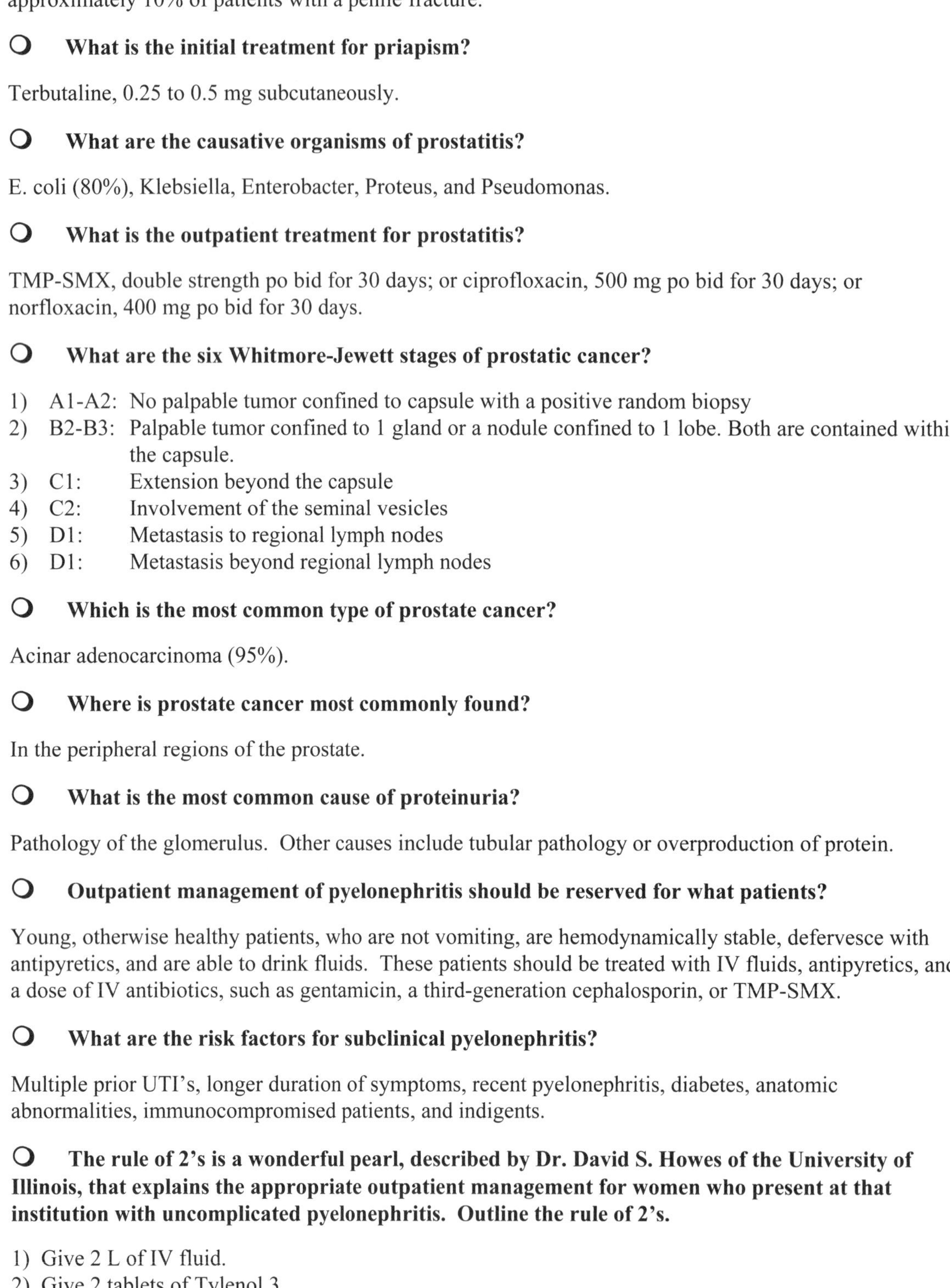

tunica albuginea. It occurs as a result of a blunt trauma to the erect penis. Urethral injury occurs in approximately 10% of patients with a penile fracture.

❍ **What is the initial treatment for priapism?**

Terbutaline, 0.25 to 0.5 mg subcutaneously.

❍ **What are the causative organisms of prostatitis?**

E. coli (80%), Klebsiella, Enterobacter, Proteus, and Pseudomonas.

❍ **What is the outpatient treatment for prostatitis?**

TMP-SMX, double strength po bid for 30 days; or ciprofloxacin, 500 mg po bid for 30 days; or norfloxacin, 400 mg po bid for 30 days.

❍ **What are the six Whitmore-Jewett stages of prostatic cancer?**

1) A1-A2: No palpable tumor confined to capsule with a positive random biopsy
2) B2-B3: Palpable tumor confined to 1 gland or a nodule confined to 1 lobe. Both are contained within the capsule.
3) C1: Extension beyond the capsule
4) C2: Involvement of the seminal vesicles
5) D1: Metastasis to regional lymph nodes
6) D1: Metastasis beyond regional lymph nodes

❍ **Which is the most common type of prostate cancer?**

Acinar adenocarcinoma (95%).

❍ **Where is prostate cancer most commonly found?**

In the peripheral regions of the prostate.

❍ **What is the most common cause of proteinuria?**

Pathology of the glomerulus. Other causes include tubular pathology or overproduction of protein.

❍ **Outpatient management of pyelonephritis should be reserved for what patients?**

Young, otherwise healthy patients, who are not vomiting, are hemodynamically stable, defervesce with antipyretics, and are able to drink fluids. These patients should be treated with IV fluids, antipyretics, and a dose of IV antibiotics, such as gentamicin, a third-generation cephalosporin, or TMP-SMX.

❍ **What are the risk factors for subclinical pyelonephritis?**

Multiple prior UTI's, longer duration of symptoms, recent pyelonephritis, diabetes, anatomic abnormalities, immunocompromised patients, and indigents.

❍ **The rule of 2's is a wonderful pearl, described by Dr. David S. Howes of the University of Illinois, that explains the appropriate outpatient management for women who present at that institution with uncomplicated pyelonephritis. Outline the rule of 2's.**

1) Give 2 L of IV fluid.
2) Give 2 tablets of Tylenol 3.
3) Give 2 g of ceftriaxone.
4) If the patient can tolerate 2 glasses of water and his or her fever decreases by 2 degrees, give TMP-SMX double strength bid for 2 weeks and plan a follow-up in 2 days.

Editor's note: We provide 1 g of ceftriaxone or use other IV antibiotics.

❍ **What is the most common cause of chronic renal failure?**

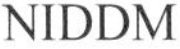
NIDDM.

❍ **When are renal insufficiency symptoms displayed?**

When 90% of the nephrons have been destroyed. Hypertension, diabetes mellitus, glomerulonephritis, polycystic kidney disease, tubulointerstitial disease, and obstructive uropathy are all causes of chronic renal failure.

❍ **What is the most common cause of intrinsic renal failure?**

Acute tubular necrosis (80 to 90%), resulting from an ischemic injury (the most common cause of ATN) or from a nephrotoxic agent. Less frequent causes of intrinsic renal failure (10 to 20%) include vasculitis, malignant hypertension, acute GN, or allergic interstitial nephritis.

❍ **What is an abnormal ultrasound finding that suggests chronic renal failure?**

Kidneys < 9 cm in length are abnormal. A difference in length between the two kidneys of > 1.5 cm suggests unilateral kidney disease. Kidneys with a small or absent renal cortex are also indicative of chronic renal failure.

❍ **What is the life expectancy of chronic renal patients after the disease has progressed to dialysis?**

Patients younger than 60 have a 4 to 5 year life expectancy. Patients over 60 have a 2 to 3 year life expectancy.

❍ **If a urine dipstick is positive for blood, but a urine analysis is negative for RBCs, what is the probable disease?**

Rhabdomyolysis. Severe muscle damage can result in free myoglobin in the blood. Very high levels can lead to acute renal failure.

❍ **What is the most common neoplasm in men under 30?**

Seminomas. This is also the most common type of testicular neoplasm. The peak incidence is between the ages 20 and 40 with a smaller peak occurring below age 10. 90-95% are germinal tumors. However, only 60-70% are germinal in children. Cryptorchidism is a significant risk factor for this cancer.

❍ **What is the best tumor marker for testicular cancer?**

Placental alkaline phosphatase (PLAP). 70-90% of patients with testicular cancer have elevated PLAP. Other tumor markers are α-fetoprotein and beta-HCG.

❍ **Testicular torsion is most common in which age group?**

14 year-olds. Two-thirds of the cases occur in the second decade. The next most common group is newborns.

❍ **T/F: Testicular torsion frequently follows a history of strenuous physical activity or occurs during sleep.**

True.

❍ **T/F: Forty percent of patients with testicular torsion have a history of similar pain in the past that resolved spontaneously.**

True.

❍ **What is the definitive treatment for testicular torsion?**

Bilateral orchiopexy in which the testes are surgically attached to the scrotum.

❍ **What is an important difference between testicular teratomas in children and adults?**

In children, teratomas are benign lesions. In adults, they may metastasize.

❍ **What is the most common cause of urethritis in males?**

Neisseria gonorrhea, gonococcal urethritis, or Chlamydia trachomatis, nongonococcal urethritis. Gonorrhea presents with a purulent discharge from the urethra, whereas chlamydia is generally associated with a thinner, white mucous discharge. Treatment should cover both gonorrhea and chlamydia because there is a high incidence of coinfection. Ceftriaxone, for gonorrhea, and doxycycline or tetracycline, for chlamydia, are the drugs of choice.

❍ **What is the most common cause of urinary tract infections (UTI's)?**

E. coli (80%). E. coli is also the most common cause of pyelonephritis and pyelitis because of its ascension from the lower urinary tract. Staphylococcus saprophyticus accounts for 5-15% of UTI's.

❍ **What patients with UTI's are candidates for single dose or short-course, i.e., 3 days, antibiotic therapy with TMP-SMX?**

Nonpregnant women without risk factors for subclinical pyelonephritis, such as prolonged symptoms, recurrent UTI's, diabetes mellitus, urinary tract abnormalities, or recurrent pyelonephritis. Follow-up within 1 week is mandatory.

❍ **Varicoceles are most common in which side of the scrotum?**

The left. Varicoceles are a collection of veins in the scrotum. These patients have a higher incidence of infertility, presumably because of the increased temperature of the testes surrounded by the warm blood of the varicocele. Incidentally, the left testis is the first to descend and also hangs lower than the right in the majority of men. Hernias are also more common on the left side, as well.

❍ **One to two percent of the affected patients will have a recurrence of the Wilms' tumor. Where is this recurrence most likely to be?**

The chest.

❍ **What is the recommended course of action for a patient with gross hematuria?**

Hospitalize and run the following tests: CBC, BUN/Cr, 24 hr creatinine/protein/calcium, urine culture, serum C3, and anti-DNAse B titer. If these do not lead to a diagnosis, get an ultrasound or IVP to look for structural abnormalities.

❍ **You still have not reached a diagnosis for the patient with hematuria. Should you get a biopsy?**

Yes. If the patient has unexplained gross hematuria, that is an indication in itself. A biopsy is also indicated for patients with persistent microscopic hematuria with associated hypertension, proteinuria, or decreased renal function.

❍ **The labs from a patient with hematuria show depressed levels of C3. What etiologies should you suspect?**

Chronic infection, lupus, post-streptococcal glomerulonephritis or membranoproliferative glomerulonephritis.

❍ **What is the classic presentation of post-streptococcal glomerulonephritis (PSGN)?**

Sudden development of gross hematuria, hypertension, edema and renal insufficiency following a throat or skin infection with group A beta-hemolytic streptococcus. Patients frequently also have generalized complaints of fever, malaise, lethargy, abdominal pain, etc.

❍ **How early in the development of "strep throat" will antibiotic therapy decrease the risk for PSGN?**

Antibiotics have not been found to decrease the risk for PSG.

❍ **What lab test best confirms PSGN as the diagnosis?**

Anti-DNAse B antibody titer

❍ **What is the most common form of lupus nephritis?**

Diffuse proliferative nephritis (WHO class IV). Unfortunately, this is also the most severe form.

❍ **The biopsy of the kidney from a 24 year-old male with nephrotic syndrome shows increased mesangial cells and, on immunofluorescence, C3 deposits in the mesangium. What is the man's diagnosis and prognosis?**

This man has membranoproliferative glomerulonephritis (a type of chronic glomerulonephritis). Prognosis is poor, with many patients progressing to end-stage renal failure.

❍ **What is the most common manifestation of Goodpasture's disease?**

Hemoptysis. These patients usually develop pulmonary hemorrhage before any signs of renal failure develop.

❍ **What is the diagnostic triad of the nephrotic syndrome?**

Edema, hyperlipidemia, and proteinuria with hypoproteinemia.

❍ **How is renal tubular acidosis (RTA) classified?**

Into one of three types: Type 1-distal RTA, Type II-proximal RTA, or Type IV-mineralocorticoid deficiency. There is no type III.

❍ **What are the mechanisms for the different types of RTA?**

In Type I, there is a deficiency in the secretion of the hydrogen ion by the distal tubule and collecting duct. In Type II, there is a decrease in the bicarbonate reabsorption in the proximal tubule.

❍ **Which isolated form of RTA will be most likely to lead to renal failure?**

Distal (Type I), though most cases of Type I RTA have an excellent prognosis.

❍ **What two common medications can induce nephrogenic diabetes insipidus?**

Lithium and amphotericin B.

❍ **A patient with nephrogenic diabetes insipidus has a serum sodium level of 117 mEq/l. How do you determine how much NaCl to administer to keep the risk of cerebral edema at a minimum?**

Amount of NaCl to add (in mEq/l)=0.6 x wt. (in kg) x (140 - serum sodium).

❍ **What percentage of kidney transplants donated from a relative (usually a parent) are still functional after three years?**

75-80%.

❍ **Patients born with what disease is more likely to have horseshoe kidneys?**

Turner's syndrome.

❍ **What type of RTA usually presents as an isolated condition?**

Type I - distal RTA.

❍ **What are the characteristic acid-base/electrolyte abnormalities associated with type I and type II RTA?**

Hypokalemic, hyperchloremic metabolic acidosis.

❍ **What are the characteristic acid-base/electrolyte abnormalities associated with type IV RTA?**

Hyperkalemic, hyperchloremic metabolic acidosis.

❍ **What is the underlying cause of type IV RTA?**

Decreased sodium reabsorption secondary to lack of aldosterone effect.

❍ **What diseases are associated with type IV RTA?**

Diseases of the adrenal gland; most commonly Addison's disease and Congenital Adrenal Hyperplasia.

❍ **What is the most common cause of acute obstructive uropathy in older men?**

Prostatic enlargement.

❍ **What is the antihypertensive of choice in patient with chronic diabetic nephropathy?**

Angiotensin-converting enzyme inhibitors are preferred.

❍ **What is the etiology of acute renal failure seen a few weeks after cardiac catheterization?**

Acute renal failure, occurring one day after a vascular procedure, suggests cholesterol emboli syndrome.

❍ **What treatments are used to ameliorate bleeding in a uremic patient?**

Dialysis may lessen bleeding as may DDAVP, cryoprecipitate or even platelet transfusions. Estrogens may lessen bleeding from angiodysplasia.

❍ **What medications are likely to cause acute renal failure with interstitial nephritis?**

Beta-lactam antibiotics, cimetidine, NSAIDs, Dilantin, Rifampin are but a few.

❍ **What are the common causes of acute renal failure seen after repair of abdominal aneurysm?**

Acute tubular necrosis with aortic cross clamping.

❍ **What glomerular diseases likely to recur in allograft post transplant patients?**

Usually focal glomerulosclerosis and membranoproliferative GN have a high risk of recurrence.

❍ **What medications may be associated with hemolytic uremic syndrome?**

Mitomycin, estrogens and cyclosporin are known culprits.

❍ **What is the therapy of choice for a patient with chronic renal failure and pericarditis?**

These patients benefit from prompt dialysis.

❍ **What are the causes of advanced chronic renal failure and large kidneys?**

Amyloidosis, Polycystic kidney disease, diabetic nephropathy, HIV-ATN (AIDS nephropathy) and multiple myeloma

❍ **What does acute renal failure in a patient with alcoholic cirrhosis and a urine sodium of less than 10 suggest?**

Pre-renal azotemia or hepatorenal syndrome.

❍ **Acute renal failure caused by Wegener's granulomatosis may respond best to what treatments?**

This is usually rapidly progressive GN and responds to high dose steroids and cyclophosphamide.

❍ **Total and persistent anuria with renal failure should prompt a work up for what?**

These patients are presumed to be obstructed until proven otherwise.

❍ **Aminoglycosides are likely to cause what type of acute renal failure?**

Non-oliguric ATN.

❍ **A renal biopsy in a patient with acute renal failure, hematuria and red cell casts will most likely reveal what lesion?**

A proliferative glomerulonephritis, usually with crescents.

❍ **Anemia of chronic renal failure is likely to respond to what agent?**

Erythropoetin given either by vein or subcutaneous injection.

❍ **What are the most common etiologies of chronic renal failure leading to dialysis in the U.S.?**

Hypertensive and diabetic renal diseases are the most likely causes.

❍ **What are the major causes of erythropoietin resistance seen in patients with CRF?**

Iron deficiency, chronic inflammatory states, folate deficiency, and sclerosed bone marrow.

❍ **What continuous modes of renal replacement therapy used in ARF?**

CVVH and peritoneal dialysis. Hemodialysis is an intermittent therapy.

❍ **What are the first line oral phosphate binders used in CRF?**

Calcium carbonate and calcium acetate. Aluminum containing agents are best avoided.

❍ **What co-morbid factors are likely to increase the risk of contrast induced ATN?**

Azotemia, diabetic nephropathy, CHF, multiple myeloma, dehydration.

❍ **What are the causes of high levels of PTH in CRF?**

Hyperphosphatemia, hypocalcemia due to deficiency of vitamin D, parathyroid receptor resistance.

❍ **What is the major predictor of future diabetic nephropathy in a diabetic patient?**

Microalbuminuria.

❍ **What is the etiology of CRF associated with cerebral berry aneurysms?**

Adult Polycystic kidney disease is associated with cerebral berry aneurysms.

❍ **What is the emergent treatment of severe hyperkalemia in patient with CRF?**

Infusion of calcium gluconate followed by hypertonic dextrose and insulin and sodium bicarbonate. Dialysis may also be initiated. Kayexalate, given orally, takes hours to start to work.

❍ **What medications have been proven to decrease the mortality in ATN?**

Unfortunately, no medication has been proven to improve overall outcome in ATN.

❍ **What are the indications for emergent dialysis in ARF?**

Intractable acidosis, intractable hyperkalemia, intractable volume overload, BUN over 80-100, encephalopathy, pericarditis, uremic bleeding and certain intoxications.

❍ **At what GFR will patients with CRF due to diabetes need to start dialysis?**

Dialysis usually begun at GFR of 10-15 cc/min.

❍ **What are some major long term complications seen with the use of aluminum containing phosphate binders?**

Aluminum induced osteomalacia, anemia and rarely dementia.

❍ **What is the major therapy used to treat allergic interstitial nephritis not responding to discontinuation of the culprit medication?**

Corticosteroids

❍ **Sudden ARF, seen after initiation of ACE inhibitors, should prompt a work up for what diseases?**

ACE inhibitors are likely to cause ARF in patients with bilateral renal artery stenosis or renal artery stenosis in a solitary kidney.

❍ **What type of ARF is usually seen with rhabdomyolysis?**

Acute tubular necrosis.

❍ **Chronic renal failure with hypertension, small shrunken kidneys and gout at an early age should suggest what?**

Lead nephropathy should be considered.

❍ **What pathology is usually seen in patients with CRF, nephrotic syndrome and AIDS?**

Usually focal segmental glomrulosclerosis is seen at biopsy.

❍ **What factors predispose to acute papillary necrosis?**

Analgesic abuse, sickle cell disease, diabetes mellitus, and alcoholism are usual predisposing factors.

❍ **Carpal tunnel syndrome often seen in patients on long-term hemodialysis have what etiology of CRF?**

Amyloidosis due to the deposition of B2 microglobulin.

❍ **What major renal toxicity's seen with amphotericin B?**

Tubulointerstitial disease with a distal hypokalemic renal tubular acidosis and hypomagnesemia.

❍ **What are some of the major adverse effects of chronic elevation of PTH seen in CRF?**

Parathyroid bone disease, bone pain and pathologic fractures. Myoneuropathy may also be a feature.

❍ **Acute renal failure seen after use of cocaine may be due to what?**

Cocaine may cause rhabdomyolysis with ATN. It may also lead to acute in blood pressure.

❍ **What are some commonly used immunosuppressive agents given to patients with CRF at time of renal transplantation?**

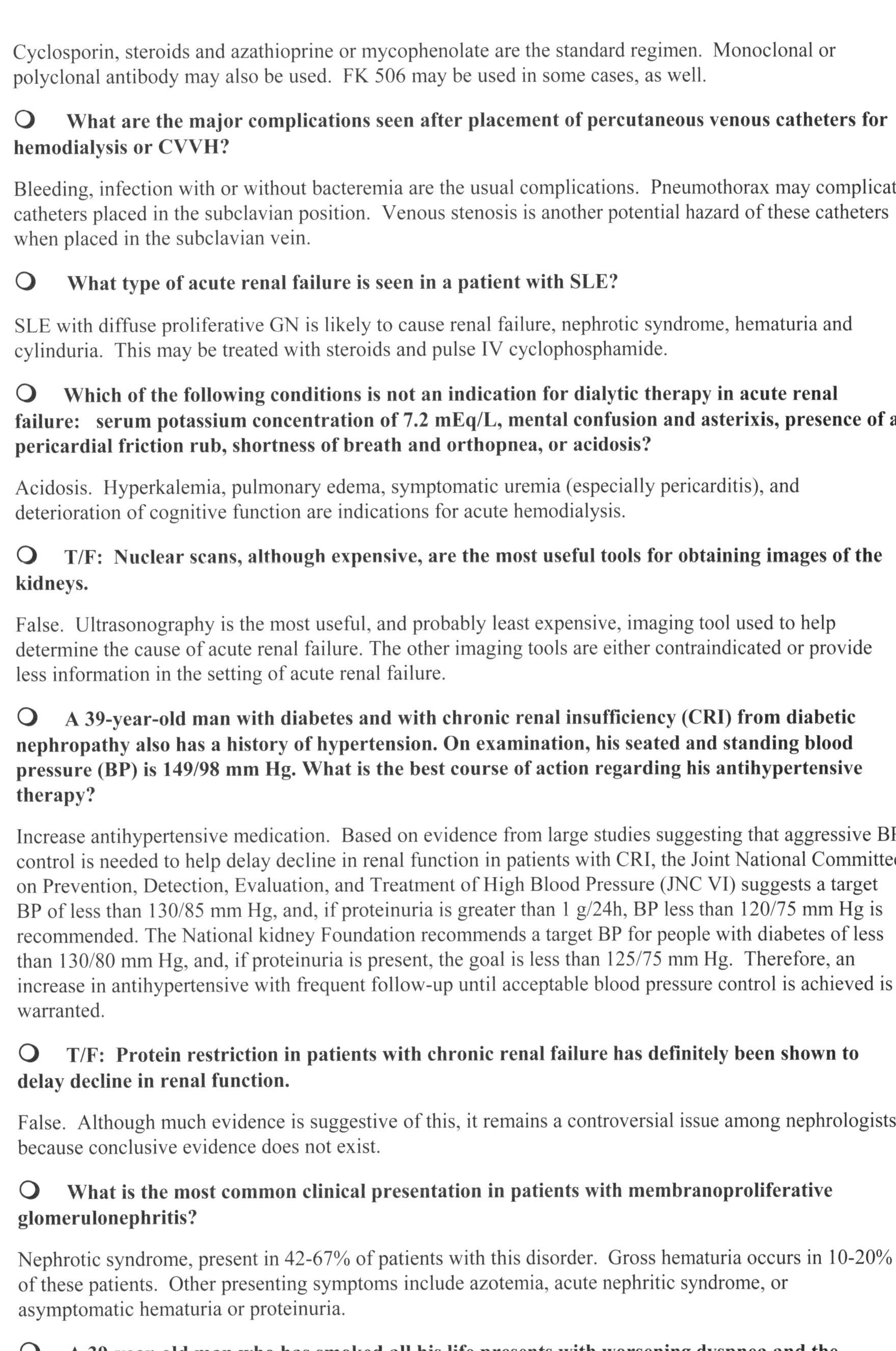

Cyclosporin, steroids and azathioprine or mycophenolate are the standard regimen. Monoclonal or polyclonal antibody may also be used. FK 506 may be used in some cases, as well.

❍ **What are the major complications seen after placement of percutaneous venous catheters for hemodialysis or CVVH?**

Bleeding, infection with or without bacteremia are the usual complications. Pneumothorax may complicate catheters placed in the subclavian position. Venous stenosis is another potential hazard of these catheters when placed in the subclavian vein.

❍ **What type of acute renal failure is seen in a patient with SLE?**

SLE with diffuse proliferative GN is likely to cause renal failure, nephrotic syndrome, hematuria and cylinduria. This may be treated with steroids and pulse IV cyclophosphamide.

❍ **Which of the following conditions is not an indication for dialytic therapy in acute renal failure: serum potassium concentration of 7.2 mEq/L, mental confusion and asterixis, presence of a pericardial friction rub, shortness of breath and orthopnea, or acidosis?**

Acidosis. Hyperkalemia, pulmonary edema, symptomatic uremia (especially pericarditis), and deterioration of cognitive function are indications for acute hemodialysis.

❍ **T/F: Nuclear scans, although expensive, are the most useful tools for obtaining images of the kidneys.**

False. Ultrasonography is the most useful, and probably least expensive, imaging tool used to help determine the cause of acute renal failure. The other imaging tools are either contraindicated or provide less information in the setting of acute renal failure.

❍ **A 39-year-old man with diabetes and with chronic renal insufficiency (CRI) from diabetic nephropathy also has a history of hypertension. On examination, his seated and standing blood pressure (BP) is 149/98 mm Hg. What is the best course of action regarding his antihypertensive therapy?**

Increase antihypertensive medication. Based on evidence from large studies suggesting that aggressive BP control is needed to help delay decline in renal function in patients with CRI, the Joint National Committee on Prevention, Detection, Evaluation, and Treatment of High Blood Pressure (JNC VI) suggests a target BP of less than 130/85 mm Hg, and, if proteinuria is greater than 1 g/24h, BP less than 120/75 mm Hg is recommended. The National kidney Foundation recommends a target BP for people with diabetes of less than 130/80 mm Hg, and, if proteinuria is present, the goal is less than 125/75 mm Hg. Therefore, an increase in antihypertensive with frequent follow-up until acceptable blood pressure control is achieved is warranted.

❍ **T/F: Protein restriction in patients with chronic renal failure has definitely been shown to delay decline in renal function.**

False. Although much evidence is suggestive of this, it remains a controversial issue among nephrologists because conclusive evidence does not exist.

❍ **What is the most common clinical presentation in patients with membranoproliferative glomerulonephritis?**

Nephrotic syndrome, present in 42-67% of patients with this disorder. Gross hematuria occurs in 10-20% of these patients. Other presenting symptoms include azotemia, acute nephritic syndrome, or asymptomatic hematuria or proteinuria.

❍ **A 39-year-old man who has smoked all his life presents with worsening dyspnea and the presence of bilateral infiltrates on his chest radiograph. He has a hemoglobin of 9 g/dL and a serum creatinine of 3.8 mg/dL. Urinalysis reveals red blood cells and proteinuria. The serum anti–glomerular basement membrane (anti-GBM) is positive. What is the most likely diagnosis?**

This patient has a pulmonary-renal syndrome secondary to anti-GBM disease, or Goodpasture syndrome. Pulmonary-renal syndromes may be caused by Goodpasture syndrome, Wegener granulomatosis, systemic lupus erythematosus, or other vasculitides. The anti-GBM antibodies correlate with disease activity and are diagnostic of Goodpasture syndrome. A male predominance in the occurrence of Goodpasture disease exists. The pulmonary hemorrhage may occur without overt hemoptysis. Anemia is common and is due to chronic blood loss. Treatment includes plasmapheresis, corticosteroids, and immunosuppressive drugs. Renal function may be recovered; this is unlikely to occur once advanced renal dysfunction is present.

❍ **A 28-year-old African American man with biopsy-proven HIV nephropathy presents with a rising creatinine level. His initial creatinine level at presentation was 2.2 mg/dL and is now 3.1 mg/dL. He is losing his appetite, has difficulty sleeping, and is nauseous. His leg swelling is increased, his blood pressure is 124/82 mm Hg, and his heart rate is 88 beats per minute. He is afebrile and has a rales and rhonchi and a breathing rate of 24 breaths per minute. He is already taking prednisone. What is best immediate step in the treatment of this patient?**

Discuss immediate access placement for dialysis. The patient has symptoms of uremia warranting consideration for a discussion regarding access placement for hemodialysis. Increasing his prednisone dose and starting cyclosporine may be effective, but improvement from this treatment, if it occurs, takes time.

❍ **T/F: Patients with HIV nephropathy are normotensive.**

True. Unlike patients with other causes of renal insufficiency, patients with HIV nephropathy are normotensive.

HEMATOLOGY AND ONCOLOGY

Hypochondria is the only disease I haven't got.
Anonymous

❍ **What four types of blood loss indicate a bleeding disorder?**

1) Spontaneous bleeding from many sites
2) Bleeding from non-traumatic sites
3) Delayed bleeding several hours after trauma
4) Bleeding into deep tissues or joints

❍ **What is the most common type of thyroid carcinoma?**

Papillary carcinoma (60 to 70% of tumors). It's a good thing too! Papillary carcinoma has the best prognosis; the 10-year survival rate is 89%. Other thyroid carcinomas are follicular (10 to 20%, common in older patients), anaplastic (3 to 5%), and medullary (2 to 5%, often occurring with familial multiple endocrine neoplasia).

❍ **What common drugs have been implicated in acquired bleeding disorders?**

Ethanol, ASA, NSAID's, warfarin, and antibiotics.

❍ **Mucocutaneous bleeding, including petechiae, ecchymoses, epistaxis, GI, GU, and menorrhagia, indicate what coagulation abnormalities?**

Qualitative or quantitative platelet disorders.

❍ **Delayed bleeding and bleeding into joints or potential spaces, such as the retroperitoneum, suggest what type of bleeding disorder?**

Coagulation factor deficiency.

❍ **What is primary hemostasis?**

The platelet interaction with the vascular subendothelium that results in the formation of a platelet plug at the site of injury.

❍ **What four components are required for primary hemostasis?**

1) Normal vascular subendothelium (collagen)
2) Functional platelets
3) Normal Von Willebrand factor (connects the platelet to the endothelium via glycoprotein Ib)
4) Normal fibrinogen (connects platelets to each other via glycoprotein IIB-IIIA)

❍ **What is the end product of secondary hemostasis (coagulation cascade)?**

Cross-linked fibrin.

❍ **What mechanism limits the size of the fibrin clots that are formed?**

The fibrinolytic system.

❍ **What is the principle physiologic activator of the fibrinolytic system?**

Tissue plasminogen activator (tPA). Endothelial cells release tPA, which converts plasminogen, absorbed in the fibrin clot, to plasmin. Plasmin degrades fibrinogen and fibrin monomer into fibrin degradation products (FDP's, once called fibrin split products) and cross-linked fibrin into D-dimers.

❍ **Below what platelet count is spontaneous hemorrhage likely to occur?**

< 10,000/mm^3.

❍ **It is generally agreed that most patients with active bleeding and platelet counts < 50,000/mm^3 should receive platelet transfusion. How much will the platelet count be raised for each unit of platelets infused?**

10,000/mm^3.

❍ **What patients with thrombocytopenia are unlikely to respond to platelet infusions?**

Those with platelet antibodies (ITP or hypersplenism).

❍ **How can an overdose of warfarin be treated? What are the advantages and disadvantages of each treatment?**

Fresh frozen plasma (FFP) or Vitamin K. However, if there are no signs of bleeding, temporary discontinuation may be all that is necessary. Treatment depends on the severity of symptoms, not the degree of prolongation of the prothrombin time (PT).
FFP advantages: Rapid repletion of coagulation factors and control of hemorrhage
FFP disadvantages: Volume overload, possible viral transmission
Vitamin K advantages: Ease of administration
Vitamin K disadvantages: Possible anaphylaxis when given IV; delayed onset of 12 to 24 hours; effects may last up to 2 weeks, making anticoagulation of the patient difficult or impossible.

❍ **What is the only coagulation factor not synthesized by hepatocytes?**

Factor VIII.

❍ **Which four hemostatic alterations are seen in patients with liver disease?**

1) Decreased protein synthesis leading to coagulation factor deficiency
2) Thrombocytopenia
3) Increased fibrinolysis
4) Vitamin K deficiency

❍ **What five treatments are available to bleeding patients with liver disease?**

1) Transfusion with PRBCs (maintains hemodynamic stability)
2) Vitamin K
3) Fresh frozen plasma
4) Platelet transfusion
5) DDAVP (Desmopressin)

❍ **What hemostasis test is most often prolonged in patients with uremia?**

Bleeding time.

❍ **What treatment options are available to patients with renal failure and coagulopathy?**

1) Dialysis
2) Optimize hematocrit (by recombinant human erythropoietin or transfusion with PRBCs)
3) Desmopressin
4) Conjugated estrogens

Cryoprecipitate and platelet transfusions if hemorrhage is life threatening.

❍ **What are the clinical complications of DIC?**

Bleeding, thrombosis, and purpura fulminans.

❍ **Which three laboratory studies are most helpful in diagnosing DIC?**

1) Prothrombin time (prolonged)
2) Platelet count (usually low)
3) Fibrinogen level (low)

❍ **What are the most common hemostatic abnormalities in patients infected with HIV?**

Thrombocytopenia and acquired circulating anticoagulants (causes prolongation of aPTT).

❍ **What is the pentad of Thrombotic thrombocytopenic purpura (TTP)?**

1) Fever
2) Thrombocytopenia
3) Neurologic symptoms
4) Renal insufficiency
5) Microangiopathic hemolytic anemia (MAHA)

❍ **What is the leading cause of death in hemophiliacs?**

AIDS.

❍ **How much will 1 unit of factor VIII concentrate raise the circulating factor VIII level?**

2%.

❍ **How much will 1 unit of factor IX concentrate raise the circulating factor IX level?**

1%.

❍ **What is the most common inherited bleeding disorder?**

Von Willebrand disease.

❍ **Seventy to eighty percent of patients with Von Willebrand disease have type I. What is current approved mode of therapy for bleeding in these patients? What is the dose?**

DDAVP, 0.3 μg/kg IV or subcutaneously every 12 hours for 3 to 4 doses.

❍ **What is the most common hemoglobin variant?**

Hemoglobin S (valine substituted for glutamic acid in the sixth position on the beta-chain).

❍ **Which clinical crises are seen in patients with sickle-cell disease?**

1) Vasoocclusive (thrombotic)
2) Hematologic (sequestration and aplastic)
3) Infectious

❍ **Which is the most common type of sickle-cell crisis?**

Vasoocclusive (average: 4 attacks/year).

❍ **What percentage of patients with sickle-cell disease have gallstones?**

75% (only 10% are symptomatic).

❍ **What is the only painless type of vasoocclusive crisis?**

CNS crisis (most commonly cerebral infarction in children and cerebral hemorrhage in adults).

❍ **What are the four mainstays of therapy for a patient in sickle-cell crisis?**

1) Hydration
2) Analgesia
3) Oxygen (only beneficial if patient is hypoxic)
4) Cardiac monitoring (if patient has history of cardiac disease or is having chest pain)

❍ **What is the most commonly encountered sickle hemoglobin variant?**

Sickle-cell trait.

❍ **What is the most common human enzyme defect?**

Glucose-6-phosphate dehydrogenase (G-6-PD) deficiency.

❍ **What drugs should be avoided in patients with G-6-PD deficiency?**

1) Drugs that induce oxidation
2) Sulfa
3) Antimalarials
4) Pyridium
5) Nitrofurantoin

❍ **What is the most useful test to ascertain hemolysis and a normal marrow response?**

The reticulocyte count.

❍ **What is the most common morphologic abnormality of red cells in hemolytic states?**

Spherocytes.

❍ **What is the most common clinical presentation of TTP (thrombotic thrombocytopenic purpura)?**

Neurologic symptoms including headache, confusion, cranial nerve palsies, coma, and seizures.

❍ **What malignancy is most frequently associated with MAHA?**

Gastric adenocarcinoma.

❍ **What is the most common worldwide cause of hemolytic anemia?**

Malaria.

❍ **What components of whole blood are used for transfusion?**

1) RBCs
2) Platelets
3) Plasma
4) Cryoprecipitate

❍ **How much will the infusion of 1 unit of PRBCs raise the hemoglobin and hematocrit in a 70-kg patient?**

Hemoglobin: 1 g/dl. Hematocrit: 3%.

❍ **What are the three conditions under which the transfusion of PRBCs should be considered?**

1) Acute hemorrhage (blood loss > 1500 ml)

2) Surgical blood loss > 2 L
3) Chronic anemia (Hgb < 7 to 8 g/dl, symptomatic, or with underlying cardiopulmonary disease)

❍ **What five factors indicate the need to type and cross-match blood in the emergency department?**

1) Evidence of shock from any cause
2) Known blood loss > 1,000 ml
3) Gross GI bleeding
4) Hgb < 10; Hct < 30
5) Potential of surgery with further significant blood loss

❍ **What are the five contents of cryoprecipitate?**

1) Factor VIII C
2) Von Willebrand factor
3) Fibrinogen
4) Factor XIII
5) Fibronectin

❍ **What is the first step in treating all immediate transfusion reactions?**

Stop the transfusion.

❍ **What infection carries the highest risk for transmission by blood transfusion?**

Hepatitis C (1/3300 units).

❍ **What is the current recommended emergency replacement therapy for massive hemorrhage?**

Type-specific, uncrossmatched blood. Type O negative, whereas immediately life-saving in certain situations, carries the risk of life-threatening transfusion reactions.

❍ **In current practice, what blood components are routinely infused along with PRBCs in a patient receiving a massive transfusion?**

None. The practice of routinely using platelet transfusion and fresh frozen plasma is costly, dangerous, and unwarranted.

❍ **What is the only crystalloid fluid compatible with PRBCs?**

Normal saline.

❍ **What condition should be suspected in a patient with multiple myeloma who presents with paraparesis, paraplegia, and urinary incontinence?**

Acute spinal cord compression. This condition occurs primarily with multiple myeloma and lymphoma, and it is also encountered with carcinomas of the lung, breast, and prostate.

❍ **What are the two most common neoplasms that cause pericardial effusion and tamponade?**

Carcinoma of the lung and breast.

❍ **A 48 year-old male smoker presents with a headache, swelling of the face and arms, and a feeling of fullness in his face and neck. He is noted to have JVD upon physical examination and papilledema upon funduscopic examination. What is the most likely diagnosis?**

Superior vena cava syndrome.

❍ **What is the most common cause of hyperviscosity syndrome?**

Waldenstrom's macroglobulinemia (IgM myeloma).

❍ **What should be considered in a patient who presents in a coma, and has anemia and Rouleaux formation on the peripheral blood smear?**

Hyperviscosity syndrome.

❍ **What are the major causes of GI bleeding in cancer patients?**

Hemorrhagic gastritis and peptic ulcer disease.

❍ **What are the vitamin K-dependent factors of the clotting cascade?**

X, IX, VII and II. Remember 1972.

❍ **An adult patient receives a major head injury. He also suffers from classic hemophilia. What treatment should be given?**

Give factor VIII, 50 U/kg.

❍ **What is Von Willebrand's disease?**

An autosomal dominant disorder of platelet function. It causes bleeding from mucous membranes, menorrhagia, and increased bleeding from wounds. Patients with Von Willebrand's disease have less (or dysfunctional) Von Willebrand's factor.

Von Willebrand's factor is a plasma protein secreted by endothelial cells and serves 2 functions: 1) it is required for platelets to adhere to collagen at the site of vascular injury, which is the initial step in forming a hemostatic plug. 2) it forms complexes in plasma with factor VIII, which are required to maintain normal factor VIII levels.

❍ **What is appropriate treatment for a life-threatening level of hypercalcemia of 16 mg per deciliter?**

Give the patient 0.9 NS at 5 to 10 liters per day. In addition, administer furosemide, the typical dose being 40-80 mg IV every 1 to 2 hours. Watch out for hypokalemia. Consider glucocorticoids if the patient is obtunded or comatose. One may also administer agents, e.g., calcitonin and mithramycin, to counteract parathyroid hormone. Newer agents, such as pamidronate are effective in reducing serum calcium levels when the other treatments are ineffective.

❍ **What factors are deficient in classic hemophilia, Christmas disease, and Von Willebrand's disease, respectively?**

Classic hemophilia:Factor VIII

Christmas disease:Factor IX

Willebrand's disease: Factor VIIIc and Von Willebrand's cofactor

❍ **What pathway involves factors VIII and IX?**

Intrinsic pathway.

❍ **What effect does deficiency of factors VIII and IX have on PT and on PTT?**

Deficiency leads to an increase in PTT.

❍ **What pathway does the PT measure? What factor is unique to this pathway?**

Extrinsic pathway. Factor VII.

❍ **Can hemophilia A be clinically distinguished from hemophilia B?**

No.

❍ **What blood product is given when the coagulation abnormality is unknown?**

Fresh frozen plasma.

❍ **What agent can be used to treat mild hemophilia A and Von Willebrand's disease type 1?**

D-Amino-8. D-arginine vasopressin (DDAVP) induces a rapid rise in factor VIII levels.

❍ **Where is a parotid gland tumor most likely to develop?**

The superficial lobe, which is located just below the ear lobe. Forty percent of parotid gland tumors are malignant. All tumors, benign or malignant, should be removed.

❍ **What is the most common type of malignant parotid gland tumor?**

Mucoepidermoid carcinoma. Other types of malignant tumors are acinic cell carcinoma, adenocarcinoma, malignant mixed tumor, adenoid cystic carcinoma, and epidermoid carcinoma.

❍ **What age and ethnic group is at greatest risk for esophageal cancer?**

Elderly African-Americans. Their risk is four times higher than in elderly Caucasian-Americans. Other ethnic groups at higher risk include Chinese, Iranians, and South Africans.

❍ **Which are the most common cancer cell types of the esophagus?**

Squamous carcinoma, occurring most frequently in African-Americans, while adenocarcinoma is most common type in Caucasian-Americans.

❍ **Where does esophageal cancer most commonly metastasizes?**

lungs, liver, and bones.

❍ **Which types of cancer metastasize to bone?**

Prostate, thyroid, breast, lung, and kidney. (Remember: "P.T. Barnum Loves Kids").

❍ **A hard mass in the upper outer quadrant of the right breast of a 45 year-old woman is detected. What are the next steps?**

Mammogram followed by an excision biopsy. A negative needle aspiration alone cannot rule out malignancy. False negative rates for fine-needle biopsy are 3-30%.

❍ **What is the most common histologic type of breast cancer?**

Infiltrating ductal carcinoma (70-80%). Subtypes are colloid, medullary, papillary, and tubular.

❍ **A 30 year-old female comes to you worried that she has breast cancer in both breasts. She is concerned because of a yellowish, green discharge from her nipples, soreness in the upper outer quadrants of her breasts, what she calls a "lumpy" feeling upon self-examination, and mild swelling that seems to come and go. Further questioning reveals that her pain begins 1 week before she menstruates, then disappears when her menses is over. Understandably concerned, your patient wants to know when she can start chemotherapy. What do you tell her?**

Hold off on the chemo! She most likely has fibrocystic breast changes. Put her mind at rest, and let her know that fibrocystic changes are not a pre-malignant syndrome.

❍ **Which is the most common type of non-cystic breast tumor?**

Fibroadenomas. These are most common in women under 25. These tumors are painless, small, mobile and round.

❍ **What does a high cathepsin D level indicate in a woman with breast cancer?**

A high risk of metastasis.

❍ **What is the most common lung cancer in non-smokers?**

Adenocarcinoma. Smoking is a great risk factor for all lung cancers, with the exception of adenocarcinoma.

❍ **A 44 year-old gentleman presents with a deep, dull pain in the center of his abdomen that radiates to his back and will not go away. He states he has not "felt like himself" for a few weeks and that he has been kind of depressed. He also notes that he has lost a lot of weight-about 30 pounds in 3 weeks. On physical examination, you palpate an enlarged liver and an abdominal mass in the epigastrium. What is your diagnosis?**

Most likely pancreatic cancer. The ability to palpate a mass suggests that the disease has progressed too far to be surgically resectable. Carcinoma of the pancreas can only be resected in 20% of patients. Depression often occurs before the onset of other symptoms.

❍ **Where is the most common anatomic and histologic location of pancreatic cancer?**

Head of the pancreas (80%). Pancreatic cancer is generally adenocarcinoma and located in the ducts.

❍ **What gender and age group most commonly presents with pancreatic cancer?**

Middle aged men.

❍ **Is there a genetic marker for adenocarcinoma of the pancreas?**

Yes. Ninety percent of patients with adenocarcinoma of the pancreas have a mutation of the Ki-ras oncogene on codon 12.

❍ **What is the 5-year survival rate for pancreatic carcinoma?**

2 to 5%. Symptoms generally do not show up until the tumor has metastasized or spread to local structures.

❍ **What is the most common endocrine tumor of the pancreas?**

An insulinoma. However, only 10% are malignant. Gastrinomas are the second most common and have a malignancy rate of 50%. Vipomas and glucagonomas are also endocrine tumors of the pancreas.

❍ **Glucagonomas arise from which type of cells?**

Alpha cells. The majority are malignant. Increased plasma glucagon is diagnostic.

❍ **What is the typical size of an adrenal carcinoma when diagnosed?**

Ninety percent are larger than 6 cm in diameter.

❍ **Pheochromocytomas produce what compounds?**

Catecholamines. This group of chemicals result in increased blood pressure, perspiration, heart palpitations, anxiety, and weight loss.

❍ **If vanillylmandelic acid, normetanephrine, and metanephrine are detected in the urine, what is the likely cause?**

Pheochromocytoma.

❍ **Where are the majority of pheochromocytomas located?**

Ninety percent are found in the adrenal medulla. The remainder are located in other tissues originating from neural crest cells.

❍ **What is the pheochromocytoma rule of 10's?**

10% are malignant; 10% are multiple or bilateral; 10% are extra-adrenal; 10% occur in children; 10% recur after surgical removal; 10% are familial.

❍ **What is the most common benign liver tumor?**

Cavernous hemangioma.

❍ **All types of hepatomas are associated with underlying liver disease except one. Which is it?**

Fibrolamellar hepatomas. These are single nodules in non-cirrhotic livers.

❍ **Where does hepatic cancer most commonly metastasizes?**

The lungs (bronchiogenic carcinoma).

❍ **Clinically, how is right-sided colon cancer differentiated from left-sided?**

Right-sided lesions present with occult bleeding, weakness, anemia, dyspepsia, palpable abdominal mass, and dull abdominal pain. Left-sided lesions present with visible blood, obstructive symptoms, and noticeable changes in bowel habits. Pencil-thin stools are also common.

❍ **Adenocarcinoma develops from adenomatous polyps. What percent of asymptomatic patients have adenomatous polyps when a routine colonoscopy is performed?**

25%. Prevalence increases with age: 50-30%; 60-40%; 70-50%; and 80-55%. The risk for adenomatous polyps is greater in patients with a history of breast cancer.

❍ **The advancement to adenocarcinoma of the colon from adenoma is size dependent. What is the risk of developing cancer if a 1.5 cm polyp is found upon colonoscopic examination?**

10%. The risk for developing adenocarcinoma is 1% if the polyp is less than 1 cm, 10% if it is 1 to 2 cm, and 45% if the polyp is greater than 2 cm.

❍ **Is a villous, tubulovillous, or tubular adenoma more likely to become malignant?**

40% of villous adenomas will become malignant, compared to 22% of tubulovillous adenomas and 5% of tubular adenomas.

❍ **Which are more likely to turn malignant, pedunculated or sessile lesions?**

Sessile.

❍ **Where are the majority of colorectal cancers found?**

In the rectum (30%), ascending colon (25%), sigmoid colon (20%), descending colon (15%), and transverse colon (10%).

❍ **Where are soft tissue sarcomas most often found?**

In the lower extremities. They are fairly rare. The most common sarcomas are liposarcomas, leiomyosarcomas, fibrosarcomas, rhabdomyosarcomas, and malignant fibrous histiocytomas.

❍ **What percentage of those with familial polyposis will go on to develop colorectal carcinoma?**

100%. Due to the imminent development of cancer, such patient should be advised to have a total colectomy and ileostomy.

❍ **A 64 year-old male presents with jaundice, upper GI bleeding, anemia, a palpable non-tender gallbladder, a palpable liver, and rapid weight loss. What is your diagnosis?**

This is the clinical picture of a tumor of the ampulla of Vater.

❍ **Which cell markers can be used to follow the progression of germinal tumors of the testes?**

Serum α-fetoprotein or human chorionic gonadotropin. HCG may be elevated in both seminomas and non-seminomas, but α-fetoprotein will never be elevated in seminomas.

❍ **Serum acid phosphatase is a common cell marker used to follow prostate cancer. What other diseases can cause the serum acid phosphatase level to rise?**

Benign prostatic hypertrophy, bone tumors, multiple myeloma, and urinary retention.

❍ **What lab result indicates bony metastasis?**

Increased alkaline phosphatase.

❍ **What percentage of palpable prostate nodules are malignant?**

50%. Surgical cure of patients who present with asymptomatic nodules and no metastasis is attempted with radical prostatectomy or radiation therapy.

❍ **Why are red cell transfusions are rarely required to treat iron deficiency anemia?**

Nucleated red blood cells and reticulocytes appear in the blood stream within 72 hours after starting oral iron replacement.

❍ **What are the three major proteins that inhibit clotting?**

Antithrombin III, Protein C, and Protein S.

❍ **What does deficiency of antithrombin III, protein C or protein S increases the risk of?**

Venous thrombosis.

❍ **Why should warfarin, as an <u>initial</u> treatment for venous thrombosis secondary to protein C deficiency, be avoided?**

It may, by inhibiting the synthesis of protein C, lead to paradoxical hypercoagulability. Always treat with heparin before warfarin.

❍ **What is the most important aspect of treating DIC?**

Attempting to correct the underlying disorder (usually septic shock).

❍ **What is the most common agent causing bacterial sepsis post-splenectomy?**

Streptococcus pneumoniae.

❍ **What are the most important factors of managing post-splenectomy sepsis?**

1) Pneumococcal, H. influenzae and meningococcal vaccines.
2) Prophylactic antibiotics.
3) Early detection and treatment.

❍ **What is the characteristic bone marrow finding in Idiopathic thrombocytopenic purpura (ITP)?**

Increased or normal megakaryocytes.

❍ **What are the potential treatment modalities for ITP?**

Gammaglobulins, steroids, radioactive phosphorus, fresh frozen plasma and plasmapheresis.

❍ **How do gamma globulin and steroids work in the treatment of ITP?**

They block the uptake of antibody-coated platelets by splenic macrophages.

❍ **Under what circumstances is a bone marrow aspirate crucial in the diagnosis and treatment of ITP?**

If treatment with steroids is planned, a bone marrow aspirate must be performed to rule out leukemia. Steroid treatment can delay the diagnosis of an occult leukemia.

❍ **Which patients with ITP and mild head trauma, without neurological findings, should be treated with gamma globulin?**

Patients whose platelet count < 20,000/mm3, who have signs of easy or spontaneous bleeding, who are within one week of diagnosis, and whose follow-up is uncertain.

❍ **What is the typical presentation of renal papillary necrosis secondary to sickle cell vaso-occlusion?**

Painless hematuria that may worsen the anemia.

Red blood cells without casts in urine sediment.

❍ **What are the typical signs and symptoms of central nervous system infarction secondary to sickle cell vaso-occlusion?**

Mild, fleeting TIA-like symptoms
Seizures
Hemiparesis
Coma
Death

❍ **What is the treatment of central nervous system vaso-occlusive crisis?**

1.5-2 volume exchange transfusion as soon as blood is ready.

❍ **What are the signs and symptoms of splenic sequestration crisis?**

Pallor, weakness, lethargy, disorientation

Shock, decreased level of consciousness, enlarged spleen.

❍ **What is the treatment of splenic sequestration crisis?**

Rapid infusion of saline and transfusion of red cells or whole blood.

❍ **Increased levels of hemoglobin A2 are found in what conditions?**

Thalassemia trait, megaloblastic anemias secondary to vitamin B12, and folic acid deficiency

❍ **In anemia, which way is the oxygen dissociation curve shifted?**

The right (affinity of hemoglobin for oxygen is decreased).

❍ **What are the factors contributing to the pathophysiology of anemia of chronic disease?**

Decreased red cell life span (hyperactive reticuloendothelial system), hypoactive bone marrow, erythropoietin production inadequate for degree of anemia, and abnormal iron metabolism.

❍ **One unit of platelets will typically raise the platelet count by how much?**

5,000/mm^3.

❍ **What causes of coagulopathy are fresh frozen plasma used to treat?**

Unknown factor deficiencies, DIC, chronic liver disease, and warfarin toxicity.

❍ **What is the formula for calculating the proper volume of red cells to transfuse in an anemic patient?**

Desired hemoglobin (gm/dl)=Observed hemoglobin (gm/dl) x weight (kg) x 3.

❍ **A patient receiving a transfusion of packed red cells abruptly develops fever, chills, chest pain, dyspnea and tachycardia. What is the most likely cause?**

Acute hemolytic transfusion reaction due to ABO incompatibility.

❍ **The most important aspect of the treatment of anemia of chronic disease is:**

Correction of the underlying disorder.

❍ **What test is used to assess vitamin B_{12} absorption?**

The Schilling test.

❍ **What test provides a relatively accurate estimate of body iron stores in the absence of inflammatory disease?**

Serum ferritin.

❍ **What is the progression of biochemical and hematological events in iron deficiency anemia?**

Decreased serum ferritin, then decreased serum iron and total iron binding capacity, followed by a fall in MCV and MCH, and a rise in RDW. Thrombocytosis may occur.

❍ **What are the most common sites for bleeding in patients with hemophilia?**

Joints, muscles, and subcutaneous tissue.

❍ **A hemophiliac presents with a headache after a minor head trauma. What should your management include?**

CT of the brain

Factor replacement

❍ **In Von Willebrand's disease, what protein is decreased or defective?**

Von Willebrand's factor (VFW) which, when combined with factor VIII procoagulant protein (factor VIIIc), forms factor VIII.

❍ **How is Von Willebrand's disease typically transmitted genetically?**

An autosomal dominant trait.

❍ **What are typical lab findings in Von Willebrand's disease?**

Normal platelet count, normal prothrombin time, normal or increased partial thromboplastin time, and increased bleeding time.

❍ **There is simultaneous activation of coagulation and fibrinolysis in what pathologic condition?**

Disseminated intravascular coagulation.

❍ **What is the predominant symptom in DIC?**

Bleeding.

❍ **What are some common ischemic complications of DIC?**

Renal failure, seizures, coma, pulmonary infarction, and hemorrhagic necrosis of the skin.

❍ **What are the common lab findings in DIC?**

Decreased platelets, increased PT and PTT, decreased fibrinogen and increased FSP.

❍ **What is the most common familial and congenital abnormality of the red blood cell membrane?**

Hereditary spherocytosis.

❍ **What is the usual pattern of inheritance for hereditary spherocytosis?**

Autosomal dominant, but it may be autosomal recessive. There is a high rate of new mutations.

❍ **What are the major complications of hereditary spherocytosis?**

Hyperbilirubinemia in newborn period, hemolytic anemia, gallstones, and susceptibility to aplastic and hypoplastic crises secondary to viral infections.

❍ **How is the diagnosis of hereditary spherocytosis made?**

Blood smear, splenomegaly, family history, and osmotic fragility test.

❍ **Treatment of hereditary spherocytosis may include:**

Splenectomy.

❍ **Hemosiderosis from chronic transfusion therapy for thalassemia can be successfully treated with:**

Subcutaneous deferoxamine via pump.

❍ **A cure for thalassemia major is possible with what treatment?**

Bone marrow transplant.

❍ **More than 90% of individuals with thalassemia trait will have an elevation of what diagnostic test?**

Hemoglobin A2 to a level of 3.4-7%.

❍ **G-6-PD deficiency is prevalent in what ethnic groups?**

Greeks, southern Italians, Sephardic Jews, Filipinos, southern Chinese, African-Americans, and Thais.

❍ **What is the incompatibility risk of typed blood, screened blood and fully crossmatched blood?**

The risk of incompatibility of ABO/Rh-compatible blood is 0.1% if the patient has never been transfused. The risk increases to 1.0% if the patient has had a previous transfusion. Adding a negative antibody screen decreases the risk to 0.06%. Fully crossmatched blood should carry a risk less than 0.05%.

❍ **What is the most common blood group? What percentage of blood is Rh positive?**

The most common blood group is type O; 45% of whites, 49% of African-Americans, 79% of Native Americans and 40% of Orientals are blood type O. Approximately 85% of the population are Rh positive and 15% Rh negative.

❍ **Where does blood have the highest viscosity? Why?**

Blood has its highest viscosity in venules and its lowest viscosity in the aorta. Blood viscosity varies depending on the flow rates. The higher viscosity at low flow rates is partly due to red cell aggregation in slowly flowing blood.

❍ **What is oxygen delivery? What is the formula to calculate oxygen delivery?**

Tissue oxygen delivery (DO_2) is the product of blood flow and arterial oxygen content, and at the whole body level, is represented by the product of cardiac output and the arterial oxygen content.

DO_2= CO [(Hb x 1.34) SaO_2 + 0.003 PaO_2], where {CO= Cardiac output, Hb = Hemoglobin, SaO_2 = Arterial oxygen saturation, and PaO_2 = Partial pressure of oxygen in arterial blood}.

❍ **At what hematocrit level is the oxygen treatment capacity maximum?**

It occurs at a hematocrit of 30%.

❍ **What is the effect of normovolemic hemodilution on heart rate, blood pressure and cardiac output (CO) in elderly patients?**

In healthy, elderly patients, with normovolemic-hemodilution, if the hematocrit is reduced from 41 to 28%, heart rate, blood pressure and cardiac output remain unchanged. There is a reduction in oxygen delivery as a result of the failure to compensate for the lowered oxygen carrying capacity by an increased cardiac output.

❍ **Which factor could predict the increase in oxygen consumption with transfusion of red cells in septic patients?**

When septic patients are transfused, only the patients that have lactic acidosis will increase the oxygen consumption, despite the fact that oxygen delivery is increased with the transfusion. Serum concentrations of lactic acid are usually decreased following the transfusion if the patients had elevated lactate levels pre-transfusion.

❍ **What is the relationship between oxygen extraction ratio (O_2ER) and anemia?**

As the hematocrit decreases below normal, there is a decrease in systemic oxygen delivery, but the oxygen extraction ratio increases, which helps maintain a constant oxygen uptake in the tissues. The point at which the compensatory increase in oxygen extraction begins to fail corresponds to an O_2ER of 0.5(50%). This is the reason why many institutions use this value as transfusion trigger when this information is available.

❍ **What are the indications for erythrocyte transfusions?**

1) Evidence of impaired tissue oxygenation (e.g. oxygen uptake less than 100 ml min-1 m-2 or hyperlactatemia) or ongoing coronary or cerebrovascular ischemia in patients with an adequate cardiac output.
2) An O_2ER above 0.5 in patients with an adequate cardiac output.
3) Correction of hemoglobin below 7 gm/dl in patients with a history of active coronary artery disease, cerebrovascular insufficiency, or significant cardiac dysfunction.

❍ **According to the CDC-RBC panel, what are the indications for perioperative red blood cell transfusion?**

The sole indication for erythrocyte transfusion was to increase oxygen carrying capacity and that, provided normovolemia was maintained, anemia had no adverse effect on cardiovascular function, wound healing, infection, postoperative blood loss or patient well-being until the anemia became profound.

❍ **What does ProthrombinTime (PT) measure? How is it performed?**

PT measures the extrinsic and common pathways of the coagulation system. The time to clot formation is measured after the addition of thromboplastin. If the concentration of factors V, VII, IX, and X are significant lower than usual, the PT may be prolonged.

❍ **What does Activated Partial Thromboplastin Time (PTT) measure? How is it performed?**

PTT measures the intrinsic and common pathways of the coagulation cascade. After the blood sample is exposed to celite for activation and a reagent is added, the clot formation is measured. When factors II, V, VIII, IX, X, XI, XII, or fibrinogen are deficient, the PTT may be prolonged.

❍ **What are the indications for the administration of FFP?**

According to the CDC-FFP there are five indications:
1- Replacement of isolated factor deficiencies.
2- Reversal of coumadin effect.
3- Treatment of pathological hemorrhage in patients who have received massive transfusion.
4- Use in antithrombin III deficiency.
5- Treatment of immunodeficiencies.

❍ **What are the indications for cryoprecipitate administration?**

For the treatment of congenital or acquired fibrinogen, and factor VIII deficiencies. Cryoprecipitate can also be administered prophylactically for nonbleeding perioperative or peripartum patients with congenital fibrinogen deficiencies or for Von Willebrand's disease that is unresponsive to desmopressin (DDAVP).

❍ **Is it necessary to administer ABO-specific platelets?**

The administration of ABO-specific platelets is not required because platelet concentrates contain few red blood cells. However, the administration of pooled platelet components of various ABO types can transfuse plasma containing anti-A and/or anti-B, resulting in alloimmunization and a weakly positive direct antiglobulin test.

❍ **What are the indications for platelet transfusion?**

Platelets should be administered to correct thrombocytopenia or platelet dysfunction (thrombocytopathy). Perioperative factors to consider for the transfusion of platelets for counts between 50-100 x 109/L are the type of surgery, anticipated and actual blood loss, extent of microvascular bleeding, presence of medications (e.g. aspirin) and disorders (e.g. uremia) known to affect platelet function and coagulation. The prophylactic administration of platelets is not recommended in patients with chronic thrombocytopenia caused by increased platelet destruction (e.g., idiopathic thrombocytopenic purpura).

❍ **How much does the transfusion of one unit of platelets increase the platelet count?**

In the adult, it generally increases the platelet count by approximately 5-10 x 109/L.

❍ **What is the most reproducible manifestation of dilutional coagulopathy?**

Thrombocytopenia.

❍ **What is the potassium load with transfusion?**

It depends on the age of the blood. The potassium load in 1 week-old whole blood is 4.5-4.8 mEq/unit. With the transfusion of 20 units of 1 week-old whole blood, the potassium load is 60 mEq (presuming no urinary output). If these 20 units are 21 days old, the potassium load is 110 mEq.

❍ **Does a massive transfusion produce hyperkalemia?**

No, except in patients that blood replacement fails to restore perfusion and reverse the acidosis. There is a progressive fall in the serum potassium levels in a massive transfusion related to the volume transfused. Citrate is metabolized to bicarbonate producing a metabolic alkalosis, which in turn moves potassium into the cells.

❍ **What is the incidence of hepatitis transmission with transfusion?**

The majority of cases are subclinical. The incidence of hepatitis C (HCV) transmission is approximately 1 in 103,000. The incidence of hepatitis B (HBV) transmission is about 1 in 63,000. Hepatitis A, having no carrier state, is rarely seen in association with transfusion.

❍ **What is the incidence of transmission of HIV types I and II with transfusion?**

The most recent estimates are 1 in 450,000 to 1 in 600,000. Prior to the implementation of testing for HIV-I p24 antigen in 1996, approximately 18 to 27 infected donor units, not detected by testing, were made available for transfusion annually. Antigen testing reduces that number by 25%.

❍ **How are Human T-lymphotrophic virus types I and II (HTLV-I and II) transmitted and what are the clinical implications?**

The transmission of HTLV-I/II by transfusion is limited to cellular blood components. Estimated incidence of transmission is 1 in 641,000. Two diseases are associated with HTLV-I infection: 1) a chronic degenerative neurologic disease, HTLV-1-associated myelopathy (HAM) or tropical spastic paraparesis (TSP), characterized by progressive lower extremity weakness, spasticity, sensory deficits and urinary incontinence; and 2) adult T-cell leukemia/lymphoma. The lifetime risk of developing overt neurologic or neoplastic disease is thought to be less than 4 percent. The consequences of HTLV-II are less clear but may include HAM/TSP.

❍ **What is the incidence of hemolytic transfusion reactions (HTR)?**

1 in 33,000 units. The HTR is potentially life threatening and often regarded the most serious complication of transfusions. Fifty one percent of 256 transfusion-associated deaths reported to the US Food and Drug Administration between 1976 and 1985 resulted from acute hemolysis following the transfusion of ABO-incompatible blood or plasma.

❍ **What are the types of HTRs and what is the pathophysiology of each one?**

HTRs are divided in two types of reactions: 1) intravascular hemolysis and 2) extravascular hemolysis. Intravascular hemolysis occurs when the antibody-coated RBC is destroyed by the activation of the complement system. Extravascular hemolysis destroys antibody-coated RBCs via phagocytosis by macrophages in the reticuloendothelial system. In most HTRs, some RBCs are probably destroyed by both mechanisms.

❍ **What is the treatment for HTRs?**

The transfusion should be stopped immediately. Hypotension should be treated with fluids, inotropes or other blood as appropriate. Renal output should be maintained with crystalloids, diuretics or dopamine, as necessary. Component therapy should be used if DIC develops.

❍ **What causes febrile reactions to blood and what are the incidences?**

The febrile reaction is the most common mild transfusion reaction and occurs in 0.5% to 4% of transfusions. It is caused by alloantibodies (leukoagglutinins) to white blood cell, platelet or other donor plasma antigens. Fever is presumably caused by pyrogens liberated from lysed cells. It occurs more commonly in previously transfused patients.

❍ **In what patient population do anaphylactic reactions occur with transfusions?**

In immunoglobin-A (IgA) deficient patients who have developed anti-IgA antibodies. The immune complexes activate mast cells, basophils, eosinophils, and the complement system to produce severe symptoms after transfusion of red blood cells, plasma, platelets, or other components containing IgA in plasma. Future transfusions should be free of IgA.

❍ **What is transfusion-related acute lung injury (TRALI)?**

TRALI is a form of noncardiogenic pulmonary edema, occurring within 2 to 4 hours after a transfusion. This reaction should be suspected in any patient who develops pulmonary edema after a transfusion in which volume overload is thought to be unlikely. Clinical signs of respiratory distress vary from mild dyspnea to severe hypoxia. It usually resolves within 48 hours in response to oxygen, mechanical ventilation, and other forms of supportive treatments.

❍ **What is the MOPP regimen of drugs used to treat?**

Hodgkin's lymphoma. MOPP stands for Mechlorethamine, Oncovin, Prednisone, and Procarbazine.

❍ **A patient with chronic myelocytic leukemia on Busulfan therapy comes to the ED complaining of shortness of breath. What should you be suspicious of?**

Pulmonary fibrosis, a toxicity of Busulfan therapy.

❍ **A patient on chemotherapy for his cancer is experiencing severe nausea and vomiting. What can you prescribe to alleviate some of his symptoms?**

Serotonin-receptor antagonists, such as Granisetron and Ondansetron, or a combination of a phenothiazide and an antihistamine.

❍ **After a course of chemotherapy, your patient has had a course of fever, neutropenia and granulocytopenia for over a week, despite antibiotic usage. What should you do now?**

Add Amphotericin B for a presumed fungal infection while continuing your search for the source of the infection.

❍ **What is the mechanism of action of methotrexate?**

It inhibits the enzyme dihydrofolate reductase.

❍ **A patient on chemotherapy for his Burkitt's lymphoma is found to be hyperkalemic, hypocalcemic, hyperphosphatemic, and hyperuracemic. What is the presumptive diagnosis?**

Tumor lysis syndrome.

❍ **A 30-year-old man with precursor B-cell acute lymphoblastic leukemia (ALL) and t(4;11) is experiencing disease remission following standard induction chemotherapy. What is the most effective postremission therapy?**

Allogeneic bone marrow transplant. Patients with precursor B-cell ALL have an extremely poor prognosis. Essentially, following standard chemotherapy or autologous transplantation, long-term survival is not achieved. Several reports have indicated that some patients with precursor B-cell ALL and t(4;11) may have prolonged survival following allogeneic transplantation. This is, therefore, the treatment of choice.

❍ **A 76-year-old woman presents with 4-month history of bilateral neck swelling and axillae. She has an enlarged spleen upon examination. Her peripheral smear demonstrates a leukocyte count of 61,000, and more than 80% of these cells are mature-appearing lymphocytes. In addition, several smudge cells are present on the peripheral smear. What is the most common disorder that is compatible with this presentation?**

Chronic lymphocytic leukemia. Several disorders can have this presentation, but chronic lymphocytic leukemia is the most common. In chronic myelocytic leukemia, the circulating cells are myeloid in origin, not mature lymphocytes. In acute lymphocytic leukemia, the circulating cells are lymphoid blasts.

❍ **T/F: The most common type of infection observed in patients with chronic lymphocytic leukemia is *Staphylococcus aureus* sepsis.**

False. The most common type of infection is pneumococcal pneumonia.

❍ **A 69-year-old man presents after his primary physician performed a routine CBC count and found his WBC count to be 26,000 cells/mL and was concerned about 2% myeloblasts, 6% myelocytes, 3% metamyelocytes with 70% mature neutrophils, and 5% basophils in the differential. Which one single study is diagnostic for chronic myelogenous leukemia?**

Cytogenetic study revealing 90% of his cells have a typical 9;22 translocation called the Philadelphia chromosome. The Philadelphia chromosome in this setting establishes the diagnosis of this patient. All the other findings, such as increased WBC count with immature cells, high platelet count, and splenomegaly, can be observed in patients with other myeloproliferative diseases. A low leukocyte alkaline phosphatase level is suggestive but not diagnostic.

❍ **A 50-year-old woman presents with pancytopenia and an enlarged spleen. His bone marrow aspirate is dry. What test result will most likely help establish the diagnosis of hairy cell leukemia?**

Hypercellular marrow with infiltration by mononucleated cells with fried-egg appearance that stain positive for tartrate-resistant acid phosphatase (TRAP). This finding is characteristic of hairy cell leukemia.

❍ **An 84-year-old woman sought medical attention because of weakness and difficulty walking. Upon examination, she was extremely pale, had a lemon-tinted skin color, and had an abnormal gait. Her hemoglobin was 4.8 g/dL, and macroovalocytes were present in the peripheral smear. What type of anemia does this woman have?**

Megaloblastic anemia, most likely pernicious anemia. This presumptive diagnosis is based on the presence of macroovalocytes in the peripheral smear, a lemon-tinted skin color, and evidence of neurological signs.

❍ **In the above woman, which one of the following findings would not be consistent with her type of anemia: erythroid hyperplasia in bone marrow aspirates, increased indirect bilirubin, increased reticulocyte count, normal direct bilirubin, or increased lactic acid dehydrogenase (LDH)?**

The correct answer is increased reticulocyte count. The patient appears to have a megaloblastic anemia, most likely pernicious anemia. The reticulocyte count is expected to be low or normal despite the severe anemia. Megaloblastic anemia is associated with ineffective erythropoiesis. In ineffective erythrocytosis, massive destruction of red cell precursors occurs before they exit the bone marrow. Therefore, erythroid hyperplasia in the bone marrow aspirate is expected, while the reticulocyte count is normal or low. Both the indirect bilirubin and LDH are increased due to the destruction of erythrocytes in the bone marrow. Actually, the LDH is extremely high in megaloblastic anemia and can be used to monitor the response to therapy. The direct bilirubin is normal because no evidence of liver disease exists. An increased indirect bilirubin is evidence for hemolysis, while an increased direct bilirubin is evidence for liver disease.

❍ **A 25-year-old man with history of Hodgkin disease treated with Mustargen (mechlorethamine), Oncovin (vincristine), procarbazine, and prednisone (MOPP) chemotherapy and radiation 5 years ago comes to the office because of tiredness, intermittent fever, and epistaxis for 2 weeks. Upon examination, he is pale and has multiple petechiae. What is the most likely diagnosis?**

Acute myelogenous leukemia. MOPP chemotherapy has been associated with myelodysplastic syndrome and acute myelogenous leukemia.

❍ **T/F: CT scan of the brain should be included in the routine staging evaluation of patients with Hodgkin disease.**

False. Hodgkin disease almost never involves the brain; therefore, no role exists for routine brain imaging in the pretreatment evaluation.

❍ **A 52-year-old man presents with symptoms of weight loss, low-grade fever, night sweats, and body malaise for 2 months. Physical examination reveals multiple cervical and axillary lymphadenopathy and hepatosplenomegaly. CBC count shows a WBC count of 4500/mL, hematocrit of 35%, and platelets of 250,000/mL. The serum lactate dehydrogenase (LDH) was 850 U/L. The liver function test results were normal, and a CT scan of the chest, abdomen, and pelvis showed mediastinal, hilar, retroperitoneal, and pelvic lymphadenopathy. What diagnostic test is most likely to provide a definitive diagnosis?**

Peripheral lymph node excisional biopsy. This patient`s clinical picture is most consistent with lymphoma; however, other differential diagnoses (eg, infectious etiology, metastatic disease to lymph nodes) should be ruled out. A peripheral excisional lymph node biopsy is the most appropriate and least invasive procedure that is likely to provide a definitive diagnosis. Fine-needle aspiration of an enlarged lymph node is usually not sufficient for making a diagnosis of lymphoma. Bone marrow is not always involved in lymphoma, but performing a bone marrow aspiration and biopsy is necessary to complete the staging workup.

❍ **T/F: HIV-associated lymphomas are most commonly low-grade in histology.**

False. Most lymphomas observed in patients with HIV infection are of intermediate-grade (diffuse large cell) and high-grade (immunoblastic and small noncleaved) histologies, and they are usually at advanced stage at presentation.

❍ **A 54-year-old white man presents to the his primary care provider with lower back pain and progressive fatigue over the preceding 2 months. He reports two moderately severe episodes of epistaxis over the past three weeks which lasted for 25 minutes each. His past medical history is significant for a 40 pack-year smoking history but otherwise is unremarkable. Physical examination reveals that he has a subtle decrease in sensation bilaterally in his toes and feet. His chest radiograph reveals no acute cardiopulmonary disease, but a lytic lesion is observed on his clavicle. Laboratory studies reveal that his hemoglobin level is 7.4 g/dL a platelet count of 84,000, a protime of 16.3 seconds with an INR of 1.8 and his calcium level is 13.5 g/dL. What is the most likely diagnosis?**

Multiple myeloma. Anemia, thrombocytopenia, elevated protime and unexplained bleeding, along with hypercalcemia in an outpatient setting must raise suspicion for myeloma. The lytic bone lesion on his clavicle makes the diagnosis of myeloma even more likely.

❍ **A 43 year-old patient with chronic alcoholism was admitted to the hospital for treatment of delirium tremens. A macrocytic anemia (hemoglobin [Hgb] 10.5 g/dL, mean cell volume [MCV] 104 fL) was demonstrated, and the serum vitamin B_{12} value was slightly low. What is the most likely etiology for the laboratory values?**

Chronic pancreatitis. Chronic pancreatitis is the most likely diagnosis because chronic pancreatitis is common in people with chronic alcoholism. Pancreatic dysfunction reduces the proteolytic enzymes in the intestinal lumen that are necessary to release vitamin B_{12} from R binders. This interferes with B_{12} binding to intrinsic factor (IF) in the small intestine. Thus, the B_{12} is unable to bind IF receptors in the distal ileum so that the B_{12} can be absorbed.

DERMATOLOGY

He: "You have beautiful skin!"
She: "Yes, and it covers my whole body."
Woody Allen

❍ **A 76 year-old, slender female with no history of diabetes or other endocrine problem is found to have acanthosis nigricans upon routine examination. What is a probable diagnosis?**

Underlying malignancy. Acanthosis nigricans is often a marker for malignancy, especially of the GI tract. It is the velvety brown hyperpigmentation and thickening of the flexures, common in the axilla and the groin. It is also associated with obesity, diabetes, and endocrine disorders.

❍ **What is a Bartholin's cyst?**

An obstructed Bartholin's duct, resulting in an abscess.

❍ **What is the most common skin malignancy?**

Basal cell carcinoma. Eighty to ninety percent of these lesions are found on the head and neck. Basal cell carcinoma appears as a pearly telangectasia with a central ulceration. These may spread locally, but they rarely metastasize.

❍ **What percentage of patients have recurrences of basal cell carcinoma within 5 years?**

36%. Metastasis to distant sites, however, is rare.

❍ **Where are Candida albicans infections of the skin most commonly located?**

The intertriginous areas, i.e., in the folds of the skin, axilla, groin, under the breasts, etc. Candida albicans appears as a beefy, red rash with satellite lesions.

❍ **What is a carbuncle?**

A deep abscess that interconnects and extends into the subcutaneous tissue. They commonly occur in patients with diabetes, folliculitis, steroid use, obesity, heavy perspiration, and in areas of friction.

❍ **Patients with untreated orbital or central facial abscesses are at risk for developing what serious complication?**

Cavernous sinus thrombosis.

❍ **What are the most common causes of allergic contact dermatitis?**

Poison ivy, poison sumac, poison oak, ragweed, topical medications, nickel, chromium, rubber, glue, cosmetics, and hair dyes.

❍ **A mother brings her 17 year-old boy to you a week after you prescribed ampicillin for his pharyngitis. Mom says he developed a rash over his torso, arms, legs, and even the palms of his hands. Upon examination, the patient has an erythematous, maculopapular rash. What might the child have other than pharyngitis?**

Infectious mononucleosis. In almost 95% of patients with Epstein-Barr viruses that are treated with ampicillin, a rash will develop. The rash and subsequent desquamation will last about a week.

❍ **Ecthyma most commonly presents on what body parts?**

The lower legs. Ecthyma is similar to impetigo but can also be associated with a fever and lymphadenopathy. The most common infecting agent is Staphylococcus aureus. This infection is most prevalent in moist, warm climates.

❍ **What is the most common bullous disease?**

Erythema multiforme. The typical erythema multiforme lesion is the iris lesion (a gray center with a red rim). These lesions are symmetrical and most frequently found on the distal extremities, spreading proximally. Patients may also develop plaques, papules, and bullous lesions. The disease is most common in children and young adults.

❍ **What is the most common cause of erythema multiforme?**

Repetitive minor herpes simplex infections (90%). Drug reactions are the second most common cause for erythema multiforme. The rash generally erupts 7 to 10 days after a bout of herpes.

❍ **Where is the most common location of erythema nodosum?**

The shins. They can also be found on the extensor surfaces of the forearms. Erythema nodosum are erythematous subcutaneous nodules that result from inflammation of subcutaneous fat and small vessels.

❍ **A patient presents with a raised, red, small, and painful plaque on the face. Upon examination, a distinct, sharp, advancing edge is noted. What is the cause?**

Erysipelas, which is caused by group A streptococci. When the face is involved, the patient should be admitted.

❍ **What type of reaction is erythema multiforme (EM)?**

Hypersensitivity. Bullae are subepidermal, the dermis is edematous, and a lymphatic infiltrate may be present around the capillaries and venules. In children, infections are the most important cause; in adults, drugs and malignancies are common causes. EM is often noted during epidemics of adenovirus, atypical pneumonia, and histoplasmosis.

❍ **What are the causes of exfoliative dermatitis?**

Chemicals, drugs, cutaneous or systemic diseases. Usually scaly erythematous dermatitis involves most or all of the surface skin. It can be recognized by erythroderma with epidermal flaking or scaling. Acute signs and symptoms include low-grade fever, pruritus, chills, and skin tightness. The chronic condition may produce dystrophic nails, thinning of body hair, and patchy hyperpigmentation or hypopigmentation. Cutaneous vasodilation may result in increased cardiac output and high-output cardiac failure. Splenomegaly suggests leukemia or lymphoma.

❍ **What is a furuncle?**

A deep-inflammatory nodule that grows out of superficial folliculitis.

❍ **What is hidradenitis suppurativa?**

Chronic suppurative abscesses located in the apocrine sweat glands of the groin and/or axilla. Proteus mirabilis overgrowth is common.

❍ **Your neighbor brings her 16 year-old daughter to you because she has a terrible rash. The child's face is patched with vesiculopustular lesions covered in a thick, honey-colored crust. Just 2 days ago, these lesions were small red papules. What is your diagnosis?**

Impetigo contagiosa. This is most common in children and usually occurs on exposed areas of skin. Treat the child by removing the crusts, cleansing the bases, and prescribing systemic antibiotics (erythromycin, cephalosporin, or dicloxacillin).

❍ **Which organism is probably responsible for the above patient's infection?**

50 to 90% of impetigo contagiosa cases are caused by Staphylococcus aureus. Beta-hemolytic Streptococcus is the second most common infecting agent. This latter organism is the sole affecting agent in 10% of cases. It can also be coinfecting with Staphylococcus aureus.

❍ **What are the ABCDEs of melanomas?**

Asymmetry
Border irregularity
Color variation
Diameter > 6 millimeters
Elevation above skin

❍ **What age group has the highest incidence of melanoma?**

30 to 50-year-olds.

❍ **A melanoma that is only in the epidermis is at what level in Clark's classification?**

Level I Clark's classification is based on how invasive a tumor is.
Level I: Epidermis
Level II: Loose papillary zone of dermis
Level III: Expands the papillary dermis
Level IV: Reticular dermis
Level V: Subcutaneous tissue

❍ **A patient has dysplastic nevus syndrome and is concerned because her aunt has just been diagnosed with melanoma. What is the patient's risk of also developing melanoma?**

100%.

❍ **What are the most common locations of melanomas in African-Americans? In Caucasian-Americans?**

African-Americans: hands, feet, and nails. Caucasian-Americans: back and lower legs.

❍ **Differentiate between pigmented and dysplastic nevi.**

Pigmented nevi are benign moles that are uniform in appearance. They are most common in sun exposed areas and warrant biopsy if they grow suddenly, change color, bleed, or begin to hurt.

Dysplastic nevi are not uniform in appearance and are frequently as large as 5 to 12 mm in diameter. 50% of malignant melanomas originate from the melanocytes in moles.

❍ **What are the most common causes of onychomycosis?**

Trichophyton rubrum and Trichophyton mentagrophytes.

❍ **What is a pilonidal abscess?**

An abscess that occurs in the gluteal fold as a result of a disruption of the epithelial surface.

❍ **Where does a perirectal abscess originate?**

Anal crypts and burrows through the ischiorectal space. They may be perianal, perirectal, supralevator, or ischiorectal. Perianal abscesses that involve the supralevator muscle, ischiorectal space, or rectum require operative drainage.

❍ **How should steroids be prescribed in patients with poison ivy?**

Prednisone, 40 to 60 mg/day tapered over 2 to 3 weeks. Short courses may result in rebound.

❍ **How quickly will people react to the Toxicodendron antigen?**

Contact dermatitis typically develops within 2 days of exposure. Cases have been reported from 8 hours to 10 days post-exposure. Lesions appear in a linear arrangement of papulovesicles or erythema. Fluid from vesicles does not contain the antigen and cannot transmit the dermatitis.

❍ **What is the most common cause of secondary pyodermia?**

Similar to impetigo and ecthyma, this superinfection of the skin is caused predominantly by Staphylococcus aureus (80 to 85%). Other responsible organisms are Streptococcus, Proteus, Pseudomonas, and E. coli.

❍ **A 17 year-old female has a rash on her elbows and knees. Upon examination you find several clearly demarcated erythematous plaques covered with silvery scales that can be removed with scraping. These lesions are on her extensor surfaces only in the areas previously mentioned. Examination of her nails reveals pitting in the nailbed. What is her diagnosis?**

Psoriasis. This is an intermittent disease that may either spontaneously disappear or be life long. There may be associated arthritis in the distal interphalangeal joints; otherwise, the disease is limited to the skin and nails. Treat with skin-hydration therapy and by topical mid-potency steroids. Remember: "Silvery scales and pitting nails".

❍ **A 60 year-old patient presents with greasy, red, scaly, plaques in his eyebrows, eyelids, and nose that are spreading to the naso-labial folds. In what population is this disease most likely to occur?**

The above patient has seborrheic dermatitis. This condition can occur in anyone, but it is a common problem in patients with HIV and Parkinson's disease. The infant form of the disease is cradle cap.

❍ **A 72 year-old female has a painful red rash with crops of blisters on erythematous bases in a band-like distribution on the right side of her lower back, which spreads down and out towards her hip. What is your diagnosis?**

Shingles or herpes zoster. This is due to the reactivation of a dormant varicella virus in the sensory root ganglia of a patient with a history of chicken pox. The rash is in the distribution of the dermatome, in this case, L5. It is most common in the elderly population or in patients who are immunocompromised. Treatment is with acyclovir and oral analgesics.

❍ **Where is the most common site of herpes zoster eruption?**

The thorax. Unlike chicken pox, shingles can recur.

❍ **A patient with shingles extending to the tip of his nose is at risk for what?**

Corneal ulceration and scarring. Lesions on the tip of the nose indicate that the nasociliary branch of the ophthalmic nerve is affected and the cornea is at risk. This is a medical emergency and needs immediate referral.

❍ **Which of the following is the premalignant lesion that can lead to squamous cell carcinoma: seborrheic keratosis or actinic keratoses?**

Actinic keratosis. The two can be differentiated:

Actinic keratosis: An isolated red-brown macule or papule with a rough yellow-brown scale over it.

Seborrheic keratosis: A benign, well-circumscribed, brownish papule with a greasy, warty appearance.

❍ **What are the two distinct causes of toxic epidermal necrolysis (scalded skin syndrome)?**

Staphylococcal infection and drugs or chemicals. Both begin with appearance of patches of tender erythema followed by loosening of the skin and denuding to glistening bases. Staphylococcal scalded skin syndrome is commonly found in children younger than 5, and is due to toxin that cleaves within the epidermis under the stratum granulosum.

❍ **What areas do staphylococcal scalded skin syndrome (SSSS) usually affect?**

The face around nose and mouth, neck, axillae, and groin. The disease commonly occurs after upper respiratory tract infections or purulent conjunctivitis. Nikolsky's sign is present when lateral pressure on the skin results in epidermal separation from the dermis.

❍ **How can SSSS be distinguished from scalded skin syndrome that is caused by drugs or chemicals?**

In drug or chemical etiologies, the skin separates at the dermoepidermal junction. Drug-induced TEN carries up to 50% mortality as a result of fluid loss and secondary infection. Upon microscopic examination of SSSS, intraepidermal cleavage occurs, and a few acantholytic keratinocytes can be seen. In the non-staphylococcal type, cellular debris, inflammatory cells, and basal cell keratinocytes are present.

❍ **What is the treatment for SSSS?**

Oral or IV penicillinase-resistant penicillin, baths of potassium permanganate or dressings soaked in 0.5% silver nitrate, and fluids. Corticosteroids and silver sulfadine are contraindicated.

❍ **A patient presents with fever, myalgias, malaise, and arthralgias has bullous lesions of the lips, eyes, and nose. The patient indicates that eating is painful. What is your diagnosis?**

Stevens-Johnson syndrome. This syndrome has a mortality of 5 to 10% and may have significant complications, including corneal ulceration, panophthalmitis, corneal opacities, anterior uveitis, blindness, hematuria, renal tubular necrosis, and progressive renal failure. Scarring of the foreskin and stenosis of the vagina can occur. Treatment in a burn unit is supportive. Steroids may provide symptomatic relief, but they are not of proven value and may be contraindicated.

❍ **What is the most common cause of Stevens-Johnson syndrome?**

Drugs, most commonly sulfa drugs. Other causes are responses to infections with Mycoplasma pneumonia and herpes simplex virus. The disease is self-limiting but severely uncomfortable.

❍ **What is the treatment of a tetanus prone wound?**

Surgical debridement, 3000 to 10,000 units of human tetanus immune globulin (TIG) IM (do not inject into wound), and penicillin G or metronidazole.

❍ **What is the danger of giving tetanus toxoid boosters in a pleonastic fashion (e.g., in 9-month intervals)?**

Arthus-type hypersensitivity reaction, with onset about 4 to 6 hours after injection. History of a severe hypersensitivity reaction or of a severe neurologic reaction is the only contraindications to tetanus toxoid.

❍ **A patient who was born with a diffuse capillary hemangioma in the distribution of the ophthalmic division of the trigeminal nerve will have what neurological findings?**

Epilepsy (usually generalized seizures), mental retardation, and/or hemiparesis. This is Sturge-Weber syndrome. The patient is born with a hemangioma of the ophthalmic nerve and ipsilateral angiomas of the pia matter and cortex (most commonly in the parieto-occipital area).

❍ **What is Tinea capitis?**

Tinea capitis is a fungal infection of the scalp that begins as a papule around one hair shaft and then spreads to other follicles. The infection can cause the hairs to break off, leaving little black dot stumps and patches of alopecia. Trichophyton tonsurans is responsible for 90% of the cases. Wood's lamp examination will fluoresce only Microsporum infections, which are responsible for the remaining 10%. This is also called "ringworm of the scalp".

❍ **What organisms most commonly cause tinea pedis and tinea manuum?**

Trichophyton rubrum and Trichophyton mentagrophytes.

❍ **What are the three most common causes of acute urticaria?**

1) Medicine
2) Arthropod bites
3) Infection

Urticaria, also known as hives or wheels, is a localized swelling due to a cytokine-mediated increase in vascular permeability.

❍ **What is the most common cause of physical urticaria?**

Dermatographism. In this case, urticaria develops after firm, rapid stroking of the skin with a blunt surface. Such urticaria generally resolves within the hour.

❍ **Where is the most common location of verrucae vulgaris?**

The back of the hands or fingers. Common warts are caused by HPV.

❍ **Xanthomas are associated with which metabolic disorder?**

Hyperlipidemia. Xanthomas are yellow plaques surrounded by erythematous rings. They are most common on the extensor surfaces of the extremities. However, eruptive xanthomas are most common on the buttocks.

❍ **How can the development of decubitus ulcers be prevented?**

Change the patient's position every 2 hours, keep the skin clean and dry, use protective padding at potential sites of ulceration, i.e., heel pads or ankle pads, and keep patients on egg crate mattresses or the equivalent. For diabetics, encourage daily foot examination.

❍ **What organism is the most common cause of bullous impetigo?**

Coagulase positive Staph. aureus.

❍ **What is the best treatment for impetigo?**

Oral erythromycin mupirocin (Bactroban) topical lotion.

❍ **What is the treatment for atopic dermatitis?**

Oral antihistamines, topical steroids, emollients, and avoidance of irritants.

❍ **Elevations of which immunoglobulin is common in atopic dermatitis?**

IgE.

❍ **What are the two main organisms responsible for Tinea capitis?**

Microsporum canis and Trichophyton tonsurans. Of these two, T. tonsurans is the most contagious.

❍ **How do you make the diagnosis of Tinea versicolor?**

Examination under a Wood's lamp would show yellow fluorescence. Also, a KOH prep is useful in confirming diagnosis.

❍ **What is the recommended therapy for Tinea capitis?**

Oral Griseofulvin (15-20 mg/kg/day) and shampooing twice a week with 2.5% Selenium Sulfide.

❍ **What is the causative agent of Tinea versicolor?**

Pityrosporum orbiculare (Malassezia furfur), a fungus.

❍ **Patients with what conditions are more likely to develop vitiligo?**

Diabetes mellitus, Addison's disease, thyroid disorders and pernicious anemia.

❍ **Which areas of the body are normally most affected by vitiligo?**

Areas that are normally hyperpigmented (i.e. face, areolae) and areas subject to friction (i.e. hands, elbows).

❍ **What is another name for erythema multiforme major?**

Stevens-Johnson syndrome.

❍ **What pattern of hair loss can be observed with trichotillomania?**

Asymmetric hair loss.

❍ **A patient presents with red and tender lateral nailfold on his big toe with a small abscess. What is the diagnosis?**

Paronychia.

❍ **Who is more likely to present with pediculosis capitis, Caucasians or African-Americans?**

Caucasians are 30% more likely to acquire this organism.

❍ **What is the drug of choice for head lice?**

Permethrin (Nix).

❍ **Where is the best place to get a scraping to rule out scabies?**

The web spaces between the fingers and toes.

❍ **What is the treatment of choice for scabies?**

5% Permethrin cream.

❍ **Psoriatic arthritis classically attacks which joints?**

The DIP joints of the hands and feet.

❍ **An 31 year-old female presents with a maculopapular rash on her trunk and upper legs. The rash is in lines along the long axis of the ovoid lesions. The patient states that one week ago, she had only one lesion, which was round and "about as wide as a golf ball". What is your diagnosis?**

Pityriasis rosea.

❍ **What is the distribution of the rash in pityriasis rosea?**

"Christmas tree" pattern with parallel rows of lesions on the trunk.

❍ **Can vitiligo be treated with topical steroids?**

Yes, though it may not be fully effective.

❍ **Is vitiligo congenital or acquired?**

Acquired.

❍ **Patients on which antibiotic are most likely to have photoallergic drug reaction?**

Tetracycline and sulfonamides.

❍ **What is the average amount of time required after contact with poison ivy to develop cutaneous lesions?**

2-4 days.

❍ **An obese 18 year-old male with a history of IDDM reports dark patches in groin and axilla. What is the most likely diagnosis?**

Acanthosis nigrans, which may be caused by insulin resistance.

❍ **What is the treatment for scalp lesions of seborrheic dermatitis?**

Antiseborrheic shampoo (i.e. coal tar, selenium sulfide).

❍ **Which responds more rapidly to topical steroids - seborrheic dermatitis or atopic dermatitis?**

Seborrheic dermatitis. This is used when the lesions are inflamed.

GERIATRICS

Do not resist growing old-many are denied the privilege.
Anonymous

❍ **According to the 1990 census, what percentage of Americans are over 65?**

12.6%

❍ **What percentage of the elderly are ambulatory?**

90%.

❍ **What percentage of the elderly live in nursing homes?**

10%.

❍ **How do the sleep patterns of the elderly differ from those of younger age groups?**

The elderly spend less time asleep. They have an increased number of nocturnal awakenings and decreased REM. They also fall asleep earlier and wake up earlier than their younger counterparts.

❍ **What may result from the administration of aminoglycoside or cephalosporins to an elderly patient who is dehydrated?**

Acute renal failure secondary to tubulointerstitial injury. This may also occur if the above mentioned drugs are given to an elderly patient on furosemide or with preexisting renal disease.

❍ **What is the most common cause of hearing loss in the elderly?**

Presbycusis. Other causes include neoplasms, noise exposure, ototoxic drugs, and otosclerosis.

❍ **Presbycusis is a hearing loss at which end of the audible range?**

The high end (4000 to 8000 Hz).

❍ **What is the most common form of incontinence in the elderly?**

Urge incontinence. It is more common in females and is due to detrusor hyperreflexia or decreased sensory capabilities.

❍ **Is the incidence of epidural and subdural hematomas higher or lower in elderly patients?**

Epidural hematomas are less common and subdural hematomas are more common.

❍ **What geriatric population is at greatest risk for esophageal cancer?**

Elderly African-Americans have a risk 4 times that of elderly Caucasian-Americans. Other populations at risk include Chinese, Iranians, and South Africans.

❍ **Who has a higher rupture rate in appendicitis, the very young or the very old?**

The very old. The rupture rate for geriatric patients is 65 to 90% with an associated mortality of 15%. The pediatric population has a rupture rate of 15 to 50% and an associated mortality rate of 3%.

❍ **What are the symptoms of sundown syndrome?**

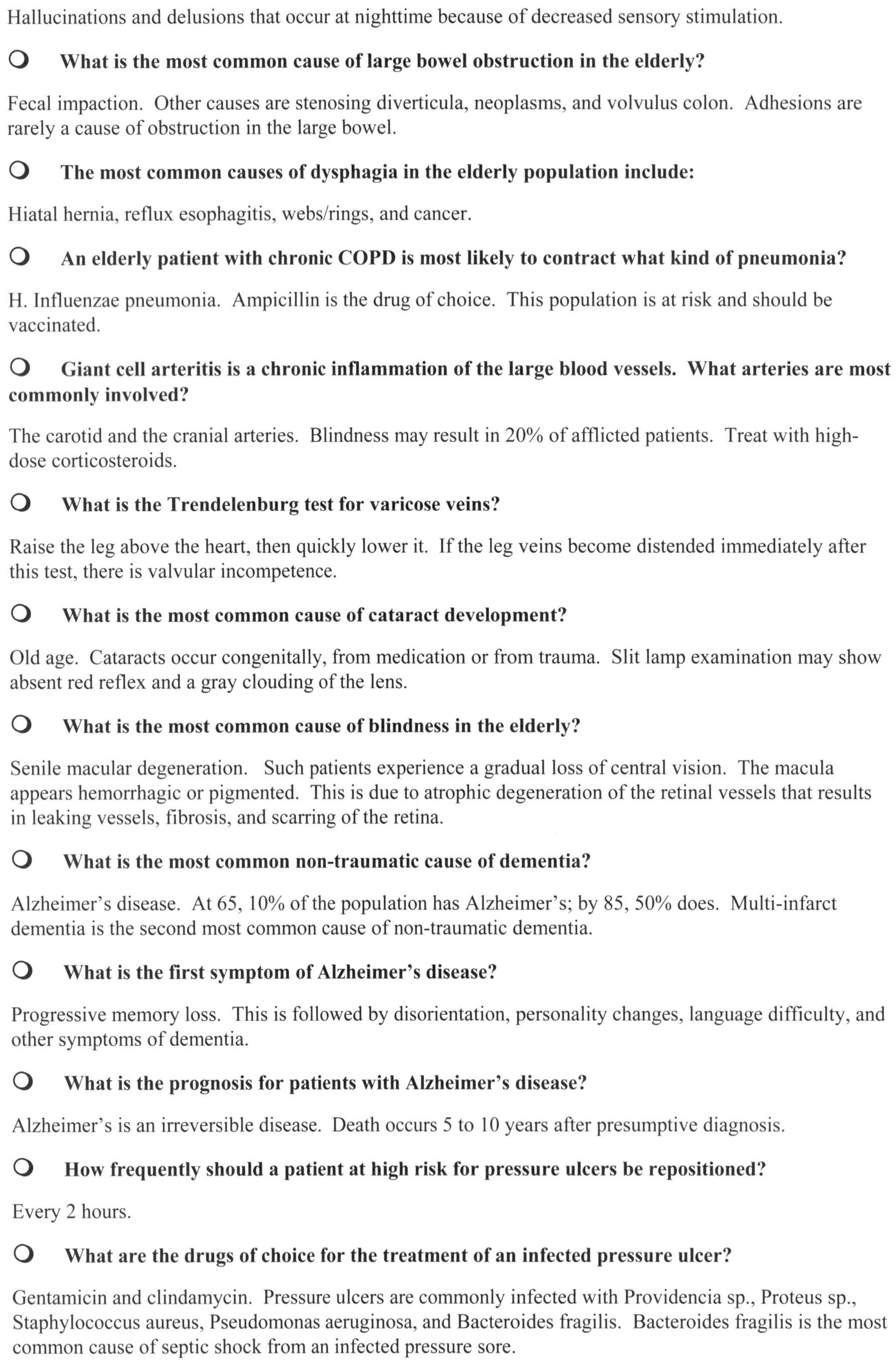

Hallucinations and delusions that occur at nighttime because of decreased sensory stimulation.

❍ What is the most common cause of large bowel obstruction in the elderly?

Fecal impaction. Other causes are stenosing diverticula, neoplasms, and volvulus colon. Adhesions are rarely a cause of obstruction in the large bowel.

❍ The most common causes of dysphagia in the elderly population include:

Hiatal hernia, reflux esophagitis, webs/rings, and cancer.

❍ An elderly patient with chronic COPD is most likely to contract what kind of pneumonia?

H. Influenzae pneumonia. Ampicillin is the drug of choice. This population is at risk and should be vaccinated.

❍ Giant cell arteritis is a chronic inflammation of the large blood vessels. What arteries are most commonly involved?

The carotid and the cranial arteries. Blindness may result in 20% of afflicted patients. Treat with high-dose corticosteroids.

❍ What is the Trendelenburg test for varicose veins?

Raise the leg above the heart, then quickly lower it. If the leg veins become distended immediately after this test, there is valvular incompetence.

❍ What is the most common cause of cataract development?

Old age. Cataracts occur congenitally, from medication or from trauma. Slit lamp examination may show absent red reflex and a gray clouding of the lens.

❍ What is the most common cause of blindness in the elderly?

Senile macular degeneration. Such patients experience a gradual loss of central vision. The macula appears hemorrhagic or pigmented. This is due to atrophic degeneration of the retinal vessels that results in leaking vessels, fibrosis, and scarring of the retina.

❍ What is the most common non-traumatic cause of dementia?

Alzheimer's disease. At 65, 10% of the population has Alzheimer's; by 85, 50% does. Multi-infarct dementia is the second most common cause of non-traumatic dementia.

❍ What is the first symptom of Alzheimer's disease?

Progressive memory loss. This is followed by disorientation, personality changes, language difficulty, and other symptoms of dementia.

❍ What is the prognosis for patients with Alzheimer's disease?

Alzheimer's is an irreversible disease. Death occurs 5 to 10 years after presumptive diagnosis.

❍ How frequently should a patient at high risk for pressure ulcers be repositioned?

Every 2 hours.

❍ What are the drugs of choice for the treatment of an infected pressure ulcer?

Gentamicin and clindamycin. Pressure ulcers are commonly infected with Providencia sp., Proteus sp., Staphylococcus aureus, Pseudomonas aeruginosa, and Bacteroides fragilis. Bacteroides fragilis is the most common cause of septic shock from an infected pressure sore.

❍ What drugs are used to treat stress incontinence?

Alpha-adrenergic agonists and estrogen.

❍ **Strokes, Parkinson's disease, and Alzheimer's disease are most commonly associated with which type of incontinence?**

Stress incontinence.

❍ **What are, by order of initiation, the drugs used for the treatment of Parkinson's disease?**

Start with amantadine (Symmetrel) and trihexyphenidyl (Artane). If this fails, use a combination of levodopa and carbidopa. Pergolide and bromocriptine can be used to treat episodes of immobility.

❍ **A 65 year-old African-American has hypertension and gout. What medications should be prescribed?**

Although diuretics are the most effective drugs for the treatment of hypertension in this race, the patient has gout, which will be exacerbated by the use of diuretics. ACE inhibitors or calcium channel blockers are better choices for this patient.

❍ **What is the most common complication of a pressure ulcer?**

Sepsis.

❍ **What is the mortality rate for geriatric patients who have sustained a hip fracture?**

25% will die in the first year following the fracture.

❍ **How do you clinically differentiate between polymyalgia rheumatica and polymyositis?**

In polymyositis, there is proximal muscle pain, weakness, and tenderness, and elevated muscle enzymes. In contrast, polymyalgia rheumatica presents with an elevated sedimentation rate (also seen in giant cell arteritis, which is associated with polymalgia rheumatica).

❍ **Which vitamin is effective for the treatment of pressure ulcers?**

Vitamin C.

❍ **What agent should be used for cleaning an infected pressure ulcer?**

Saline.

❍ **What are the two pathologic findings used to confirm the diagnosis of Alzheimer's disease?**

The quantity of neurofibrillary tangles and senile plaques. Other findings include neuronal loss and amyloid degermation.

❍ **What is the most common cause of UTI's in uncatheterized elderly patients?**

E. coli.

❍ **What is the most common cause of relapsing UTI's in elderly patients?**

Chronic bacterial prostatitis, caused by E. coli, Proteus, Klebsiella pneumoniae, and enterococci.

❍ **In the elderly, what is a common side effect of verapamil?**

Constipation.

❍ **What is the most common pathophysiologic cause of delirium?**

Acetylcholine deficiency.

❍ **Parkinson-like side effects are common with which class of drugs?**

Neuroleptics. Parkinson-like side effects can develop with perphenazine, chlorpromazine, reserpine, haloperidol, metoclopramide, and the illicit meperidine analog MPTP.

❍ **In the elderly, what is the most common cause of death resulting from community acquired infections? Institutional? Nosocomial?**

In the community and institutions, it is bacterial pneumonia; in hospitals, it is UTI's.

❍ **What is the most common cause of drug-induced hallucinations in the geriatric population?**

Propranol.

❍ **What percentage of patients with primary Alzheimer's disease will present with secondary depression?**

30 to 35%.

❍ **What is the most common cause of recurrent abdominal pain in the elderly?**

Constipation.

❍ **What is the most common risk factor for Alzheimer's disease?**

A family history of dementia.

❍ **An elderly female presents with high blood pressure and a history of CHF. What is the antihypertensive drug of choice?**

ACE inhibitors. They will reduce both preload and afterload.

❍ **What diagnostic test should be performed on a patient with delirium?**

EEG. Other tests should be ordered dependent upon the patient's history and a physical examination.

❍ **What percentage of the elderly suffer from urinary incontinence?**

5 to 15% in the community and 50% in nursing homes. Incontinence is the second most common cause of admission to long-term care facilities.

❍ **Patients with which type of apolipoprotein are more likely to acquire Alzheimer's disease?**

Type 4, apolipoprotein E.

❍ **An elderly male presents with high blood pressure and a history of NIDDM. What is the antihypertensive drug of choice?**

ACE inhibitors. They have renal protective properties.

❍ **What are the common neurologic signs and symptoms of giant cell arteritis?**

Amaurosis fugax, deafness, depression, and paralysis. Amaurosis fugax is the most dangerous because it can lead to permanent monocular or binocular blindness.

❍ **What is the major risk of tricyclic antidepressants in the elderly?**

Orthostatic hypotension, because this can lead to falls.

❍ **An elderly African-American male presents with high blood pressure and a history of angina. What is the antihypertensive drug of choice?**

Calcium channel blockers.

❍ **Which type of laxative is most associated with long-term side effects in the elderly?**

Stimulant laxatives.

❍ **What are the most common sources of sepsis in the elderly?**

Respiratory > urinary > intra-abdominal.

❍ **Describe the common findings of benign essential tremors?**

Tremulousness of speech and nodding of head. This is an action tremor that is usually familial and is often treated with atenolol, propranolol, diazepam, and alcohol.

❍ **Narcotic drugs are associated with which type of urinary incontinence?**

Overflow. Anticholinergic, beta-blockers, and calcium channal blockers also commonly cause overflow incontinence.

❍ **What lab values increase with age?**

BUN/Cr, sedimentation rate, thyroxine (T4), and calcium (in females).

❍ **What lab values decrease with age?**

Leukocyte count and creatinine phosphokinase.

❍ **What lab values are not affected by age?**

Bicarb, bilirubin, chloride, coagulation tests, hemoglobin, magnesium, RBC indices, and sodium.

❍ **What is the most typical complaint for a patient over 85 with an acute MI?**

Shortness of breath. The classic presentation is only present in 20% of elderly patients.

❍ **What are the most common ECG abnormalities in an elderly patient?**

Degenerative changes in the heart's conduction system.

❍ **What is the incidence of morbidity and mortality in patients over 60 who present with syncope?**

1 in 5 will suffer significant morbidity or mortality within 6 months.

❍ **What percentage of septic elderly patients do not present with a fever?**

25%.

❍ **What drugs are most commonly associated with ARDS in the elderly?**

Analgesics, cardiovascular, and psychotropic drugs.

❍ **What are the common adverse drug interactions of cimetidine in the elderly?**

Inhibits the metabolism of phenytoin, coumadin, and theophylline.

❍ **What are the common adverse drug interactions of coumadin?**

Metabolism is inhibited by allopurinol, trimethoprim-sulfamethoxazole, metronidazole, and quinolones.

❍ **What are the most common mechanisms of injury in the elderly?**

Falls > motor vehicle accidents > burns > assaults.

❍ **What is the most common cause of acute abdominal pain in the elderly?**

Acute cholecystitis. Approximately 50% of patients over 65 have gallstones.

❍ **Describe the clinical features of appendicitis in the elderly?**

The elderly account for 50% of the deaths as a result of appendicitis. Half of elderly patients with appendicitis have normal white counts upon presentation. Anorexia and vomiting are less common, and migration of the pain to the RLQ is absent in up to 60% of elderly patients.

CLINICAL EPIDEMIOLOGY

Logic is the art of going wrong with confidence.
Joseph Wood Krutch

❍ **How do you <u>define</u> the sensitivity of a diagnostic test?**

Out of all the people known to have disease, how many have a positive (or abnormal) test result. It is the likelihood of a positive test result in patients known to have disease.

❍ **How do you <u>calculate</u> the sensitivity of a diagnostic test?**

The sensitivity is equal to the true positive rate of a diagnostic test and can be calculated as the number of True Positives divided by all those who have disease (i.e. the number of True Positives plus the False Negatives). Sensitivity (or True Positive rate) = A/(A+C).

		DISEASE		
		Present	Absent	
TEST	**Positive**	A (True Positives)	B (False Positives)	A + B
	Negative	C (False Negatives)	D (True Negatives)	C + D
		A + C	B + D	A + B + C + D

❍ **What is the clinical <u>utility</u> of a highly sensitive test?**

A highly sensitive test is most useful when it is negative or normal. It is good for "ruling out" disease. A positive or abnormal test result may or may not indicate the patient has the disease of interest.

❍ **How do you <u>define</u> the specificity of a diagnostic test?**

Out of all the people without disease, how many have a negative (or normal) test result. It is the likelihood of a negative test result in patients known to be free of disease.

❍ **How do you <u>calculate</u> the specificity of a diagnostic test?**

The specificity is equal to the true negative rate of a diagnostic test and can be calculated as the number of True Negatives divided by all those who do not have disease (i.e. the number of True Negatives plus the False Positives). Specificity (or True Negative rate) = D/(B+D)

		DISEASE		
		Present	Absent	
TEST	**Positive**	A (True Positives)	B (False Positives)	A + B
	Negative	C (False Negatives)	D (True Negatives)	C + D
		A + C	B + D	A + B + C + D

❍ **What is the clinical <u>utility</u> of a highly specific test?**

A highly specific test is most useful when it is positive or abnormal. It is good for "ruling in" disease. A negative or normal test result may or may not indicate the patient does not have the disease of interest.

❍ **<u>Case 1</u>: The "classical clinical triad" of pheochromocytoma includes headaches, palpitations, and excessive perspiration. In one study, 2585 patients were referred to a hypertensive clinic. Of these, 11 patients were eventually diagnosed with pheochromocytoma and 10 had the clinical triad. Of the 2574 remaining patients without pheochromocytoma, 160 had the clinical triad. What is the sensitivity of the "classical clinical triad" for pheochromocytoma**

		Pheochromocytoma		
		Present	Absent	
Clinical **Triad**	**Positive**	10 (True Positives)	B (False Positives)	A + B
	Negative	1 (False Negatives)	D (True Negatives)	C + D
		11	B + D	2585

Sensitivity = True Positives/All Pheochromocytoma Patients = TP/(TP + FN) = 10/11 = 91%

❍ **<u>Case 1</u>: Using the same information given above, what is the specificity of the "classical clinical triad" for pheochromocytoma?**

		Pheochromocytoma		
		Present	Absent	
Clinical **Triad**	**Positive**	10 (True Positives)	160 (False Positives)	A + B
	Negative	1 (False Negatives)	2414 (True Negatives)	C + D
		11	2574	2585

Specificity = True Negatives/All Patients without Pheochromoctyoma = TN/(TN + FP) = 2414/2574 = 94%

❍ **How do you <u>define</u> the false negative rate of a diagnostic test?**

Out of all the people known to have disease, how many have a negative (or normal) test result. It is the likelihood of a negative test result in patients known to have disease.

❍ **How do you <u>calculate</u> the false negative rate of a diagnostic test?**

The false negative rate can be calculated as the number of False Negatives divided by all those who have disease (i.e. the number of True Positives plus the False Negatives). False Negative rate = C/(A+C) which is also equal to 1 - Sensitivity.

		DISEASE		
		Present	Absent	
TEST	**Positive**	A (True Positives)	B (False Positives)	A + B
	Negative	C (False Negatives)	D (True Negatives)	C + D
		A + C	B + D	A + B + C + D

❍ **What is the clinical <u>utility</u> of the false negative rate of a diagnostic test?**

Note that both sensitivity and the false negative rate of a diagnostic test describe how such tests perform in patients known to have the disease.

❍ How do you <u>define</u> the false positive rate of a diagnostic test?

Out of all the people without disease, how many have a positive (or abnormal) test result. It is the likelihood of a positive test result in patients known to be free of disease.

❍ How do you <u>calculate</u> the false positive rate of a diagnostic test?

The false positive rate can be calculated as the number of False Positives divided by all those who do not have disease (i.e. the number of True Negatives plus the False Positives). False Positive rate = B/(B+D) which is equal to 1 - Specificity

		DISEASE		
		Present	Absent	
TEST	**Positive**	A (True Positives)	B (False Positives)	A + B
	Negative	C (False Negatives)	D (True Negatives)	C + D
		A + C	B + D	A + B + C + D

❍ What is the clinical <u>utility</u> of the false positive rate of a diagnostic test?

Note that both specificity and the false positive rate of a diagnostic test describe how such tests perform in patients known to be free of disease.

❍ <u>Case 1</u>: The "classical clinical triad" of pheochromocytoma includes headaches, palpitations, and excessive perspiration. In one study, 2585 patients were referred to a hypertensive clinic. Of these, 11 patients were eventually diagnosed with pheochromocytoma and 10 had the clinical triad. Of the 2574 remaining patients without pheochromocytoma, 160 had the clinical triad. What is the False Negative Rate of the "classical clinical triad" for pheochromocytoma?

		Pheochromocytoma		
		Present	Absent	
Clinical **Triad**	**Positive**	10 (True Positives)	B (False Positives)	A + B
	Negative	1 (False Negatives)	D (True Negatives)	C + D
		11	B + D	2585

False Negative Rate = False Negatives/All Pheochromocytoma Patients = FN/(TP + FN) = 1/11 = 9%. (Note that the False Negative Rate is also equal to 1 - sensitivity or 1 - .91 = 0.09 or 9%.)

❍ <u>Case 1</u>: Using the same information given above, what is the False Positive Rate of the "classical clinical triad" for pheochromocytoma?

		Pheochromocytoma		
		Present	Absent	
Clinical **Triad**	**Positive**	10 (True Positives)	160 (False Positives)	A + B
	Negative	1 (False Negatives)	2414 (True Negatives)	C + D
		11	2574	2585

False Positive Rate = False Positives/All Patients without Pheochromoctyoma = FP/(TN + FP) = 160/2574 = 6%. (Note that the False Positive Rate is also equal to 1 -specificity or 1 - 0.94 = 0.06 or 6%.)

❍ **How do you define the prevalence of disease in a particular population?**

Out of all the people studied, how many have the disease of interest.

❍ **How do you calculate the prevalence of disease in a particular population?**

The prevalence of disease is calculated by the number of patients with disease divided by the total number of patients in the population being studied. Prevalence of Disease = (A+C)/(A+B+C+D

		DISEASE		
		Present	Absent	
TEST	**Positive**	A (True Positives)	B (False Positives)	A + B
	Negative	C (False Negatives)	D (True Negatives)	C + D
		A + C	B + D	A + B + C + D

❍ **What is the clinical utility of the prevalence of disease in a particular population?**

In a patient or population being studied, this is the baseline probability of having the disease (i.e. often called the "pre-test probability" of disease). Additional tests, signs, or symptoms are useful only if they lower or raise this initial probability.

❍ **Case 1: The "classical clinical triad" of pheochromocytoma includes headaches, palpitations, and excessive perspiration. In one study, 2585 patients were referred to a hypertensive clinic. Of these, 11 patients were eventually diagnosed with pheochromocytoma and 10 had the clinical triad. Of the 2574 remaining patients without pheochromocytoma, 160 had the clinical triad. What is the Prevalence of pheochromocytoma in the study population?**

		Pheochromocytoma		
		Present	Absent	
Clinical **Triad**	**Positive**	10 (True Positives)	160 (False Positives)	A + B
	Negative	1 (False Negatives)	2414 (True Negatives)	C + D
		11	2574	2585

Prevalence = All those with pheochromocytoma/Total number of patients in the study population = 11/2585 = 0.004 = 0.4%.

❍ **How do you calculate the positive predictive value of a diagnostic test?**

The positive predictive value can be calculated as the number of True Positives divided by all those who have a positive test result (i.e. the number of True Positives plus the False Positives). Positive Predictive Value = A/(A+B)

		DISEASE		
		Present	Absent	
TEST	**Positive**	A (True Positives)	B (False Positives)	A + B
	Negative	C (False Negatives)	D (True Negatives)	C + D
		A + C	B + D	A + B + C + D

❍ **What is the clinical utility of the positive predictive value of a test?**

Most clinicians are interested in the predictive value of a diagnostic test. However, it is important to remember that the prevalence of disease critically affects the post-test result interpretation. When the prevalence of the disease is high in the suspected population, a positive (or abnormal) test result tends to confirm the actual presence of disease. When the prevalence of the suspected disease is low, however, a positive (or abnormal) test may be a false positive test result.

❍ **How do you define the negative predictive value of a diagnostic test?**

Out of all the people with a negative (or normal) test result, how many do NOT have the disease. It is the likelihood a negative test results indicates the absence of disease among all patients with a negative test result.

❍ **How do you calculate the negative predictive value of a diagnostic test?**

The negative predictive value can be calculated as the number of True Negatives divided by all those who have a negative test result (i.e. the number of True Negatives plus the False Negatives). Negative Predictive Value = D/(C+D)

		DISEASE		
		Present	Absent	
TEST	**Positive**	A (True Positives)	B (False Positives)	A + B
	Negative	C (False Negatives)	D (True Negatives)	C + D
		A + C	B + D	A + B + C + D

❍ **What is the clinical utility of the negative predictive value of a test?**

Most clinicians are interested in the predictive value of a diagnostic test. However, it is important to remember that the prevalence of disease critically affects post-test result interpretation. When the prevalence of the disease is low in the suspected population, a negative (or normal) test result tends to confirm the absence of disease. When the prevalence of the suspected disease is high, however, a negative (or normal) test may be a false negative test result.

❍ **Case 1: The "classical clinical triad" of pheochromocytoma includes headaches, palpitations, and excessive perspiration. In one study, 2585 patients were referred to a hypertensive clinic. Of these, 11 patients were eventually diagnosed with pheochromocytoma and 10 had the clinical triad. Of the 2574 remaining patients without pheochromocytoma, 160 had the clinical triad. What is the Positive Predictive Value of the "classical clinical triad" for pheochromocytoma?**

		Pheochromocytoma		
		Present	Absent	
Clinical **Triad**	**Positive**	10 (True Positives)	160 (False Positives)	170
	Negative	1 (False Negatives)	2414 (True Negatives)	2415
		11	2574	2585

Positive Predictive Value = True Positives/All patients who test positive = TP/(TP + FP) = 10/170 = 6%. (Note when the prevalence of the suspected disease is low, as in this situation equal to 0.4%, even a test with a high sensitivity and specificity often yields a false positive test result. Of all those who have a positive "classical clinical triad" for pheochromocytoma, only 6% will indeed turn out to actually have a pheochromocytoma, whereas 94% of those with the "classical clinical triad" will NOT have a pheochromocytoma.)

❍ **Case 1: Using the same information given above, what is the Negative Predictive Value of the "classical clinical triad" for pheochromocytoma?**

		Pheochromocytoma		
		Present	Absent	
Clinical Triad	**Positive**	10 (True Positives)	160 (False Positives)	170
	Negative	1 (False Negatives)	2414 (True Negatives)	2415
		11	2574	2585

Negative Predictive Value = True Negatives/All patients who test negative = TN/(TN + FN) = 2414/2415 = 99.9%. (Note when the prevalence of the suspected disease is low, as in this equal to 0.4%, a negative test results tends to confirm the absence of disease in more than 99% of the time.)

❍ **How do you define the accuracy of a diagnostic test?**

This is the proportion of all test results that are correct, both positive and negative, for a disease in a given population being studied.

❍ **How do you calculate the accuracy of a diagnostic test?**

The accuracy of a diagnostic test is calculated by the number of True Positives plus True Negatives divided by the total number of patients in the population being studied. Accuracy = (A+D)/(A+B+C+D)

		DISEASE		
		Present	Absent	
TEST	**Positive**	A (True Positives)	B (False Positives)	A + B
	Negative	C (False Negatives)	D (True Negatives)	C + D
		A + C	B + D	A + B + C + D

❍ **What is the clinical utility of the accuracy of a diagnostic test**

The accuracy of a diagnostic test is the overall value of the test. However, this summary term is often too crude to be useful clinically because specific information about the component parts (e.g. sensitivity, specificity, positive and negative predictive values, etc.) - often that part which which physicians most need - are lost when they are aggregated into a single index.

❍ **Case 2: In a recent publication describing the utility of the physical examination in predicting ascites, the following information was presented (JAMA 1992;267:2645-8):**

PHYSICAL FINDING	SENSITIVITY (%)	SPECIFICITY (%)
Bilateral Bulging Flanks	81	59
Fluid Wave	62	90
Shifting Dullness	77	72
Puddle Sign	45	73
Everted Navel	33	88
Pedal Edema	87	77
Ballotable Liver	27	93

Which single bedside physical exam maneuver is best at ruling *out* ascites?
A highly sensitive test when negative (or absent) is best at ruling out disease. In this case, the *absence* of pedal edema is the single best physical exam sign to predict the absence of ascites.

❍ Case 2: Which single bedside physical exam maneuver is best at ruling *in* ascites?

A highly specific test when positive (or present) is best at ruling in disease. In this case the *presence* of a ballotable liver is the single best bedside test to confirm the presence of ascites.

❍ Case 3: In a recent publication describing the utility of the physical examination in predicting lumbar disc herniation as a cause of low back pain, the following information was presented (JAMA 1992;268:760-5):

PHYSICAL FINDING	SENSITIVITY (%)	SPECIFICITY (%)
Ipsilateral Straight Leg Raising	80	40
Crossed Straight Leg Raising	25	90
Ankle Dorsiflexion Weakness	35	75
Impaired Patellar Reflex	50	---
Impaired Ankle Reflex	50	60
Sensory Loss	50	50

Which single bedside physical exam maneuver is best at ruling *out* disc herniation as a cause of low back pain?

A highly sensitive test when negative (or absent) is best at ruling out disease. In this case, the *absence* of pain on ipsilateral straight leg raising is the best physical exam sign to predict the absence of disc herniation.

❍ Case 3: Which single bedside physical exam maneuver is best at ruling *in* disc herniation as a cause of low back pain?

A highly specific test when positive (or present) is best at ruling in disease. In this case the *presence* of a pain on crossed straight leg raising is the single best bedside test to confirm the presence of disc herniation.

❍ Case 4: A 25-year old woman presents for an insurance examination that requires HIV testing. She is in good health and has a normal physical exam. She enjoys a monogamous sexual relationship with her husband and has no risk factors for HIV. Her HIV ELISA (enzyme-linked immunosorbent assay) test is positive. Based on available information from your hospital's laboratory, the ELISA test has a sensitivity and specificity of 98%. The pretest prevalence of HIV infection in similar patients at your hospital is estimated to be 1 in 10,000. Before confirmation, with a Western blot test, what is the post-test probability this patient actually has a true HIV infection?

		HIV Infection		
		Present	Absent	
ELISA **Test**	**Positive**	.98 (True Positives)	199.98 (False Positives)	200.96
	Negative	.02 (False Negatives)	9799.02 (True Negatives)	9799.04
		1	9,999	10,000

Note: for test taking purposes, the math can be "simplified" as follows:

		HIV Infection		
		Present	Absent	
ELISA **Test**	**Positive**	1 (True Positives)	200 (False Positives)	200
	Negative	0 (False Negatives)	9800 (True Negatives)	9800
		1	10,000	10,000

This question is asking for the positive predictive value of the ELISA test for HIV infection. The positive predictive value is calculated by the TP/(TP + FP) = 1/201 = 0.5%. Simply, stated even after a positive ELISA test, this woman has only a 0.5% chance of truly being infected with HIV.
This example illustrates an important axiom to remember in the interpretation of a diagnostic test: when the prevalence of the suspected disease is low, a positive (or abnormal) test is often times a false positive test result.

❍ **<u>Case 4</u>: If the same patient's ELISA test for HIV returned negative, what is the likelihood she actually does not have HIV infection ?**

		HIV Infection		
		Present	Absent	
ELISA **Test**	**Positive**	.98 (True Positives)	199.98 (False Positives)	200.96
	Negative	.02 (False Negatives)	9799.02 (True Negatives)	9799.04
		1	9,999	10,000

Note: for test taking purposes, the math can be "simplified" as follows:

		HIV Infection		
		Present	Absent	
ELISA **Test**	**Positive**	1 (True Positives)	200 (False Positives)	200
	Negative	0 (False Negatives)	9800 (True Negatives)	9800
		1	10,000	10,000

This question is asking for the negative predictive value of the ELISA test for HIV infection. The negative predictive value is calculated by the TN/(TN + FN) = 9800/9800 = 100% (or actually 9799.02/(9799.02 + 0.02) = 99% Simply, stated after a negative ELISA test, this woman has a very, very small chance of being infected with HIV. This example illustrates an important axiom to remember in the interpretation of a diagnostic test: when the prevalence of the disease is low in the suspected population, a negative (or normal) test result tends to confirm the absence of disease.

❍ **<u>Case 5</u>: A 25-year old man presents to a sexually transmitted disease (STD) clinic for treatment of chlamydia. The clinic routinely screens all patients with an HIV test. He is in good health and has a normal physical exam. His HIV ELISA (enzyme-linked immunosorbent assay) test is positive. Based on available information from your hospital's laboratory, the ELISA test has a sensitivity and specificity of 98%. The pretest prevalence of HIV infection in similar patients at your hospital is estimated to be 3 in 10. Before confirmation, with a Western blot test, what is the post-test probability this patient actually has a true HIV infection?**

		HIV Infection		
		Present	Absent	
ELISA **Test**	**Positive**	294 (True Positives)	14 (False Positives)	308
	Negative	6 (False Negatives)	686 (True Negatives)	692
		300	700	1000

This question is asking for the positive predictive value of the ELISA test for HIV infection. The positive predictive value is calculated by the TP/(TP + FP) = 294/(294 +14) = 95.5%. Simply, stated, this man has more than a 95% chance of truly being infected with HIV. This example illustrates an important axiom to remember in the interpretation of a diagnostic test: when the prevalence of the disease is high in the suspected population, a positive (or abnormal) test result tends to confirm the actual presence of disease. Note that the characteristics of the ELISA test (i.e. sensitivity and specificity) have remained the same, only the prevalence of disease has changed from the previous example. Prevalence of disease can markedly affect the interpretation of post-test probabilities of disease.

❍ **What is the definition of absolute risk?**

The absolute risk is the number of patients with the risk factor and disease of interest divided by all patients with the risk factor present

❍ **How do you calculate the absolute risk?**

The absolute risk is equal to the True Positives divided by all those who have the risk factor (i.e. the number of True Positives plus the False Positive) = A/(A+B)

		DISEASE		
		Present	Absent	
RISK **FACTOR**	**Positive**	A (True Positives)	B (False Positives)	A + B
	Negative	C (False Negatives)	D (True Negatives)	C + D
		A + C	B + D	A + B + C + D

❍ **What is the clinical utility of absolute risk?**

Absolute risk indicates the likelihood patients with a particular risk factor will develop the disease studied. Unfortunately, this measure does not assess the risk of disease in those who do not possess the risk factor and the lack of this information can be deceptive in interpreting the risk of disease.

❍ **What is the definition of attributable risk?**

Attributable risk (or absolute risk reduction or risk difference) is defined as the difference in disease (or outcome event) between the absolute risk of those without the risk factor from the absolute risk of those with the risk factor.

❍ **How do you calculate the attributable risk?**

Attributable risk is calculated as (True Positive/[True Positives + False Positives]) - (False Negatives/[True Negatives + False Negatives]) = (A/[A+B]) - (C/[D+C])

		DISEASE		
		Present	Absent	
RISK **FACTOR**	**Positive**	A (True Positives)	B (False Positives)	A + B
	Negative	C (False Negatives)	D (True Negatives)	C + D
		A + C	B + D	A + B + C + D

❍ **What is the clinical utility of attributable risk?**

Attributable risk quantifies the contribution of the risk factor under study in producing disease in a study population. It can be helpful in predicting impact on the population health if the risk factor were treated or removed. Unfortunately, the expression as a decimal fraction or percentage may not seem sensible to the practicing physician and may therefore be difficult to remember and incorporate into clinical practice.

❍ **What is the definition of relative risk?**

Relative risk is the likelihood that disease will occur among patients with a particular risk factor compared to the likelihood that the disease will occur among patients without the same risk factor.

❍ **How do you calculate the relative risk?**

(Incidence of diseased subjects with the risk factor divided by all subjects positive for the risk factor) divided by the (incidence of diseased subjects without the risk factor divided by all subjects without the risk factor) = (A/[A+B])/(C/[C+D})

		DISEASE		
		Present	Absent	
RISK FACTOR	**Positive**	A (True Positives)	B (False Positives)	A + B
	Negative	C (False Negatives)	D (True Negatives)	C + D
		A + C	B + D	A + B + C + D

❍ **What is the clinical utility of relative risk?**

Relative risk does provide comparative information of the incidence of disease in the presence of absence of a particular risk factor. However, relative risk does not reveal the magnitude of the absolute risk. In clinical decision making, the relative risk will tend to either overestimate or underestimate the absolute impact of treatment when the adverse events in untreated patients are either very rare or very common respectively.

❍ **What is the definition of number needed to treat (NNT)?**

The number needed to treat (NNT) is the number of patients who must be treated in order to prevent one adverse event.

❍ **How do you calculate the number needed to treat (NNT)?**

The NNT is equal to the reciprocal of the attributable risk (or absolute risk reduction).

❍ **What is the clinical utility of number needed to treat (NNT)?**

The NNT allows comparisons of the efforts to prevent or treat other events in patients with other disorders.

❍ **Case 6: In a comparative study of the safety of US airlines, airline A was found to incur a risk of death 1 in every 1 million flights, while airline B was found to incur a risk of death 1 in every 15 million flights. What is the absolute risk of dying when flying airline A? when flying airline B?**

The absolute risk of dying on airline A is 1/1,000,000 = 0.000001 = 0.0001%. Similarly, the risk of dying on airline B is 1/15,000,000 = 0.00000067 = 0.000067%.

❍ **Case 6: What is the attributable (or excess) risk of dying when flying airline A compared to airline B?**

The excess risk attributable to flying airline A compared to airline B is 1/1,000,000 - 1/15,000,000 = 15/15 million - 1/15 million = 14/15 million = 14/15,000,000 = 0.00000093 = 0.000093%. Note that this measure of expression of risk in either a fraction or percentage is somewhat difficult to remember and incorporate into every day clinical practice.

❍ **Case 6: What is the relative risk of death for flying airline A compared to airline B?**

Relative risk of flying airline A compared to airline B equals (1/1,000,000) / (1/15,000,000) = (15/15 million) / (1/15 million) = 15/1 = 15. Simply stated one has a 15 times greater risk of dying when flying airline A compared to airline B.

❍ **<u>Case 6</u>: What is the "number needed to treat" (NNT) for flying airline A compared to airline B?**

The NNT = 1/Attributable Risk = 1/0.00000093 = 1,075,269. Simply stated one would have to fly airline A over 1 million times before incurring the risk of one added death compared to airline B. Note that while all these measures of risk (absolute risk, attributable risk, relative risk) are correct, the number needed to treat is readily understandable and easier to incorporate into clinical decision making. While the relative risk is high (i.e. 15 times greater), the absolute risk still remains very low and this is reflected in the very large "number needed to treat."

❍ **<u>Case 7</u>: In a large randomized double-blind study (N Engl J Med 1996;335:1001-9), pravastatin was used to lower cholesterol in a group of patients who previously had a myocardial infarction. Of the 2078 patients in the placebo group, 274 had a cardiac end point after five years compared to 212 cardiac events in the 2081 treated patients after five years. What is the absolute risk of incurring a cardiac event in the placebo group? the group treated with pravastatin?**

The absolute risk of a cardiac event after five years in the placebo group is equal to 274/2078 = 0.13 or 13%. The absolute risk of a cardiac event after five years in the treated group is equal to 212/2081 = 0.10 or 10%.

❍ **<u>Case 7</u>: What is the absolute risk reduction in the treated group compared to the placebo group?**

The absolute risk reduction (or attributable risk) is 0.13 -0.10 or 0.03 or 3%

❍ **<u>Case 7</u>: What is the relative risk of a cardiac event in the treated group compared to the placebo group?**

The relative risk of a cardiac event after five years in the treated group compared to the placebo group is 0.10/0.13 = 0.77 or 77%. The relative risk reduction is (0.13 - 0.10)/0.13 = 0.23 or 23%. Simply stated there is a 23% less chance of having an adverse cardiac event after 5 years with treatment compared to placebo.

❍ **<u>Case 7</u>: What is the number needed to treat (NNT)?**

The number needed to treat is equal to 1/0.03 = 33. Simply stated, one has to treat 33 individuals with medication to prevent one cardiac event over the next 5 years.

❍ **What is the <u>definition</u> of a likelihood ratio?**

Likelihood ratios indicate how much a given diagnostic test will either raise or lower the pretest odds (i.e. probability) of a particular disease. A positive likelihood ratio is the frequency of positive results in patients with disease divided by the frequency of positive results in patients without disease. A negative likelihood ratio is the frequency of negative results in patients with disease divided by the frequency of negative results in patients without disease.

❍ **How do you <u>calculate</u> likelihood ratios?**

A positive likelihood ratio equals the True Positive Rate (or Sensitivity) divided by the False Positive Rate (or 1 - Specificity) = (A/[A+C]) / (B/[B+D])

		DISEASE		
		Present	Absent	
TEST	**Positive**	A (True Positives)	B (False Positives)	A + B
	Negative	C (False Negatives)	D (True Negatives)	C + D
		A + C	B + D	A + B + C + D

A negative likelihood ratio equals the False Negative Rate (or 1 - Sensitivity) divided by the True Negative Rate (or Specificity) = (C/[A+C]) / (D/[B+D])

		DISEASE		
		Present	Absent	
TEST	**Positive**	A (True Positives)	B (False Positives)	A + B
	Negative	C (False Negatives)	D (True Negatives)	C + D
		A + C	B + D	A + B + C + D

❍ **What is the clinical <u>utility</u> of likelihood ratios?**

Likelihood ratios are a powerful tool in converting pre-test odds into post-test odds. Like sensitivity and specificity, likelihood ratios need not change with changes in the prevalence of the disease. Likelihood ratios can be calculated for several levels of a particular sign, symptom, or laboratory test result. Its major disadvantage is the necessity of calculating and switching back and forth between probabilities and odds.

❍ **<u>Case 8</u>: A 65 year-old gentleman presents with atypical chest pain undergoes further diagnostic testing with an exercise treadmill test (ETT). It is estimated in the population seen at your clinic that approximately 1/2 individuals with atypical chest pain truly have coronary artery disease. The following information is provided you about the test characteristics of exercise treadmill testing:**

Exercise Treadmill Test (ETT) Characteristics				
Criterion - **ST Depression**	Sensitivity	Specificity	+ Likelihood Ratio	- Likelihood Ratio
≥ 0.5 mm	0.86	0.77	3.74	0.18
≥ 1.0 mm	0.65	0.89	5.91	0.39
≥ 1.5 mm	0.42	0.98	21.00	0.59
≥ 2.0 mm	0.33	0.99	33.00	0.66
≥ 2.5 mm	0.20	0.995	40.00	0.80

What is the likelihood that this individual truly has coronary artery disease if he has a positive ETT at 1 mm ST segment depression?

The question is asking for the post-test probability of coronary artery disease after a positive ETT. One can calculate this in two different methods. One could calculate the positive predictive value as follows: TP/(TP + FP) = 65/76 = 86%. Simply stated the individual has an 86% chance of actually having coronary artery disease after a positive ETT.

		DISEASE		
		Present	Absent	
TEST	**Positive**	65 (True Positives)	11 (False Positives)	76
	Negative	35 (False Negatives)	89 (True Negatives)	124
		100	100	200

Another method would be to use the likelihood ratio in the following manner:

1) Determine the pretest probability of disease: in this case = 50%
2) Convert the pretest probability into a pretest odds by the following formula: Pretest odds = probability of disease divided by 1 - the probability of disease = 0.5/(1.-0.5) = 1/1
3) Multiply the pretest odds by the appropriate likelihood ratio which for 1 mm = 5.91 x 1/1 = 5.91/1

4) Convert the post-test odds back to probability by the following formula: numerator of odds divided by numerator + denominator of odds = 5.91/(5.91 + 1) = 86%.

While this may seem more laborious initially, one advantage of likelihood ratios can be seen in the table above noting the progressive increase in magnitude of the positive likelihood ratio with each increment of 0.5 mm ST depression. This is not intuitively obvious by just examining the specificity column alone. For example, if the gentleman instead had 1.5 mm ST depression rather than 1.0 mm ST depression, his post-test probability of coronary artery disease can simply be recalculated as follows: Pre-test odds x appropriate likelihood ratio = 1/1 x 21 = 21/1. Converting back to post-test probability using the above formula = 21/(21 + 1) = 95%. Another advantage of likelihood ratios can be illustrated below.

❍ **Case 9: A 45 year-old gentleman with a long history of alcoholism present with increasing abdominal "fullness" and you suspect he has a 30% chance of having ascites based on his history. On physical exam you find he has bilateral bulging flanks, shifting dullness, and absent pedal edema and absent everted navel. What would you estimate is his likelihood of having ascites after your physical exam?**

PHYSICAL FINDING	**SENSITIVITY (%)**	**SPECIFICITY (%)**	**+ Likelihood** Ratio	**- Likelihood Ratio**
Bilateral Bulging Flanks	81	59	1.98	0.32
Fluid Wave	62	90	6.20	0.42
Shifting Dullness	77	72	2.75	0.32
Puddle Sign	45	73	1.67	0.75
Everted Navel	33	88	2.75	0.76
Pedal Edema	87	77	3.78	0.19
Ballotable Liver	27	93	3.86	0.78

The question asks for the post-test probability of ascites after the physical examination. Using odds and likelihood ratios, combining all the above information, the positive likelihood ratios for bulging flanks and shifting dullness = 1.98 and 2.75 respectively. The negative likelihood ratios for pedal edema and everted navel are 0.19 and 0.76 respectively. The post-test probability =

1) Pre-test odds = Probability of disease divided by 1 - Probability of disease = 0.3/(1-0.3) = 0.3/0.7 = 3/7
2) Multiply the pre-test odds by the appropriate likelihood ratios = 3/7 x 1.98 x 2.75 x 0.19 x 0.76 = 2.4/7
3) Converting odds back to probability = numerator of odds divided by numerator plus the denominator of odds = 2.4/(2.4 + 7) = 26%.

Note how using likelihood ratios enables one to easily combine all available clinical information into one calculation.

PREOPERATIVE EVALUATION OF THE SURGICAL PATIENT

The best way to stop smoking, is to carry wet matches..
Anonymous

❍ **Case 1: A 76-year gentleman is seen by vascular surgery who plans to repair an asymptomatic abdominal aortic aneurysm. His only medical problems are hypertension (treated with a thiazide diuretic), diabetes (treated with insulin), and degenerative arthritis of the hips which limit his ability to walk more than two blocks. What is the most important test for reducing this patient's perioperative risk?**

The most important "test" in assessing and minimizing this patient's perioperative risk is a thorough history and physical examination. The history should focus on the patient's functional capacity (or exercise tolerance), control and complications of his hypertension and diabetes, prior history of bleeding disorders, and concomitant medical conditions (e.g. smoking and cardiac disease). Only after a thorough history and physical exam should further laboratory or diagnostic tests be considered.

❍ **Case 1: On physical examination, what particular findings are you focusing on?**

Evidence of poorly controlled congestive heart failure (e.g. S3 gallop, jugular venous distention, crackles in the lungs, etc.) would carry the greatest risk for a perioperative complication.

❍ **Case 1: After completing the history and physical examination, what additional laboratory tests would you order?**

While many individuals order a "battery" of preoperative laboratory tests, most such tests in otherwise healthy patients have little justification. In this patient the following are recommended: complete blood count (since the surgery could entail significant blood loss); glucose, electrolytes, blood urea nitrogen and creatinine (since the patient has a history of hypertension treated with a diuretic and diabetes); chest radiography (since the patient is > 60 years and undergoing a major abdominal surgery); and an electrocardiogram (since the patient >50 and undergoing a high risk surgery).

❍ **How accurate are electrocardiograms (EKGs) in predicting perioperative cardiac complications?**

EKGs by themselves are poor predictors of ischemic heart disease (sensitivity 27%, positive predictive value 1%) in othrwise young, health patients undergoing surgery.

❍ **Case 1: After completing the history and physical examination, what additional laboratory "bleeding studies" would you order?**

"Bleeding studies" (e.g. PTT, PT, bleeding times) are not necessary in most patients who have normal histories and physical examinations since these are better predictors of perioperative blood loss. Laboratory bleeding studies may be helpful with those with a history of bleeding disorders, leukemias, hepatic disease or anticoagulant use.

❍ **Case 1: After completing the history, physical exam, and initial blood and laboratory tests, what other tests (if any) would you order to further assess this patient's perioperative risk?**

Because this patient is undergoing a "high risk" vascular surgery (i.e. perioperative cardiac complication is greater than 5%), the patient has associated conditions for cardiac complications, and his functional capacity is limited by his degenerative joint disease, even if the patient has no complaints, he should undergo additional evaluation with a non-invasive test to assess his risk for coronary artery disease. The most well studied test in this situation is a dipyridamole-thallium test. Measurement of left ventricular function (i.e. ejection fraction) does NOT seem to give additional information beyond the history, physical exam, and other non-invasive studies.

❍ **After completing a normal history and physical exam, what additional laboratory tests would you order for a 35-year old man about to undergo elective repair of a torn medial collateral ligament of the right thumb?**

Surgery on a distal extremity is very "low risk" (i.e. perioperative cardiac complication rate is less than 1%), and in view of a normal history and physical examination, it is unlikely that any further additional laboratory tests are necessary.

❍ **After completing a normal history and physical exam, what additional laboratory tests would you order for a 55-year old man about to undergo left knee replacement ?**

Since most orthopedic surgeries (as well as head and neck, prostate, and intra-abdominal surgeries) are "intermediate" risk (i.e. perioperative cardiac complication rate between 1-5%), the decision for additional diagnostic tests will depend on other factors such as the patient' functional status (or exercise tolerance).

❍ **What is the perioperative death rate in the first 48 hours for a healthy patient undergoing general anesthesia?**

The estimated death rate in the first 48 hours after surgery in a healthy patient is about 0.3%. Of all the deaths, 10% occur during anesthesia induction, 35% occur intraoperatively, and 55% in the remaining 48 hours.

❍ <u>Case 1</u>**: What is the most likely perioperative complication in this patient?**

As with most surgeries for peripheral vascular disease, acute myocardial infarction is the most common perioperative complication and cause of death.

❍ **In a patient with a prior myocardial infarction, when is it advised to safely perform an elective surgical procedure?**

Waiting at least 6 months after an acute myocardial infarction is advised before performing any elective surgical procedure. This applies to both Q wave and non-Q wave infarctions. More recent studies suggest that with careful patient selection and aggressive perioperative hemodynamic monitoring, some patients may undergo surgery within 3 months of an acute myocardial infarction.

❍ **When do most perioperative myocardial infarctions occur?**

Most perioperative infarctions occur post-operatively. Non-Q wave infarctions tend to occur within the first 48 hours after surgery, while Q wave infarctions tend to occur around the third to fifth post-operative days.

❍ **What is the most common symptom of perioperative myocardial infarction in an elderly patient?**

In the elderly, more than 50% of perioperative infarctions are NOT accompanied by typical anginal chest pain. Any postoperative complaint of dyspnea, unexplained tachycardia, hypotension, new onset congestive heart failure, new onset dysrrhythmia, or change in mental status should raise the clinical suspicion of a perioperative myocardial infarction.

❍ **What are the most common causes of death within the first 48 hours of surgery?**

In decreasing order of frequency, myocardial infarction, peritonitis, congestive heart failure, sepsis, and pulmonary embolism.

❍ **Case 1: On the evening of this patient's surgery, his electrocardiogram (EKG) shows occasional premature ventricular contractions (PVCs). The anesthesiologist is concerned that the patient may go into a ventricular dysrrhythmia and asks for a medicine consult. What do your recommend?**

Asymptomatic PVCs do NOT require treatment. The general rule of thumb for pre-operative rhythm disturbances is to "treat only those dysrrhythmias that would ordinarily be treated even if the patient were not going to surgery."

❍ **Case 1: This patient's electrocardiogram also reveals right bundle branch block and left axis deviation. What are your recommendations?**

Asymptomatic bifasciular block (including left bundle branch block) does NOT require treatment. The risk of developing acute heart block during surgery is well less than 1%. The general rule of thumb is "temporary pacemakers are indicated in those situations that usually warrant a permanent pacemaker even if the patient were not gong to surgery."

❍ **Case 1: The anesthesiologist asks you whether general or spinal anesthesia is safer in this patient?**

Spinal and/or epidural anesthesias have NOT been shown to be safer alternatives than general anesthesia in high risk cardiac patients.

❍ **Which valvular heart disease is associated with the highest perioperative complication rate?**

Aortic stenosis

❍ **In the original Goldman's Multifactorial Index for predicting cardiac risk in non-cardiac surgery, what two factors when present carried the worst prognosis?**

Poorly controlled congestive heart failure (manifested by the presence of an S-3 gallop or abnormal jugular venous distention) and a previous myocardial infarction in the last 6 months prior to surgery.

❍ **Case 1: A 76-year gentleman is seen by vascular surgery who plans to repair an asymptomatic abdominal aortic aneurysm. His only medical problems are hypertension (treated with a thiazide diuretic), diabetes (treated with insulin), and degenerative arthritis of the hips which limit his ability to walk more than two blocks. On the morning of his surgery you are consulted by the anesthesiologist who notes his blood pressures from the evening before have consistently been 158/105 mm Hg. You are asked whether or not to delay his surgery.**

While optimal blood pressure control is always desirable, elective surgeries need NOT be postponed for diastolic blood pressures less than 110 mmHg. (While systolic blood pressures also predict perioperative complications, no well defined cutoff has been determined. Recommendations for delaying elective surgeries based on systolic blood pressure limits have ranged anywhere from ≥ 160 to 200 mm Hg.)

❍ **Case 1: The same 76-year old gentleman instead presents with blood pressures consistently around 185/115. How would you manage his hypertension?**

While it may be tempting to lower this patient's blood pressure quickly by the administration of a sublingual or IV anti-hypertensive medication, this approach may actually worsen the patient's perioperative cardiac risk. For elective operations, the patient should be discharged home and his chronic anti-hypertensive regimen adjusted over the course of the next several weeks.

❍ **Case 1: What medication would you choose to treat this patient's elevated blood pressure prior to his abdominal aortic aneurysm repair?**

While there are several classes of anti-hypertensive agents available, beta-blockers have been the most well studied in reducing perioperative and long term mortality.

❍ **What is the major perioperative risk in a patient with hypertension?**

The most important perioperative risk in a hypertensive patient is the potential for wide variations in blood pressure. A 50% drop in blood pressure at anytime perioperatively or a 33% drop in blood pressure sustained for 10 minutes or more is associated with a 15-20% incidence of cardiac complications such a myocardial infarction or congestive heart failure.

❍ **When does the rebound exacerbation of angina and hypertension occur with the abrupt withdrawal of beta blockers?**

The abrupt withdrawal of beta blockers can precipitate a rebound angina and hypertension 24 to 48 hours after stopping the medication.

❍ **Case 1: A 76-year old gentleman is seen by vascular surgery who plans to repair an asymptomatic abdominal aortic aneurysm. His only medical problems are hypertension (treated with a thiazide diuretic), diabetes (treated with NPH insulin 30 units in the morning and 10 units in the evening), and degenerative arthritis of the hips which limit his ability to walk more than two blocks. What is the best method of controlling this patient's blood sugar intraoperatively?**

For major prolonged operations, the preferred method of controlling diabetic patients' intraoperative blood sugars is to use *two* separate intravenous infusions, one containing insulin and another containing glucose to allow for independent adjustments of each infusion rate.

❍ **Case 1: What time of the day should a major operation in a diabetic be scheduled?**

Ideally diabetic should be schedule early in the morning to allow close monitoring of blood sugars intraoperatively and post-operatively.

❍ **Case 2: A 48-year old diabetic patient is about to undergo elective hernia repair. She is treated with a combination of two oral agents, glyburide and metformin. What recommendations would you make regarding her medications?**

Both glyburide and metformin should be stopped 1-2 days prior to her surgery, her blood sugars should be monitored carefully perioperatively, and small doses of subcutaneous regular insulin may be administered for increase blood sugars.

❍ **What if the same patient were instead on chlorpropamide?**

Of all the sulfonylureas, chlorpropamide has the longest half life and should be stopped 3-4 days prior to any elective surgery to avoid the risk of perioperative hypoglycemia. Most other sulfonylureas can be stopped the day prior to surgery.

❍ **Case 3: A 32-year old type I diabetic patient is scheduled to deliver her second baby. Her insulin dose the past month has been 40 units of NPH and 10 unit of regular every morning and 20 units of NPH and 5 units of regular every evening. What insulin orders would you write for on the day of her planned delivery?**

Following delivery, insulin requirements drop precipitously in pregnant women and this patient's dose of insulin on the day of delivery should not exceed half her usual dose prior to deliver.

❍ **What is the best management strategy for a type I diabetic patient presenting with diabetic ketoacidosis and an acute abdomen?**

Diabetic ketoacidosis can mimic the signs and symptoms of an acute abdomen and it is best to delay surgery as safely as possible (e.g. 4-6 hours) to correct the fluid and electrolyte disorders as much as possible to reduce perioperative morbidity and mortality.

❍ **What associated physical exam finding may place the diabetic patient at particularly high perioperative complications?**

Diabetic patients who have evidence of autonomic neuropathy may be at particularly high risk for perioperative complications (e.g. blood pressure swings) and need to be closely monitored.

❍ **Case 4: A 58-year old gentleman with chronic obstructive pulmonary disease (COPD) is scheduled for elective repair of an asymptomatic 10 cm lower abdominal ventral hernia. His only current medication is a beta agonist inhaler which he takes three times a day. He continues to smoke but has significantly cut down the last year to one-half pack a day. The anesthesiologist asks you whether spinal anesthesia is safer than general anesthesia in this patient?**

Spinal and/or epidural anesthesia have NOT been shown to be safer alternatives than general anesthesia in patients with chronic lung disease.

❍ **Case 4: What time of the day should this patient's operation be scheduled?**

Ideally patients with chronic bronchitis should be schedule later in the day to allow them to mobilize and cough up any morning secretions.

❍ **Case 4: As a predictor of perioperative pulmonary complications, when should pre-operative pulmonary function tests be ordered in this patient?**

Routine pulmonary function tests best predict perioperative complications in patients undergoing lung resection and *perhaps* for those patient undergoing major cardiothoracic and upper abdominal surgeries. Very little evidence exits to support the use of routine pulmonary function tests in asymptomatic, non-smoking patients undergoing other types of surgery.

❍ **Case 4: For this elective operation, how long would you advise this patient to stop smoking prior to his surgery?**

Smokers should be advised to discontinue their cigarette use at least 6-8 weeks prior to an elective surgery to minimize perioperative pulmonary complications.

❍ **Case 4: This same patient reports a history of chronic steroid use (20 mg qd) up until the last 3 months. How would you assess this patient's perioperative need for steroid replacement?**

A Cortrosyn (ACTH) stimulation test can be performed: a plasma cortisol is drawn as a baseline value, 250 mcg of ACTH is administered parenterally (IV or IM), and 30 to 60 minutes later, a second cortisol level is drawn - a peak cortisol level of $\geq$ 20 mcg/dl is considered normal.

❍ **Case 4: If there is insufficient time for the laboratory to measure the cortisol levels, what recommendations would you make?**

If the Cortrosyn (ACTH) stimulation test cannot be performed and there is the suspicion of adrenal suppression, a short course of corticosteroid is relatively safe and free of long term side effects (e.g. 100 mg of IV hydrocortisone on call to the operating room, 50 mg of hydrocortisone q6-8 hours on Day 1, 25 mg q6-8 hours on Day 2, 25 mg q 6-8 hours on Day 3, and gradually tapering over the next 2-5 days).

❍ **Case 4: The same patient relates that he had an acute exacerbation of his chronic bronchitis about one week age but feels fine now. What recommendation would you make regarding repair of his ventral hernia?**

Patients with chronic obstructive lung disease and a recent exacerbation should wait at least three weeks after the episode before undergoing any elective operation.

❍ **Which patients have a higher perioperative pulmonary complication rate - those with obstructive lung disease or those with restrictive lung disease?**

Obstructive lung disease carries a greater risk than restrictive lung disease for perioperative pulmonary complications.

❍ **Is a smoker who is otherwise healthy, takes no medications, and has normal spirometry at increase risk for perioperative pulmonary complications?**

Even in the absence of symptoms or normal pulmonary function tests, smokers continue to have higher risks for periperative pneumonias.

❍ **What type of surgeries carry the greatest risk for pulmonary complications?**

Thoracic and upper abdominal surgeries carry the greatest risk for perioperative pulmonary complications. The lowest risk surgeries are those involving the distal extremities.

❍ **In a patient about to undergo lung resection for a suspected tumor, which preoperative spirometric test best separates those who can be successfully operated upon versus those who are inoperable patients?**

It is very important to remember that no single spirometric number, percent, or category will absolutely separate operable from inoperable surgical patients.

❍ **In a patient recently diagnosed with hyperthyroidism, when can the patient safely undergo an elective knee surgery?**

For elective surgeries, hyperthyroid patients should be brought to the euthyroid state prior since surgery can precipitate thyroid storm with associated perioperative mortality rates as high as 20% to 40%. This usually takes at least 2 to 3 months when anti-thyroid medications are administered.

❍ **In a patient recently diagnosed with hypothyroidism, when can the patient safely undergo an elective ventral hernia repair?**

For elective surgeries hypothyroid patients should be brought to the euthyroid state prior since surgery can precipitate myxedema coma. This usually takes at least 2 to 3 months to achieve optimal replacement.

❍ **For stable patients on oral thyroid replacement, what recommendations would you make regarding the perioperative administration of the thyroid medication?**

Ideally, administering the thyroid replacement on the morning of surgery and resuming postoperatively once the patient can eat. However, because levothyroxine has such a long half life (approximately 7 days), withholding a dose or two will not usually have any adverse effects.

❍ <u>Case 5</u>: **A 62-year old gentleman with end stage renal disease on chronic hemodialysis is about to undergo repair of a dislocated shoulder under general anesthesia. The patient's hemoglobin is 8 and the anesthesiologist consults medicine to see whether the patient should have a blood transfusion prior to the operation. What would be your recommendation?**

In general, patients with chronic renal failure are well adapted to lower hemoglobins than normal and do NOT routinely require blood transfusions unless signs and symptoms of anemia are present or significant blood loss is anticipated.

❍ <u>Case 5</u>: **When should this patient's surgery be scheduled for in relationship to his regular dialysis?**

For elective operations, dialysis should be completed at least six hours prior to an elective surgery and can be resumed 24 to 48 hours after the operation.

❍ **In a patient with chronic renal failure, what is the most important factor in estimating perioperative surgical risk?**

The degree of glomerluar filtration rate (GFR) reduction is more important in estimating surgical risk than the actual type of renal disease.

❍ **In a patient with normal renal function, what is the best predictor of postoperative acute renal failure?**

The strongest predictor of acute renal failure is intraoperative hypotension. Other predictors include diabetes, poorly controlled heart failure, and jaundice. Certain operations are more often accompanied by acute renal failure such as cardiothoracic surgery, repair of abdominal aortic aneurysm, and biliary tract surgery in the presence of jaundice.

❍ **What is the most common causes of death in patients on chronic hemodialysis undergoing elective surgery?**

Sepsis and myocardial infarction.

❍ **In a patient who has been recently diagnosed with acute viral hepatitis, how long should any elective operation be reasonably postponed?**

Following an acute episode of viral hepatitis, most elective operations should be postponed at least one month following the return to normal of the liver function tests.

❍ **In a patient with chronic hepatitis, what criteria do you use to send a patient to an elective surgery?**

Any patient with chronic hepatitis should be stable for at least 3 months prior to any elective surgery. Patients in Child-Pugh class A (normal bilirubin, albumin prothrombin time, and nutritional status in the absence of ascites and encephalopathy) can safely undergo most surgical operations.

❍ **What are the major perioperative complications in a liver diseased patient undergoing non-hepatic surgery?**

The major complications in patients with liver disease are worsening encephalopathy, jaundice, gastrointestinal bleeding, and renal failure.

❍ **What is the most common non-obstetrical surgical problem seen during pregnancy?**

An acute abdomen most commonly caused by acute appendicitis.

❍ **Premature labor most commonly complicates what type of non-obstetrical surgery?**

While premature labor is a rare complication in most non-obstetrical surgeries (<1%), in pelvic or lower abdominal surgeries premature labor may occur as high as 4-6% of the time.

❍ **In a pregnant patient about to undergo surgery, what analgesics for pain control can be safely administered to the patient?**

Acetaminophen, meperidine and morphine appear to be safe drugs when administered for short periods of time for perioperative pain. Codeine and aspirin have been associated with certain fetal complications and probably are best avoided.

❍ **What recommendation would you make to a women on oral contraceptive pills prior to an elective operation?**

Because of the increase risk of deep venous thrombosis associated with most surgeries and the potential of oral contraceptives to further increase this risk, many authorities recommend advising women to stop taking their oral contraceptives if possible for 3 to 4 weeks prior to an elective operation.

❍ **What percentage of all post-operative deaths occur among the elderly?**

Even though the elderly account for approximately 15% of the general population, the elderly account for 20-40% of all surgeries, 50% of emergency procedures, and 75% of all post-operative deaths.

❍ **Among the elderly, what are the best predictors of perioperative complications?**

More important than the absolute chronological age of the patient are the presence of coexisting medical conditions and patients' exercise (or functional) capacity in predicting perioperative complication rate

❍ **In an elderly patient about to undergo partial colectomy for a mass, what is the appropriate management of an asymptomatic carotid bruit?**

In general asymptomatic carotid bruits in the elderly do not predict an increase in perioperative stroke except *possibly* in those patients undergoing coronary artery bypass surgery.

❍ **When should preoperative chest radiographs be ordered?**

In general routine chest radiographs should be ordered when patients have pulmonary signs and symptoms, risk factors for lung diseases, or is expected to undergo cardiothoracic or upper abdominal surgery.

❍ **What types of operations are associated with the highest risk of perioperative deep venous thromboses?**

Hip surgeries and knee repairs.

❍ **In a patient undergoing abdominal surgery, what type of thromboembolism prophylaxis would you recommend?**

Low-dose heparin (5000 units subcutaneously every 8 - 12 hours)

❍ **In a patient undergoing hip surgery, what type of thromboembolism prophylaxis would you recommend?**

Either low molecular weight heparin or oral anticoagulants, adjusting the prothrombin time to an INR of 2 - 3 for the latter.

❍ **In a patient undergoing a neurosurgical operation, what type of thromboembolism prophylaxis would you recommend?**

Intermittent pneumatic compression devices applied to the lower extremities.

❍ **In a patient undergoing knee surgery, what type of thromboembolism prophylaxis would you recommend?**

Low molecular weight heparin or possibly intermittent pneumatic compression devices combined with low-dose heparin.

❍ **For most patients undergoing surgery, how long should thromboembolism prophylaxis continue?**

Prophylaxis against perioperative deep venous thrombosis should continue as long as the patient is at risk and this often means until the end of hospitalization.

❍ **For patients undergoing hip surgery, how long should thromboembolism prophylaxis continue?**

Recent studies suggest that patients undergoing orthopedic hip surgeries may be at particularly high risk and prophylaxis against perioperative deep venous thrombosis should continue for 4-6 weeks *after* hospital discharge.

❍ **In a patient who has recently undergone surgery and notices unilateral leg swelling 5 days later, what is the best means of diagnosing deep venous thrombosis?**

The best test to make the diagnosis of deep venous thrombosis post-operatively is venography. Most non-invasive tests have a particularly low sensitivity and therefore a normal result does NOT exclude the diagnosis of venous thrombosis.

❍ **In a patient with documented perioperative deep venous thrombosis, how long would you recommend oral anticoagulation with warfarin?**

In this situation in which presumably the surgery is the precipitating factor and assuming the patient is now fully ambulatory, most authors recommend treatment with oral anticoagulants for a total of only 4-6 weeks duration.

❍ **In a pregnant patient with a documented deep venous thrombosis following delivery of her baby, how long would you recommend oral anticoagulation with warfarin?**

In this situation therapeutic oral anticoagulation should be given for at least 3 months after delivery.

❍ **In a patient with atrial fibrillation on therapeutic doses of oral anticoagulants about to undergo repair of a torn right medial meniscus, what would you recommend?**

Assuming the patient's INR is therapeutic (INR = 2-3), stop the warfarin 4-5 days prior and resume the usual warfarin dose 1-3 days after surgery.

❍ **In a patient with a prosthetic mechanical heart valve who is therapeutically anticoagulated about to undergo repair of a torn left medial meniscus, what would you recommend?**

Since mechanical heart valves have a high risk for thromboembolism, one could recommend stopping the warfarin prior to surgery, replacing this with full dose intravenous heparin until 6 hours prior to surgery, and then resuming the heparin 12-24 hours after the operation and restarting the warfarin 1-2 days after the operation.

❍ **In a patient known to have mitral valve prolapse and mitral regurgitation, what kind of endocarditis prophylaxis would you recommend prior to a dental cleaning?**

Amoxicillin 2.0 gms orally one hour before the procedure

❍ **In a penicillin allergic patient known to have hypertrophic cardiomyopathy, what kind of endocarditis prophylaxis would you recommend prior to a dental cleaning?**

According to the American Heart Association, either one of the three following choices are recommended: (1) Clindamycin 600 mg orally one hour before the procedure; OR (2)cephalexin or cefadroxil 2.0 gms orally one hour before the procedure; OR (3)azithromycin or clarithromycin 500 mg one hour before the procedure

❍ **In a penicillin allergic patient known to have hypertrophic cardiomyopathy, what kind of endocarditis prophylaxis would you recommend prior to a cardiac catheterization?**

No prophylaxis for endocarditis is required for patients undergoing cardiac catheterization.

❍ **In a patient who has had coronary artery bypass surgery, what endocarditis prophylaxis would you recommend prior to a dental cleaning?**

No prophylaxis for endocarditis is required for patients who have had coronary artery bypass surgery.

❍ **In a high risk patient known to have had rheumatic heart disease and unable to take oral medications, what kind of endocarditis prophylaxis would you recommend prior to an esophageal dilatation?**

Intravenous (IV) or intramuscular (IM) ampicillin 2.0 gms plus gentamicin 1.5 mg/kg (not to exceed 120 mg), within 30 minutes of starting the procedure; 6 hours later, either ampicillin 1 gm IM/IV OR amoxicillin 1 gm orally.

❍ **In a high risk patient known to have had rheumatic heart disease, allergic to penicillin and unable to take oral medications, what kind of endocarditis prophylaxis would you recommend prior to cystoscopy?**

Intravenous vancomycin 1.0 gm over 1-2 hours completing the infusion within 30 minutes of starting the procedure.

❍ **In a patient with a past history of endocarditis, what prophylaxis would you recommend prior to a vaginal hysterectomy.**

According to the most recent recommendations by the American Heart Association, prophylaxis is optional for high-risk patients prior to a vaginal hysterectomy. If one choose to give antibiotics then intravenous (IV) or intramuscular (IM) ampicillin 2.0 gms plus gentamicin 1.5 mg/kg (not to exceed 120 mg), within

30 minutes of starting the procedure; 6 hours later, either ampicillin 1 gm IM/IV OR amoxicillin 1 gm orally.

❍ **In a patient with a past history of endocarditis, what prophylaxis would you recommend prior to a Cesarean section?**

No prophylaxis for endocarditis is required for patients undergoing Cesarean section.

❍ **What kind of wound infection prophylaxis would you recommend for a patient about to have a pacemaker placed?**

Cefazolin 1-2 gms intravenously just prior the operation

❍ **What antibiotic regimen would you recommend for a patient about to have emergency surgery for a ruptured appendicitis?**

Cefoxitin 1-2 grams intravenously prior to the operation and every 6 hours for 7 - 10 days. Note that this is treatment for an infection and not wound prophylaxis.

❍ **What antibiotic regimen would you recommend for a patient about to have an elective colectomy for ulcerative colitis?**

Oral neomycin 1 gm and erythromycin 1 gm every 8 hours for 3 doses the day before surgery.

❍ **What can the medical consultant do to enhance compliance with the recommendations made?**

Limit the number of recommendations to five or fewer. Make recommendations as specific as possible (e.g. specify exact dose, route of administration, and duration of recommended). Identify key recommendations as “critical” or “crucial.” Directly communicate with the referring physician.

❍ **If there is a conflict of opinion between the referring physician and consultant, how should this be resolved.**

Conflicts of opinion can be resolved by a second consultant or withdrawal of the consultant; however, the consultant may express his opinion to the patient in the presence of the referring physician.

SURGICAL PEARLS

After the game, the king and the pawn go into the same box.
Italian proverb

MEDICAL CARE OF THE SURGICAL PATIENT

A good surgeon operates with his hand, not with his heart.
Alexandre Dumas

❍ **How long does an area of abraded skin or a laceration need to be kept out of the sun?**

For at least 6 months. Abraded skin can develop permanent hyperpigmentation when exposed to the sun.

❍ **What organisms are most common in wound infections?**

Staphylococci.

❍ **A patient who develops a reddish brown exudate within 6 hours of an appendectomy most likely has a wound infected with what?**

Clostridium. Necrotizing fasciitis, dehiscence, and sepsis may result if not treated promptly.

❍ **What is the most likely cause of a postoperative fever which occurs: (1) the day of the operation, (2) 1 to 2 days postoperative, (3) 3 to 5 days postoperative, (4) 5 to 7 days postoperative, and (5) 2 weeks postoperative?**

Metabolic abnormalities
Atelectasis,
UTI
(4) wound infection
(5) DVT or PE

(Remember: "What-Wind-Water-Wound-Walk-Wonder-drugs")

❍ **Normal saline and Ringer's lactate have how many mEq/L of sodium, respectively?**

154 mEq/L, 130 mEq/L.

❍ **What solutes determine serum osmolality?**

Sodium, glucose, and urea. $\text{Osmolality} = 2\,\text{Na}^+ + \frac{\text{glucose}}{18} + \frac{\text{BUN}}{2.8}$

❍ **What are the laboratory criteria for placing a patient on mechanical ventilation?**

$pO_2 < 70$ on 50% O_2
$pO_2 < 55$ on room air
$pCO_2 > 50$

pH < 7.25

❍ **What negative pressure must be generated by an intubated patient for weaning to be successful?**

At least -20 cm of H_2O. Other important factors include paO_2, arterial saturation, pH, respiratory rate, minute volume, tidal volume, A-a oxygen tension, and dead space to tidal volume ratio.

❍ **What fungal infection is most common in transplant patients?**

Candida albicans.

❍ **What transplant organ can be preserved the longest?**

The kidney. Kidneys can be preserved in cold storage for up to 48 hours, the pancreas and liver for 8 hours, and the heart for 4 hours. Viability can be extended by using cold storage solutions, such as Collins solution and UW-Belzer solution.

❍ **What is the caloric requirement of a 100-kg firefighter who was burned over 20% of his body?**

3300 Kcal (25 Kcal/kg of body weight + 40 Kcal/1% burned surface).

❍ **What is the 24 hour fluid resuscitation requirement for the above patient?**

4 L in the first 8 hours (500 ml/hour) and 4 L in the next 16 hours (250 ml/hour). The Parkland formula gives the requirement as 4 ml × body weight in kg × % burned (4 ml × 100 kg × 20 = 8L). Give half the volume in the first 8 hours and the other half in the next 16 hours. Management after this should be based on clinical judgement. Urine output should be maintained at 50 ml/hour in adults and 0.5 to 1 ml/kg/hour in children.

❍ **At what percentage of an airway obstruction will inspiratory stridor become evident?**

70% occlusion.

❍ **What is the initial treatment for a tension pneumothorax?**

Large bore IV catheter placed in the anterior second intercostal space (not a chest tube).

❍ **What is the most important cause of hypoxia in a patient with flail chest?**

Underlying lung contusion.

❍ **How much fluid must collect in the chest to be detected on decubitus or upright chest x-rays?**

200 to 300 ml. If supine, greater than 1 L may be necessary to be seen on AP CXR.

❍ **A patient presents with fever and shoulder pain 4 days following a splenectomy. What is the most probable postoperative complication?**

Subphrenic abscess. This condition can cause fever as well as irritation to the diaphragm and to the branch of the phrenic nerve that innervates it.

❍ **What organisms are most commonly responsible for overwhelming postsplenectomy sepsis?**

Encapsulated organisms: pneumococcal (50%); meningococcal (12%); E. coli (11%); H. influenza (8%); staphylococcal (8%); and streptococcal (7%).

❍ **What is a sentinel loop?**

A distended loop of bowel detected by x-ray that lies near a localized inflammatory process. A sentinel loop often is associated with an underlying inflammatory process adjacent to the distended bowel. The possibility of pancreatitis or appendicitis should be considered.

❍ **What is a delphian node?**

A palpable node on the trachea which is just above the thyroid isthmus. It heralds thyroid malignancy or a thyroiditis.

❍ **Are epidural hematomas and subdural hematomas more or less common among elderly patients?**

Epidural hematomas are less common, and subdural hematomas are more common.

❍ **When does a subdural hematoma become isodense?**

One to three weeks after the bleed. However, it may not be detectable by CT unless contrast is used.

❍ **What is the sensory innervation to the nipple, umbilicus, and perianal region?**

Nipple: T4
Umbilicus: T10
Perianal: S2-S4

❍ **A 44 year-old female comes to your office complaining of a mass in the center of her neck near the hyoid bone. It is tender and raises if she sticks her tongue out. What is your diagnosis?**

An infected thyroglossal duct cyst. This is a remnant from the embryological descent of the thyroid in the neck. Thyroid tissue is actually found in 10 to 45% of these cysts. Treatment includes antibiotics, drainage, and then excision once the inflammation subsides. If the cyst were found in a noninfected state elective surgery would also be the treatment of choice as most of these cysts eventually become infected.

❍ **Inability to pass a nasogastric tube in a trauma victim suggests damage to what organ?**

Diaphragm, usually on the left.

❍ **What is the most common acute surgical condition of the abdomen?**

Acute appendicitis.

❍ **Why would you order a chest x-ray in a case of "acute abdomen"?**

Air under the diaphragm, which is an indication of a ruptured viscous, can be detected with greater ease by a chest x-ray. In addition, subdiaphragmatic abscesses or pancreatitis can cause pleural effusions that are evident on chest x-rays. Lastly, lower lobe pneumococcal pneumonia can present as abdominal pain.

❍ **What might be visible on abdominal films in a patient with appendicitis?**

Sentinel loops with air fluid levels in the RLQ, a gas filled appendix. A barium enema may show a partially filled appendix, a mass effect on the medial/inferior boarder of the cecum, and mucosal changes on the terminal ileum.

❍ **What is the most common cause of appendicitis?**

Fecaliths. Fecaliths are found in 40% of uncomplicated appendicitis cases, 65% of cases involving gangrenous appendices that have not ruptured, and 90% of cases involving ruptured appendices. Other causes of appendicitis include lymphoid tissue hypertrophy, inspissated barium, foreign bodies, and strictures.

❍ **How does retrocecal appendicitis most commonly present?**

Dysuria and hematuria (due to the proximity of the appendix to the right ureter). Poorly localized abdominal pain, anorexia, nausea, vomiting, diarrhea, mild fever, and peritonitis are also common signs.

❍ **What percentage of patients with a pre-operative diagnosis of appendicitis actually have appendicitis?**

85%. Other postoperative diagnoses commonly include acute mesenteric lymphadenitis, PID, epiploic appendicitis, ruptured graafian follicle, acute gastroenteritis, and twisted ovarian cysts.

❍ **Which type of antibiotic should be given to a patient with a perforated appendix prior to surgery?**

A broad-spectrum antibiotic effective on both aerobic and anaerobic enteric organisms. Intraoperative cultures can guide further antibiotic therapy. Antibiotics may be continued for 7 days post-op. If the patient has an uncomplicated appendicitis, i.e. no perforation or gangrene, then 1 preoperative dose of a broad-spectrum antibiotic such as cefoxitin or cefotetan is sufficient.

❍ **What kind of wound closure should be used in a patient with a perforated appendix?**

Delayed primary closure with direct drainage of the infection. Wound infection occurs in 20% of patients with perforated appendices.

❍ **A 27 year-old man who smokes heavily complains of tingling in his fingers. On examination he has cyanotic digits with ulcers forming. What is the diagnosis?**

Thromboangiitis obliterans or Buerger's disease. This is a disease that effects young smokers (males three times more often than females). Inflammatory changes in the small- to medium-sized vessels cause occlusions. Patients must stop smoking!

❍ **Where is the most common site of intracranial aneurysms?**

The circle of Willis (most common in the anterior communicating artery). A ruptured aneurysm presents as a headache followed by altered consciousness.

❍ **What are the clinical signs of CSF leakage?**

Raccoon eyes, bruises behind the ears (Battle's sign), otorrhea, and rhinorrhea.

❍ **What are the most common microorganisms found in brain abscesses?**

The enteric Gram-negative bacilli, anaerobes, nocardia, staphylococci, streptococci, and toxoplasma.

❍ **How many minutes of cerebral anoxia will result in irreversible brain injury?**

Over 8 minutes.

❍ **What is Westermark's sign?**

Decreased vascular markings on chest x-ray, indicative of pulmonary embolism.

❍ **What is Courvoisier's law?**

The gallbladder is smaller than its normal size if a gallstone is blocking the common bile duct and larger than its normal size if the bile duct is blocked by something else, most commonly cancer of the pancreas.

❍ **What do muffled heart tones, hypotension, and distended neck veins indicate?**

Pericardial tamponade. This is Beck's triad.

❍ **What are Grey-Turner's and Cullen's signs?**

Flank ecchymosis indicative of pancreatic disease.

Grey-Turner's sign: Periumbilical ecchymosis indicative of pancreatic hemorrhage.

Cullen's sign: Flank ecchymosis indicative of pancreatic hemorrhage

Both are caused by dissection of blood into the retroperitoneal cavity.

❍ **Which type of operation is associated with a higher incidence of common bile duct injury, laparoscopic cholecystectomy or conventional cholecystectomy?**

Laparoscopic.

❍ **What is the two-year survival rate for patients with liver cancer who have had a liver transplant?**

25 to 30%.

❍ **Where will colorectal cancer most commonly metastasize?**

The liver.

❍ **α-Fetoprotein (AFP) will be elevated in which types of tumors?**

Primary hepatic neoplasms and endodermal sinus or yolk sac tumors of the ovaries and testes. AFP is present in 30% of patients with primary liver cancer. It is not associated with metastatic tumors to the liver, but it is used as a cellular marker in the above-mentioned tumors.

❍ **Laparoscopic cholecystectomy is the procedure of choice for removal of gallstones. What is the most common complication associated with this surgery?**

Injury to the bile duct.

❍ **A patient presents with acute cholecystitis. Should the cholecystectomy be performed immediately or only after the inflammation has subsided?**

Early cholecystectomy should be performed unless surgery is contraindicated.

❍ **After a cholecystectomy, can gallstones reform?**

Yes. They can recur in the bile ducts.

❍ **Where is the most common site for fibromuscular dysplasia?**

The right renal artery. Fibromuscular dysplasia is an arterial disease that causes areas of stenosis and dilation; the artery appears as a link of sausage. Women are more commonly affected than men.

❍ **Where are most hernias located?**

In the groin (75%). Incisional and ventral hernias account for 10%, and umbilical hernias account for 3%.

❍ **Differentiate between reducible, incarcerated, strangulated, Richter, and complete hernias.**

Reducible: Contents of hernia sac return to the abdomen spontaneously or with slight pressure when the patient is in a recumbent position.

Incarcerated: Contents of the hernia sac are irreducible and cannot be returned to the abdomen.

Strangulated: Sac and its contents turn gangrenous.

Richter: Only part of the hernia sac and its contents becomes strangulated. This hernia may spontaneously reduce and be overlooked.

Complete: An inguinal hernia that passes all the way into the scrotum.

❍ **What are the boundaries of Hesselbach's triangle?**

The triangle is medial to the inferior epigastric artery, superior to the inguinal ligament, and lateral to the rectus sheath. Hesselbach's triangle is the site through which direct hernias pass.

❍ **A direct hernia is due to a weakness in what tissue?**

The transversalis fascia that makes up the floor of Hesselbach's triangle. Direct hernias do not pass through the inguinal canal and are often called pantaloon hernias.

❍ **Indirect inguinal hernias occur secondary to what defect?**

A failure of the processus vaginalis to close. The resulting hernia can then pass through the inguinal ring.

❍ **Which type of hernias are most common in females?**

Direct hernias. Direct hernias are the most common hernias in both women and men.

Note: While femoral hernias are more common in females than in males, they are still less common than direct hernias.

❍ **Of all hernias in the groin area, which is most likely to strangulate?**

A femoral hernia. Femoral hernias occur in the femoral canal, an unyielding space between the lacunar ligament and the femoral vein.

❍ **Which are more common, sliding or paraesophageal hiatal hernias?**

Sliding hiatal hernias account for 95% of hiatal hernias.

❍ **In paraesophageal hiatal hernias, does the stomach herniate to the left or to the right of the esophagus?**

Most frequently to the left. Paraesophageal hiatal hernias have a high rate of strangulation that can quickly lead to death. These hernias should be surgically repaired. Treat sliding hernias with antacids, H^+ blockers, and changes in eating and sleeping habits. Surgery should only be used as a last resort.

❍ **What are the most common causes of small bowel obstruction in adults?**

Adhesions (70%), followed by strangulated groin hernia and neoplasm of the bowel. Twenty percent of acute abdominal surgical admissions are due to obstructions.

❍ **Volvulus of the colon most frequently involves which segment?**

The sigmoid (65%), cecum (30%), transverse colon (3%), and splenic flexure (2%). Volvulus is the cause of 5 to 10% of all large bowel obstructions.

❍ **Where is the most common site of intestinal obstruction secondary to gallstones?**

The terminal ileum. Fifty-five to 60% will have associated air in the biliary tree.

❍ **What is the differential diagnosis for a 65 year-old man who has abdominal pain and bloody diarrhea a few days after the repair of an abdominal aortic aneurysm?**

Ischemic colitis is most probable. This condition occurs secondary to a decreased blood flow to the inferior mesenteric artery during the operation. Other differentials include pseudomembranous colitis (assuming the patient was receiving antibiotics) and aorto-enteric fistulas (generally a later development).

❍ **Is colovesicular fistula between the colon and the urinary tract more common among men or women?**

Men (3:1) more than women because a woman's uterus lies between her colon and bladder.

❍ **What is Osler-Weber-Rendu syndrome?**

Hereditary hemorrhagic telangiectasias found in the small intestine, mucosal membranes and skin with A-V malformations, most notably in the lung.

❍ **What is the surgical treatment of choice for a bleeding peptic ulcer?**

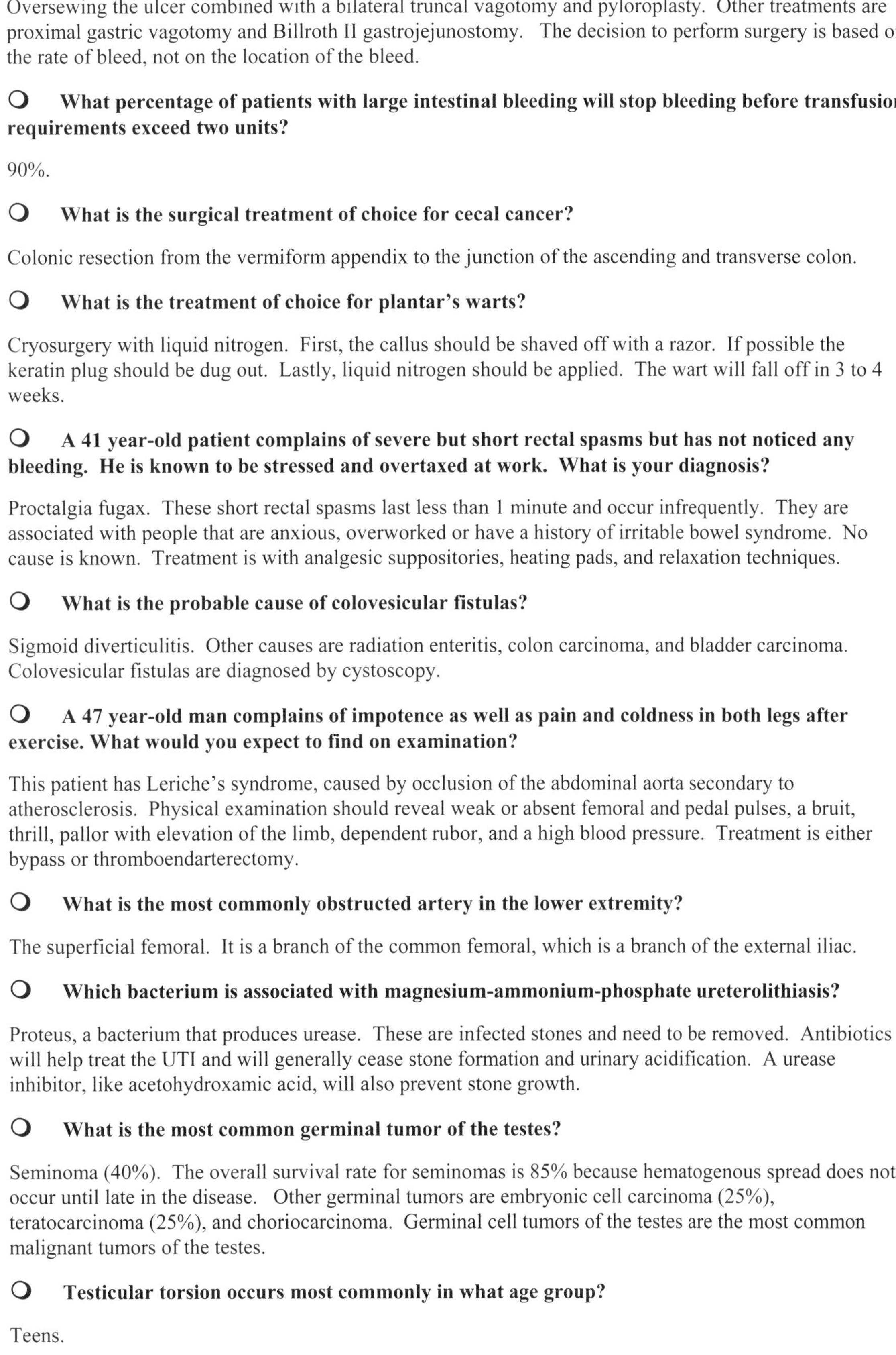

Oversewing the ulcer combined with a bilateral truncal vagotomy and pyloroplasty. Other treatments are proximal gastric vagotomy and Billroth II gastrojejunostomy. The decision to perform surgery is based on the rate of bleed, not on the location of the bleed.

❍ **What percentage of patients with large intestinal bleeding will stop bleeding before transfusion requirements exceed two units?**

90%.

❍ **What is the surgical treatment of choice for cecal cancer?**

Colonic resection from the vermiform appendix to the junction of the ascending and transverse colon.

❍ **What is the treatment of choice for plantar's warts?**

Cryosurgery with liquid nitrogen. First, the callus should be shaved off with a razor. If possible the keratin plug should be dug out. Lastly, liquid nitrogen should be applied. The wart will fall off in 3 to 4 weeks.

❍ **A 41 year-old patient complains of severe but short rectal spasms but has not noticed any bleeding. He is known to be stressed and overtaxed at work. What is your diagnosis?**

Proctalgia fugax. These short rectal spasms last less than 1 minute and occur infrequently. They are associated with people that are anxious, overworked or have a history of irritable bowel syndrome. No cause is known. Treatment is with analgesic suppositories, heating pads, and relaxation techniques.

❍ **What is the probable cause of colovesicular fistulas?**

Sigmoid diverticulitis. Other causes are radiation enteritis, colon carcinoma, and bladder carcinoma. Colovesicular fistulas are diagnosed by cystoscopy.

❍ **A 47 year-old man complains of impotence as well as pain and coldness in both legs after exercise. What would you expect to find on examination?**

This patient has Leriche's syndrome, caused by occlusion of the abdominal aorta secondary to atherosclerosis. Physical examination should reveal weak or absent femoral and pedal pulses, a bruit, thrill, pallor with elevation of the limb, dependent rubor, and a high blood pressure. Treatment is either bypass or thromboendarterectomy.

❍ **What is the most commonly obstructed artery in the lower extremity?**

The superficial femoral. It is a branch of the common femoral, which is a branch of the external iliac.

❍ **Which bacterium is associated with magnesium-ammonium-phosphate ureterolithiasis?**

Proteus, a bacterium that produces urease. These are infected stones and need to be removed. Antibiotics will help treat the UTI and will generally cease stone formation and urinary acidification. A urease inhibitor, like acetohydroxamic acid, will also prevent stone growth.

❍ **What is the most common germinal tumor of the testes?**

Seminoma (40%). The overall survival rate for seminomas is 85% because hematogenous spread does not occur until late in the disease. Other germinal tumors are embryonic cell carcinoma (25%), teratocarcinoma (25%), and choriocarcinoma. Germinal cell tumors of the testes are the most common malignant tumors of the testes.

❍ **Testicular torsion occurs most commonly in what age group?**

Teens.

❍ **What is the maximum amount of time a testicle can remain torsed without being irreversibly damaged?**

4 to 6 hours.

❍ **What are mycotic aneurysms?**

Mycotic aneurysms are true aneurysms that have become infected or false aneurysms that have occurred because of an arterial infection. The femoral artery is the most common site for such aneurysms.

❍ **Where is mesenteric ischemia more serious, in the small or the large bowel?**

The small bowel. Embolization in the superior mesenteric artery affects the entire small bowel. Mortality from small bowel ischemia is 60%. Embolization to the large bowel is not as serious due to collateral circulation. Ischemia of the large bowel rarely results in a full thickness injury or perforation.

❍ **Is venous thrombosis more common in the upper or the lower extremities?**

The lower. There is less fibrinolytic activity in the lower extremities as compared to the upper extremities.

❍ **Where do glomus tumors develop?**

In the hands, more specifically under the fingernails. These tumors are composed of blood vessels and unmyelinated nerves. Benign yet very painful, they should be surgically removed.

❍ **A trauma patient presents with a decreasing level of consciousness and an enlarging right pupil. What is your diagnosis?**

Probable uncal herniation with oculomotor nerve compression.

❍ **The corneal reflex tests what nerves?**

The ophthalmic branch (V_1) of the trigeminal (fifth) nerve (afferent), and the facial (seventh) nerve (efferent).

❍ **Name 5 clinical signs of basilar skull fracture.**

1) Periorbital ecchymosis (raccoon's eyes)
2) Retroauricular ecchymosis (Battle's sign)
3) Otorrhea or rhinorrhea
4) Hemotympanum or bloody ear discharge
5) First, second, seventh, and eighth CN deficits

❍ **A trauma patient presents with anisocoria, neurological deterioration, and/or lateralizing motor findings. What should be the immediate treatment?**

Immediate intubation and hyperventilation. Unless the patient is hypovolemic, infuse mannitol 1 g/kg rapidly. Elevate the head of the bed 30 °. Some authors still recommend dexamethasone, 10 mg, and phenytoin, 18 mg/kg at 20 mg/min.

❍ **Define increased intracranial pressure.**

ICP > 15 mm Hg.

❍ **Amputation is often required after vascular injuries to what artery?**

Popliteal artery. Injuries to arteries below the adductor hiatus lead to a loss of limb more frequently than injuries elsewhere.

❍ **How do you clinically differentiate between acute compartment syndrome, neuropraxia, and arterial occlusion?**

The patient will have normal pulses in neuropraxia, decreased pulses in compartment syndrome, and no pulses in arterial occlusion. Stretching the muscles will cause great pain in compartment syndrome but not in neuropraxia.

❍ **What is Finkelstein's test?**

A test used to determine whether a patient has de Quervain's disorder (an entrapment syndrome caused by tenosynovitis of the abductor pollicis longus and extensor pollicis brevis). If pain is elicited when the patient grasps his thumb with the fingers of the same hand and deviates his wrist in the ulnar direction, the test is positive.

❍ **What is the most common type of peripheral nerve compression?**

Carpal tunnel syndrome. This syndrome is more often diagnosed in female patients than male. Clinically, the patient will have pain and weakness which worsen at night. Moderate relief will come by shaking the hands. Wrist supports or hydrocortisone and Xylocaine injections may provide relief. If conservative measures do not work, surgical decompression can be performed.

❍ **What fingers are most often affected by carpal tunnel syndrome?**

The third and fourth digits. The sensory nerves to these digits are closest to the volar carpal ligament, which compresses the structures in the carpal tunnel.

❍ **Describe Tinel's and Phalen's tests.**

Both test for carpal tunnel syndrome.

Tinel's: Tapping the volar aspect of the wrist over the median nerve produces paresthesias that extend along the index and long finger.

Phalen's: Full flexion at the wrist for 1 minute leads to paresthesia along distribution of median nerve.

❍ **Where is the most common site of osteomyelitis of the vertebral column?**

The lumbar spine.

❍ **What is the most common cause of pyogenic osteomyelitis of the vertebral column?**

Staphylococcus aureus, secondary to hematogenous spread.

❍ **What population is most likely to develop osteoid osteoma?**

Males under 30 years of age. Osteoid osteoma is a benign musculoskeletal tumor. It is characterized by intense localized pain that is relieved by aspirin. Definitive treatment is surgery.

❍ **What are the four muscles of the rotator cuff?**

Supraspinatus, infraspinatus, teres minor, and subscapularis.

❍ **A 43 year-old female complains that her left knee hurts when she walks down stairs or when she bends her knee too far. There has been no trauma or new exercise. What is the probable diagnosis?**

Chondromalacia, which is degeneration of the cartilage of the patella. The cause is unknown.

HEAD AND NECK

In the country of the blind, the one-eyed man is king.
Erasmus

❍ **What are cotton wool spots?**

White patches on the retina that are observed upon fundiscopic examination. These patches are due to ischemia of the superficial nerve layer of the retina. They are most commonly associated with hypertension but also occur in patients with diabetes, anemia, collagen vascular disease, leukemia, endocarditis, and AIDS.

❍ **Do visual changes in chronic open-angle glaucoma patients begin centrally or peripherally?**

Peripherally. Patients with chronic glaucoma experience a gradual and painless loss of vision. Those with acute or subacute angle glaucoma will have either dull or severe pain, blurry vision, lacrimation, and even nausea and vomiting. The pain may be more severe in the dark.

❍ **Which is more common, chronic open-angle glaucoma or acute closed-angle glaucoma?**

Chronic open-angle glaucoma (90%). Four percent of the population over age 40 has glaucoma.

❍ **What is the most common cause of chronic open-angle glaucoma?**

Outflow obstruction through the trabecular meshwork. Other causes are obstruction of Schlemm's canal and excess secretion of aqueous fluid.

❍ **What is the normal range of intraocular pressure?**

10 to 23 mm Hg. Patients with acute angle-closure glaucoma generally have pressures elevated to 40 to 80 mm Hg.

❍ **Topical steroids for the eyes are absolutely contraindicated in what cases?**

If the patient has a herpetic infection. Herpetic lesion in the eye are often seen as dendritic patterns of fluoroxein uptake upon slitlamp examination.

❍ **What is the most common finding upon fundiscopic examination of a patient with AIDS?**

Cotton wool spots due to disease of the microvasculature. Other findings are hemorrhage, exudate, or retinal necrosis.

❍ **What percentage of the elderly are hard of hearing?**

What? Twenty-nine percent of people over the age of 65 and 36% of people over the age of 75 suffer hearing loss sufficient to interfere with normal conversation.

❍ **What is the most common type of hearing loss in the elderly?**

Presbycusis. This is an idiopathic, insidious, symmetrical decline in hearing that is associated with aging.

❍ **What is the prognostic significance of vertigo in a patient with sudden sensorineural hearing loss?**

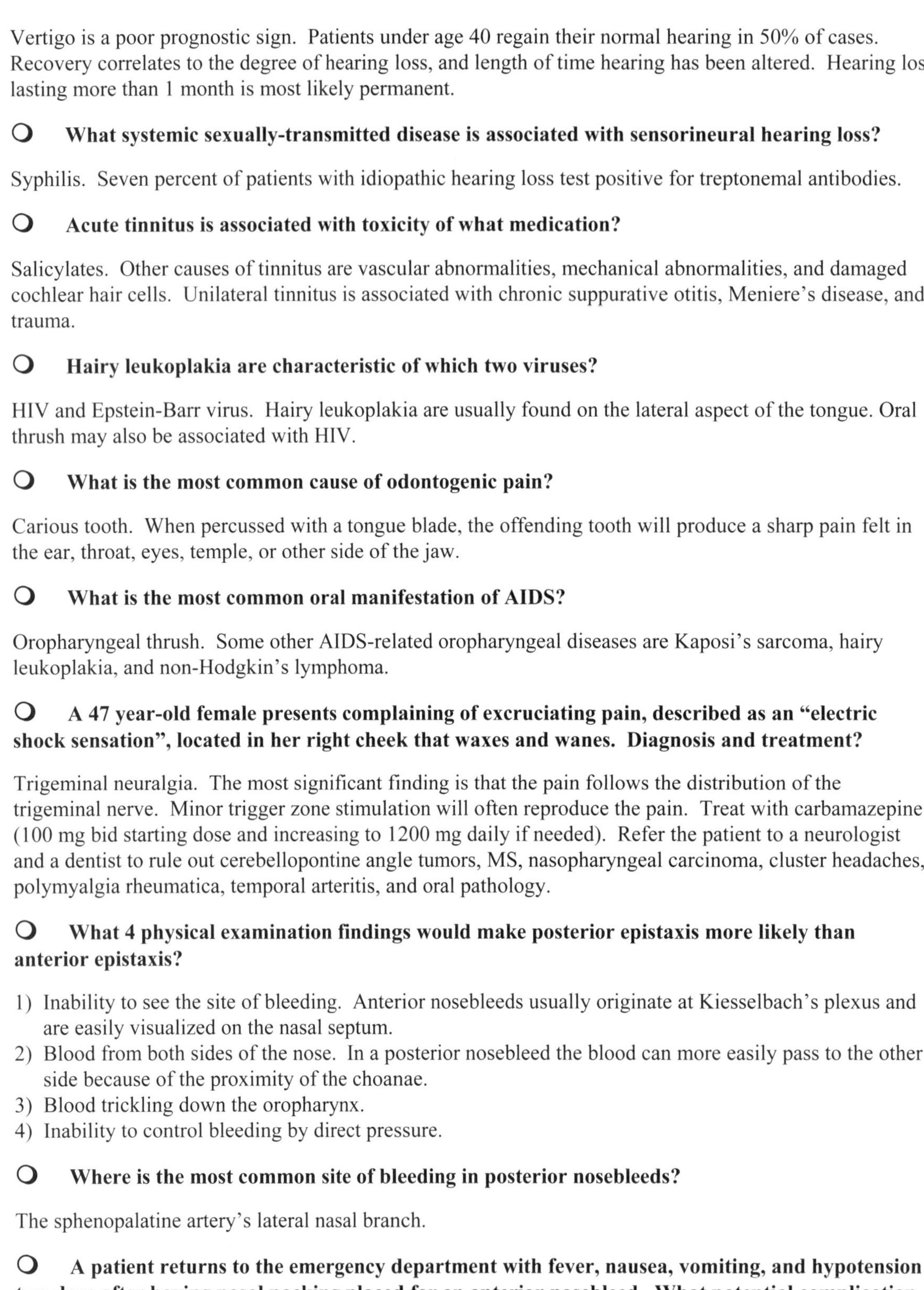

Vertigo is a poor prognostic sign. Patients under age 40 regain their normal hearing in 50% of cases. Recovery correlates to the degree of hearing loss, and length of time hearing has been altered. Hearing loss lasting more than 1 month is most likely permanent.

❍ **What systemic sexually-transmitted disease is associated with sensorineural hearing loss?**

Syphilis. Seven percent of patients with idiopathic hearing loss test positive for treptonemal antibodies.

❍ **Acute tinnitus is associated with toxicity of what medication?**

Salicylates. Other causes of tinnitus are vascular abnormalities, mechanical abnormalities, and damaged cochlear hair cells. Unilateral tinnitus is associated with chronic suppurative otitis, Meniere's disease, and trauma.

❍ **Hairy leukoplakia are characteristic of which two viruses?**

HIV and Epstein-Barr virus. Hairy leukoplakia are usually found on the lateral aspect of the tongue. Oral thrush may also be associated with HIV.

❍ **What is the most common cause of odontogenic pain?**

Carious tooth. When percussed with a tongue blade, the offending tooth will produce a sharp pain felt in the ear, throat, eyes, temple, or other side of the jaw.

❍ **What is the most common oral manifestation of AIDS?**

Oropharyngeal thrush. Some other AIDS-related oropharyngeal diseases are Kaposi's sarcoma, hairy leukoplakia, and non-Hodgkin's lymphoma.

❍ **A 47 year-old female presents complaining of excruciating pain, described as an "electric shock sensation", located in her right cheek that waxes and wanes. Diagnosis and treatment?**

Trigeminal neuralgia. The most significant finding is that the pain follows the distribution of the trigeminal nerve. Minor trigger zone stimulation will often reproduce the pain. Treat with carbamazepine (100 mg bid starting dose and increasing to 1200 mg daily if needed). Refer the patient to a neurologist and a dentist to rule out cerebellopontine angle tumors, MS, nasopharyngeal carcinoma, cluster headaches, polymyalgia rheumatica, temporal arteritis, and oral pathology.

❍ **What 4 physical examination findings would make posterior epistaxis more likely than anterior epistaxis?**

1) Inability to see the site of bleeding. Anterior nosebleeds usually originate at Kiesselbach's plexus and are easily visualized on the nasal septum.
2) Blood from both sides of the nose. In a posterior nosebleed the blood can more easily pass to the other side because of the proximity of the choanae.
3) Blood trickling down the oropharynx.
4) Inability to control bleeding by direct pressure.

❍ **Where is the most common site of bleeding in posterior nosebleeds?**

The sphenopalatine artery's lateral nasal branch.

❍ **A patient returns to the emergency department with fever, nausea, vomiting, and hypotension two days after having nasal packing placed for an anterior nosebleed. What potential complication of nasal packing should be considered?**

Toxic shock syndrome.

❍ **An ill-appearing patient presents with a fever of 103° F, bilateral chemosis, third nerve palsies, and untreated sinusitis. What is the diagnosis?**

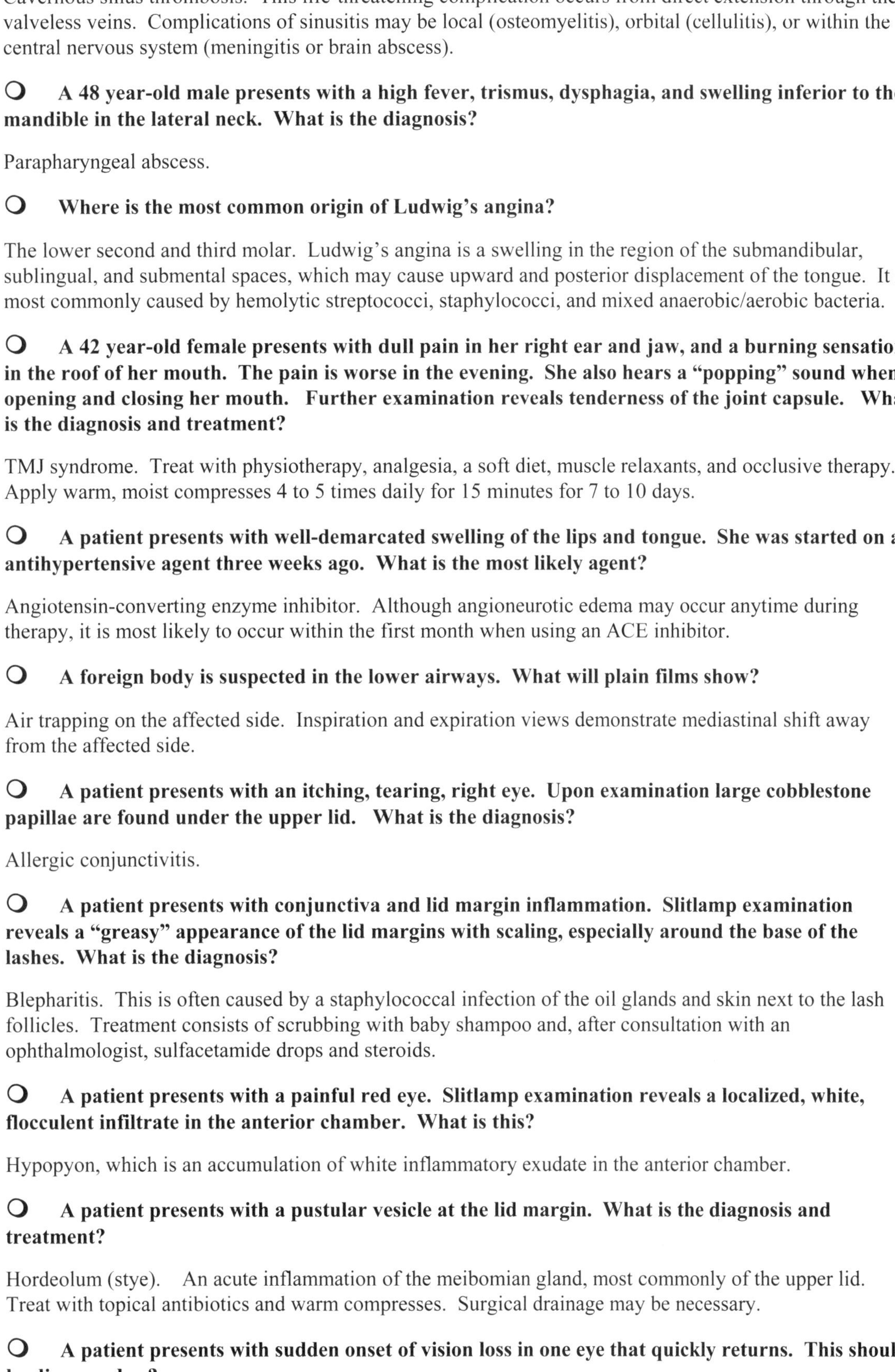

Cavernous sinus thrombosis. This life-threatening complication occurs from direct extension through the valveless veins. Complications of sinusitis may be local (osteomyelitis), orbital (cellulitis), or within the central nervous system (meningitis or brain abscess).

❍ **A 48 year-old male presents with a high fever, trismus, dysphagia, and swelling inferior to the mandible in the lateral neck. What is the diagnosis?**

Parapharyngeal abscess.

❍ **Where is the most common origin of Ludwig's angina?**

The lower second and third molar. Ludwig's angina is a swelling in the region of the submandibular, sublingual, and submental spaces, which may cause upward and posterior displacement of the tongue. It is most commonly caused by hemolytic streptococci, staphylococci, and mixed anaerobic/aerobic bacteria.

❍ **A 42 year-old female presents with dull pain in her right ear and jaw, and a burning sensation in the roof of her mouth. The pain is worse in the evening. She also hears a "popping" sound when opening and closing her mouth. Further examination reveals tenderness of the joint capsule. What is the diagnosis and treatment?**

TMJ syndrome. Treat with physiotherapy, analgesia, a soft diet, muscle relaxants, and occlusive therapy. Apply warm, moist compresses 4 to 5 times daily for 15 minutes for 7 to 10 days.

❍ **A patient presents with well-demarcated swelling of the lips and tongue. She was started on an antihypertensive agent three weeks ago. What is the most likely agent?**

Angiotensin-converting enzyme inhibitor. Although angioneurotic edema may occur anytime during therapy, it is most likely to occur within the first month when using an ACE inhibitor.

❍ **A foreign body is suspected in the lower airways. What will plain films show?**

Air trapping on the affected side. Inspiration and expiration views demonstrate mediastinal shift away from the affected side.

❍ **A patient presents with an itching, tearing, right eye. Upon examination large cobblestone papillae are found under the upper lid. What is the diagnosis?**

Allergic conjunctivitis.

❍ **A patient presents with conjunctiva and lid margin inflammation. Slitlamp examination reveals a "greasy" appearance of the lid margins with scaling, especially around the base of the lashes. What is the diagnosis?**

Blepharitis. This is often caused by a staphylococcal infection of the oil glands and skin next to the lash follicles. Treatment consists of scrubbing with baby shampoo and, after consultation with an ophthalmologist, sulfacetamide drops and steroids.

❍ **A patient presents with a painful red eye. Slitlamp examination reveals a localized, white, flocculent infiltrate in the anterior chamber. What is this?**

Hypopyon, which is an accumulation of white inflammatory exudate in the anterior chamber.

❍ **A patient presents with a pustular vesicle at the lid margin. What is the diagnosis and treatment?**

Hordeolum (stye). An acute inflammation of the meibomian gland, most commonly of the upper lid. Treat with topical antibiotics and warm compresses. Surgical drainage may be necessary.

❍ **A patient presents with sudden onset of vision loss in one eye that quickly returns. This should be diagnosed as?**

Amaurosis fugax. Usually caused by central retinal artery emboli from extracranial atherosclerosis.

❍ **A patient presents with painless vision loss in one eye, described as a wall slowly developing in the visual field. What finding do you expect upon examination?**

A gray, detached retina. The patient may also complain of flashing lights in the peripheral visual field or spider webs in the visual field. Inferior detachment is treated with the patient sitting up. Superior detachment is treated with the patient lying flat.

❍ **Three hours ago, a patient experienced sudden, painless visual loss in her right eye. Central retinal artery occlusion is suspected. What findings are expected upon eye examination? What is the prognosis?**

Afferent pupillary defect, pale gray retina, and a small cherry red dot near the fovea. This dot is the choroidal vasculature being seen at the macula where the retina is the thinnest. After 2 hours the prognosis is extremely poor for visual recovery. Digital massage or anterior chamber paracentesis may dislodge the clot. Immediate ophthalmic consultation is necessary.

❍ **What conditions have been associated with central retinal vein occlusion?**

Hyperviscosity syndromes, diabetes, and hypertension. Fundiscopic examination shows a chaotically streaked retina with congested dilated veins. There are superficial and deep retinal hemorrhages, cotton wool spots, and macular edema.

❍ **A patient presents with traumatic pain behind the left eye, a left pupil afferent defect, central visual loss, and a left swollen disc. What is the diagnosis and potential causes?**

Optic neuritis. This may be idiopathic or may be associated with multiple sclerosis, Lyme disease, neurosyphilis, lupus, sarcoid, alcoholism, toxins, or drug abuse.

❍ **After entering a dark bar, a patient developed eye pain, nausea, and vomiting and blurred vision; also, he sees halos around lights. Why would this patient be given mannitol, pilocarpine, and acetazolamide?**

This patient has acute narrow angle glaucoma. The goal of treatment is to decrease intraocular pressure. To accomplish this, one should:

1) Decrease the production of aqueous humor with carbonic anhydrase inhibitor.
2) Decrease intraocular volume by making the plasma hypertonic to the aqueous humor with glycerol or mannitol.
3) Constrict the pupil with pilocarpine, allowing increased flow of the aqueous humor out through the previously blocked canals of Schlemm.

❍ **A patient's cornea fluoresces prior to instillation of fluorescein. What should be considered?**

Pseudomonal infection. Several species fluoresce on their own.

❍ **A patient presents with a ptosis and ipsilateral miosis of the pupil and has pain in the ipsilateral arm. Where is the lesion?**

The clinical diagnosis is Horner's syndrome. This can be confirmed with topical pharmacologic testing with cocaine drops. If the involved pupil does not dilate, the patient has an ipsilateral Horner's syndrome. The presence of arm pain suggests that the lesion involves the sympathetic chain at the level of the brachial plexus. An apical lung tumor (Pancoast tumor) should be suspected in this setting.

❍ **A patient with normal vision presents with bilateral small, irregular pupils that do not react to light but constrict normally to convergence effort. What is the diagnosis?**

This patient demonstrates light near dissociation of the pupils. Tertiary syphilis causing Argyll-Robertson pupils should be suspected and syphilis serology should be ordered.

❍ **A 55 year-old patient with diplopia presents with an inability to elevate, depress, or adduct the left eye. The ipsilateral lid is ptotic and the pupil is not reactive to light. There are no other neurologic signs or symptoms. Where is the lesion and what is the evaluation?**

The diagnosis is an isolated pupil-involved third nerve palsy. This patient should undergo an evaluation to exclude an aneurysm of the posterior communicating artery including cerebral arteriography.

❍ **A patient with diplopia has an inability to elevate, depress, abduct or adduct the left eye. The left pupil is smaller than the right pupil. The left eyelid is ptotic. Where is the lesion?**

This patient has a third, fourth, and sixth nerve paresis. The pupil is smaller due to presumed involvement of the oculosympathetic pathway within the cavernous sinus. Neuroimaging studies should be directed to this location.

❍ **An obese, white female presents with headaches, normal visual acuity, an enlarged blind spot bilaterally, and bilateral optic disc edema. What is the most appropriate evaluation?**

Any patient with bilateral optic disc edema should be presumed to have increased intracranial pressure until proven otherwise. Neuroimaging, on an emergent basis, should be performed, and if negative, should be followed by a lumbar puncture with cerebrospinal fluid analysis and measurement of the intracranial pressure. Patients with normal neuroimaging, normal cerebrospinal fluid contents, signs and symptoms only related to increased intracranial pressure (i.e. headache, papilledema), and an elevated opening pressure have the clinical diagnosis of pseudotumor cerebri.

❍ **A 60 year-old white male with hypertension and diabetes develops acute painless unilateral loss of vision and an ipsilateral swollen optic nerve. What is the evaluation and treatment?**

The patient has anterior ischemic optic neuropathy. Giant cell arteritis should be considered and the patient should be asked about symptoms such as jaw claudication, weight loss, headache, scalp tenderness or polymyalgia rheumatica. An erythrocyte sedimentation rate should be performed. The eye should be examined for the structural "disc at risk" appearance of a small cup to disc ratio.

❍ **A 75 year-old patient develops acute onset of a markedly constricted visual field to 10 degrees in each eye. The remainder of the ocular exam is normal. A tangent screen at 1 and 2 meters demonstrates an organic and appropriate expansion of the visual field. What is the next most appropriate evaluation?**

This patient could have cortical visual impairment and a neuroimaging study should be performed. A cerebrovascular accident would be the most likely etiology.

❍ **A 23 year-old female presents with an irregular, 6 mm right pupil that does not respond to light stimulus but reacts briskly to convergence effort. There is a sector paresis of the iris sphincter and pilocarpine 1/8% constricts the right pupil but not the left pupil. What is the most likely diagnosis?**

Adie's tonic pupil. There is a 4% chance per year of bilateral involvement. The condition is benign and usually requires no therapy.

❍ **A 45 year-old patient presents with painless variable diplopia and ptosis. There is moderate weakness of eyelid closure bilaterally. The pupils and the remainder of the exam are normal. What is the next most appropriate evaluation?**

Myasthenia gravis may mimic any pupil-spared, non-proptotic, painless ophthalmoplegia. It may occur with or without ptosis. An edrophonium (Tensilon) test may reverse the ptosis and ophthalmoplegia, but a positive Tensilon test is not pathognomonic for the disorder nor does a negative test exclude myasthenia.

❍ **A 55 year-old diabetic patient develops acute onset of proptosis, chemosis, and ophthalmoplegia. A black eschar is seen on the palate. What is the most likely diagnosis?**

An acute ophthalmoplegia with orbital signs in a diabetic patient is Mucormycosis until proven otherwise. Early recognition is crucial as the disease may be life-threatening.

❍ **A 22 year-old female presents with acute onset of severe headache and a bitemporal hemianopsia. What is the most likely diagnosis?**

Pituitary apoplexy.

❍ **A 23 year-old patient with a ventriculoperitoneal shunt develops an upgaze paresis, light near dissociation of the pupils, and convergence retraction nystagmus in attempted upgaze. Where is the lesion? What is the significance of the finding?**

The lesion is at the level of the dorsal midbrain. In a patient with a shunt the constellation of findings consistent with the Parinaud's dorsal midbrain syndrome suggest shunt malfunction.

❍ **A 40 year-old patient develops diplopia. There is an adduction deficit in the right eye with abducting nystagmus in the left eye on attempted gaze to the left. The remainder of the eye exam is normal. Where is the lesion? What is the most likely etiology?**

This patient has an internuclear ophthalmoplegia (INO) on the right. The most likely etiologies are demyelinating disease in a young person and stroke in an elderly person, but other entities involving the medial longitudinal fasciculus including neoplasm, infection or inflammation may cause an INO.

❍ **An 80 year-old white female develops acute loss of vision. Ophthalmoscopy reveals a non-embolic central retinal artery occlusion. In addition to embolic disease, what systemic vasculopathy should be considered high on the differential diagnosis?**

Giant cell arteritis should be suspected in any non-embolic branch or central retinal artery occlusion.

❍ **What is the structural appearance of the "disc at risk" for the development of non-arteritic anterior ischemic optic neuropathy?**

The "disc at risk" is a small disc with a small crowded appearance and a small cup to disc ratio.

❍ **What are the demographics for patients with pseudotumor cerebri?**

Pseudotumor cerebri is a disease of obese, young females. The diagnosis should be considered one of exclusion in thin, elderly, and/or male patients.

❍ **A 40 year-old patient develops the acute onset of intermittent "shimmering" or "fluttering" of the right eye, lasting seconds to minutes at a time. Examination during the episode demonstrates fine intorsion movements of the right eye. The remainder of the exam is normal. What is the most likely diagnosis?**

Superior oblique myokymia.

❍ **The pupils in a patient with anisocoria react normally to light. What are the possible causes of the anisocoria?**

Anisocoria with normally active pupils may be due to essential anisocoria or Horner's syndrome. The two can be differentiated by instilling 10% cocaine drops into both eyes. The Horner pupil will not dilate while the essential anisocoria pupils will dilate well.

❍ **A patient is knocked unconscious when hit in the forehead by a baseball bat. After the injury, he complains of binocular vertical diplopia. On examination, there is a right hypertropia on left gaze and a left hypertropia in right gaze. Head tilt to the right reveals a right hypertropia and head tilt to the left reveals a left hypertropia. What has happened?**

The patient has developed bilateral fourth nerve palsies. The long course of the fourth nerve around the midbrain, near the edge of the tentorium, makes this nerve particularly vulnerable, and a severe blow to the forehead may cause a contrecoup contusion of one or both fourth nerves against the rigid tentorium. Severe frontal trauma may also cause bilateral fourth nerve palsies by contusion of the anterior medullary velum where both nerves cross.

❍ **A patient with Graves' ophthalmopathy (thyroid eye disease) is noted to be exotropic. Is this from the Graves' disease?**

Unlikely. Graves' disease mainly affects the inferior rectus, medial rectus, and superior rectus muscles, in that order, and causes a restrictive myopathy. Lateral rectus muscle involvement is very rare and, thus, an exotropia should raise the possibility of associated myasthenia gravis with medial rectus paresis. There is an increased risk of myasthenia gravis in patients with Graves' disease.

❍ **A 24 year-old woman develops acute visual loss in the right eye. Examination reveals decreased acuity and decreased color vision in the affected eye with a relative afferent pupillary defect. Fundiscopic exam revealed disc swelling in the right eye with a macular star and 2+ vitreous cells. The left eye was normal. What entities should be considered? What is the patient's chance of developing multiple sclerosis in the future?**

The patient has neuroretinitis or optic disc edema with a macular star (ODEMS). The clinical features include sudden visual loss, swelling of the optic disc, peripapillary and macular exudates which may occur in a star pattern, and cells in the vitreous. Although usually idiopathic, infectious etiologies for this syndrome, especially syphilis, Lyme disease, cat scratch disease, and toxoplasmosis, should be considered. The macular exudate likely results from primary optic nerve disease and not from inflammation in the retina. Patients who demonstrate acute papillitis with a normal macula should be reevaluated within two weeks for the development of a macular star. Unlike optic neuritis, the presence of a macular star militates strongly against the subsequent development of multiple sclerosis.

❍ **A 28 year-old obese woman describes headaches for three months and episodes lasting "seconds" of unilateral or bilateral loss of vision. The episodes of visual loss occur 20 to 30 times per day and occasionally are precipitated by sudden changes in posture. Fundiscopic examination reveals papilledema. What is the cause of the episodes of transient visual loss (TVL)?**

Episodes of TVL lasting less than 60 seconds may occur in patients with papilledema secondary to increased intracranial pressure. These transient obscurations of vision may occur in one or both eyes (individually or simultaneously) and typically last only a few seconds. The episodes may be precipitated by changes in position and are thought to be related to the effects of increased intracranial pressure on the flow of blood to the eye, perhaps where the central retinal artery penetrates the optic nerve sheath to enter the substance of the nerve.

❍ **A 75-year-old man describes two recent episodes of monocular TVL lasting 15 minutes and also complains of recent jaw pain induced by chewing or talking. The fundi are normal with no retinal emboli evident. What is the diagnosis?**

Jaw claudications are very characteristic of giant cell arteritis, which may present with episodes of TVL or transient diplopia. The patient needs immediate steroid therapy and should undergo a temporal artery biopsy.

❍ **A middle-age woman develops acute onset of mild eyelid swelling, conjunctival chemosis, proptosis, and dilated conjunctival vessels. She also complains of pulsatile tinnitus. Vision is normal. What etiology is likely?**

The clinical findings are suggestive of a spontaneous dural carotid-cavernous sinus fistula. Cerebral angiography is indicated.

❍ **After a brainstem stroke, a patient complains of diplopia. On examination he can move neither eye to the left. On attempted right gaze, abduction is full in the right eye but there is no adduction of left eye. What has happened?**

The patient has one-and-a-half syndrome. In the one-and-a-half syndrome, there is a conjugate gaze palsy to one side ("one") and impaired adduction on looking to the other side ("and-a-half"). As a result, the only horizontal movement remaining is abduction of one eye, which may exhibit nystagmus in abduction. Patients with the one and a half syndrome often have exotropia of the eye opposite the side of the lesion (paralytic pontine exotropia) because, due to the gaze palsy, the eyes tend to drift to the side opposite the lesion.

❍ **A 58 year-old man has had four recent episodes of TVL followed by headache. The episodes are stereotyped and consist of loss of vision in both eyes, always in the left hemifield, followed by right occipital headache. Neuro-ophthalmologic exam reveals a left scotomatous central homonymous field defect. Is this a migraine?**

The presence of a small area of bilateral visual loss or a mild bilateral disturbance of vision that progressively increases over 15 or more minutes is highly characteristic of migraine. However, any patient with abnormalities on visual field examination suggesting a retrochiasmal lesion or any patient with atypical migraine-like phenomena, especially patients with visual symptoms that are brief, episodic, unformed, and not associated with the angular, scintillating figures that occur with migraine, requires neuroimaging to investigate the possibility of occipital arteriovenous malformation (AVM), venous sinus thrombosis, or tumor. The patient had a right occipital AVM.

❍ **A 58 year-old man develops a unilateral complete third nerve palsy, except the pupil is completely normal. Is an aneurysm likely?**

Third nerve palsy with a normal pupillary sphincter and completely palsied extraocular muscles is almost never caused by aneurysms. This type of third nerve palsy is most commonly caused by ischemia, especially related to diabetes (see above).

❍ **A 30 year-old man with a history of chronic lymphocytic leukemia (CLL) complains of painless, bilateral visual impairment. Acuity and color vision are diminished bilaterally, the pupillary reaction is sluggish bilaterally, but the discs are normal. What should be considered?**

Progressive visual loss from optic nerve infiltration may be a clinical manifestation of leukemia, including CLL. The discs may be normal or swollen and progressive optic atrophy with loss of acuity and visual fields often occurs. MR imaging with gadolinium may reveal optic nerve involvement, and meningeal involvement and spinal tap to document meningeal infiltration by the leukemia is warranted. Optic nerve irradiation may result in improvement.

❍ **A 40 year-old woman has a history of bilateral lid retraction, mild bilateral proptosis, and vertical diplopia secondary to thyroid ophthalmopathy (Graves' disease). She now complains of unilateral progressive visual loss for the last 2 weeks. Acuity is 20/40 and 20/30, respectively, color vision is depressed on the left, a left relative afferent pupillary defect is evident, and the discs are normal bilaterally. The anterior segment appears normal. What is causing the visual impairment?**

The patient has optic neuropathy secondary to her thyroid ophthalmopathy. Optic neuropathy with thyroid ophthalmopathy is usually caused by apical compression of the optic nerve by enlarged extraocular muscles and can cause permanent visual loss. The discs may be swollen, normal, or atrophic. Treatment possibilities include high doses of oral or intravenous corticosteroids, orbital irradiation, orbital decompression, or a combination of these procedures.

❍ **A 40 year-old horse-racing jockey, weighing 105 lbs., was brought to the emergency room because of slowly progressive confusion and imbalance of several days duration. He is disoriented and confused and frequently repeated himself and has an unsteady gait. He has a full range of eye motion and has no ocular misalignment. However, he had a primary position upbeat nystagmus, which became downbeating with convergence, and mild horizontal end gaze nystagmus. What is the likely etiology for his confusion and eye findings?**

The patient probably has Wernicke's encephalopathy caused by thiamine deficiency. Although most often seen with nutritional deprivation associated with chronic alcoholism, the disorder may also be seen with eating disorders, bulimia, hyperemesis gravidorum, and maintaining low weight (e.g., jockeys). Characteristic findings include the classic triad of ophthalmoplegia (bilateral lateral rectus weakness), ataxia, and mental changes. The ocular motor signs are quite varied in Wernicke's disease and include bilateral abducens palsies, gaze-evoked or primary position vertical nystagmus, various combinations of horizontal and vertical gaze palsies and internuclear ophthalmoplegia, convergence disorders and ocular bobbing. Thiamine therapy must be urgently instituted.

❍ **What two organisms are most commonly associated with late onset endophthalmitis associated with glaucoma filtering blebs?**

Streptococcal species and Hemophilus influenzae.

❍ **When does severe acute endophthalmitis caused by S. aureus, Streptococcus species, or gram-negative bacteria usually present?**

1-4 days after surgery. Endophthalmitis, from less virulent organisms, may present much later.

❍ **What is the appropriate treatment of chronic Propionibacterium endophthalmitis?**

Removal of involved capsular and residual lens material through pars plana vitrectomy and intravitreal vancomycin.

❍ **What retinal findings characterize HIV retinopathy?**

Cotton-wool spots, retinal hemorrhages, and microaneurysms. HIV retinopathy is the most common ocular finding in AIDS patients and usually does not cause significant vision problems.

❍ **What is the most common sight-threatening ocular infection in AIDS patients?**

Cytomegalovirus (CMV) retinitis occurs in 15-40% of AIDS patients.

❍ **What clinical findings characterize ocular histoplasmosis syndrome?**

Multiple peripheral chorioretinal scars, peripapillary atrophic scars, and no vitritis. Maculopathy with choroidal neovascularization may also occur.

❍ **Which is the more common cause of posterior uveitis, toxoplasmosis or toxocariasis?**

Toxoplasmosis. Although there is a high prevalence of exposure to toxocariasis, clinical disease is uncommon.

❍ **What are the ocular manifestations of Lyme disease?**

Uveitis, keratitis, and optic neuritis.

❍ **"River blindness", a major cause of blindness worldwide, characterized by uveitis, chorioretinal changes and optic atrophy is caused by what organism?**

Microfilariae of Onchocerca volvulus cause this disease, also known as onchocerciasis.

❍ **What is the most common cause of endogenous fungal endophthalmitis?**

Candida species.

❍ **What are the two major risk factors for ocular candidiasis?**

Indwelling venous catheters and intravenous drug abuse.

❍ **Are patients with acute retinal necrosis (ARN) syndrome usually immunosuppressed or not?**

Patients with ARN are otherwise healthy and not immunosuppressed.

❍ **What systemic bacterial infection is associated with granulomatous uveitis and yellow-white choroidal nodules?**

Tuberculosis.

❍ **When are topical steroids used in treating herpetic keratitis?**

For stromal keratitis, once epithelial disease has been treated. Concurrent antivirals should be used.

❍ **Which is the more effective therapy for corneal epithelial herpes simplex keratitis, topical or systemic antivirals?**

Topical antivirals.

❍ **Treatment with oral acyclovir has been shown to be most effective in treating which disease, recurrent herpes simplex keratitis or herpes zoster ophthalmicus?**

Herpes Zoster ophthalmicus.

❍ **Extended wear contact lenses worn overnight increase the risk of infectious keratitis by how much compared to daily wear?**

Approximately 10-fold.

❍ **What type of conjunctivitis is caused by adenovirus?**

Acute follicular conjunctivitis.

❍ **Are topical antivirals effective in the treatment of adenoviral keratoconjunctivitis?**

No.

❍ **What are the ocular signs of cat-scratch disease?**

Follicular conjunctivitis with granulomatous nodules on the palbebral conjunctiva, swollen preauricular or submandibular lymph nodes.

❍ **How is chlamydial inclusion conjunctivitis transmitted?**

Sexual contact.

❍ **What are the most common causes of chronic follicular conjunctivitis?**

Chlamydial inclusion conjunctivitis, trachoma, molluscum contagiosum, toxicity from topical medications, parinaud's oculoglandular conjunctivitis.

❍ **A patient with chronic follicular conjunctivitis is found to have several smooth, centrally umbilicated papules on the eyelids. What is the most likely diagnosis?**

Molluscum contagiosum.

❍ **Is it likely for an untreated corneal ulcer caused by Pseudomonas aeruginosa to progress to a corneal perforation?**

Yes.

❍ **What retinal involvement can be associated with infectious mononucleosis (Epstein-Barr Virus)?**

Macular edema, retinal hemorrhages, chorioretinitis, punctate outer retinitis, multifocal chorioretinitis and panuveitis.

❍ **What two organisms are most likely to cause endogenous bacterial endopthalmitis in a host not otherwise predisposed to infection?**

Neisseria meningitidis and Haemophilus influenzae.

❍ **What is the most frequent condition associated with orbital cellulitis ?**

Sinusitis.

❍ **What is the mortality rate of orbital mucormycosis with aggressive treatment?**

Approximately 30%.

❍ **A 35 year old patient with chronic conjunctivitis, erythematous lid margins with telangiectatic vessels, and malar pustules most likely has what diagnosis?**

Acne rosacea.

❍ **Progressive outer retinal necrosis is associated with what disease and caused by what virus?**

This is associated with AIDS and is a form of varicella zoster retinitis.

❍ **What is the appropriate treatment for chlamydial conjunctivitis?**

Oral doxycycline, tetracycline, or erythromycin.

❍ **What would be the best therapy for a methicillin-resistant Staphylococcus aureus corneal ulcer, unresponsive to fortified topical cefazolin and gentamicin?**

Fortified topical vancomycin.

❍ **What is the treatment for severe or vision-threatening ocular toxoplasmosis?**

Pyrimethamine (with folinic acid), and sulfadiazine. Clindamycin and trimethoprim/sulfamethoxazole are alternative treatments. Prednisone may be added after antibiotic therapy has begun. Periocular steroid injections are contraindicated.

❍ **Interstitial keratitis and a "salt-and-pepper" chorioretinitis are characteristic of what ocular infection?**

Syphilis.

❍ **What sexually transmitted disease would be the most likely cause of an optic neuritis in a 25-year old male?**

Acquired syphilis.

❍ **How does acetazolamide increase the risk of renal stones?**

By reducing urinary citrate excretion.

❍ **Is mannitol contraindicated in diabetic patients?**

No. Unlike glycerol, mannitol is not metabolized and poses no hyperglycemic threat to diabetics.

❍ **What are the most common side effects associated with systemic gancyclovir therapy?**

Myelosuppression is most common. Elevated liver enzymes, skin rash, GI and CNS toxicity may also occur. In children, carcinogenicity and reproductive toxicity are also issues of concern.

❍ **What is the initial treatment regimen for HSV retinitis (acute retinal necrosis)?**

Oral and IV acyclovir. If no response and the lesions are sight-threatening, add foscarnet and/or gancyclovir.

❍ **A patient with traumatic hyphema is treated with aminocaproic acid to prevent secondary hemorrhage. What side effects should you monitor for?**

Nausea and vomiting (25% of patients), and dizziness and hypotension (20% of patients).

❍ **An elderly woman with macular degeneration reports high-dose vitamin supplementation in an effort to slow the progression of her disease. What are your concerns?**

High zinc levels can cause copper deficiency anemia and decreased HDL. High vitamin E levels can lead to fatigue, muscle weakness and decreased thyroid function.

❍ **A 22 year-old female presents with a two day history of preseptal cellulitis. What germs are you worried about and what antibiotic coverage is appropriate?**

Common bugs include Staph and Strep species, as well as H. flu and some anaerobes. Amoxicillin-clavulanic acid or a second-generation cephalosporin would be adequate coverage.

❍ **A 28 year-old male presents with conjunctivitis and urethritis. Inclusion bodies are seen on conjunctival smear. The diagnosis of chlamydial inclusion conjunctivitis is made. What treatment is appropriate?**

Systemic (oral) administration of tetracycline to the patient and his partner(s).

❍ **What adverse reactions to chloramphenicol led to its disuse despite its broad spectrum of activity?**

Aplastic anemia, optic atrophy, peripheral neuritis, and gray syndrome (vomiting, cyanosis, gray stools, ashen skin color, tachypnea, vasomotor collapse, and a 40% mortality rate).

❍ **What is the mechanism of action of the fluoroquinolones?**

They are bactericidal via inhibition of DNA gyrase.

❍ **A hypertensive patient, on oral propranolol, undergoes routine dilated fundiscopic exam, and winds up in the ER later that night in hypertensive crisis. Why?**

Beta-blockers may enhance the vasopressor effect of phenylephrine by inhibiting vasodilation.

❍ **Chronic management of myasthenia gravis depends on direct-acting cholinergic agents--true or false?**

False. The agents of choice are indirect-acting cholinergics (cholinesterase inhibitors).

❍ **Rank the following steroids in terms of potency (lowest to highest): methylprednisolone, prednisone, dexamethasone, cortisone, hydrocortisone.**

Cortisone, hydrocortisone, prednisone, methylprednisolone, dexamethasone.

❍ **A 28 year-old woman is diagnosed with pigmentary glaucoma and betaxolol is prescribed. She mentions she is two months postpartum and breastfeeding. Is your management still appropriate?**

No. Betaxolol is secreted in breast milk in high enough concentration to cause systemic beta-blockade in the infant. Timolol achieves lower breast milk concentrations and is deemed safe, by the American Academy of Pediatrics, for breastfeeding mothers.

❍ **Why must the anesthesiologist be informed, prior to general anesthesia, that a patient is taking echothiophate?**

Phospholine Iodide inhibits plasma pseudocholinesterase (as well as acetylcholinesterase), the enzyme responsible for metabolism of succinylcholine. Intraoperative administration of succinylcholine might lead to cardiovascular collapse and respiratory shut-down.

❍ **Which of the alpha-2 agonists (clonidine, apraclonidine, brimonidine) is most likely to produce CNS side effects such as drowsiness and fatigue? Which is least likely?**

Clonidine is most likely; apraclonidine is least likely.

❍ **A 62 year-old woman, with 2 mm of left ptosis and unilateral glaucoma OS, has uncontrolled IOP with timolol and dorzolamide. What might you consider as a third agent and why?**

Apraclonidine can cause 1.4mm (average) lid retraction, presumably due to sympathetic stimulation of Mueller's muscle.

❍ **The two most common adverse reactions reported with dorzolamide are?**

Transient ocular surface irritation (33%) and bitter taste (26%).

❍ **What aspect of intracellular acyclovir activation gives the drug exquisite specificity for HSV- or VZV-infected cells?**

Acyclovir is a prodrug, and is activated by a viral (rather than a cellular) enzyme; thus activity is only achieved in infected cells.

❍ **What options are available for the CMV retinitis patient who is systemically intolerant to gancyclovir (GCV) therapy?**

GCV intraocular implant or periodic intravitreal GCV injections; systemic foscarnet; intravitreal or systemic cidofovir.

❍ **An African immigrant, from a region where river blindness is endemic, presents with uveitis and the diagnosis of onchocerciasis is made. What is the treatment of choice, and what is its mechanism of action?**

Ivermectin, which paralyzes nematodes by enhancing signal transmission in peripheral nerves of microfilaria but not in adult worms.

❍ **What is the clinical spectrum of activity of polymyxin B?**

Gram negative rods (except Proteus, Serratia, Brucella). No gram-positive organisms, gram-negative cocci, or fungi.

❍ **A 22 year-old contact lens wearer presents with a red eye, pain, and a ring-shaped stromal infiltrate after swimming in a pond. You diagnose acanthamoeba infection. What are your medical management options?**

Propamidine (only available in United Kingdom); neosporin (polymyxin B, neomycin, gramicidin); pentamidine (use transiently while waiting for a colleague in England to send you propamidine); miconazole/ketaconazole/clotrimazole; polyhexamethylene biguanide; sulindac.

❍ **A 29 year-old man is treated for idiopathic anterior uveitis with topical prednisolone acetate, and presents, during treatment, with mild ptosis of the treated eye, as well as 1mm of anisocoria (the treated eye having the larger pupil). What's going on?**

These transient findings have been attributed to the steroid vehicle, and resolve with cessation of therapy.

❍ **A 36-year-old male psychiatric patient presents with blurred vision after eating his cat raw, and is found to have active chorioretinitis with adjacent satellite scars. What is the probable diagnosis and appropriate treatment for the ocular disease?**

Toxoplasmosis chorioretinitis. Treatment includes sulfonamides, clindamycin, and steroids.

PSYCHIATRY PEARLS

Roses are red, violets are blue. I'm a schizophrenic, and so am I.
Frank Crow

❍ **According to our best knowledge, what is the frequency of rape?**

The 1987 Uniform Crimes Report states that at least 1 in 8 women have been raped. It is estimated that only 25% of all rapes are reported.

❍ **What is the definition of domestic abuse?**

A pattern of assaultive and coercive behaviors including physical, sexual, and psychological abuse designed to gain power and control over an intimate partner.

❍ **What is the epidemiology of domestic violence?**

95% of the victims are women. An estimated 4 million women are battered each year. Domestic abuse is the number one cause of injuries to women. More than half of all women murdered in the US are killed by their intimate partner.

❍ **What are the clinical clues for domestic violence?**

1) Any evidence of injury during pregnancy or late entry into prenatal care; 2) injuries presenting after significant delay or in various stages of healing--especially to the head, neck, breasts, abdomen, or areas suggesting a defensive posture, such as bruises on the forearms; 3) vague complaints or unusual injuries, such as bites, scratches, burns, or rope marks; and 4) suicide attempts and rapes.

❍ **What is the prevalence of alcoholism in the US?**

Ten to fifteen percent is the lifetime prevalence. Ten percent of men and 3.5% of women are alcoholic.

❍ **What age range has the highest prevalence of drinking problems?**

Clearly, 1 to 2 year-olds are known to spill and drool the most when drinking. However, if we are talking about alcoholic drinking problems, 18 to 29 year-olds have the greatest prevalence.

❍ **What laboratory changes are suggestive of alcoholism?**

Look for an increase in ALT, AST, alkaline phosphatase, amylase, bilirubin, cholesterol, GGT, LDH, MCV, prothrombin time, triglycerides, and uric acid; look for a decrease in BUN, calcium, coagulopathy, hematocrit, magnesium, phosphorus, platelet count, and protein.

❍ **Describe the symptoms of alcohol withdrawal and their temporal relations.**

Hallucinations: Auditory, visual, and tactile occur 24 hours after patient's last drink.

Autonomic hyperactivity: Tachycardia, hypertension, tremors, anxiety, and agitation occur 6 to 8 hours after patient's last drink.

Global confusion: Occurs 1 to 3 days after patient's last drink.

❍ **What is the difference in treatment methods between alcohol withdrawal and sedative-hypnotic withdrawal?**

Alcohol withdrawal is treated with benzodiazepene, carbamazepine, or paraldehyde. Sedative-hypnotic withdrawal is treated with the substitution of a long-acting barbiturate.

❍ **What is the most common mental illness in large cities?**

Substance abuse. Substance abuse is prevalent in rural communities as well but the addiction percentages are lower. Incidentally, opiates are predominantly a city drug, while marijuana, alcohol, and amphetamines are found in both rural and urban settings.

❍ **A patient presents with tearing eyes, a runny nose, tachycardia, hair-on-end, abdominal pains, nausea, vomiting, diarrhea, insomnia, pupillary dilation, and leukocytosis. What is the diagnosis?**

Opiate and/or opioid withdrawal. Treat with methadone or dolophine.

❍ **What is the most effective long-term treatment program for alcoholism?**

Alcoholics Anonymous.

❍ **What is the difference between methadone and heroin?**

Methadone causes analgesia, but does not cause euphoria. Habituation occurs with both drugs. The withdrawal symptoms of methadone are less severe, but they last longer.

❍ **What are the two most common behavior problems seen by physicians?**

Anxiety and depression.

❍ **Describe a patient with generalized anxiety disorder.**

Patients afflicted with this disorder appear apprehensive, restless, irritable, and are easily distracted. Patients can also experience muscle tension and fatigue, as well as various autonomic symptoms, such as palpitations, shortness of breath, chest tightness, nausea, or diffuse weakness and numbness.

❍ **What are a few substances that might mimic generalized anxiety when ingested?**

Nicotine, caffeine, amphetamines, cocaine, and anticholinergics. Alcohol and sedative withdrawal can also mimic this disorder.

❍ **What are eight common medical causes of anxiety or anxiety attacks?**

(1) Alcohol withdrawal, (2) thyrotoxicosis, (3) caffeine, (4) stroke, (5) cardiopulmonary emergencies, (6) hypoglycemia, (7) psychosensory/psychomotor epilepsy, and (8) pheochromocytoma.

❍ **Match the aphasia with the anatomy involved.**

1) Broca's aphasia a) Superior temporal gyrus, posterior third
2) Global aphasia b) Arcuate fasciculus near the dominant parietal lobe
3) Wernicke's aphasia c) Middle cerebral artery occlusion
4) Conduction aphasia d) Left frontal lobe posterior inferior region

Answers: (1) d, (2) c, (3) a, and (4) b.

❍ **A sibling to a female patient with ADHD is at a higher risk for what other disorders?**

Conduct, mood, anxiety, and antisocial disorders, substance abuse, and, of course, ADHD. Relatives of females with ADHD are at higher risk for these disorders compared to relatives of males.

❍ **What effect does ADHD have on sleep?**

ADHD causes restless sleep and decreases REM latency, the time from the onset of sleep to REM sleep.

❍ **What are the side effects of Ritalin?**

Depression, headache, hypertension, insomnia, and abdominal pain. Ritalin (methylphenidate) is a psychostimulant used to treat ADHD.

❍ **Bereavement generally lasts how long?**

6 months. Full melancholic syndrome, hallucinations, and suicidal ideation are not common in bereavement.

❍ **Which has an earlier onset, bipolar disorder or unipolar disorder?**

Bipolar. Onset of bipolar disorder is usually in the patient's twenties or thirties; onset of unipolar disorder is usually between ages 35 and 50.

❍ **Differentiate between bipolar I, bipolar II, and hypomania.**

Bipolar I: Mania and major depression
Bipolar II: Hypomania and major depression
Hypomania: Mania without severe impairment or psychotic features

❍ **Are the majority of affective disorder patients bipolar or unipolar?**

Unipolar (80%).

❍ **Which is most commonly the first episode of bipolar disease, mania or depression?**

Mania. Depression is rarely the first symptom. In fact, only 5 to 10% of patients who develop depression first, go on to have manic episodes.

❍ **First degree relatives of bipolar patients have a greater risk for which mental illnesses?**

Unipolar disorders and alcoholism.

❍ **Other than classic mania, what can lithium be used to treat?**

Bulimia, anorexia nervosa, alcoholism in patients with mood disorders, leucocytosis in patients on antineoplastic medication, cluster headaches, and migraine headaches.

❍ **Postural tremor is a major side effect of lithium. How is this side effect controlled?**

Minimize the dose during the workday and give small doses of beta-blockers.

❍ **Should people who are physically active have their lithium dosage increased or decreased?**

Increased. Lithium, a salt, is excreted more than sodium in sweat.

❍ **T/F: A patient starting lithium will be expected to gain weight.**

True. All psychotropic medications cause weight gain, hence lithium's usefulness in combating anorexia nervosa.

❍ **What is the potential complication associated with treating manic depression and congestive heart failure simultaneously?**

Lithium toxicity. A low salt diet and/or sodium-losing diuretics can cause lithium retention and toxicity.

❍ **Lithium toxicity begins at what level?**

14 mg/L. Above this level nausea, diarrhea, vomiting, rigidity, tremor, ataxia, seizures, delirium, coma, and death can occur.

❍ **Why can a patient taking lithium experience polyuria?**

Long-term lithium ingestion can cause nephrogenic diabetes.

What findings in a female patient who presents with parotid gland swelling and eroding tooth enamel might you expect?

Bulimia, which is associated with elevated serum amylase and hypokalemia.

What are some common laboratory findings associated with eating disorders?

Hyponatremia, hypokalemia, hypocalcemia, hypophosphatemia, anemia, hypoglycemia, starvation ketoacidosis, abnormal glucose tolerance, hypothyroidism due to low T3 levels, persistently elevated cortisol due to starvation, low FSH, LH and estrogens, and elevated growth hormone.

What is conversion disorder?

An internal psychological conflict that manifests itself through somatic symptoms. Voluntary motor or sensory functions are affected. Examples include weakness, imbalance, dysphagia, and changes in vision, hearing, or sensation. These symptoms are not feigned or intentionally produced. They are also not fully explained by medical conditions.

Name some over-the-counter and "street" drugs that may produce delirium or acute psychosis.

Salicylates, antihistamines, anticholinergics, alcohols, phencyclidine, LSD, mescaline, cocaine, and amphetamines.

What are eight common medical causes of depression?

(1) Stroke, (2) viral syndromes, (3) corticosteroids, (4) Cushing's disease, (5) antihypertensive medication, (6) SLE, (7) multiple sclerosis, and (8) subcortical dementias such as Huntington's and Parkinson's diseases and HIV encephalopathy.

What are some vegetative symptoms?

Loss of appetite, lack of concentration, chronic fatigue, agitation, restlessness, inability to sleep, and weight loss.

What is dysthymia?

Dysthymia is a chronic disorder that last for more than 2 years. The severe symptoms of depression, such as delusions and hallucinations, are absent. Patients with dysthymia have some good days, they react to their environment, and they have no vegetative signs. 10% of patients with dysthymia develop major depression.

Matching:

1) Hypomania	a) One or more hypomanias plus one or more major depressive symptoms
2) Melancholia	b) A mild manic episode
3) Bipolar II	c) Deep depression and vegetative characteristics
4) Unipolar mania	d) Manic episodes only
5) Cyclothymia	e) Many mild episodes of hypomania and depression

Answers: (1) b, (2) c, (3) a, (4) d, and (5) e.

What percentage of melancholic episodes are associated with hallucinations and/or delusions?

20%.

Wild and abundant dreams may result from the withdrawal of what drugs?

Antidepressants. Other side effects of withdrawal are anxiety, akathesia, bradykinesia, mania, and malaise.

What is a dystonic reaction?

A very common side effect of neuroleptics . It involves muscle spasms of the tongue, face, neck, and back. Severe laryngospasm and extraocular muscle spasms may also occur. Patients may bite their tongues, leading to an inability to open the mouth, to tongue edema, or to hemorrhage.

❍ **How do you treat a dystonic reaction?**

Diphenhydramine (Benadryl), 25 to 50 mg IM or IV, or benztropine (Cogentin), 1 to 2 mg IV or PO. Remember that dystonias can recur acutely.

❍ **What are the five Kubler-Ross stages of dying?**

1) Denial
2) Anger
3) Bargaining
4) Depression
5) Acceptance

Patients may undergo all or only a few of these stages.

❍ **What psychiatric disease is the most hereditary?**

Idiopathic enuresis. If one parent has enuresis, there is a 44% chance that the child will also have the disease. If both parents have it, the likelihood increases to 77%.

❍ **A 24 year-old male presents complaining of pleuritic pain, palpitations, dyspnea, dizziness, and tingling in his arms and legs. What is your diagnosis?**

Hyperventilation syndrome. This is frequently associated with anxiety. The tingling is caused by decreased carbonate levels in the blood.

❍ **Hallucinogens affect what neurotransmitter?**

Serotonin.

❍ **Who is at a greater risk for mood disorders, men or women?**

Women (7:3).

❍ **What is an extreme case of factitious disorder?**

Munchausen's syndrome. These patients may actually try to cause harm to themselves (e.g., by injecting feces into their veins) and are very accepting/seeking of invasive procedures. Munchausen by proxy is another example. In this disease, the patient seeks medical care for another, usually a child.

❍ **A 27 year-old male arrives somnolent with vitals of P: 130, R: 26, BP: 170/80, and T: 105° F. You note diffuse muscular rigidity and intermittent focal muscle twitching and/or jerking that lasts for 1 to 2 seconds. As you "work him up", your nurse returns from the waiting area with news from the family that the patient has had a progressive decline of mental status for the last 2 days, after seeing his psychiatrist. The patient has had a history of psychosis for almost a year. What process should be included in your differential diagnosis at this time?**

Neuroleptic malignant syndrome (NMS).

❍ **What labs would you expect to be elevated for the above patient?**

CPK is usually elevated, which correlates with a higher risk of fatality due to myoglobinuria. Serum alkaline phosphatase and serum aminotransferases are elevated. Leukocytosis with a left shift, hyponatremia, and hypokalemia are also present. Treatment for NMS is with dopaminergic agents, muscle relaxants, discontinuation of the neuroleptics, and supportive therapy. The mortality rate is 20%.

❍ **What is the difference between low potency and high potency neuroleptics?**

Low potency neuroleptics have greater sedative, postural hypotensive, and anticholinergic effects. High potency neuroleptics have greater extrapyramidal effects.

❍ **Neuroleptic medications come in low, medium, and high potency. What are some of these medicines and their categories?**

Low potency: Chlorpromazine (Thorazine)
Medium potency: Perphenazine (Trilafon)
High potency: Haloperidol, droperidol (Inapsine), thiothixene (Navane), fluphenazine (Prolixin), trifluoperazine (Stelazine)

❍ **Why shouldn't 600 mg/day of thioridazine (Mellaril) be exceeded?**

Exceeding this dosage causes retinitis pigmentosa. Thioridazine is a piperidine phenothiazine with low frequency extrapyramidal effects.

❍ **Why is Haloperidol one of the preferred neuroleptics?**

It can be used IM in emergencies plus it has few side effects. It does, however, have a high frequency of extrapyramidal effects.

❍ **What psychiatric disorder is associated with carcinoma of the pancreas?**

Depression.

❍ **What is the only neuroleptic with tardive dyskinesia as a side effect?**

Clozapine. Unfortunately, patients taking clozapine can develop agranulocytosis and are at a higher risk for seizures than patients on other neuroleptics. Other side effects include hypotension, anticholinergic symptoms, and oversedation.

❍ **You are considering chemical restraint. What are your options?**

Benzodiazepines: 1) Lorazepam (Ativan), 1 to 2 mg IV, 2 to 6 mg orally every 30 minutes
2) Midazolam (Versed), 2 to 4 mg IV every 30 minutes
3) Diazepam (Valium), 5 mg IV or orally every 30 minutes
Sedative hypnotics: 1) Haloperidol (Haldol), 1 to 5 mg IM/IV, titrate to clinical response
2) Droperidol (Inapsine), 1 to 2 mg IV every 30 minutes
Benzodiazepines may be given in combination with the sedative hypnotics above to both hasten and potentiate their effect. Titrate to effect and monitor appropriately.

❍ **A patient has ingested a phenothiazine and arrives hypotensive. What intervention(s) may be considered?**

IV crystalloid boluses usually suffice. Severe cases are best managed with norepinephrine (Levophed) or metaraminol (Aramine). These pressors stimulate α-adrenergic receptors preferentially. Beta-agonists, such as isoproterenol (Isuprel), are contraindicated due to the risks of beta-receptor-stimulated vasodilation.

❍ **What happens when ethanol is combined with an anxiolytic (benzodiazepine)?**

Death due to their combined respiratory depressive effects.

❍ **Name another contraindication to benzodiazepine use.**

Known hypersensitivity, acute narrow-angle glaucoma, and pregnancy, especially in the first trimester.

❍ **What should be used to treat a hypertensive crisis caused by the combination of MAO inhibitors with a known toxin?**

An α- and beta-adrenergic antagonist, such as labetalol. Also consider nifedipine or nitroglycerin. If unsuccessful, consider IV phentolamine or sodium nitroprusside.

❍ **Name some drugs contraindicated in a patient on MAO inhibitors.**

Meperidine (Demerol) and dextromethorphan can cause toxic reactions, such as excitation and hyperpyrexia. The effects of indirect-acting adrenergic drugs are potentiated, including ephedrine, sympathomimetic amines in cold remedies, amphetamines, cocaine, and methylphenidate (Ritalin).

❍ **Name the three common MAO inhibitors (chemical and brand name).**

1) Phenelzine (Nardil).
2) Isocarboxazid (Marplan).
3) Tranylcypromine (Parnate).

❍ **Obsessive compulsive disorders generally begin before what age?**

25.

❍ **What are some common obsessions?**

Dirt and contamination, order and symmetry, religion and philosophy, daily decisions. Unfortunately, compulsion does not relieve the anxiety of the obsession. Serotonin reuptake inhibitors and exposure therapy can be helpful.

❍ **What is organic brain syndrome?**

A reversible or irreversible mental condition believed to be caused by either disease or the use of a substance that interrupts normal anatomical, physiological, or biochemical brain functions.

❍ **A 20 year-old female complains of sudden episodes of palpitations, diaphoresis, lightheadedness, a fear of losing control, a sense of being choked, tremors, and paresthesias. What is the diagnosis?**

Panic disorder. Panic disorders need not be linked to any events, although they are commonly associated with agoraphobia, social phobia, mitral valve prolapse, and late non-melancholic depression.

❍ **What percentage of patients with panic disorder also suffer from major depression?**

50%. Patients who suffer from panic attacks generally have a low self-esteem.

❍ **Cite an example for each of the following perceptual disturbances: illusion, complete auditory hallucination, functional hallucination, and extracampine hallucination.**

Illusion: A kitten is perceived as a dragon. (The patient misinterprets reality.)

Complete auditory hallucination: The patient claims to hear people talking when no one is around. (Clear voices are reportedly heard. They are perceived as being external to the patient.)

Functional hallucination: The patient hears voices only when cars honk their horns. (Hallucinations occur only after sensory stimulus in the same category as the hallucination.)

Extracampine hallucination: The patient can see people waving from the top of the Eiffel Tower--even though she is in Chicago. (Hallucinations are external to the patient's normal range of senses.)

❍ **What is the most common phobia in men?**

Social phobia.

❍ **Can a person acquire posttraumatic stress disorder (PTSD) if they did not actually witness a disturbing event?**

Yes. According to the DSM-IV, one can experience PTSD if an event, such as a violent personal assault, a serious accident, or the serious injury of a close friend or family member, is learned of indirectly. PTSD can also occur after a person hears of a life-threatening disease affecting a friend or family member.

❍ **A 28 year-old female, who was raped 6 months ago, has been psychologically sound thus far. She now suddenly develops recurrent flashbacks of the rape, nightmares, intense fear, avoidance of all men, a diminished memory of the rape, and an exaggerated startle response. Is this woman experiencing PTSD?**

Yes. This is delayed-onset PTSD. The onset of symptoms occurs at least 6 months after the provoking event.

❍ **List some life-threatening causes of acute psychosis.**

WHHHIMP
Wernicke's encephalopathy.
Hypoxia.
Hypoglycemia.
Hypertensive encephalopathy.
Intracerebral hemorrhage.
Meningitis/encephalitis.
Poisoning.

❍ **What signs and symptoms suggest an organic source for psychosis?**

Acute onset, disorientation, visual or tactile hallucinations, age under 10 or over 60, and any evidence suggesting overdose or acute ingestion, such as abnormal vital signs, pupil size and reactivity, or nystagmus.

❍ **When are women at the greatest risk for psychiatric illness?**

The first few weeks postpartum. A psychiatric illness most often occurs in patients who are primiparous, have poor social support, or have a history of depression.

❍ **When does postpartum psychosis begin?**

Within a week to 10 days following childbirth. A second, smaller peak occurs 5 to 7 weeks later, correlating with the first menses postpartum. The risk of psychosis is lowest during pregnancy.

❍ **What is the difference between schizophrenia and schizophreniform disorder?**

Schizophreniform disorder implies the same signs and symptoms as schizophrenia, yet these symptoms have been present for less than 6 months. The impaired functioning in schizophreniform disorder is not consistent. Schizophreniform disorder is generally a provisional diagnosis with schizophrenia following.

❍ **What are some characteristics of schizophrenia?**

Delusional disorder, hallucinations (usually auditory), disorganized thinking, loosening of associations, disheveled appearance, and the inability to realize thoughts and behavior are abnormal.

❍ **What are the five first rank symptoms of Schneider?**

1) Experiences of influence.
2) Thought broadcasting.
3) Experiences of alienation.
4) Complete auditory hallucinations.
5) Delusional perceptions.

First-rank symptoms occur in 60 to 75% of schizophrenics. They also develop in patients with affective disorder, more commonly during manic stages.

❍ **What are the five criteria for diagnosing schizophrenia?**

1) Psychosis.
2) Emotional blunting.
3) Absence of affective features or episodes.
4) Clear consciousness.
5) Absence of coarse brain disease, systemic illness, and drug abuse.

❍ **What percentage of patients with schizophrenia become chronically ill?**

60 to 80%. Males are at a greater risk for chronic illness.

❍ **The onset of schizophrenia generally occurs by what age?**

Eighty percent of schizophrenics develop the disease before their early twenties. The disease is very rare after 40.

❍ **What are five causes of schizophrenia?**

1) Viral infection in the CNS.
2) Problem during pregnancy that affects the neuronal development.
3) Head injury.
4) Seizure disorder.
5) Street drugs.

❍ **Are first degree relatives of schizophrenics more likely to have schizoidia or schizophrenia?**

Schizoidia (3:1).

❍ **A patient who is unable to express his anger, has few close friends, is indifferent to praise from others, is absent-minded, and is emotionally cold and aloof, probably has which kind of personality disorder?**

Schizoidia.

❍ **What is the body's largest sex organ?**

The skin. It is also the body's largest overall organ.

❍ **What are eight classes of drugs that decrease sexual desire?**

(1) Antidepressants, (2) antihypertensives, (3) anticonvulsants, (4) neuroleptics, (5) digitalis, (6) cimetidine, (7) clofibrate, and (8) high doses or chronic ingestion of alcohol or street drugs.

❍ **What are four medical causes of sexual arousal disorder?**

(1) Leriche syndrome, (2) diabetes, (3) perineal surgery, and (4) transection of the spinal chord.

❍ **A child reared by a homosexual couple will most likely have what sexual orientation?**

Heterosexual.

❍ **Which populations have the greatest incidence of insomnia?**

Women and the elderly. Insomnia can involve trouble falling asleep or trouble staying asleep. It is generally initiated by a stressor in the patient's life.

❍ **In which stage of sleep do we spend the most time?**

Stage 2 accounts for 50% of our sleep. This stage is characterized by sleep spindles and K complexes on EEG. REM accounts for only 25% of our sleep.

❍ **Narcolepsy is a disorder of which sleep cycle?**

REM. Attacks of sleep, dreams, and paralysis last anywhere from 10 minutes to 1 hour. Amphetamines and planned naps throughout the day can help.

❍ **A 30 year-old female complains of calf pain, a headache, shooting pain when flexing her right wrist, random epigastric pain, bloating, and irregular menses, all of which cannot be explained after medical examination. What is the diagnosis?**

Somatization disorder--many unexplained medical symptoms involving multiple systems. In order to diagnose a patient with somatization disorder, one must have 4 or more unexplained pain symptoms. Symptoms generally begin in childhood and are fully developed by age 30. This is more common in women than men.

❍ **Who is more successful at suicide, men or women?**

Males (3:1). However, women attempt suicide 3 times as often as men.

❍ **Major depression and bipolar affective disorder account for what percentage of suicides?**

50%. Another 25% are due to substance abuse, and another 10% are attributed to schizophrenia.

❍ **What psychiatric problems are associated with violence?**

Acute schizophrenia, paranoid ideation, catatonic excitation, mania, borderline and antisocial personality disorders, delusional depression, posttraumatic stress disorder, and decompensating obsessive/compulsive disorder.

❍ **What are the prodromes of violent behavior?**

Anxiety, defensiveness, volatility, and physical aggression.

GYNECOLOGY PEARLS

To my embarrassment I was born in bed with a lady.
Wilson Mizner

❍ **What is the most common non-gynecologic condition presenting with lower abdominal pain?**

Appendicitis.

❍ **What is secondary amenorrhea?**

No menstruation for 6 months or more in a women who previously had regular menses.

❍ **What is the most common cause of secondary amenorrhea?**

Yes, the obvious: pregnancy. The second most common cause is hypothalamic hypogonadism, which can be due to weight loss, anorexia nervosa, stress, excessive exercise, or hypothalamic disease.

❍ **A 26 year-old with secondary amenorrhea and an essentially normal work-up is given an IM injection of 100 mg of progesterone and responds with a normal menstrual period. What does this tell you?**

She has a functional endometrium and a normal production of estrogen. Patients producing less than 40 pg/ml of estrogen will not bleed. This test is called the progesterone challenge.

❍ **What are the 2 major differential diagnoses in the above patient?**

Premature ovarian failure and hypothalamic dysfunction. Premature ovarian failure can be diagnosed if the serum LH level is greater than 25 mIU/ml; otherwise, the diagnosis is most likely hypothalamic dysfunction.

❍ **A patient with secondary amenorrhea fails the progesterone challenge and has a high FSH level. What is the problem?**

Gonadal failure. A low FSH level would be more indicative of hypothalamic dysfunction.

❍ **What is the treatment of choice for a Bartholin gland abscess?**

Marsupialization with the placement of a word catheter. This prevents recurrences.

❍ **A patient presents with pain in her eyes, chancre sores in her mouth, and sores and scars in her genital area. What is the diagnosis?**

Behcet's disease. This is a rare disease involving ocular inflammation, oral apthous ulcers, and destructive genital ulcers (generally on the vulva). No cure is known, but remission may occur with high estrogen levels.

❍ **What is the most common type of benign breast tumor?**

Fibroadenomas. These are usually solitary, mobile masses with distinct borders; they are more prevalent in women under age 30.

❍ **What medicines are contraindicated in breast-feeding mothers?**

Tetracycline, warfarin, and chloramphenicol.

❍ **What are the most common cancers in women?**

Lung cancer > Breast cancer > Colorectal cancer.

❍ **What are the most deadly cancers in women?**

Lung cancer > breast cancer > colorectal cancer.

❍ **Are the majority of breast cancers in the ducts or in the lobes?**

Invasive ductal tumors account for 90% of all breast cancers. Only 10% are lobular.

❍ **What is the most common invasive ductal tumor?**

Nonspecific infiltrating ductal carcinoma.

❍ **A 53 year-old female presents with a hard, barely palpable lump in the upper, outer quadrant of her left breast. The lump is mobile and causes no pain. The patient has noted blood oozing from her nipple. What is the most likely diagnosis?**

Benign intraductal papilloma. Intraductal papillomas are the most common cause of bleeding from the nipple. Growths usually develop just before or during menopause, and they are rarely palpable.

❍ **What are the American Cancer Society's 1996 recommendations for mammography?**

Every 1 to 2 years after age 40. Annually after age 50.

❍ **What are the risk factors for breast cancer, and how do they compare with the risk factors for endometrial cancer?**

Risk factors for both cancers include nulliparity, early menarche, late menopause, significant amounts of unopposed estrogen, and prior ovarian, endometrial, or breast cancer. Unopposed estrogen is a much greater risk in endometrial cancer than in breast cancer. Risk factors specific to breast cancer include family history, age over 40, high fat intake, radiation of the breast, or cellular atypia in fibrocystic disease.

❍ **Geographically, where is breast cancer most common?**

North America and northern Europe have an incidence and mortality rate 5 times that of most Asian and African countries. However, while Asians and Africans who immigrate to North America or northern Europe maintain a lower rate of incidence, their offspring quickly assume a higher one. This points to environmental and dietary factors.

❍ **What is the surgical treatment of choice for breast cancer?**

Modified radical mastectomy--removal of the breast tissue, pectoralis minor, and axilla. (A radical mastectomy includes the pectoralis major). For small primary tumors, a partial mastectomy may be performed. This is a local lumpectomy with axillary node dissection and postoperative irradiation of the breast. It has not been shown that radiation following a modified radical mastectomy improves survival.

❍ **Which types of chemotherapy are most commonly used against breast cancer?**

Cyclophosphamide (C), adriamycin (A), methotrexate (M), and 5-fluorouracil (F). Combinations are most effective: CMF or AC. Chemotherapy increases the chance of survival for pre-menopausal patients by about 15%.

❍ **Who have higher incidences of estrogen receptor positive tumors, pre-menopausal or postmenopausal women?**

Post-menopausal (60%). If the tumors are both estrogen and progesterone sensitive, then the anti-estrogen drug tamoxifen is 80% effective. Otherwise, it is 40 to 50% effective.

❍ **What is the most accurate prognostic indicator of breast cancer?**

Axillary node involvement, which is related to the size of the tumor, not the location. 40 to 50% of patients have axillary node involvement when diagnosed.

❍ **A patient presents with crusty erosion of the nipple and no discharge. What is the possible diagnosis?**

Paget's disease. This rare cancer occurs in 3% of breast cancer patients. It involves the excretory ducts of the breast.

❍ **What is peau d'orange?**

French for skin of the orange. It is the dimpling and thickening of the breast in breast cancer.

❍ **What are the American Cancer Society's 1996 recommendations for Pap smears?**

Annually for 3 years, starting at age 18, or when the patient becomes sexually active, and every 1 to 3 years, thereafter.

❍ **What percentage of cervical cancers are squamous cell?**

85%.

❍ **Where does cervical cancer most commonly metastasize?**

The liver.

❍ **When is a woman most likely to get choriocarcinoma?**

50% of choriocarcinoma cases occur in conjunction with molar pregnancies. The remaining half can occur with normal, aborted, or ectopic pregnancies. If there are any signs of metastasis (e.g. vaginal bleeding, dyspnea, rectal bleeding, or hemoptysis) in a woman who has recently been pregnant, strongly consider gestational choriocarcinoma.

❍ **What are the rates of pregnancy with the following forms of birth control: (1) surgical sterilization, intrauterine devices, or oral contraceptives; (2) coitus interruptus and rhythm method; (3) condoms; and (4) foams, jellies, sponges, or diaphragms?**

(1) 0.2 to 2%; (2) 10%; (3) 12%; and (4) 18 to 20%.

❍ **How long after the removal of Norplant capsules must patients wait to become pregnant?**

Ovulation usually occurs within 3 months.

❍ **What chemical changes may predispose patients taking oral contraceptives to weight gain?**

Increases in low-density lipoproteins, decreases in high-density lipoproteins, and sodium retention.

❍ **A 66 year-old woman presents with vaginal bleeding. What is your provisional diagnosis?**

Endometrial cancer. 15% of women with postmenopausal bleeding have endometrial cancer. 30% of these tumors are due to exogenous estrogens, 30% are due to atrophic endometriosis or vaginitis, 10% are due to cervical polyps, and 5% are due to endometrial hyperplasia. Most tumors are caught in stage I.

❍ **What are the risk factors of endometrial cancer?**

Endometrial cancer correlates highly with estrogen levels. Early menarche, late menopause, obesity, nulliparity, anovulation in the reproductive years, and unopposed estrogen are all risk factors. Diabetes, gallbladder disease, and breast, colon and ovarian cancers are additional risk factors.

❍ **What percentage of the female population has endometriosis?**

More than 15%. 7% of these women have it during their reproductive years.

❍ **What is the most common site of endometriosis?**

The ovaries (60%).

❍ **What is the drug of choice for treating endometriosis?**

Danazol.

❍ **Can ecclampsia occur postpartum?**

Yes. It can occur up to 2 weeks postpartum.

❍ **Where do enteroceles, due to a herniation, most commonly occur?**

The pouch of Douglas.

❍ **Spontaneous labor will occur within 3 weeks of fetal death in what percentage of patients?**

80%. It may be helpful to induce labor with vaginal suppositories due to the psychological effects of carrying a dead baby.

❍ **What is the treatment for gestational diabetes?**

Diet, insulin, and exercise. Do not give patients oral hypoglycemics because these cross the blood-brain barrier.

❍ **When should you be most concerned about a pregnant patient with heart disease?**

During weeks 18 to 24, when the female body experiences a maximal increase in cardiac output (40%).

❍ **What is the most common heart problem in pregnant women?**

Congenital heart disease.

❍ **How much blood does a standard size pad absorb?**

20 to 30 ml. This is useful to know when trying to estimate blood loss.

❍ **In hyperprolactinemia, the serum prolactin level is higher than:**

400 ng/ml. Hyperprolactinemia is caused by pituitary adenomas, hypothyroidism, or drugs, such as reserpine, methyldopa, phenothiazine, or oral contraceptives. Clinically, patients do not menstruate, and they have galactorrhea.

❍ **What percentage of American couples are infertile?**

15%. 20% of women in the US above 35 are infertile.

❍ **What are the numbers for a normal semen analysis?**

> 1 ml in volume (> 20,000,000 sperm) with > 50% motility.

❍ **What percentage of infertility is due to the male factor?**

40%. Problems with the cervix, uterus, fallopian tubes, peritoneum, or ovulation account for the remaining 60%.

❍ **A breast-feeding mother presents to your office complaining of fever, chills, and a swollen, red breast. What is the most likely causative organism?**

Staphylococcus aureus is the most common cause of mastitis. Mastitis is seldom present in the first week postpartum. It is most often seen 3 to 4 weeks postpartum.

❍ **Matching--time to keep those M's straight:**

1) Menorrhagia a) Bleeding between menstrual periods
2) Metrorrhagia (hypermenorrhea) b) Excessive amount of blood or duration
3) Menometrorrhagia c) Excessive amount of blood at irregular frequencies

Answers: (1) b, (2) a, and (3) c.

❍ **Matching--101 more ways to describe menstrual bleeding:**

1) Hypermenorrhea a) Menstrual periods > 35 days apart
2) Oligomenorrhea b) Menstrual periods < 21 days apart
3) Polymenorrhea c) Menorrhagia

Answers: (1) c, (2) a, and (3) b.

❍ **If a woman has ascites, what is the most likely tumor to be found?**

An ovarian carcinoma. This is part of Meigs' syndrome.

❍ **What is Meigs' syndrome?**

Ascites and hydrothorax in the presence of an ovarian tumor.

❍ **What levels of FSH and LH would you expect in a 63 year-old woman who is not on estrogen replacement therapy?**

High levels of both FSH and LH. The ovarian response to FSH and LH is decreased in menopause. Consequently, there is less estrogen and progesterone being produced, hence, no negative feedback inhibits the rising FSH and LH.

❍ **What are some causes of premature menopause?**

Smoking, radiation, chemotherapy, and anything else that limits the ovarian blood supply.

❍ **Morning sickness is due to increased levels of what?**

Beta-HCG.

❍ **What is the most common complication of ovarian cysts?**

Torsion of the ovary. Torsion is more common in small to medium-sized tumors. Emergency surgery is required.

❍ **What are the most common sites for metastasis of ovarian carcinoma?**

The peritoneum and omentum.

❍ **T/F: A woman with pelvic inflammatory disease (PID) is likely to have an exacerbation of symptoms when she menstruates.**

True. The breakdown of the cervical mucus antibacterial barrier allows bacteria to ascend from the lower tract to the upper tract. Pelvic examination, intercourse, and exercise can all exacerbate symptoms.

❍ **What two organisms cause most cases of PID?**

Neisseria gonorrhea and Chlamydia trachomatis.

❍ **Which patients with PID should be admitted?**

Admit patients who are pregnant, have a temperature > 38° C (100.4° F), are nauseated or vomiting (which prohibits oral antibiotics), have pyosalpinx or tubo-ovarian abscess peritoneal signs, have IUCD, show no response to oral antibiotics, or for whom diagnosis is uncertain.

❍ **What are the criteria for diagnosis of PID?**

All of the following must be present: (1) adnexal tenderness, (2) cervical and uterine tenderness, and (3) abdominal tenderness. In addition, one of the following must be present: (1) temperature > 38° C, (2) endocervix Gram's stain positive for gram-negative intracellular diplococci, (3) leukocytosis > 10,000/mm^3, (4) inflammatory mass on ultrasound or pelvic examination, or (5) WBC's and bacteria in the peritoneal fluid.

❍ **What kind of changes occur in the cardiovascular system of a pregnant patient?**

Plasma volume increases 50%, pulse increases 12 to 18 beats per minute, stroke volume increases 25%, and hematocrit drops, due to hemodilution.

❍ **What causes dependent and non-dependent edema in pregnant women?**

Compression of veins by the growing uterus cause dependent edema, whereas hypoalbuminemia can cause non-dependent edema.

❍ **What is pregnancy-induced hypertension?**

An increase in the systolic pressure > 30 mm Hg or an increase in diastolic pressure > 15 mm Hg over base line, measured on 2 separate occasions, at least 6 hours apart.

❍ **What is Sheehan's syndrome?**

Anterior pituitary necrosis following postpartum hemorrhage and hypotension. It results in amenorrhea, decreased breast size, and decreased pubic hair.

❍ **What predisposes a woman to yeast infections?**

Diabetes, oral contraceptives, and antibiotics.

❍ **What is the most common cause of vaginitis?**

Candida albicans.

❍ **A patient presents with a 2 day history of vaginal itching and burning. On examination, you note a thin, yellowish, green bubbly discharge and petechiae on the cervix (also known as a "strawberry cervix"). What test do you perform, and what do you expect to find?**

Mix the discharge with saline and view under a microscope. If you see Trichomonas vaginalis (mobile and pear-shaped protozoa with flagella), then the patient should be treated with Metronidazole (Flagyl).

❍ **A 20 year-old sexually active female presents to your office complaining of a heavy thin discharge with an unpleasant odor. Adding 10% KOH to the discharge produces a fishy odor. What would you expect to see on microscopic examination?**

"Clue cells", which are epithelial cells with bacilli attached to their surfaces. This patient has Gardnerella vaginitis. The patient and her partner should both be treated with Metronidazole (Flagyl).

❍ **When should you avoid treating a woman with Flagyl?**

If she is in her first trimester, Metronidazole may have teratogenic effects. Clotrimazole (Gyne-Lotrimin) may be used instead. Side effects of Flagyl include nausea, vomiting, and metallic tastes. It acts similarly to disulfiram (Antabuse), and therefore, should not be taken with alcohol.

❍ **A 30 year-old female complains of a painful sore on her vulva that resembled a pimple at first. On examination, you find an ulcer with vague borders and a gray base. What is the probable diagnosis?**

Gram's stain, culture, and biopsy (used in combination because of the high false-negative rates) should show that this woman has chanchroid, caused by Haemophilus ducreyi. Treatment is erythromycin or ceftriaxone.

❍ **Condylomata acuminata frequently occurs in combination with what other STD?**

Trichomonas vaginitis.

❍ **What is the most common cause of septic arthritis in young adults?**

Disseminated gonococcal infection.

❍ **What is the treatment for gonorrhea?**

Ceftriaxone and doxycycline. The latter is given because half of the patients infected with gonorrhea are simultaneously infected with chlamydia.

❍ **What is the predominant organism in a healthy female's vaginal discharge?**

Lactobacilli (95%).

❍ **A 34 year-old female presents with a maculopapular rash on her palms and soles. She complains of headaches and general weakness. On examination, you find she has multiple condyloma lata and lymphadenopathy. What is the diagnosis?**

Secondary syphilis. This develops 6 to 9 weeks after the syphilitic chancre, which will have resolved by this time. If it goes untreated, tertiary syphilis will develop. This can affect all the tissues in the body, including the CNS and the heart. Treatment is with penicillin G.

❍ **Is the Stein-Leventhal syndrome a unilateral or bilateral phenomenon?**

Bilateral. Both ovaries are cystic and enlarged with a thickened and fibrosed tunica. Patients are often infertile, obese, and hirsute.

❍ **What is the number one cause of UTI's in males?**

Chlamydia trachomatis.

❍ **Chlamydia only invades what kind of epithelium?**

Columnar epithelium.

❍ **What are some common teratogens?**

Alcohol, anticonvulsants, Coumadin, DES, isotretinoin, lithium, methimazole, and propylthiouracil.

❍ **What causes toxic shock syndrome (TSS)?**

An exotoxin, composed of certain strains of Staphylococcus aureus. Other organisms that cause toxic shock syndrome are group A streptococci, Pseudomonas aeruginosa, and Streptococcus pneumoniae. Tampons, IUD's, septic abortions, sponges, soft tissue abscesses, osteomyelitis, nasal packing, and postpartum infections all can house these organisms.

❍ **What dermatological changes occur with TSS?**

Initially, the patient will have a blanching erythematous rash that lasts for 3 days. After 10 days from the start of the infection, there will be a full thickness desquamation of the palms and soles.

❍ **What criteria are necessary for the diagnosis of TSS?**

All of the following must be present: T > 38.9° C (102° F), rash, systolic BP < 90, orthostasis, involvement of 3 organ systems (GI, renal, musculoskeletal, mucosal, hepatic, hematologic, or CNS), and negative serologic tests for diseases such as RMSF, hepatitis B, measles, leptospirosis, VDRL, etc.

❍ **How should a patient with TSS be treated?**

Fluids, pressure support, fresh frozen plasma or transfusions, vaginal irrigation with iodine or saline, and anti-staphylococcal penicillin or cephalosporin with anti-beta-lactamase activity (nafcillin or oxacillin). Rifampin should be considered to eliminate the carrier state.

❍ **A 42 year-old woman complains of painful urination and bleeding and "leaking a bit" after she urinates. On pelvic examination, you feel a small mass under the urethra that emits a purulent discharge from the urethral meatus when compressed. What is the diagnosis?**

Urethral diverticulum.

❍ **What is the most common type of urinary fistula?**

Vesico-vaginal fistulas. They most commonly occur after surgical procedures, but they can also occur with invasive cervical carcinoma or radiotherapy due to cervical cancer.

❍ **What is the number one cause of urinary tract infections?**

E. coli. Other causative agents are also gram-negative.

❍ **What causes condylomata acuminata (venereal warts)?**

Human papilloma virus types 6 and 11.

❍ **A 24 year-old female presents with fever, aches and pains, and painful sores that looked like blisters before they popped and began to hurt. What would you expect to find on culture of the vesicular fluid?**

Multinucleated giant cells by Giemsa stain. This patient most likely has HPV type 2

❍ **What subtypes of HPV are associated with cervical cancer?**

HPV types 16, 18, and 31 are risk factors for cervical dysplasia, which can lead to cervical cancer. Multiple sexual partners and early onset of sexual activity are also risk factors for cervical cancer.

❍ **Tumors of the vulva most commonly occur in which population?**

Postmenopausal women.

❍ **What is the precursor of epidermoid carcinoma of the vulva?**

Leukoplakia.

❍ **Describe the effect pregnancy has on (1) cardiac output, (2) BP, (3) heart rate, (4) coagulation, (5) sedimentation rate, (6) leukocytes, (7) blood volume, (8) tidal volume, (9) bladder, (10) BUN/Cr, and (11) GI.**

1) Cardiac output:	Increases (moving the uterus off the IVC increases cardiac output 25%)
2) BP:	Falls in second trimester; returns to normal in third
3) Heart rate:	Increases
4) Coagulation:	Factors 7, 8, 9, and 10 and fibrinogen increase; others remain unchanged
5) Sed rate:	Elevates
6) Leukocytes:	Increase (up to 18,000)
7) Blood volume:	Increases; no change in RBC; dilutional "anemia" is physiologic
8) Tidal volume:	Increases 40%
9) Bladder:	Displaces superiorly and anteriorly

10) BUN/Cr:	Decreases because of increased GFR and renal blood flow
11) GI:	Gastric emptying and GI motility decrease; alkaline phosphatase increases; peritoneal signs such as rigidity and rebound are diminished or absent

❍ **What anticoagulant should be used in pregnant patients?**

Heparin. It does not cross the placenta.

❍ **What antiemetic should be used in pregnant patients?**

Prochlorperazine (Compazine) or trimethobenzamide (Tigan).

❍ **What is the most common surgical complication during pregnancy?**

Appendicitis. Cholecystitis is the second most common.

❍ **Is appendicitis more common during pregnancy?**

No. (Occurs in 1 out of 850 pregnancies). However, the outcome is worse. The WBC count usually does not increase beyond the normal value of 12,000 to 15,000. In a pregnant patient, pyuria with no bacteria suggests appendicitis. Pregnant patients may lack GI distress, and fever may be absent or low-grade.

❍ **How is the appendix displaced during pregnancy?**

Superiorly and laterally. Diagnosis of appendicitis in pregnant patients may be further complicated by the fact that a normal pregnancy can itself cause an increased WBC. Prompt diagnosis is important because the incidence of perforation increases from 10% in the first trimester to 40% in the third.

❍ **What viral or protozoal infections require extensive work-up during pregnancy?**

ToRCH
Toxoplasma gondii
Rubella
Cytomegalovirus
Herpes genitalis

❍ **Can iodinated radiodiagnostic agents be used in pregnant patients?**

No. They should be avoided because concentration in the fetal thyroid can cause permanent loss of thyroid function. Nuclear medicine scans, pulmonary angiography with pelvic shielding, and impedance plethysmography are preferred.

IMAGING PEARLS

No man really becomes a fool until he stops asking questions.
Charles Steinmetz

❍ **What is an ABI, and why is it significant?**

An ankle/brachial index. The ankle systolic pressure (numerator) is compared to the higher of the 2 brachial arterial pressures (denominator). It is used to determine if arterial obstruction is present.

❍ **What technical factors can affect the accuracy of the ABI?**

Probe pressure, rapid deflation of the BP cuff, arterial wall calcifications, and probe placement, which should be longitudinal to the vessel and at a 30 to 60 degree angle to the skin surface.

❍ **What is the diagnostic test of choice for documenting DVT?**

Duplex ultrasound. The accuracy of physical examination for DVT is generally quoted to be 50%.

❍ **What are some of the advantages and disadvantages of DPL, CT, and ultrasound for assessing trauma patients?**

	Advantages	Disadvantages
DPL	Low complication rate, Done at bedside	Invasive, time-consuming, can't identify retroperitoneal injury, significant false positive rate
CT	Identifies location and extent of injury, including the retroperitoneum	Expensive, time-consuming, requires travel and interpretation expertise, patient monitoring is not optimal
US	Fast, cheap, noninvasive, done at bedside, good for hemoperitoneum	Operator-dependent, not good for identifying specific organ injurys

❍ **When is surgical repair of abdominal aortic aneurysms (AAA) is generally indicated?**

Aneurysm measuring >4 cm. Ultrasound is extremely sensitive for detecting AAA, but it is not sensitive for the detection of ruptured AAA.

❍ **What is the incidence of allergic reaction to IV contrast materials?**

Severe allergic reactions occur in approximately 1/14,000 patients; fatal reactions occur in about 1/40,000 cases.

❍ **What is the prevalence of adverse reactions to ionic and nonionic contrast materials?**

Ionic: 12.7%. Nonionic: 3.1%. Adverse reactions to nonionic contrast include hypotension, bronchospasm, arrhythmia, angioneurotic edema, urticaria, flushing, nausea, and vomiting. It is unclear whether or not nonionic materials are less nephrotoxic than ionic materials.

❍ **T/F: Oral contrast should be avoided in patients with marginal renal function.**

False. Little nephrotoxic iodine is absorbed with oral contrast administration. When barium is used, it is inert and not absorbed.

❍ **What contraindicates oral iodine or barium contrast?**

Barium cannot be given when complete colon obstruction exists or intestinal perforation is suspected. Severe allergy to iodine is the only contraindication to oral iodine-containing preparations.

❍ **T/F: IV contrast material is contraindicated in chronic renal failure.**

False. The contrast material can be dialyzed, and the kidney is already maximally impaired.

❍ **What is the typical shape and vessel origin of a subdural hematoma (SDH) and an epidural hematoma (EDH) on CT scan?**

An SDH is typically crescent-shaped. It can be arterial in origin but is most often caused by the tearing of bridging veins. An acute SDH is hyperdense relative to the brain and becomes isodense to the brain in 1 to 3 weeks. An EDH is biconvex (lenticular) and usually arterial in origin. An EDH does not cross intact skull sutures, but can cross the tentorium and the midline.

❍ **What percentage of subdural hematomas are bilateral?**

About 25%.

❍ **What is the test of choice for evaluating and staging renal trauma?**

IV contrast-enhanced CT. CT is more accurate than IVP because IVP is not sensitive for renal injuries.

❍ **The magnetic fields of an MRI can be detrimental to patients with what?**

Ferrous metal in their body or electrical equipment whose function can be disrupted by strong magnetic fields. Examples include pacemakers, metal foreign bodies in the eye (e.g., welders), ferromagnetic cerebral aneurysm clips (unless they are made of nonmagnetic steel), and cochlear implants. Relative contraindications for an MRI include certain prosthetic heart valves, implantable defibrillators, bone growth, and neurostimulators. One might also include patients who are claustrophobic.

❍ **Although bone scans are useful for detecting subtle fractures missed on x-ray, why is it not always useful in the emergency setting for recent fractures?**

Bone scans may not pick up the increased bone turnover until hours or days after trauma, because skeletal uptake is dependent on blood flow and osteoblastic activity. A positive scan demonstrates asymmetric skeletal uptake.

❍ **Are radionucleotide studies most helpful in determining the bleeding site in upper or lower GI bleeds?**

Lower.

❍ **What two studies can detect testicular torsion and differentiate it from epididymitis, orchitis, or torsion of the appendix testis?**

Technetium 99m nuclear studies and duplex ultrasound.

PREVENTIVE PEARLS

To cease smoking is the easiest thing I ever did;
I ought to know because I've done it a thousand times.
Mark Twain

❍ **When is screening the population for a disease appropriate?**

When the disease is prevalent, when failure to catch the disease results in significant morbidity, when appropriate screening tests exist, or when therapy initiated due to the early detection will significantly alter the pattern of the disease.

❍ **Matching:**

1) Sensitive	a) Actual positives/total number of positive test results
2) Specific	b) Actual positives/total number with the disease
3) Positive predictive value	c) Actual negatives/total number without the disease
4) Negative predictive value	d) Actual negatives/total number of negative test results

Answers: (1) b, (2) c, (3) a, and (4) d.

❍ **What is the equation for prevalence of a disease?**

Incidence of a disease multiplied by its duration.

❍ **What is the difference between standard error of the mean (SEM) and standard deviation (SD)?**

SEM measures the uncertainty in the estimation of the mean. It represents the mean value of a collection of several sample means and is thus closer to the true mean of a population. SD measures the variability in a given population.

❍ **What is a retrospective study?**

A study in which people who have a disease are compared to those who don't.

❍ **Match the prevention with the example that fits.**

1) Primary prevention	a) Tetanus booster shots every 10 years
2) Secondary prevention	b) Controlling blood sugar with appropriate diet and insulin
3) Tertiary prevention	c) Identifying and treating a patient with asymptomatic diabetes mellitus

Answers: (1) a, (2) c, and (3) b.

Primary prevention prevents a disease from ever occurring.
Secondary prevention prevents future problems if actions are taken during an asymptomatic period.
Tertiary prevention prevents further complications in a disease that is already present.

❍ **What are the top 10 causes of death in the US?**

1) Heart disease	6) Accidents
2) Cancer	7) Pneumonia and influenza
3) Stroke	8) Diabetes
4) HIV	9) Suicide
5) COPD	10) Homicide

❍ **What immunizations are recommended for patients with HIV?**

1) IPV and Td every 10 years
2) Influenza vaccine yearly
3) Pneumococcal vaccine once
4) Hepatitis B vaccine for at risk patients
5) Hib and MMR are optional

❍ **At what point should AZT treatment begin in an asymptomatic patient with HIV?**

When the CD-4+ count reaches 300 cells/mm^3 and 500 cells/mm^3, respectively.

❍ **What is the prophylactic regime of choice for PCP in patients with AIDS?**

Trimethoprim-sulfamethoxazole DS should be started when the CD-4+ count reaches 200 cells/mm^3.

❍ **At what point should prophylaxis treatment against mycobacterium avium-intracellulare and toxoplasmosis be started in patients with AIDS?**

When the CD-4+ count reaches 100 cells/mm^3.

❍ **What percentage of untreated group A beta-hemolytic streptococcal infections will progress to rheumatic fever?**

3%. Increased incidence of the disease is noted in lower socioeconomic areas.

❍ **What medication is the best treatment for preventing nephropathy in diabetic patients?**

ACE inhibitors. They are found to reduce endpoint renal disease, dialysis, and transplantation by 50%.

❍ **T/F: Patients with hypertension are at a greater risk for CAD and stroke than the normal population.**

True. Hypertensive patients have a 3 to 4 times greater risk of CAD and a 7 times greater risk of stroke.

❍ **What is the routine health screening for an asymptomatic 56 year-old male with no significant risk factors?**

History and physical, stool test for occult blood, serum cholesterol test, syphilis test, and a flexible sigmoidoscopy every 3 to 5 years.

❍ **People with elevated serum cholesterol have a greater risk for cardiovascular disease. Decreasing one's cholesterol by 1% reduces the risk of death due to heart disease by what percentage?**

2%.

❍ **Death rates from CAD are down 40% from 15 years ago. What is the major cause of this reduction?**

Changes in eating and exercise habits.

❍ **Match the poison with the antidote.**

1) Acetaminophen	a) Deferoxamine
2) Anticholinergics	b) Digoxin antibody
3) Arsenic	c) Dimercaptosuccinic acid or penicillamine
4) Carbon monoxide	d) Acetylcysteine (Mucomyst)
5) Digoxin	e) Oxygen
6) Iron	f) Atropine
7) Lead	g) Physostigmine
8) Mercury	h) Calcium EDTA or penicillamine

9) Methanol or ethylene glycol i) Naloxone (Narcan)
10) Narcotics j) Ethanol
11) Organophosphates k) Penicillamine

Answers: (1) d, (2) g, (3) k, (4) e, (5) b, (6) a, (7) h, (8) c, (9) j, (10) i, and (11) f.

❍ **What percentage of deaths due to CHD can be attributed to smoking?**

25%. Smokers with CHD have a 70% higher incidence of MI and death than non-smokers with CHD.

❍ **Is a nonsmoker who has lived with a smoker for 25 years at greater risk of lung cancer than a nonsmoker who has not lived with a smoker?**

Of course. The risk is 1.34 times as great as a person living in a smoke-free environment.

❍ **What percentage of smokers who quit lapse back into their smoking habits?**

85%.

❍ **What is the most common cause of blindness in the elderly?**

Cataracts.

❍ **What percentage of people over 65 live independently?**

80%. By age 85, only 54% of men and 38% of women still live independently at home.

❍ **Smoking does not increase the risk for what type of cancer?**

Thyroid cancer.

❍ **What must be checked in a patient with Down's syndrome before medical clearance can be given for participation in sports?**

Atlantoaxial instability ruled out by means of cervical roentgenograms. 10 to 20% of children with Down's syndrome have unstable atlantoaxial joints.

❍ **What percentage of teenage girls have eating disorders?**

20%.

❍ **What is used to control outbreaks of meningococcal meningitis?**

Rifampin and ceftriaxone are used as chemoprophylaxis for contacts. A vaccine for groups A, C, Y, and W-135 is available and widely used, even though most outbreaks are caused by strains A, B, C, and W-135.

❍ **How do you adjust for creatinine clearance in senior citizens?**

$$\text{Male creatinine clearance} = \frac{140 - \text{age}}{\text{serum creatinine}}$$

$$\text{Female creatinine clearance} = \frac{(140 - \text{age}) \times .85}{\text{serum creatinine}}$$

❍ **At what age can routine Pap smears be discontinued?**

Age 70, if the patient has had several negative examinations. Cervical cancer reaches a plateau, so further screening is not necessary.

❍ **A patient is brought in because she believes butterflies are landing all around her. The butterflies talk to her and tell her to love everyone. She denies suicidal ideation and any desire to**

harm herself or others. She has no record of harming people in the past. Can this person be institutionalized against her will?

No. Unless the patient is a danger to herself or others, she cannot be confined to an institution despite questionable mental status.

❍ **Geographically, where is multiple sclerosis most prevalent?**

In the northern US. Migration to warmer climates does not seem to affect the disease. People born in the north will still have a higher incidence of the disease.

❍ **What prophylactic medication would you recommend to a patient travelling to Costa Rica?**

Mefloquine, 250 mg, once a week. Treatment should begin 1 week before travel and continue 6 weeks after returning. Mefloquine, not chloroquine, is now the drug of choice due to the resistance of chloroquine in some regions. Check with the CDC for specific information.

❍ **What is the most virulent strain of malaria?**

Plasmodium falciparum. It can cause CNS changes and even death.

❍ **What preventive measures would you recommend to a patient planning a trip to Mexico?**

Avoidance of water, ice, foods prepared in water, and raw or pre-peeled fruits and vegetables. Prophylactic antibiotics are not routinely recommended. However, if they are a necessity, Ciprofloxacin is the drug of choice. Otherwise, treatment with antibiotics should begin with the onset of symptoms, as should rehydration.

❍ **A friend is headed to Benin on the West Coast of Africa. What immunizations and prophylactic treatments must she receive before departing?**

1) Hepatitis A vaccine
2) Oral polio vaccine
3) Tetanus-diptheria vaccine
4) Live oral typhoid vaccine
5) Measles vaccine
6) Yellow fever vaccine
7) Mefloquine prophylaxis for malaria

❍ **Should pregnant women abstain from intercourse?**

There is no risk to mother or fetus if mother engages in sex with no more than one orgasm at a time in the first 2 trimesters. In the third trimester, anorgasmic intercourse is safe until the 34th week. Intercourse should be avoided if there is bleeding.

❍ **What percentage of lung cancer is related to smoking?**

80%.

❍ **What types of cancer are more common in farmers?**

Cancer of the lip, Hodgkin's disease, leukemia, malignant melanoma, multiple myeloma, and prostate cancer.

❍ **What are the four most common cancers in men?**

1) Skin cancer
2) Lung cancer
3) Colorectal cancer
4) Prostate cancer

❍ **What cancer causes the most deaths in men?**

1) Lung cancer
2) Colorectal cancer

3) Prostate cancer

❍ **Overall, cancer deaths have increased 7% between 1971 and 1991. What cancers have actually shown a decrease in death rates?**

Cancer of the bladder, colon, cervix, larynx, mouth, pharynx, stomach, testes, thyroid, uterus.

❍ **What is the incubation period of the Epstein-Barr virus?**

30 to 50 days.

❍ **Why is it important to identify food service workers with furunculosis?**

Furunculosis is most commonly caused by coagulase-positive staphylococcus. Staphylococcal enterotoxin is a leading cause of food poisoning.

❍ **Ingestion of benzene, an ingredient in pesticides, detergent, and paint remover, causes dermatitis, leukemia, and aplastic anemia. How can it be identified as a causative agent in such illnesses?**

Phenol, the metabolite, can be found in the urine.

❍ **Which has a longer incubation period, staphylococci or salmonellae?**

Salmonellae. It is generally ingested in small doses and then multiplies in the GI tract. Symptoms occur 6 to 48 hours after ingestion. Staphylococcus aureus has an incubation period of just 3 hours.

❍ **What is the biggest risk factor for prostate cancer?**

Age. The median age for diagnosis of prostate cancer is 72.

❍ **Name 7 risk factors for malignant melanoma.**

1) Fair skin
2) Sensitivity to sunlight
3) Excessive exposure to the sun
4) Dysplastic moles
5) 6 or more moles > 0.5 cm
6) Prior basal or squamous cell carcinoma
7) Parental history of skin cancer

❍ **What percentage of melanomas occur in sun-exposed areas?**

Only 65%. A good screen of all surface area is important. In African American, Hispanic, and Asian patients, acral lentiginous melanomas are more common. Careful examination of subungual, palmar, and plantar surfaces is important in these populations.

❍ **What percentage of American adults are obese?**

30 to 40%.

❍ **What percentage of obesity can be attributed to genetics?**

25 to 30%.

❍ **What percentage of obesity can be attributed to organic causes?**

1%.

❍ **Which malignancies are more common in obese individuals?**

Endometrial cancer, breast cancer (post-menopausal), gallbladder cancer, biliary cancer, prostate cancer, and colorectal cancer.

❍ **What disease is found only in obese individuals?**

Pickwickian syndrome. This syndrome involves hypoventilation, right ventricular failure, secondary polycythemia, and somnolence.

❍ **Obesity is a risk factor for what common diseases?**

CAD, NIDDM, HTN, left ventricular hypertrophy, sleep apnea, cholelithiasis, pulmonary emboli, and osteoarthritis.

❍ **What is the risk of sudden death in morbidly obese patients compared to patients with normal body mass index (BMI)?**

15 to 30 times higher.

❍ **What surgical procedures may be considered for weight control in patients with morbid obesity?**

Gastroplasty or gastric bypass.

❍ **Why does moderate alcohol consumption decrease the risk of MI's?**

Moderate drinking (< 3 drinks a day) increases HDL.

❍ **What is the target heart rate during exercise for a 26 year-old?**

Between 126 and 175. The target heart rate is 65 to 90% of the maximal heart rate. Maximal heart rate is 220 minus age.

❍ **Which immunizations do healthy senior citizens need?**

Tetanus booster every 10 years, influenza vaccination every year, and a pneumococcal vaccination.

❍ **A 37 year-old carpenter has stepped on a rusty nail. His last tetanus shot was in high school. How should you immunize?**

Immediate tetanus immunoglobulin, followed by three doses of tetanus toxoid over the next year. The first two doses should be 1 month apart and the third dose should be 6 to 12 months later.

❍ **Besides aspirin, what actions can be taken to prevent stroke in patients with increased risk factors?**

Good control of the blood pressure and anticoagulation with warfarin in patients who have atrial fibrillation.

❍ **What 5 vaccines should be administered to adults?**

1) Hepatitis B vaccine: Give to high-risk patients (healthcare workers, homosexuals, and IV drug users)
2) Influenza vaccine: Give annually to elderly patients and patients with chronic illnesses
3) MR: Give to all patients without immunity (most often required by school institutions)
4) Pneumococcal vaccine: Give once to patients over 65 and patients with chronic illnesses
5) Tetanus/diphtheria: Give all adults a primary series and a booster every 10 years

❍ **Immunocompromised patients can safely be given which vaccines?**

Killed or inactivated vaccines:

1) Diphtheria
2) H. Influenzae
5) Enhanced inactivated polio
6) Hepatitis

3) Influenza 7) Pertussis
4) Pneumococcal 8) Tetanus

It may be easier to remember the vaccines that should be avoided. The following are live, attenuated vaccines:
1) Oral polio 2) MMR

❍ **Other than immunocompromised patients, who should not receive live vaccines?**

Pregnant women. Oral polio vaccine should be avoided in anyone in close contact with an immunocompromised person because of the ability of the virus to spread.

❍ **A patient comes in for vaccinations and has a URI and a fever of 37.5° C. Can you administer vaccines to this patient?**

Yes. URI or gastrointestinal illness are not contraindications to vaccination. Fever may be as high as 38° C and the vaccine can still be administered. Likewise, use of antibiotics or recent exposure to illness is not a reason to delay vaccination.

❍ **When administering the Mantoux skin test to a person with HIV, what induration indicates a postive reaction?**

$\geq$ 5 mm. In individuals with risk factors for TB, induration must be $\geq$ 10 mm. For those with no risk factors, induration must be $\geq$ 15 mm to be positive.

❍ **Influenza epidemics and pandemics are generally associated with which strain of influenza?**

Influenza A.

❍ **Amantadine is 70 to 90% effective in preventing which strain of influenza?**

Influenza A. Amantadine should be prescribed as chemoprophylaxis in immunocompromised patients who are not vaccinated or as a supplement to vaccination. It can also be given to healthy unvaccinated people who want to avoid the flu.

❍ **When should the influenza vaccine be given?**

In September or October, about 1 to 2 months before the influenza season begins. The vaccine, unlike amantadine, is protective against influenza A and B.

❍ **What is a contraindication to the administration of the influenza vaccine?**

A history of anaphylactic hypersensitivity to eggs or their products.

❍ **Which routine screenings should be performed on pregnant women?**

Hepatitis B, syphilis, rubella, gonorrhea, and other STD's. Women in high-risk categories should also be screened for HIV.

❍ **Diabetes is most common in which ethnic group?**

Hispanics. The prevalence in Hispanics is 1.7 to 2.4 times higher than in non-Hispanics, and the death rate is also twice as high. The high rate of disease in this group is attributed to increased incidence of obesity and hyperlipidemia.

❍ **If a diabetic patient on oral hypoglycemics mixes her medication with alcohol, is she more likely to become hyperglycemic or hypoglycemic?**

Hypoglycemic.

❍ **What is recommended in the prevention of hemorrhoids?**

Fiber supplements and stool softeners.

❍ **What is the diet recommended to reduce the risk of colon cancer?**

Decrease fat (especially saturated fat), increase fiber, increase cruciferous vegetables, decrease ETOH, and decrease smoked, salted, or nitrate-based foods.

❍ **What are the risk factors for colon cancer?**

Age over 50, familial polyposis (100%), ulcerative colitis, Crohn's disease, radiation exposure, benign adenomas, and previous history of colon cancer.

❍ **What percentage of patients with gonococcal genital infections have concomitant Chlamydia trichomatous infections?**

45%. This is why treatment for gonorrhea includes ceftriaxone and doxycycline to cover both infections.

❍ **A woman with condyloma acuminatum is how many times more likely to develop cervical cancer than a woman without this lesion?**

4 times more likely. These women should have yearly Pap smears and be screened for other STD's.

❍ **Patients with cirrhosis or chronic active hepatitis should have what routine testing to screen for hepatomas?**

α-Fetoprotein should be measured every 6 months, and an ultrasound should be performed at the same time. These patients are at a higher risk for developing liver cancer.

❍ **How can gallstone formation be prevented in patients undergoing rapid weight loss?**

10 mg/kg/day of ursodeoxycholic acid.

❍ **How can gallstone formation be prevented in patients on TPN for more than a month?**

Daily ingestion of 100 kcal or injection of cholecystokinin.

❍ **What are the risk factors for hernias?**

Obesity, heavy lifting, chronic cough, constipation, tumors, pregnancy, ascites, and other conditions which chronically increase intra-abdominal pressure.

❍ **What medications are likely to exacerbate angle-closure glaucoma?**

Anticholinergics, antihistamines, antidepressants, benzodiazepine, carbonic anhydrase inhibitors, CNS stimulants, phenothiazine, sympathomimetics, theophylline, and vasodilators.

❍ **Which medications put patients at risk for hearing loss?**

Aminoglycoside, antineoplastic agents, loop diuretics, and salicylates.

❍ **What nutritional deficiencies may lead to apthous ulcers?**

B_{12}, folate, and iron deficiencies.

❍ **A 22 year-old male, who has no significant medical history and is taking no medication, has a creamy white coat on his tongue. The substance easily rubs off, revealing an erythematous base. What should you be concerned about?**

HIV. In a patient who has no obvious reason for having an overgrowth of oral candida, HIV should be suspected. Other causes for oral thrush overgrowth include cancer, systemic illness, neutropenia, diabetes, adrenal insufficiency, nutritional deficiencies, or an immunocompromised state.

❍ **When should RhoGAM (anti-Rh immunoglobulin) be used?**

Within 3 days of the birth of an Rh+ child (if the mother is Rh-). It should also be used in the event of any mixing of fetal and maternal blood (e.g., trauma). RhoGAM is safe because it does not pass the placental barrier.

❍ **Why is estrogen protective against coronary artery disease?**

Estrogen increases HDL-cholesterol and decreases total cholesterol, LDL-cholesterol and VLDL-cholesterol..

❍ **What is the number one cause of death for African-American males between the ages of 10 and 24?**

Firearm injury. The overall homicide rate for young men in the US is over 7 times that of the next developed country.

❍ **Do intentional or unintentional causes account for more firearm-related deaths?**

Intentional causes account for 94% of firearm deaths, suicide for 48%, and homicide for 46%. Unintentional firearm injuries account for about 4%. Only 1% of firearm deaths occur as a result of legal intervention. The number of firearm-related fatalities has more than doubled in the last 30 years.

❍ **What are risk factors for homicide?**

Most homicide victims are killed by someone they know, someone of the same race, and usually during an argument or fight. Drugs and alcohol are important co-factors, as is the presence of a handgun.

❍ **What are the relative risks for suicide and homicide if a gun is kept in the home?**

Suicide is 5 times more likely. Homicide is 3 times more likely. The victim is 43% more likely to be a member of the family than an intruder. In the case of domestic violence, a gun at home increases the risk of homicide 20-fold.

❍ **What is the clinical significance of the increased availability of semi-automatic weapons?**

Between 1982 and 1992, the percentage of gunshot victims with multiple gunshot wounds increased from 5 to 20%, and the rate of spinal cord injuries from gunshot wounds quadrupled. This trend has resulted in an increased number of major organ injuries, complications, and surgeries, as well as in a greater severity of injury and a higher probability of death.

RANDOM PEARLS

Errors, like straws, upon the surface flow; he who would search for pearls must dive below.
John Dryden

❍ **What is the most common symptom of tularemia?**

Skin sores at the site of inoculation and lymphadenopathy (75%). Other symptoms include pneumonia, lesions in the GI system, infection of the eyes, fever, and headache.

❍ **How is tularemia most commonly transmitted?**

Ticks and rabbits. Tularemia is caused by F. tularensis.

❍ **What organism is most commonly implicated in sickle cell infections?**

Streptococcus pneumonia (60%). Daily doses of prophylactic penicillin are recommended for those individuals least resistant to encapsulated bacteria.

❍ **Which organs are most commonly damaged in sickle cell patients?**

Spleen, lung, liver, kidney, skeleton, and skin.

❍ **Contrast pneumonia due to Mycoplasma sp. with pneumonia due to Streptococcal pneumoniae.**

	S. pneumoniae	M. pneumoniae
Prodrome	Little	Mild fever, malaise, cough, HA
Onset	Rapid	Gradual
URI symptoms	Tachypnea, cough, occasional pleuritic pain	Little
Associated findings	High fever	Exanthem, arthritis, GI complaints, neurologic complications
Pleural effusion	Occasional	Rare
Lab	Leukocytosis	WBC normal or slight elevation
Treatment	Penicillin	Erythromycin

❍ **Staphylococcal pneumonia frequently develops pleural effusion or empyema. Which lung is most frequently involved?**

The right lung is involved in 65% of the cases. 80% of these pneumonias are unilateral. 25% of the patients will go on to develop pyopneumothorax.

❍ **What is the treatment for ITP patients who fail to recover with medical therapy?**

Splenectomy.

❍ **What x-ray findings are often seen in coarctation of the aorta?**

The "3" sign made up of the aortic knob and the dilated post coarctation segment of the descending aorta. The "E" sign is the same thing seen in a negative image on barium esophagram.

❍ **Coarctation of the aorta is associated with a narrowing of the aortic arch. Where is the narrowing located?**

Just distal to the origin of the left subclavian. This results in hypertensive upper extremities and normotensive lower extremities.

❍ **What drugs can cause gynecomastia?**

Marijuana, hormones, digitalis, spironolactone, cimetidine, ketoconazole, antihypertensives, antidepressants, and amphetamines.

❍ **What disease did the "Elephant Man" have?**

Neurofibromatosis, also known as Von Recklinghausen's disease. He developed large, disfiguring, stalk-like tissue tumors. Patients with neurofibromatosis should be screened for visual and hearing diseases.

❍ **What is the most common anatomical abnormality associated with chronic urinary tract infections?**

Vesicoureteral reflux.

❍ **Patients with exercise-induced asthma will most likely trigger their asthma with what kind of exercise?**

High intensity exercise for more than 5 to 6 minutes.

❍ **Which type of malignancy is most commonly associated with AIDS?**

Kaposi's sarcoma, followed by non-Hodgkin's lymphoma.

❍ **Where are Kaposi's sarcoma lesions found?**

Everywhere—inside and out. They typically occur on the face, neck, arms, back, thighs, and in the lungs, lymphatic system, and GI system.

❍ **How many years does a patient usually live after being diagnosed with HIV?**

8 to 10 years. Most patients eventually die from PCP.

❍ **A patient with AIDS presents with a grayish-white plaque on the lateral borders of her tongue that does not scrape off. What is the diagnosis?**

Hairy leukoplakia.

❍ **What parts of the pulmonary system are affected by asbestosis?**

The pleura and peritoneum. Asbestosis increases the risk of mesothelioma. It also causes pneumoconioses that invade the lungs.

❍ **What is the most common cause of hypercalcemia?**

Hyperparathyroidism. This condition accounts for 60% of ambulatory hypercalcemics.

❍ **What are the most common causes of non-gonococcal urethritis?**

Chlamydia trachomatis. Ureaplasma urealyticum is another common cause.

❍ **What is the most common clinical manifestation of disseminated gonococcal infection?**

Gonococcal arthritis-dermatitis syndrome. Arthritis, a pustular or papular rash, and tenosynovitis are exhibited with this syndrome.

❍ **What is the most common cause of epididymitis?**

Chlamydia trachomatis, in men under 35 years old. E. Coli, in prepubertal and older patients.

❍ **A patient with polyuria, a low urine osmolality, and a high serum osmolality is given vasopressin, but no change in osmolality is noted. Which type of diabetic insipidus does she have?**

Nephrogenic. Vassopressin will not help because the distal renal tubules are refractory to antidiuretic hormone. In central DI, the pathology involves a problem with the production of ADH in the posterior pituitary. An increase in urine osmolality of at least 50% will occur with vasopressin administration if the problem is central DI.

❍ **What organisms are usually implicated in the development of diverticulitis?**

E. coli and B. fragilis.

❍ **What is Hampton's hump?**

A chest x-ray finding associated with pulmonary embolisms. It is an infiltrate with a "hump" pointed toward the hilus and a clearing with a vascular distribution.

❍ **What is the most common cause of portal hypertension in adults?**

Cirrhosis of the liver.

❍ **The portal vein receives blood from what two tributaries?**

The splenic vein and the superior mesenteric vein.

❍ **Herpangina is caused by what virus?**

Coxsackie group A virus. A sore throat, fever, malaise, and vesicular lesions on the posterior pharynx or the soft palate are prevalent with this disease.

❍ **A patient presents with arms extended and fingers spread apart. Her extremities are flexing and extending in a static-kinetic tremor. This tremor can be associated with what disease?**

Hyperthyroidism.

❍ **What is the acid base disorder in the following situation?**

pH = 7.29, pCO_2 = 30, HCO^{3-} = 15, Na = 131, and Cl = 94

This is a primary metabolic acidosis with an elevated ion gap.

❍ **What is the most common cause of secondary lymphedema?**

Malignant metastases to the lymph nodes. Lymphatic fibrosis secondary to surgery is another cause.

❍ **What organisms most often induce lymphedema?**

Staphylococcal or beta-hemolytic Streptococcal.

❍ **Dermacentor andersoni (wood tick) is a pesky arthropod associated with 4 tick-borne illnesses! Name these illnesses and the cause of each.**

Rocky Mountain spotted fever is caused by Rickettsia rickettsii; Dermacentor andersoni is a vector.

Tick paralysis is caused by a neurotoxin. The symptoms, consisting of ascending paralysis with decrease or loss of DTR's, are similar to those associated with Guillain-Barré syndrome.

Q fever is caused by Coxiella burnetii (a Rickettsiae).

Colorado tick fever is caused by an arbovirus.

❍ **What is the most common cause of focal encephalitis in AIDS patients?**

Toxoplasma gondii.

❍ **What species of Plasmodium is resistant to chloroquine?**

Falciparum.

❍ **A pulmonary embolism causes which type of cyanosis?**

Central cyanosis. However, secondary shock and right-heart failure can lead to peripheral cyanosis.

❍ **What is the most common conduction disturbance in acute myocardial infarction?**

First degree AV block.

❍ **Describe Dupuytren's contracture.**

A contraction of the longitudinal bands of the palmar aponeurosis.

❍ **What is the most common form of anorectal abscess?**

Perianal abscess. Anorectal abscesses are usually mixed infections (i.e., both gram-negative and anaerobic organisms). Fistula formation is a frequent complication.

❍ **Describe the clinical characteristics of carboxyhemoglobin concentrations, specifically for ranges of 10 to 70%.**

10%: Frontal headache
20%: Headache and dyspnea
30%: Nausea, dizziness, visual disturbance, fatigue, and impaired judgment
40%: Syncope and confusion
50%: Coma and seizures
60%: Respiratory failure and hypotension
70%: May be lethal

❍ **Which organisms produce focal nervous system pathology via an exotoxin?**

Clostridium diphtheria, Clostridium botulinum, Clostridium tetani, Staphylococcus aureus plus wood and dog ticks (Dermacentor A and B).

❍ **What is the most common cause of intestinal obstruction?**

Adynamic ileus.

❍ **What are the most common causes of small bowel obstruction?**

Adhesions, followed by hernias.

❍ **What are the most common causes of large bowel obstruction?**

Carcinoma, followed by volvulus and sigmoid diverticulitis.

❍ **What layers of the bowel wall and mesentery are affected by regional enteritis?**

All layers.

❍ **What symptoms are associated with regional enteritis?**

Fever, abdominal pain, weight loss, and diarrhea. Fistulas, fissures, and abscesses may also be noted.

Ulcerative colitis, on the other hand, usually presents with bloody diarrhea.

❍ **Subacute bacterial endocarditis (SBE) most commonly affects which valve?**

The mitral valve. The aortic valve is the second most commonly involved valve. Rheumatic fever is the most probable cause of valvular damage associated with SBE. Mitral stenosis is a very common predisposing factor in SBE. Drug addicts tend to develop right-sided SBE, usually involving the tricuspid valve.

❍ **Describe the skin lesions found in a patient with disseminated gonococcemia.**

Umbilicated pustules with red halos.

❍ **Describe the skin lesions associated with a Pseudomonas aeruginosa infection.**

Pale, erythematous lesions, 1 cm in size, with an ulcerated necrotic center.

❍ **Describe the intracorporeal dissipation of the rabies virus.**

The virus spreads centripetally up the peripheral nerve into the CNS. The incubation period for rabies is usually 30 to 60 days with a range of 10 days to 1 year. Transmission usually occurs via infected secretions, saliva, or infected tissue. Stages of the disease include upper respiratory tract infection symptomatology, followed by encephalitis. The brainstem is affected last.

❍ **What animals are the most prevalent vectors of rabies in the world? In the US?**

Worldwide, the dog is the most common carrier of rabies. In the US, the skunk has become primary carrier. In descending order bats, raccoons, cows, dogs, foxes, and cats are also sources.

❍ **Describe the chest x-ray image of mycoplasma pneumonia.**

Patchy densities involving the entire lobe. Pneumatoceles, cavities, abscesses and pleural effusions can occur but are uncommon. Treat with erythromycin.

❍ **Which type of bacterial pneumonia commonly occurs secondary to viral illness?**

Staphylococcal infection.

❍ **What two types of pneumonia are often contracted during the summer months?**

Staphylococcal and Legionella pneumonia.

❍ **Describe the chest x-ray image of Legionella pneumonia.**

Dense consolidation and bulging fissures. Expect elevated liver enzymes and hypophosphatemia. Relative bradycardia is evident upon physical examination.

❍ **What are the classic symptoms of TB?**

Night sweats, fever, weight loss, malaise, cough, and greenish yellow sputum most commonly seen in the mornings.

❍ **What do chest x-rays reveal in cases of tuberculosis?**

Cavitation of the right upper lobe. Lower lung infiltrates, hilar adenopathy, atelectasis, and pleural effusion are also common.

❍ **What is the most common cause of paralytic ileus?**

Surgery.

❍ **Where is the most common site of volvulus?**

The sigmoid colon.

❍ **Describe the location of an indirect inguinal hernia.**

Lateral to the epigastric vessels, protruding through the inguinal canal.

❍ **Describe the location of a femoral hernia.**

Protrudes through the femoral canal and below the inguinal ligament.

❍ **What are the signs and symptoms of Crohn's disease?**

Fever, diarrhea, right lower quadrant pain with mass possible, fistulas, rectal prolapse, perianal fissures, and abscesses. Arthritis, uveitis, and liver disease are also associated with this condition.

❍ **What systemic diseases are associated with Crohn's disease?**

Pyoderma gangrenosum, uveitis, episclerosis, scleritis, arthritis, erythema nodosum, and nephrolithiasis.

❍ **What contrast x-ray findings are associated with Crohn's disease?**

The segmental involvement in the colon with an abnormal mucosal pattern and fistulas, often without involvement of the rectum. A narrowing of the small intestine may also be displayed.

❍ **What are the principal signs and symptoms of ulcerative colitis?**

Fever, weight loss, tachycardia, panniculitis, and 6 bloody bowel movements per day.

❍ **Does toxic megacolon commonly occur with ulcerative colitis or with Crohn's disease?**

Ulcerative colitis.

❍ **Which medications may be used for Crohn's disease but not for ulcerative colitis?**

Anti-diarrheal agents.

❍ **Does cancer more often develop with ulcerative colitis or Crohn's disease?**

Ulcerative colitis. Think of toxic megacolon and cancer. Always avoid anti-diarrheal agents in the treatment regime.

❍ **What bacterial cause of diarrhea is most commonly associated with seizures?**

Shigella.

❍ **What organism induces rose spots and watery diarrhea, as well as high fever and relative bradycardia?**

Salmonella.

❍ **What is the treatment for individuals infected with Salmonella?**

Supportive care without antibiotics. However, if a severe fever is exhibited, antibiotic therapy may be warranted.

❍ **What microbial agent is associated with mesenteric adenitis and pseudoappendicitis?**

Yersinia.

❍ **Which type of diarrhea is profuse and bloody, but does not involve vomiting?**

Entamoeba histolytica. Diarrhea which is not necessarily bloody, but can be associated with contaminated meat could be due to Clostridium perfringens.

❍ **What causes the type of diarrhea commonly seen in AIDS patients?**

Cryptosporidiosis. This agent is diagnosed by a positive acid-fast stain. Patients with this condition present with profuse, watery diarrhea that is not bloody.

❍ **What is the incubation period for hepatitis A?**

30 days. The disease is caused by a Retrovirus.

❍ **What does an elevated IgM anti-HBc indicate?**

Exposure to hepatitis B with antibody to the core antigen. High titers indicate the contagious disease, low titers suggest chronic hepatitis B.

❍ **Which type of hepatitis is caused by a DNA virus?**

Hepatitis B. The incubation period is 90 days.

❍ **What does an anti-HB indicate?**

Prior infection and immunity.

❍ **What defects cause left-to-right shunt murmurs?**

ASD, VSD, and PDA.

❍ **What is the most common cause of otitis media?**

Streptococcus pneumoniae.

❍ **What is the most common cause of orbital infections?**

Staphylococcus aureus. Periorbital infections are usually caused by H. influenzae.

❍ **How do steroids function in the treatment of asthma?**

Steroids increase c-AMP, decrease inflammation, and aid in restoring the function of beta-adrenergic responsiveness to adrenergic drugs.

❍ **What serious complication may arise from the use of valproic acid?**

Hepatic failure.

❍ **What complications may occur with phenytoin use?**

Folate deficiency, osteomalacia, neutropenia, neuropathies, lupus, and myasthenia.

❍ **What are some possible complications of sodium bicarbonate therapy?**

Hypokalemia, paradoxical CSF acidosis, impaired O_2 dissociation, and sodium overload.

❍ **What is the most common precipitating cause of thyroid storm?**

Pulmonary infection.

❍ **What is the second most common cause of hypothyroidism?**

Hashimoto's thyroiditis.

❍ **How can primary hypothyroidism be distinguished from secondary hypothyroidism?**

Primary hypothyroidism: The TSH levels are high, patients often have a history of thyroid surgery, and they may have a goiter.

Secondary hypothyroidism: the TSH levels are low or normal, there is no history of surgery, and no goiter is evident.

❍ **What drugs may worsen myxedema?**

Propranolol and phenothiazine.

❍ **What common surgical problem encountered with myxedema should be treated conservatively?**

Acquired megacolon.

❍ **What is the cause of primary adrenal insufficiency?**

Failure of the adrenal cortex, also known as Addison's disease.

❍ **Two weeks after a myocardial infarction, a patient takes warfarin and has sudden onset of hypotension, right flank pain, right CVA pain, epigastric pain, fever, nausea, and vomiting. What is the diagnosis?**

Adrenal gland hemorrhage (adrenal apoplexy).

❍ **Define Waterhouse-Friderichsen syndrome?**

Septicemia secondary to meningococcemia with associated bilateral adrenal gland hemorrhage. The patient will have a petechial rash, purpura, shaking, chills, and a severe headache.

❍ **What effect does Addison's disease have on cortisol and aldosterone levels?**

It lowers them. Low cortisol levels induce nausea, vomiting, anorexia, lethargy, hypoglycemia, water intoxication, and the inability to withstand even minor stress without shock. Low aldosterone levels cause sodium depletion, dehydration, hypotension, and syncope.

❍ **What are the signs and symptoms of Addison's disease?**

Hyperpigmentation, hyperkalemia, alopecia, and ascending paralysis secondary to hyperkalemia. Lab findings in Addison's disease indicate hypoglycemia, hyponatremia, hyperkalemia, and azotemia.

❍ **What abnormal ECG results can occur in patients with Addison's disease?**

Tall, peaked T waves in the presence of hyperkalemia.

❍ **What are the principal signs and symptoms of adrenal crisis?**

Abdominal pain, hypotension, and shock. The most common cause is withdrawal of steroids. Treat by administering hydrocortisone; 100 mg IV bolus and 100 mg added to the first liter of D_5 0.9 NS.

❍ **Does cyanide evoke cyanosis?**

No (except secondarily, when bradycardia and apnea precede asystolic arrest). If hypoxia is not present according to ABG results, consider administering cyanide to an acidotic, non-cyanotic, comatose patient.

❍ **What key lab results are expected with SIADH?**

Low serum sodium levels and high urine sodium levels (i.e., > 30).

❍ **If a lesion is in the right hemisphere, which way will the eyes deviate?**

Toward the lesion.

❍ **If a lesion is in the brain stem, which way will the eyes deviate?**

Away from the lesion in the brain stem.

❍ **Do household pets transmit Yersinia?**

Yes.

❍ **What is the most common cause of intrinsic renal failure?**

Acute tubular necrosis.

❍ **What is the most common cause of cardiac arrest in an uremic patient?**

Hyperkalemia.

❍ **What is the first cardiac finding in a cyclic antidepressant overdose?**

Sinus tachycardia.

❍ **What is the most common cause of chronic heavy metal poisoning?**

Lead. Arsenic is the most common cause of acute heavy metal poisoning.

❍ **Erythema nodosa is associated with which type of gastroenteritis?**

Yersinia.

❍ **What are some common causes of increased anion gap?**

Aspirin, methanol, uremia, diabetes, idiopathic (lactic), ethylene glycol, and alcohol.

❍ **What are the causes of normal anion gap metabolic acidosis?**

Diarrhea, ammonium chloride, renal tubular acidosis, renal interstitial disease, hypoadrenalism, ureterosigmoidostomy, and acetazolamide.

❍ **What are some common causes of respiratory alkalosis?**

Respiratory alkalosis is defined as a pH above 7.45 and a pCO_2 less than 35. Common causes of respiratory alkalosis include any process that may induce hyperventilation: shock, sepsis, trauma, asthma, PE, anemia, hepatic failure, heat stroke, exhaustion, emotion, salicylate poisoning, hypoxemia, pregnancy, and inadequate mechanical ventilation.

❍ **How should neurogenic shock be managed?**

With replacement of the volume deficit, followed by vasopressors.

❍ **What medication is most appropriate for hypertensive patients with acute aortic dissections?**

Nitroprusside and beta-blockers.

❍ **An elderly male presents with ataxia, confusion, amnesia, and ocular paralysis. He is apathetic to his situation and his neurologic examination is normal. Probable diagnosis?**

Vitamin B deficiency, associated with Wernicke-Korsakoff's syndrome.

❍ **What agent is usually responsible for the onset of endemic encephalitis?**

Arbovirus.

❍ **What is the appropriate treatment for a non-immunized individual exposed to hepatitis B?**

Immune globulin, specifically Hepatitis-B immune globulin. Consider vaccination.

❍ **What gynecological infection presents with a malodorous, itchy, white to gray and sometimes frothy vaginal discharge?**

Trichomoniasis.

❍ **What are the distinguishing characteristics of benign positional vertigo?**

Positional vertigo is usually provoked by certain head positions or movement. Nystagmus is always positional, of brief duration, and with fatigability.

❍ **What are the key features of viral labyrinthitis or vestibular neuritis?**

Severe vertigo (usually lasting 3 to 5 days), with nausea and vomiting. Symptoms generally regress over 3 to 6 weeks. Nystagmus may be spontaneous during the severe stage.

❍ **What is a major concern for a patient with unilateral Parkinsonian features?**

Intracranial tumor.

❍ **Describe signs and symptoms of acoustic neuroma.**

Unilateral high tone sensorineural hearing loss and tinnitus. Decreased corneal sensitivity, diplopia, headache, facial weakness, and positive radiographic findings may also be displayed. Vertigo usually appears late, is more often exhibited as a progressive feeling of imbalance, and can be provoked by changes in head movement. Nystagmus is frequently present and is usually spontaneous. The CSF may have elevated protein.

❍ **Describe the key features of vertebrobasilar insufficiency.**

Vertigo (nearly always positional accompanied by nystagmus). Other signs of arteriosclerosis may be found. Vertebrobasilar insufficiency is typically prevalent in older persons and may occur with other symptoms of brainstem ischemia.

❍ **What therapy should be initiated for a bleeding patient who is on warfarin and has a high PT?**

D/C warfarin, followed by a water soluble form of vitamin K. Prescribe SQ and consider a test dose. If the bleeding is severe or in a dangerous location (i.e., the brain), fresh frozen plasma containing active factors X, IX, VII, and II should be given. (Remember: 1972)

❍ **What electrolyte abnormality is commonly associated with the transfusion of packed RBCs?**

Hypocalcemia secondary to citrate toxicity. Citrate, when rapidly infused, binds ionized calcium and therefore decreases the calcium level. Hyperkalemia may also develop, especially if the patient is in renal failure or if the blood products are old.

❍ **What invasive procedure should be performed to evaluate a patient whose face, neck, and arms are swollen?**

CVP. Swelling of the face, neck and arms suggests superior vena cava syndrome. To confirm, an increased CVP pressure in the upper body and abnormal pressure in the lower extremities must be documented. A chest x-ray will detect only about 10% of the masses causing this syndrome.

❍ **Describe Leriche's syndrome.**

Impotence with buttock, calf, and back pain. It is usually occurs with aortoiliac disease.

❍ **What signs and symptoms are prevalent with post streptococcal glomerulonephritis?**

Facial edema and decreased urinary output. Urine may be dark. Other laboratory results include normochromic anemia because of hemodilution, increased sedimentation rate, numerous RBCs and WBC's in the urine with casts, and hyperkalemia. Hospitalization is advised.

❍ **Name the five major modified Jones criteria.**

1) Erythema marginatum
2) Polyarthritis
3) Subcutaneous nodules

4) Carditis
5) Chorea

Other criteria include rheumatic fever or rheumatic heart disease, arthralgias, fever, prolonged PR interval on an ECG, C reactive protein, elevated sedimentation rate, and antistreptolysin O titer.

❍ **What disorder is present when two out of the five major modified Jones criteria are met?**

Rheumatic fever.

❍ **What organism typically causes paronychia?**

Staphylococcus.

❍ **What visual deficit is typically associated with lesions at the optic chiasm?**

Bitemporal hemianopsia.

❍ **A ring lesion is noted on a CT scan of the brain of an immunocompromised patient. The patient is confused and has a lymphadenopathy, fever, and headache. What is the probable diagnosis?**

Toxoplasmosis, secondary to Toxoplasma gondii cyst. The disease is typically treated with pyrimethamine and sulfadiazine.

❍ **What are the signs and symptoms of posterior inferior cerebellar artery syndrome?**

Cerebellar dysfunction, such as vertigo, ataxia, and dizziness.

❍ **Do local anesthetics freely cross the blood brain barrier?**

Yes. Most systemic toxic reactions to local anesthetics involve the CNS or cardiovascular system.

❍ **What are the most common causes of hemoptysis in the US?**

Bronchitis and bronchiectasis.

❍ **Where is the most common site of thrombophlebitis?**

The deep muscles of the calves, particularly the soleus muscle.

❍ **How should hypercalcemia be treated?**

Administer furosemide and normal saline. Intravenous pamidronate is very effective in reducing serum calcium levels to normal for extended periods of time. Oral or intravenous steroids are also an effective alternative.

❍ **What are the potential complications of excess sodium bicarbonate?**

Cerebral acidosis, hypokalemia, hyperosmolality, and an increased binding of hemoglobin to oxygen.

❍ **What are the effects of dopamine at various doses?**

1 to 4 mg/kg:	Renal, mesenteric, coronary, and cerebral vasodilation.
5 to 10 mg/kg:	Arterial vasoconstriction from predominant alpha-adrenergic effects and little beta-adrenergic effect.
>10 mg/kg:	Arterial vasoconstriction from alpha-adrenergic effect with no beta-adrenergic effect.

❍ **What are the common presentations of a transfusion reaction?**

Myalgia, dyspnea, fever associated with hypocalcemia, hemolysis, allergic reactions, hyperkalemia, citrate toxicity, hypothermia, coagulopathies, and altered hemoglobin function.

❍ **A woman comes to your office frantic because her husband has just received a positive VDRL result. They have been happily married for 35 years and she can't believe he has been unfaithful. Is it at all possible that he has been loyal to his wife?**

Yes. False-positive tests can occur if the patient has had a viral or mycoplasma infection in the near past, if the patient is an IV drug user, or if the patient has SLE. The presence or absence of syphilis can be confirmed with the fluorescent treptonemal antibody absorption test (FTA-ABS).

❍ **A 63 year-old woman asks you about the risk-benefit ratio for estrogen therapy. What do you tell her?**

Estrogen therapy is currently recommended for postmenopausal menopausal women that are not at high risk for breast cancer. Research suggests that estrogen decreases the risk of CHD by 35%, the risk of hip fractures by 25%, and the risk of vertebral fractures by 50%. Unopposed estrogen increases the risk of endometrial cancer 8 times, yet estrogen given with progesterone eliminates this risk. A minor side effect of progesterone is weight gain.

❍ **How is hepatitis A transmitted?**

By the oral-fecal route. No carrier state exists.

❍ **Which type of gastroenteritis involves diarrhea and is associated with the consumption of seafood?**

Vibrio parahaemolyticus.

❍ **Technetium-99m–labeled studies of the gallbladder are viewed every 10 minutes for 1 hour. If the gallbladder is not visualized at the 1-hour interval, what does this signify?**

Either complete obstruction of the cystic duct, due to inflammation and stones (acute cholecystitis), or partial obstruction, with a slow filling rate, because of scaring (chronic cholecystitis). Images delayed up to 4-hours are obtained to rule out the latter possibility.

❍ **A patient who is taking oral contraceptives is concerned about the added risk of gynecological cancers. What should you tell her?**

Combined (estrogen and progesterone) oral contraceptives are not associated with a significant risk for breast cancer. In fact, they decrease the risk of ovarian and endometrial cancer. Oral contraceptives do increase the risk for thromboembolism, MI's, CVA's, hypertension, amenorrhea, cholelithiasis, and benign hepatic tumors, but they help regulate the menstrual cycle, decrease cramping, and curb the progression of endometriosis, ovarian cysts, and benign breast disease. They also decrease the incidence of ectopic pregnancy, salpingitis, and anemia, and they are therapeutic against rheumatoid arthritis.

❍ **Where are the most common sites of the hematologic spread of breast cancer?**

Lungs and liver. Other sites include bone, adrenals, ovaries, brain, and pleura.

❍ **What characteristics are associated with the best prognosis in breast cancer?**

No nodal involvement, increased age, and positive estrogen receptor tumors.

❍ **How should cholesterol be monitored in patients with a history of CHD? Without a history of CHD?**

A baseline total cholesterol and HDL-C should be obtained for all adults over 20. If the cholesterol is less than 200 mg/dl, and the HDL is greater than 35 mg/dl, then repeat monitoring can be done every 5 years. For patients with CHD, a full lipoprotein analysis should be done as a base line. If LDL-C is less than 100 mg/dl, then annual lipoprotein monitoring is sufficient. If the patient's LDL-C is greater than 100 mg/dl, then diet and/or drug intervention is required with more frequent testing.

❍ **What mnemonic can be used for remembering what drugs or conditions commonly cause seizures?**

SHAKE WITH eL SPOC.
Salicylates
Hypoxia
Anticholinergics
Carbon monoxide (CO)
EtOH withdrawal
Withdrawal
Isoniazid
Theophylline and tricyclics
Hypoglycemia
Lead, lithium, and local anesthetics
Strychnine and sympathomimetics
PCP, phenothiazine, and propoxyphene
Organophosphates
Camphor, cholinergics, carbon monoxide, and cyanide

❍ **What is a mnemonic for remembering the drugs that cause nystagmus?**

MALES TIP.
Methanol
Alcohol
Lithium
Ethylene glycol
Sedative hypnotics and solvents
Thiamine depletion and Tegretol (carbamazepine)
Isopropanol
PCP and phenytoin

❍ **What is a mnemonic for remembering drugs that are radiopaque?**

BAT CHIPS.
Barium
Antihistamines
Tricyclic antidepressants
Chloral hydrate, calcium, cocaine
Heavy metals
Iodine
Phenothiazine, potassium
Slow-release (enteric coated)

❍ **What is pernio (chilblain)?**

Exposure of an extremity for a prolonged period of time to dry, cold but above freezing temperatures. Patients develop superficial, small, painful ulcerations over the chronically exposed areas. Sensitivity of the surrounding skin, erythema, and pruritus may also develop.

❍ **What is appropriate treatment for frostbite?**

Do not use dry heat! The exposed extremity should be rewarmed rapidly by immersing the affected area in 42°C circulating water for 20 minutes or until flushing is observed. Refreezing thawed tissue greatly increases damage. Remember to provide tetanus prophylaxis. Debride white or clear blisters as toxic mediators (prostaglandin and thromboxanes) may be present. However, leave hemorrhagic blisters intact. Topical antibiotics, such as silver sulfadiazine, may be used. After admission, the patient should undergo whirlpool treatments with a warm antibiotic solution at least twice a day.

❍ **What are some common complications of frostbite?**

Rhabdomyolysis, permanent depigmentation of the extremity, and an increased probability of a subsequent injury caused by cold conditions. An x-ray, approximately 3 to 6 months after a frostbite injury, will reveal irregular, fine, punched-out lytic lesions, which may appear on the MTP, PIP, and DIP joints.

❍ **What is the most common adverse effects of AZT?**

Granulocytopenia and anemia.

❍ **What is the cause of granuloma inguinale?**

The bacterium Donovania granulomatis, recently renamed Calymmatobacterium granulomatis.

❍ **What is the cause of condylomata acuminata?**

Papilloma virus.

❍ **A patient has previous focal deficits from CVAs. Is it true that such a patient can present with confusion when afflicted with a new focal lesion?**

Yes. The presentation of a new focal lesion may be displayed with generalized or non-focal symptoms in the context of previous insults.

❍ **A patient with a dementia contracts a wound infection. Is it true that such a patient can present with a severe decrease in mental status?**

Yes. Normal minor insults can cause drastic changes in the neurologic functioning of patients with pre-existing deficits.

❍ **A patient had right arm and hand paralysis from a previous CVA. However, only residual weakness remains. If the patient has a subsequent episode of hyponatremia, can right arm and hand paralysis reoccur?**

Sure. Formerly compensated deficits may return in response to a generalized neurological insult.

❍ **RBC basophilic stippling occurs with what two disorders?**

Thalassemia and lead poisoning.

❍ **What triad is associated with Reiter's syndrome?**

Non-gonococcal urethritis, polyarthritis, and conjunctivitis. Conjunctivitis is the least common and occurs in only 30% of the patients. Acute attacks respond well to NSAIDs.

❍ **What complication of rheumatoid arthritis requires emergency treatment?**

Vasculitis. This condition should be treated promptly with systemic steroids. If treatment is delayed, irreversible neuropathy may occur.

❍ **What is Felty's syndrome?**

Rheumatoid arthritis with splenomegaly and neutropenia. It is a late complication of rheumatoid arthritis.

❍ **What is the most serious complication associated with dental infections (besides possible respiratory compromise, from Ludwig's angina)?**

Septic cavernous sinus thrombosis.

❍ **What joint is most commonly affected with gout?**

The great toe MCP joint.

❍ **What joint is most commonly affected with pseudogout?**

The knee. The causative agent is calcium pyrophosphate crystals.

❍ **What are the complications of impetigo?**

Streptococcal-induced impetigo can result in post streptococcal glomerulonephritis. However, it has not been shown to be associated with rheumatic fever. Treat with erythromycin, dicloxacillin, or cephalexin to help eliminate the skin lesions. There is no conclusive proof that treatment prevents glomerulonephritis.

❍ **A patient has had three days of diarrhea which was abrupt in onset. The patient reports slimy green, malodorous stools that contain blood. In addition, the patient is febrile. What is the most likely cause?**

Salmonella. Treat with the antibiotics Ampicillin, TMP/SMX or Chloramphenicol.

❍ **What is the treatment for Campylobacter?**

Erythromycin or tetracycline.

❍ **What is the pharmacological treatment for persistent E. coli?**

Trimethoprim with sulfamethoxazole (TMP-SMX).

❍ **What is the pharmacological treatment for Giardia lamblia?**

Quinacrine or metronidazole or furazolidone.

❍ **What is the pharmacological treatment for persistent salmonellosis?**

Ampicillin, TMP-SMX, Chloramphenicol.

❍ **What is the pharmacological treatment for Shigella sp.?**

TMP-SMX or Ciprofloxacin (if resistant).

❍ **What is the pharmacological treatment for Yersinia sp.?**

Nematode microfilaria.

❍ **What vector transmits Chagas' disease (Trypanosoma Cruzi)?**

Reduviid ("assassin" or "kissing") bug.

❍ **Cysticercosis is associated with what symptom?**

New onset seizure.

❍ **Hookworm is associated with what sort of anemia?**

Iron deficiency anemia.

❍ **Fish tapeworm (Diphyllobothrium latum) is associated with what type of anemia?**

Pernicious anemia.

❍ **Onchocerciasis (from Onchocerca volvulus) is associated with what visual deficit?**

Blindness.

❍ **Chagas' disease is associated with what pathologic condition?**

Acute myocarditis. Trypanosoma cruzi invades the myocardium resulting in myocarditis. Conduction defects may occur. The vector for this parasite is the insect Reduviid.

❍ **Roundworm is associated with what GI problem?**

Small bowel obstruction.

❍ **What is rhinocerebral phycomycosis?**

Rhinocerebral phycomycosis, also known as mucormycosis, is a fungal infection typically seen in diabetic patients with ketoacidosis and immunocompromised patients. The disease is rapidly fatal if not recognized and treated quickly. Treatment includes antifungal drugs and surgical debridement.

❍ **Magnesium containing antacids may cause what side effect?**

Diarrhea.

❍ **Aluminum containing antacids may cause:**

Constipation.

❍ **Acute testicular pain and relief of pain with elevation of the scrotum (Prehn's sign) is classically associated with:**

Epididymitis.

❍ **What is the drug of choice for treating urinary tract infection due to Proteus mirabilis?**

Ampicillin. This condition is common in young boys.

❍ **What distinguishes heat stroke from heat exhaustion?**

Heat exhaustion involves the progressive loss of electrolytes and body fluid. Therapy is rehydration. Heat stroke occurs when body temperature exceeds 42°C and enzyme systems cease to function normally. As a result, there is necrosis, denaturing, and organ failure. Heat stroke requires much more aggressive treatment than simple fluid rehydration.

Remember: in patients with an altered sensorium and a core temperature above 42°C, always suspect heat stroke. Only half of these patients will be diaphoretic.

❍ **What lab abnormalities may be found with heat stroke?**

High elevations in SGOT, SGPT, and LDH. The BUN/CR ratio will also show dehydration in many cases.

❍ **How should a patient with heat stroke be treated?**

1) Cool the patient with lukewarm water and fans.
2) Pack the axillae, neck, and groin with ice.
3) Give fluids cautiously as large boluses of fluids may precipitate pulmonary edema.
4) Treat shivering with chlorpromazine (Thorazine) 25 to 50 mg IV.

❍ **What complications can result from heat stroke?**

Renal failure, rhabdomyolysis, DIC, and seizures. Remember-Antipyretics won't help.

❍ **An elderly patient presents with sudden onset of severe abdominal pain followed by a forceful bowel movement. Probable diagnosis?**

Acute mesenteric ischemia. Keep in mind that abdominal series may be normal early in acute mesenteric ischemia. Possible late x-ray findings include: Absent bowel gas, ileus, gas in the intestinal wall, and thumb-printing of the intestinal mucosa. In most cases, films are normal or not specifically suggestive. Expect heme-positive stools. Patients especially prone to mesenteric ischemia include those with CHF and chronic heart disease.

❍ **Under what conditions does neurogenic pulmonary edema occur?**

Neurogenic pulmonary edema is commonly associated with increased intracranial pressure. It is commonly seen with head trauma, subarachnoid hemorrhage, and even with seizures.

❍ **A patient had a severe headache two days ago. The headache is now subsiding, and the physical examination is normal. Should the possibility of a subarachnoid hemorrhage be evaluated, and if so, how?**

Yes. CT.

Note: A significant percentage of scans will be negative 48 hours after intracranial hemorrhage. However, an LP done 2 to 3 days after a bleed should still be positive, and xanthochromia typically persists for 7 to 10 days.

❍ **An asthmatic patient suddenly develops a supraventricular tachycardia. Blood pressure is normal and the QRS complex is also narrow. What therapy is most appropriate?**

Verapamil. Avoid the use of adenosine as it is relatively contraindicated and may exacerbate bronchospasm in asthmatic patients. Also avoid beta-blockers.

❍ **Where is the most common site of infectious arthritis?**

The knee, followed by the hip. Staphylococcus is the most common cause.

❍ **A patient has difficulty squatting and standing. What is the most likely spinal pathology?**

L4 root compression with involvement of quadriceps.

❍ **What STD pathogens cause painful ulcers?**

Type II Genital herpes and chancroid.

STD	Ulcer	Node
Genital herpes	Painful	Painful
Chancroid	Painful	Painful
Syphilis	Painless	Less painful
Lymphogranuloma venereum	Painless	Moderately painful

❍ **A patient presents with a complaint of pain at the site of the deltoid insertion with radiation into the back of the arm (C5 distribution). On examination, there is increased pain with active abduction from 70° to 120°. X-rays reveal calcification at the tendinous insertion of the greater tuberosity. Diagnosis?**

Supraspinatus tendonitis.

❍ **A patient in the emergency department cannot recall ever having a tetanus shot. The nurse gives him a tetanus shot. Later, he develops a hypersensitivity reaction and recalls that he recently had a tetanus shot. Which type of reaction does he have?**

Type 3—an Arthus reaction caused by immune complexes or antigen-antibody complexes that activate complement and platelets forming aggregates and complexes with IgE.

❍ **A positive TB test is which type of reaction?**

Type 4. Cells are mediated, hypersensitivity is delayed, and neither complements nor antibodies are involved.

❍ **What drugs commonly cause erythema multiforme?**

Carbamazepine, penicillin, sulfa, pyrazolone, phenytoin, and barbiturates.

❍ **What causes a greenish-gray frothy vaginal discharge with mild itching?**

Trichomonas vaginitis. On physical examination, the cervix will have a strawberry appearance 20% of the time.

❍ **Describe the presentation of a patient with Gardnerella vaginitis?**

On physical examination, note a frothy, grayish-white, fishy smelling vaginal discharge. Wet mount may show clue cells (clusters of bacilli on the surface of epithelial cells).

Pulmonary: ARDS, atelectasis, mediastinal adenopathy, pneumothorax, pleural effusion, and abscess

❍ **Under what conditions should staphylococcal pneumonia be considered as a possible diagnosis?**

Although it only accounts for 1% of bacterial pneumonias, it should be considered in patients with sudden chills, hectic fever, pleurisy, and cough—especially following a viral illness, such as measles or influenza.

❍ **A patient presents with granuloma inguinale. What does it look like?**

Papular, nodular, or vesicular painless lesions. These can result in extensive destruction of local tissues. Cause is Calymmatobacterium granulomatis.

❍ **What causes chancroid?**

Hemophilus ducreyi.

❍ **Describe lesions associated with chlamydia.**

Painless, shallow ulcerations, papular or nodular lesions, and herpetiform vesicles that wax and wane.

❍ **What are the chief clinical features of ulcerative colitis?**

Bloody diarrhea and involvement of the colon and rectum. Incidence peaks between ages 20 and 30. The most common site is the rectosigmoid colon. Ulcerative colitis typically involves only the submucosal and mucosal layers. Crypt abscesses, ulcerations and pseudopolyps may also be present.

❍ **Contrast regional enteritis with ulcerative colitis.**

	Regional Enteritis	Ulcerative Colitis
Areas	Stem-to-stern, social to anti-social Segmental (skip areas) Most commonly in ileum	95% rectosigmoid Contiguous (no skip areas)
Demographics	Ages 15 to 22 and 55 to 60 Common in European Jews White > Black 10 to 15% have family history	Ages 10 to 30 15 times greater risk with first-degree relative
Bowel	All layers Thick bowel wall Narrow lumen Creeping fat (mesenteric fat over bowel wall) "Cobblestone" mucosal appearance Fissures Fistulas Abscesses	Mucosa and submucosa Mucosal ulceration Epithelial necrosis Mild: mucosa fine, granular, and friable Severe: spongy, red, and oozing ulcerations Crypt abscesses Toxic megacolon

❍ **Describe a patient presenting with Sjogren's syndrome.**

Sjogren's syndrome usually occurs in women older than 50 years of age. Symptoms often include diminished lacrimal and salivary gland secretions, salivary gland enlargement, and arthritis. Sjogren's syndrome predisposes a patient to corneal irritation, ulceration, and superimposed infection. It may complicate many rheumatic diseases or may occur independently. The most probable cause of Sjogren's syndrome is lymphatic infiltration of the lacrimal and salivary glands, which results in dry eyes and a dry mouth.

❍ **What is the most common source of arterial embolisms?**

Embolism from atheromatous plaques from the aorta. Next common is atrial thrombi originating in the presence of atrial fibrillation. Other causes include LV thrombi, post antero-apical infarction, valvular heart disease, rheumatic heart disease and SBE.

❍ **What is the most common presentation of cryptococcosis?**

Fungal meningitis with Cryptococcus neoformans.

❍ **Which general group of bacteria is most commonly found in lung abscesses?**

Anaerobic bacteria.

CARDIAC GRAPHICS

❍ What is the cardiac arrhythmia?

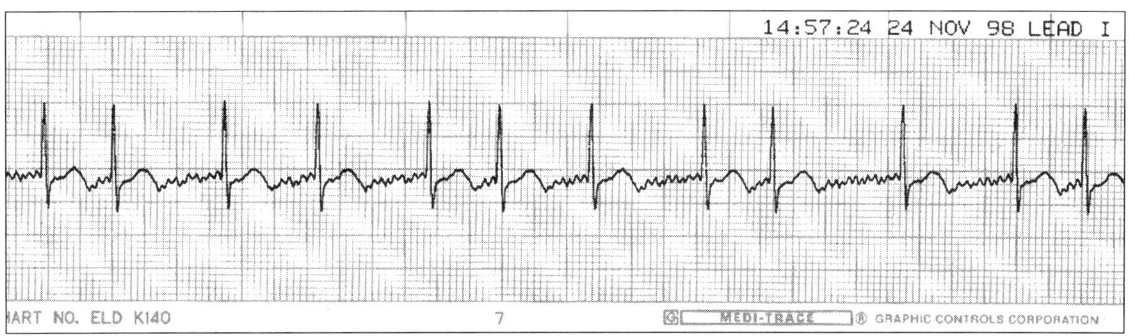

Atrial fibrillation.

❍ What is the cardiac arrhythmia?

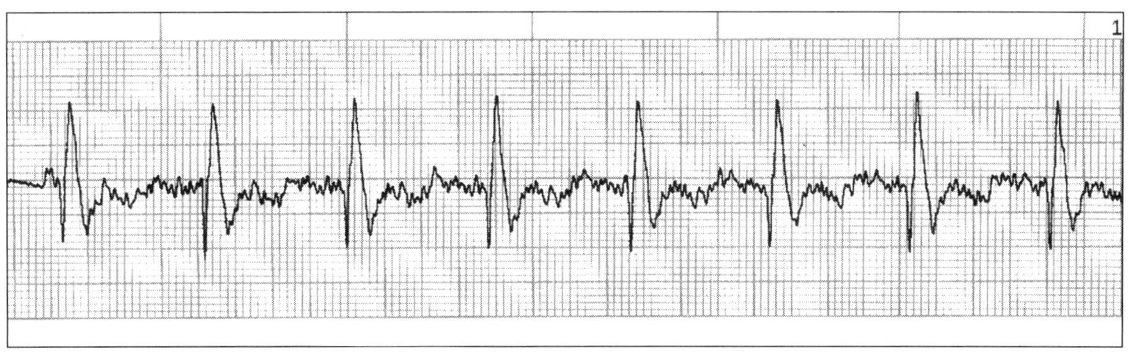

Ventricular paced rhythm with artifact.

❍ What is the cardiac arrhythmia?

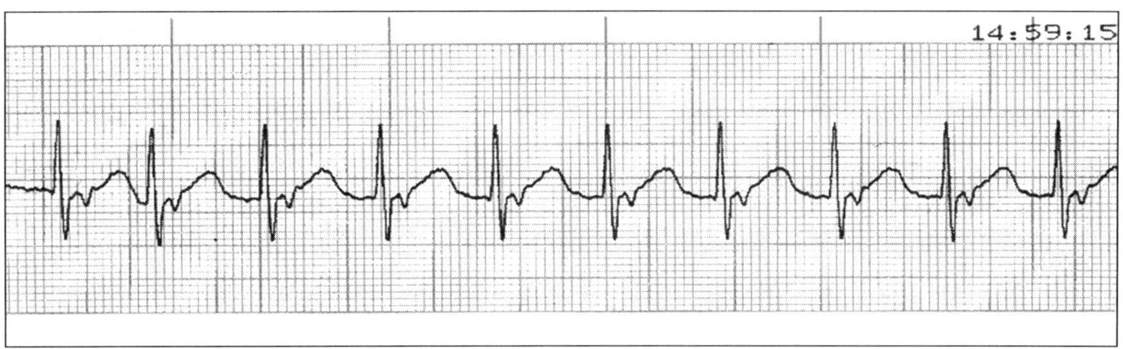

Accelerated junctional rhythm with retrograde P waves.

❍ **What is the cardiac rhythm seen below?**

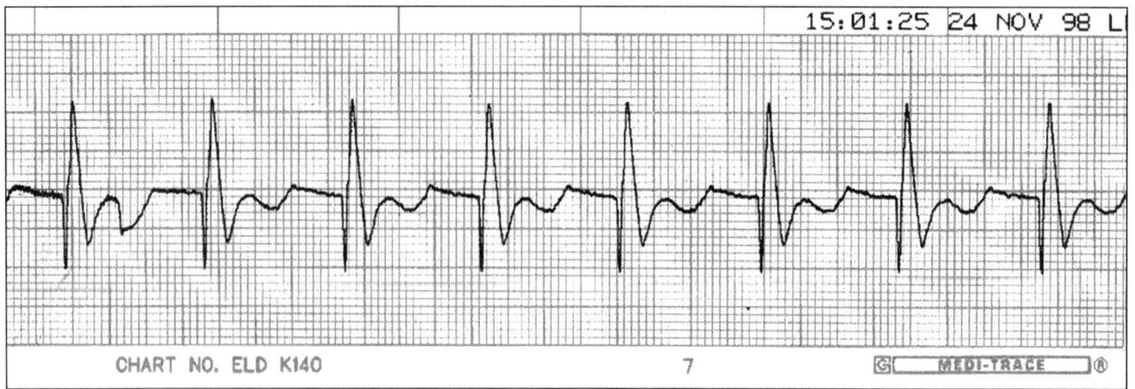

Ventricular pacemaker rhythm.

❍ **What is the ECG rhythm abnormality seen below?**

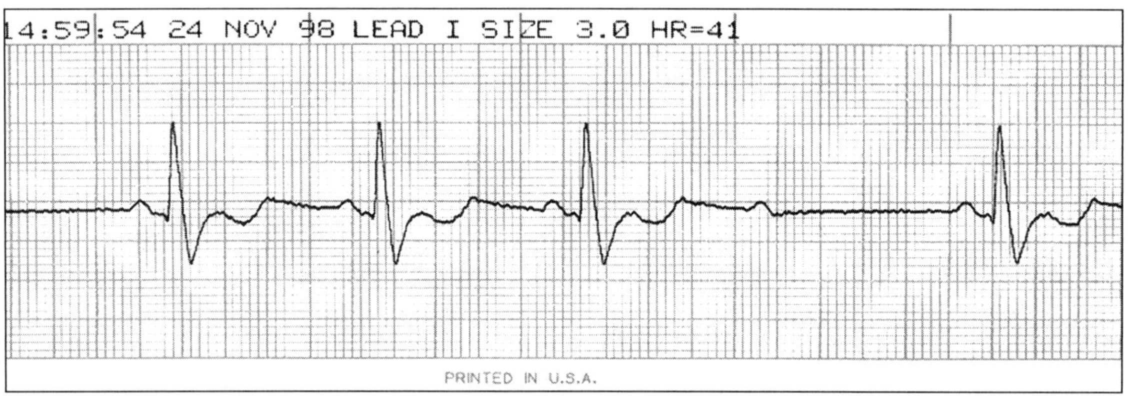

Mobitz II 2nd degree AV block.

❍ **What is the ECG rhythm abnormality seen below?**

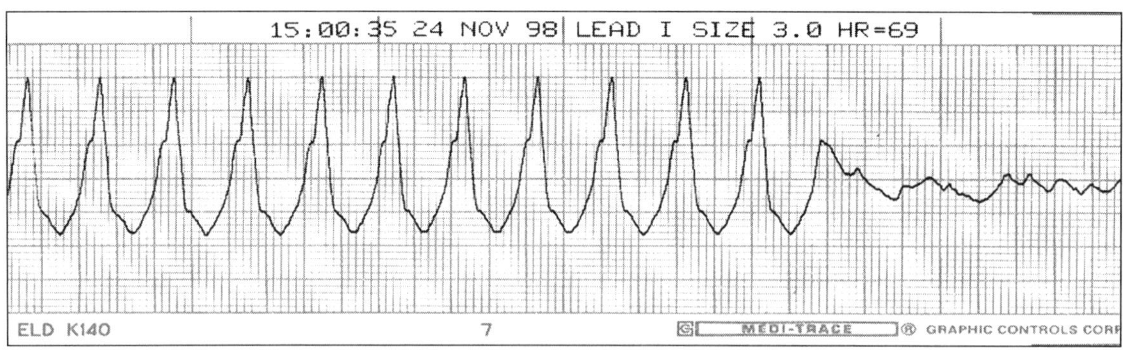

Ventricular tachycardia evolving into ventricular fibrillation.

❍ **What is the cardiac arrhythmia below?**

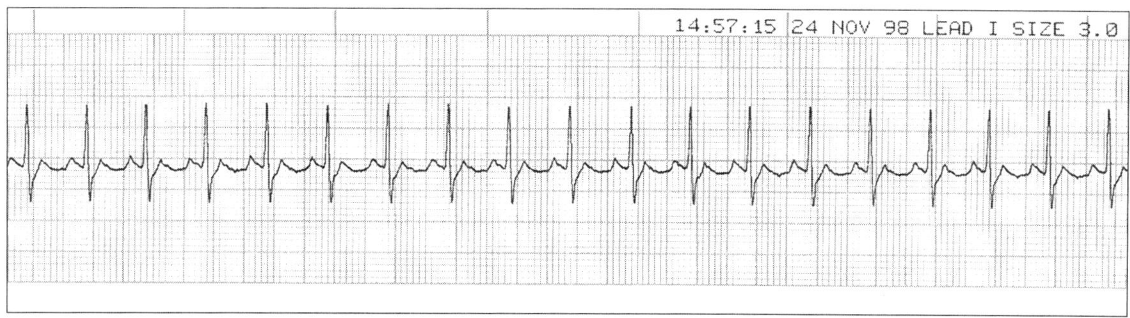

Atrial tachycardia with 2:1 conduction.

❍ **What is the abnormality in the ECG seen below?**

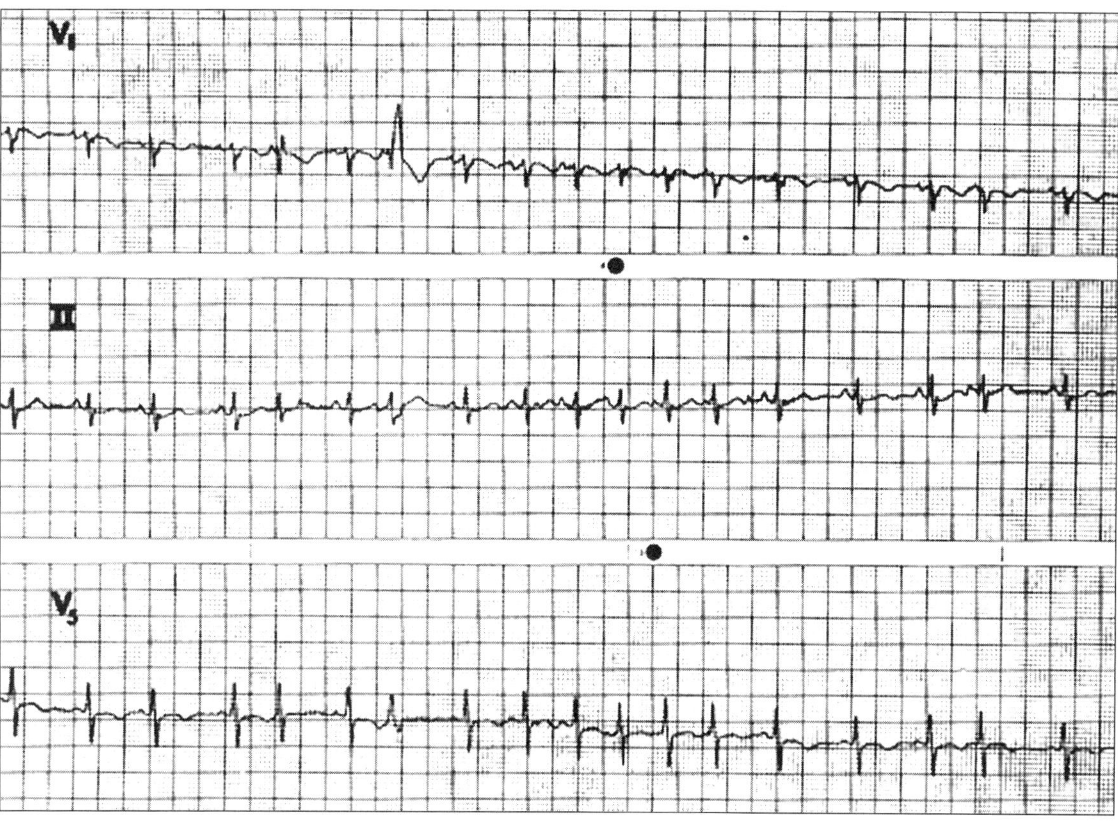

Multifocal atrial tachycardia.

❍ **What is the abnormality seen in the rhythm below?**

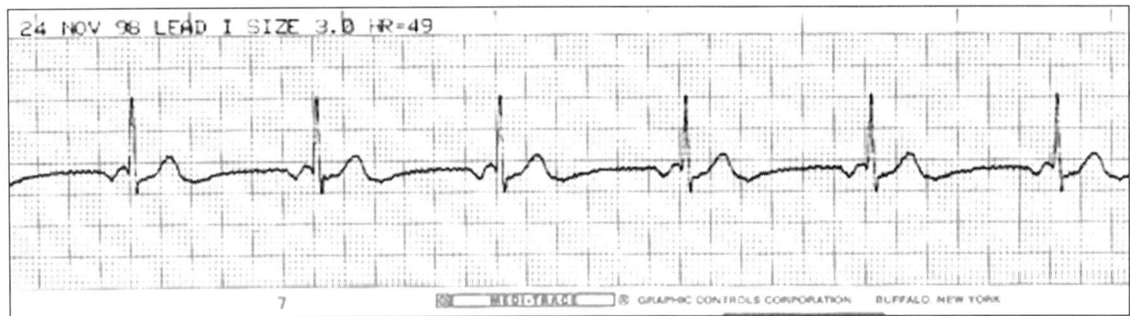

Junctional rhythm.

❍ **What is the abnormality seen in the rhythm below?**

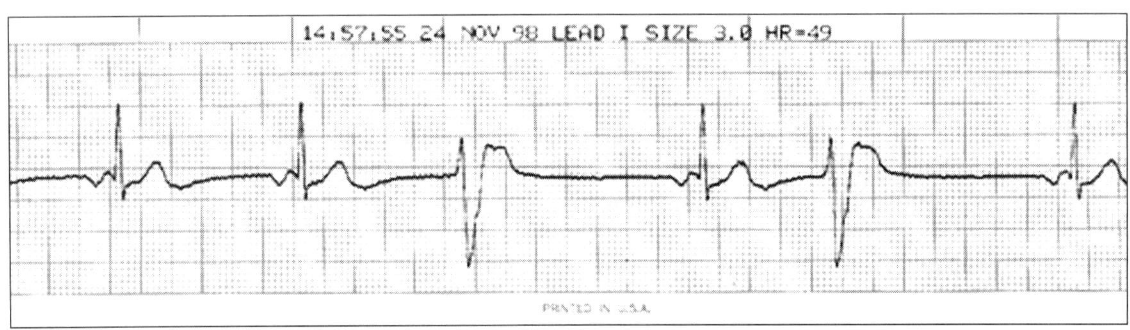

Junctional rhythm with escape ventricular beats.

❍ **What is the abnormality seen in the rhythm below?**

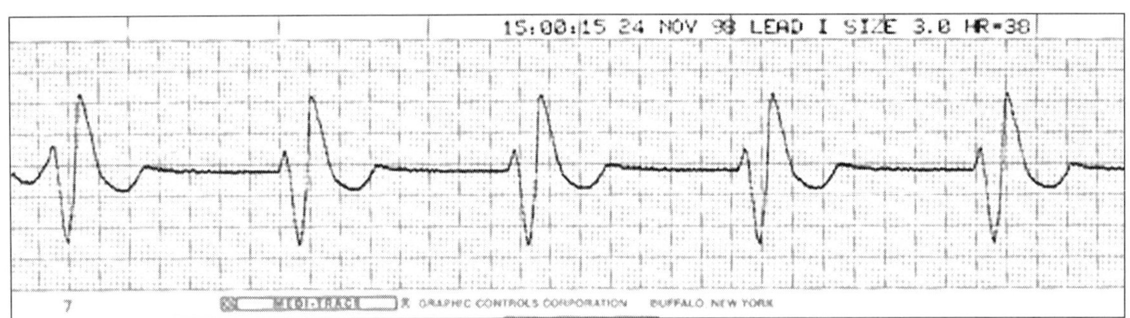

Idioventricular rhythm.

❍ **What is the abnormality seen in the rhythm below?**

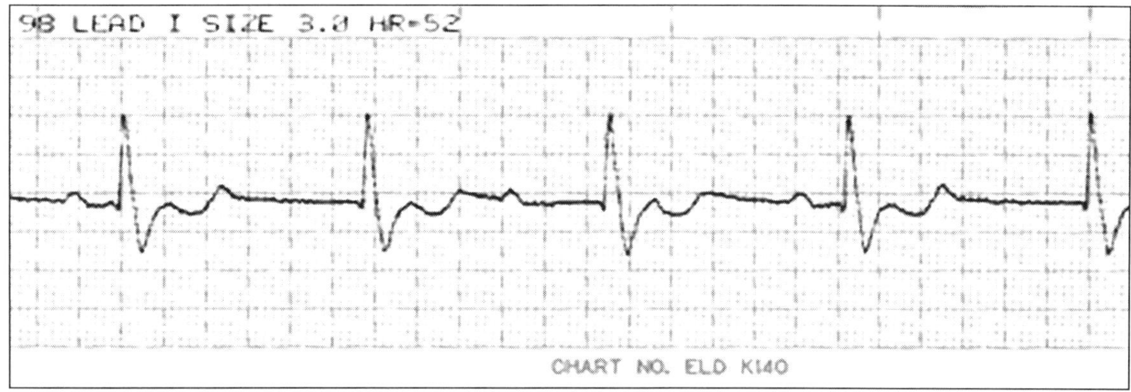

2:1 AV block.

❍ **What is the abnormality seen in the rhythm below?**

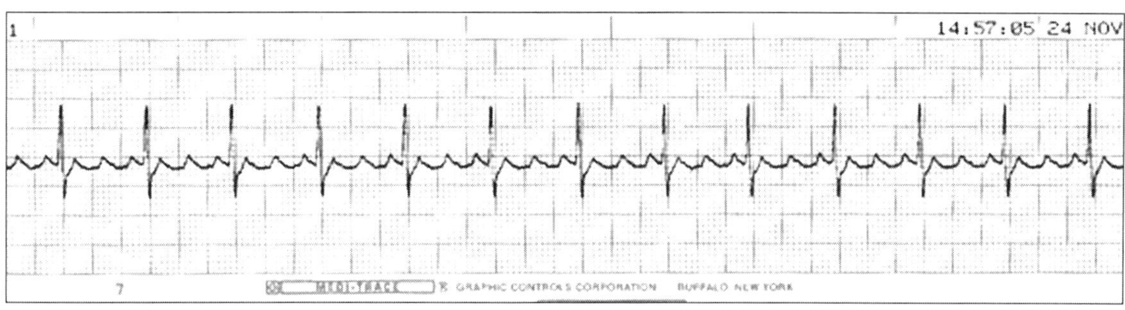

Atrial flutter.

❍ **What is the abnormality seen in the rhythm below?**

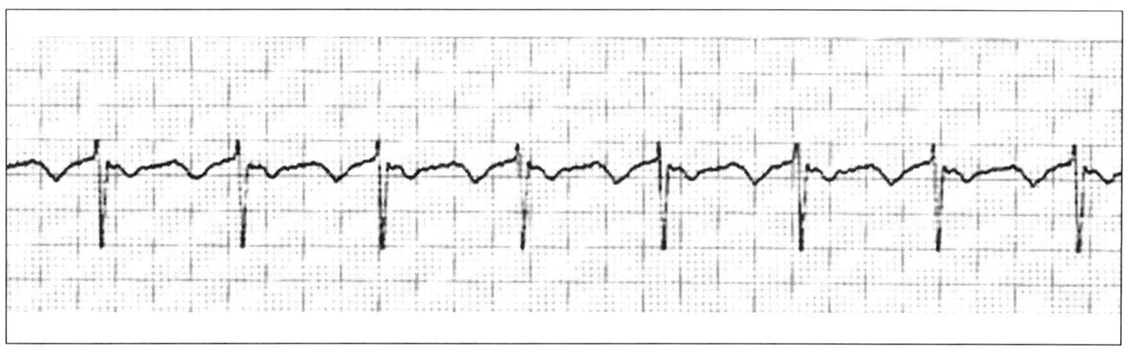

Rhythm strip erroneously mounted upside down. When viewed right-side up, it shows normal sinus rhythm.

O What is the abnormality seen in this two-dimensional echocardiogram?

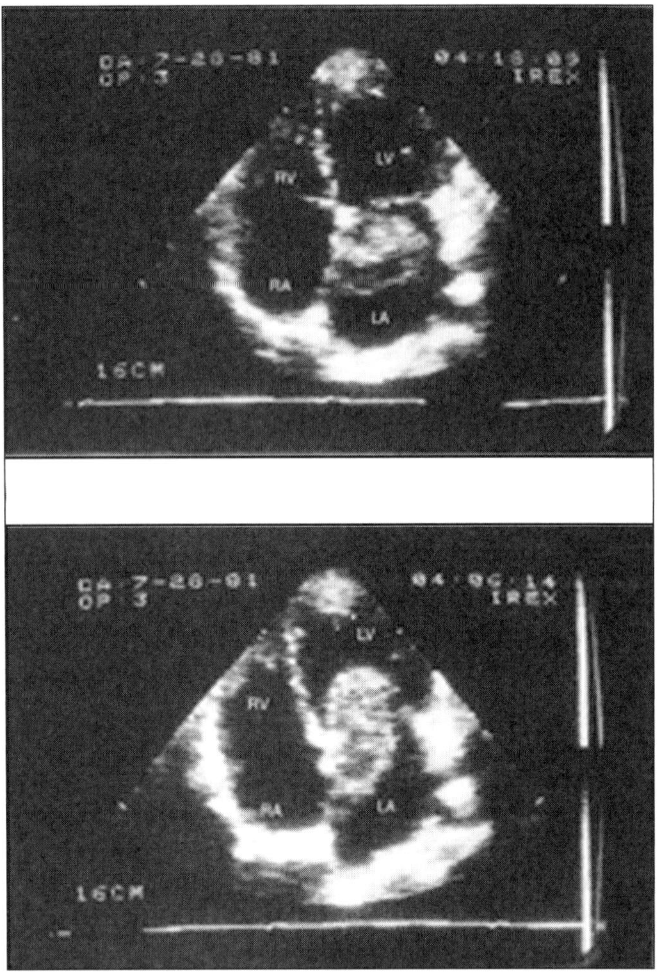

Left atrial myxoma.

O What is the rhythm seen below?

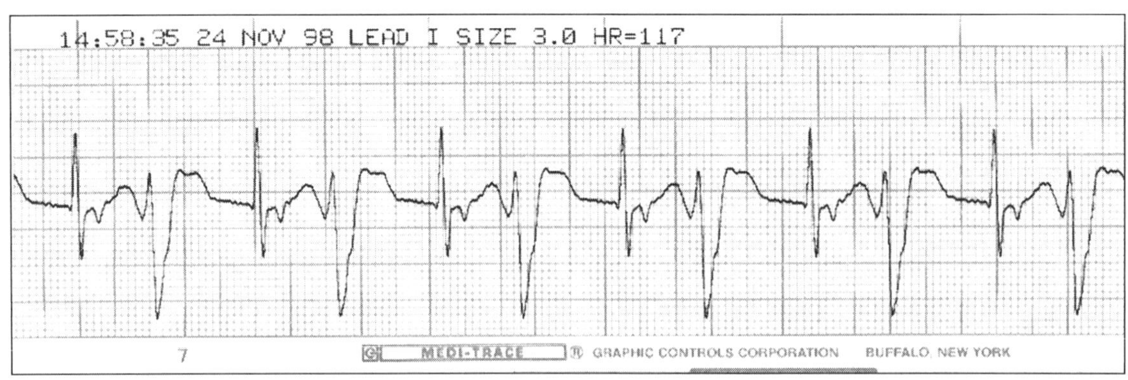

Atrial tachycardia with ventricular bigeminy.

❍ **What is the rhythm abnormality seen below?**

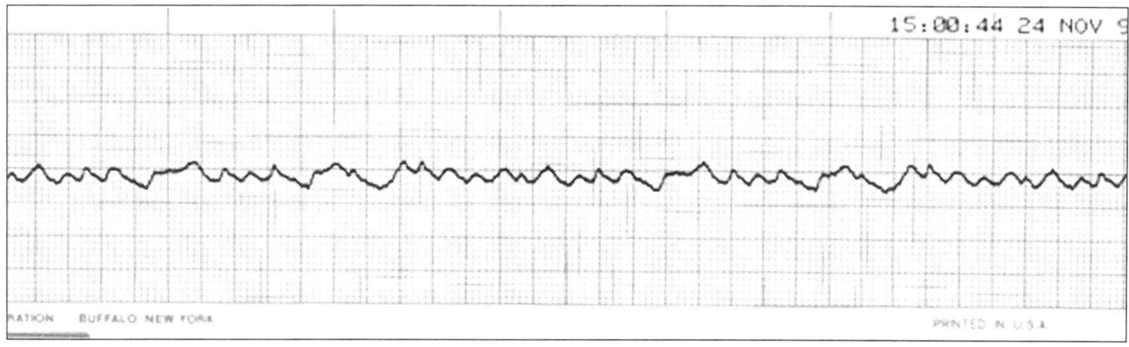

Ventricular fibrillation.

❍ **What is the rhythm abnormality seen below?**

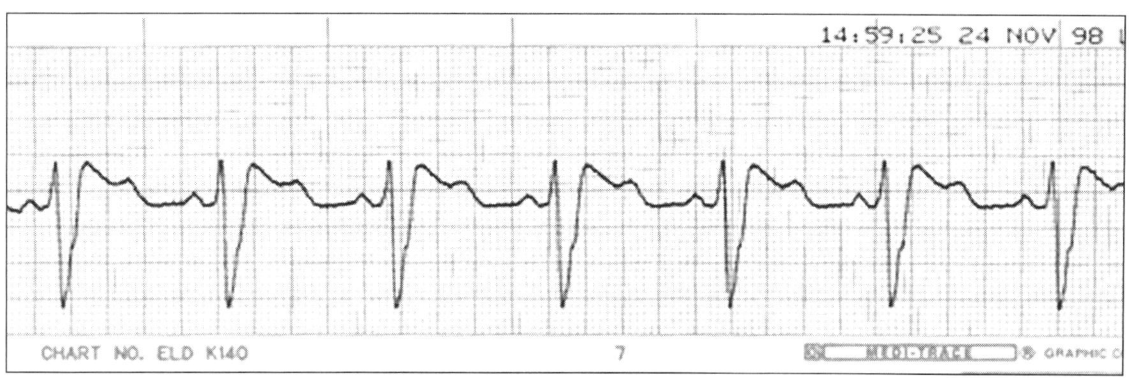

Complete heart block.

❍ **What does the Doppler echocardiogram below show?**

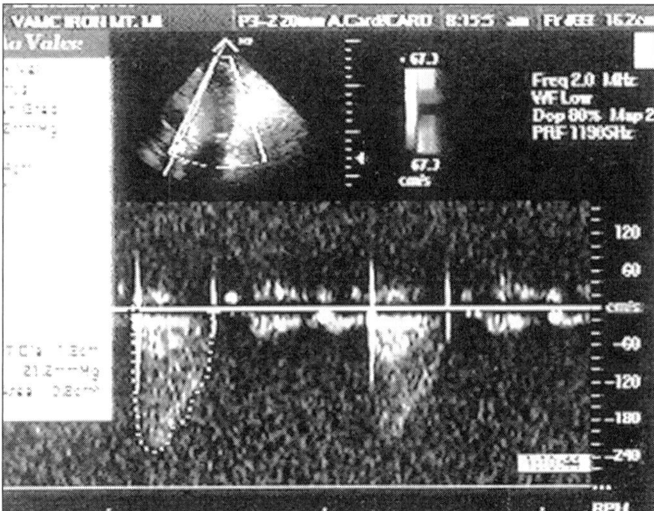

Mild aortic stenosis with a peak systolic flow velocity of 2.5 m/sec.

❍ **What does the Doppler echocardiogram below show?**

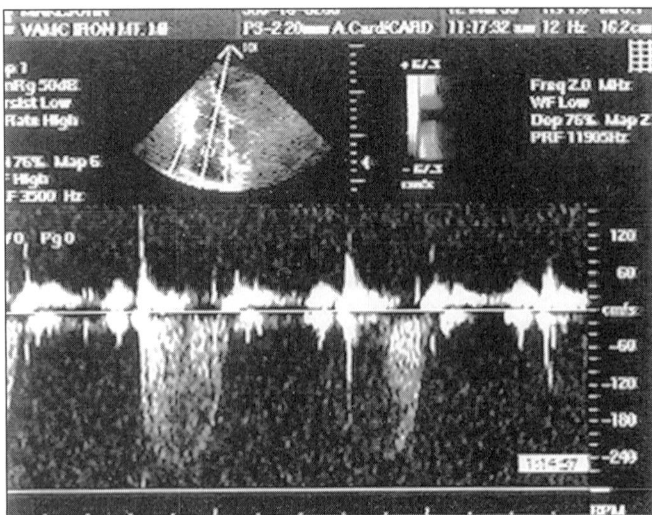

Mild tricuspid regurgitation with mild pulmonary hypertension, as evidenced by a 25 mm peak gradient across the tricuspid valve.

❍ **What does the Doppler echocardiogram below show?**

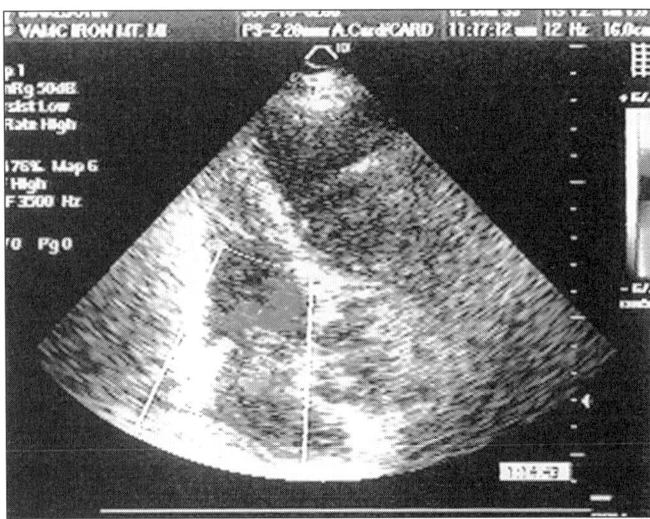

Moderate tricuspid regurgitation.

❍ **What does the Doppler echocardiogram below show?**

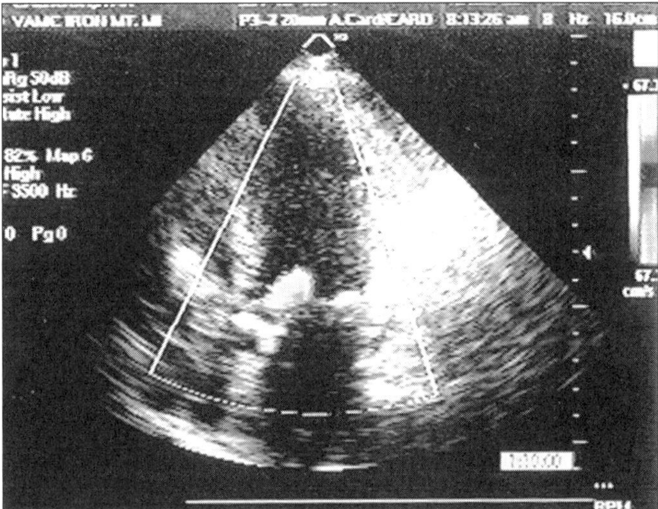

Moderate aortic regurgitation.

❍ **What does the M-mode echocardiogram below show?**

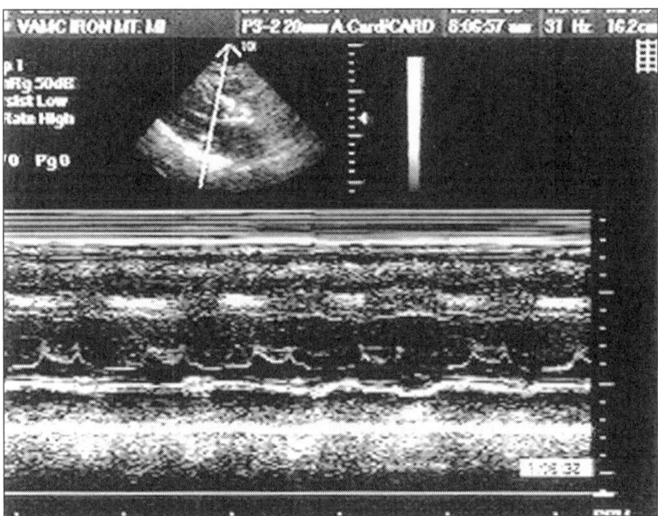

Mitral valve sclerosis with mitral annular calcification.

❍ **What does the Doppler echocardiogram below show?**

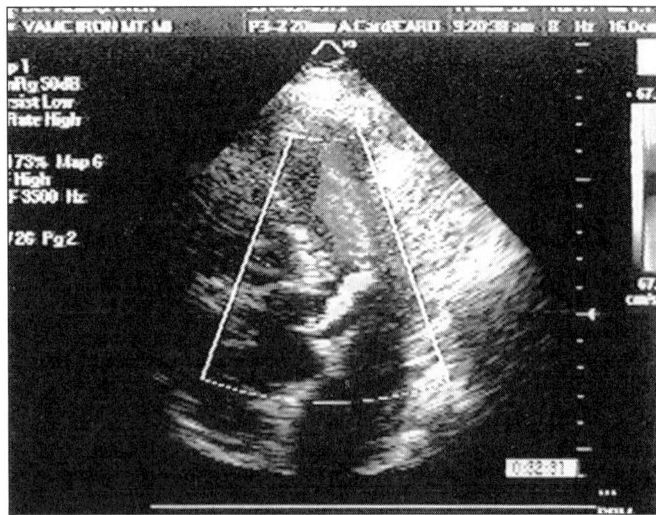

Moderate to severe aortic regurgitation.

❍ **What can you say about the LV function based on the M-mode of the aortic valve shown below?**

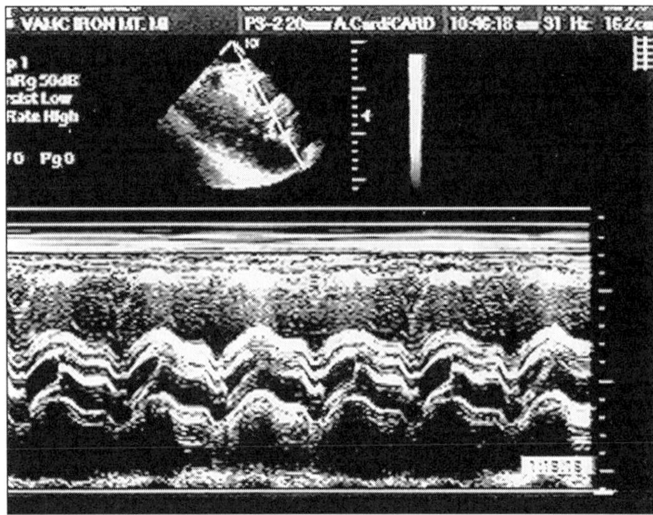

This patient has normal LV systolic function. Note the excellent aortic motion.

❍ **What does this transesophageal echocardiogram of the thoracic aorta show?**

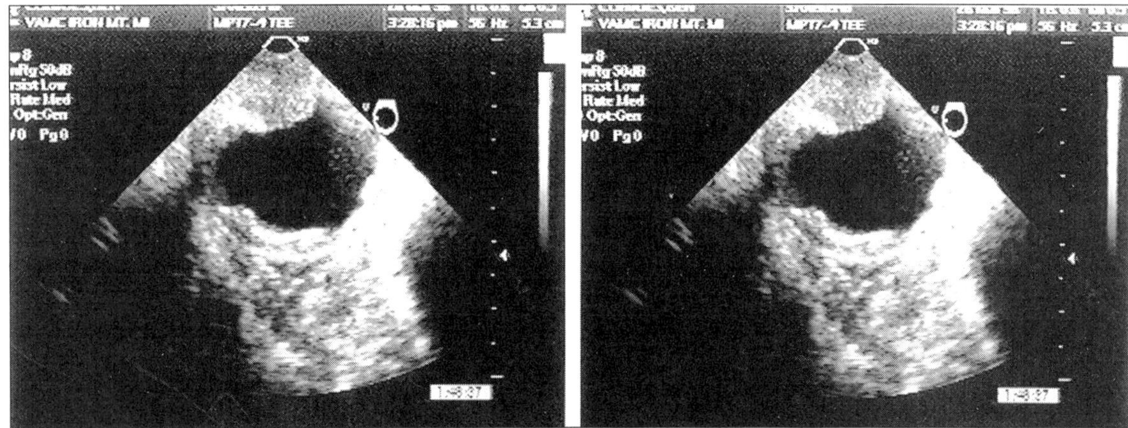

Moderate to severe aortic atherosclerosis with a large plaque in the anterior aspect of the aortic wall. Note the circumferential disease of the aorta.

❍ **What does this transesophageal echocardiogram show?**

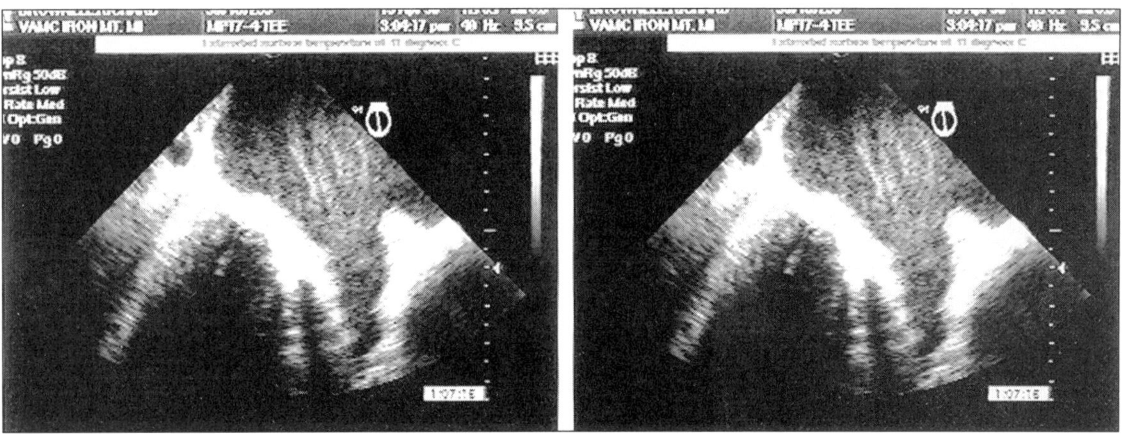

Spontaneous contrast in a large left atrium and enlarged left atrial appendage. No atrial thrombi are seen.

O What is seen in the transesophageal echocardiogram below?

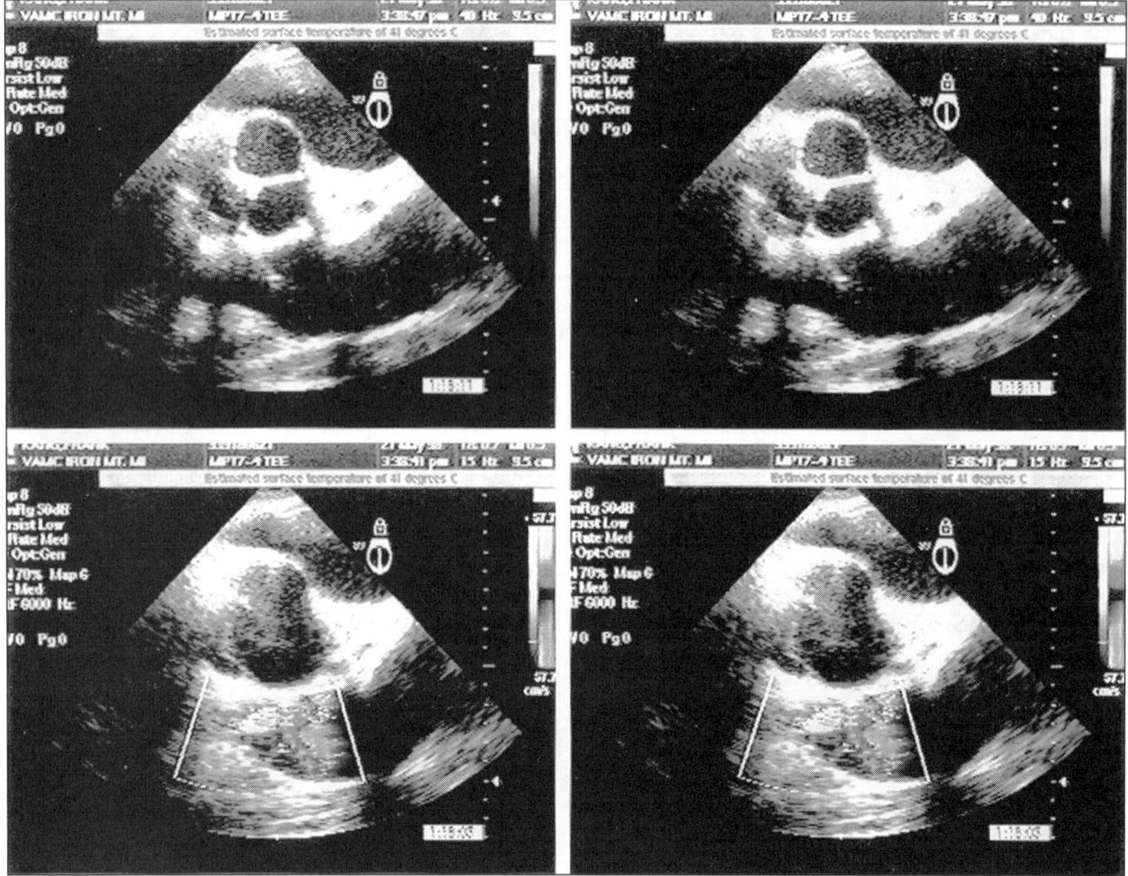

The pulmonic valve with the pulmonary artery is seen below the aorta and aortic valve. The color Doppler shows pulmonic regurgitation.

O What is seen in the transesophageal echocardiogram below?

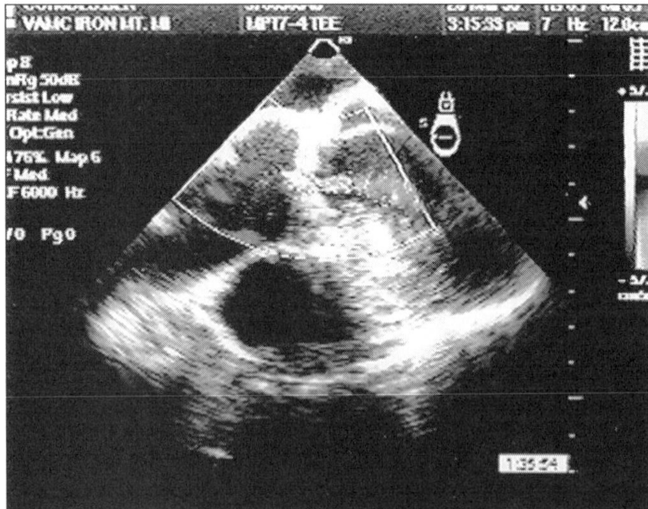

Aortic regurgitation across a very thickened aortic valve.

❍ **What is seen in this transesophageal echocardiogram shown below?**

Thickened mitral valve, mild to moderate aortic regurgitation, and mild to moderate eccentric mitral regurgitation.

❍ **What is seen in this Doppler echocardiogram shown below?**

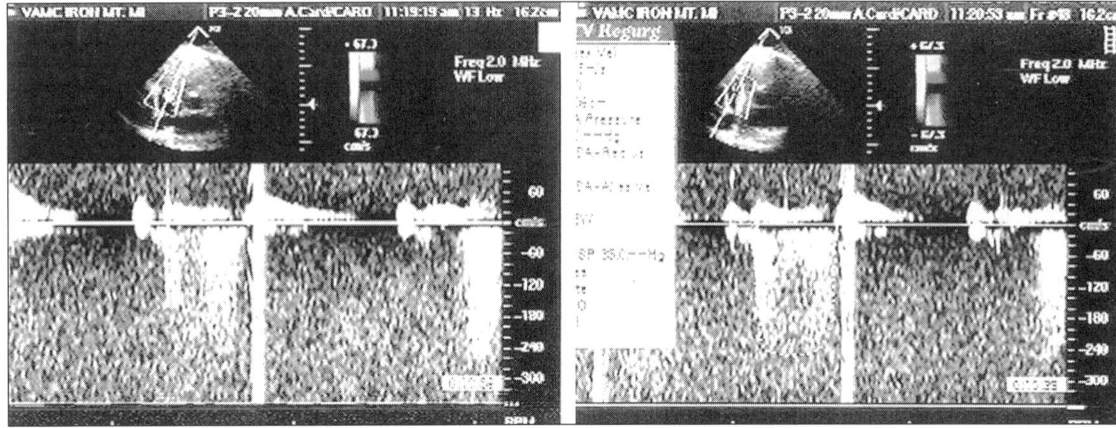

Mild to moderate tricuspid regurgitation with a peak gradient across the tricuspid valve of 36 mm Hg. This patient has mild to moderate pulmonary hypertension.

❍ **What does this M-mode echocardiogram of the LV reveal about this patient's LV systolic function?**

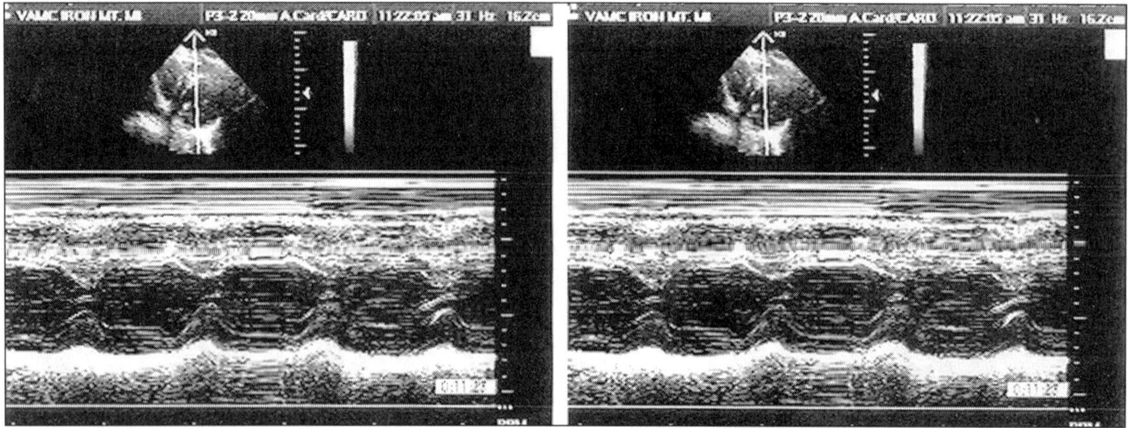

This patient's systolic function is normal.

❍ **What does this M-mode echocardiogram at the aortic valve level reveal about this patient's LV systolic function?**

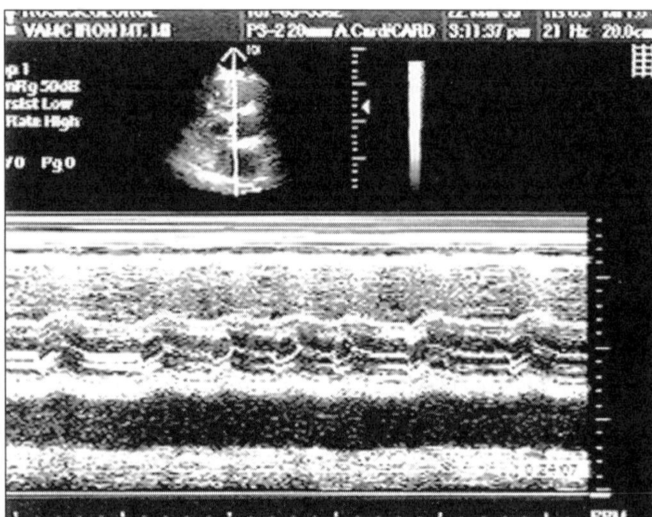

This patient's LV systolic function is poor. Note the poor motion of the aorta and the early closure of the aortic valve.

❍ **What does this M-mode echocardiogram at the LV level reveal?**

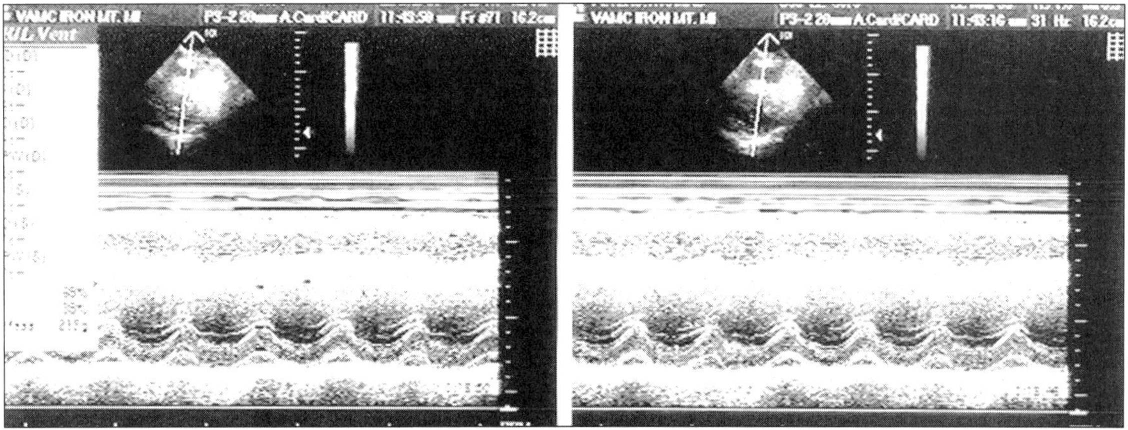

This patient has a small pericardial effusion. Note the echo-free space below the posterior wall and between the pericardium.

❍ **What does this electrophysiology study show?**

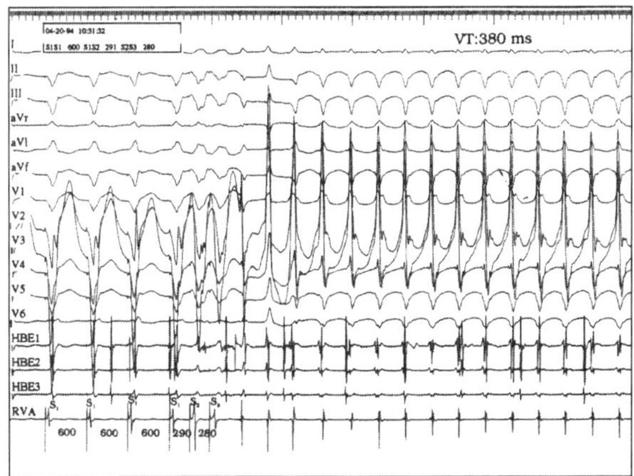

Induced sustained monomorphic ventricular tachycardia.

❍ **What is the abnormality seen on this waveform tracing taken during cardiac catheterization?**

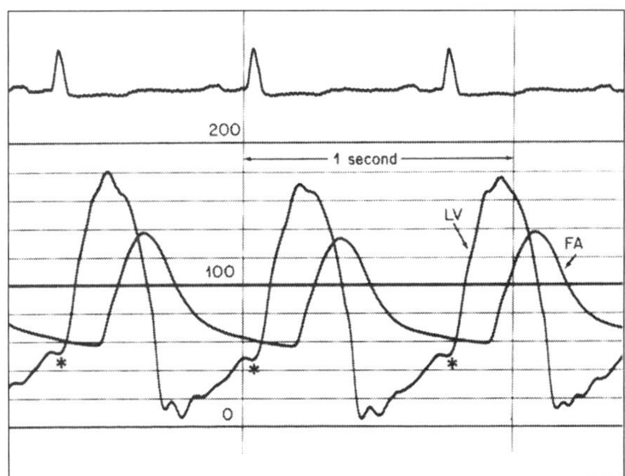

Severe aortic stenosis.

O What is the abnormality seen on this Doppler echocardiogram shown below?

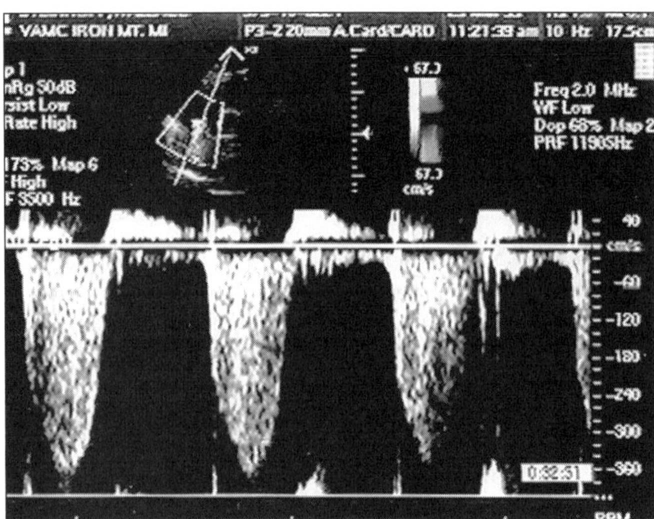

Moderate to severe tricuspid regurgitation with severe pulmonary hypertension, as evidenced by the 4 m/sec flow velocity across the tricuspid valve.

O What is the interpretation of this ECG shown below?

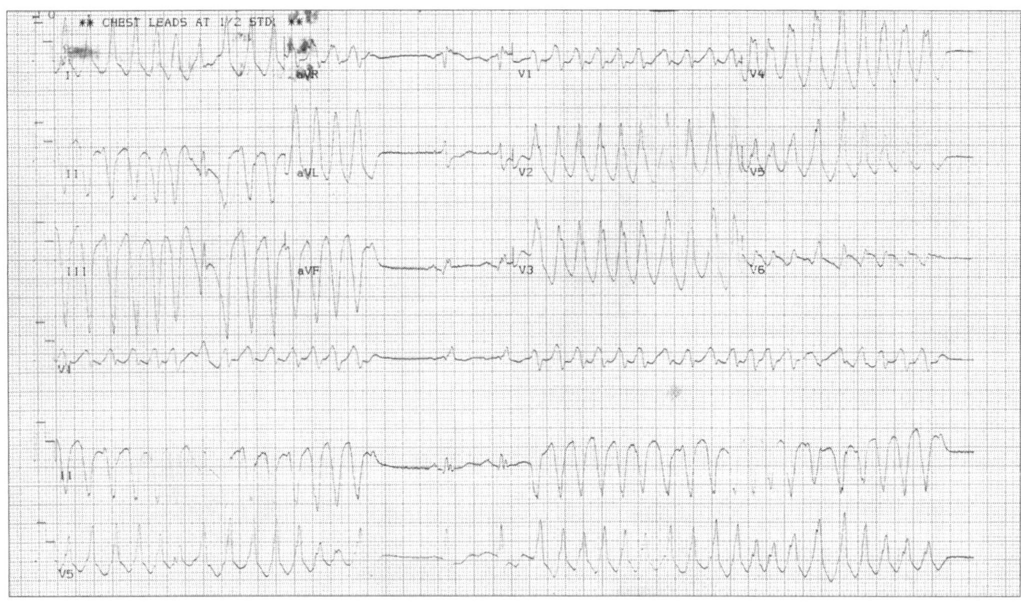

Ventricular tachycardia, most likely originating from the left ventricle.

❍ What is the interpretation of this ECG shown below?

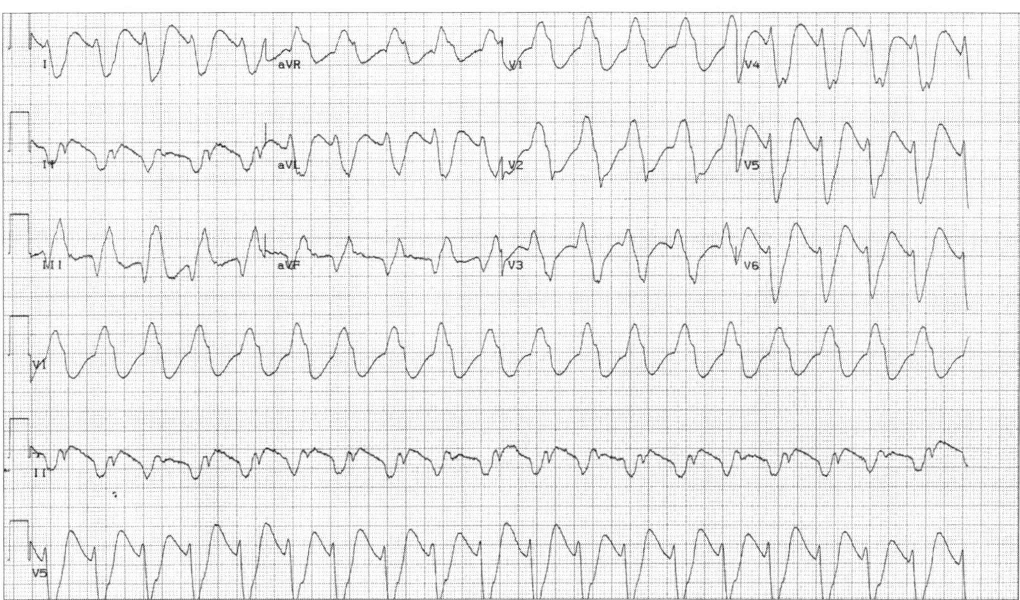

Ventricular tachycardia with hyperkalemia. Note the very wide QRS complex with the early stages of a "sine wave".

❍ What is the interpretation of the ECG shown below?

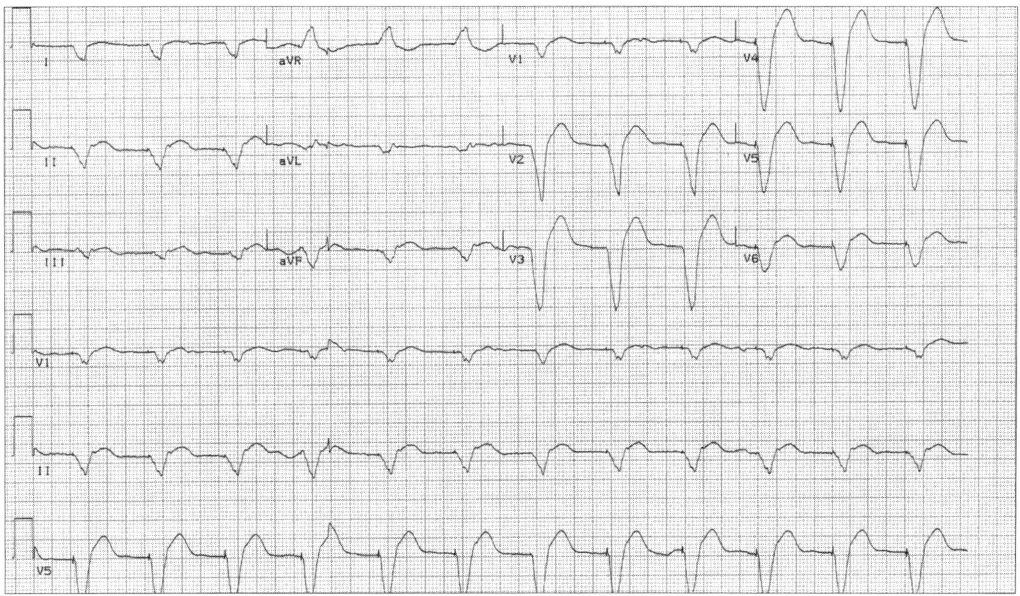

A single chamber ventricular pacemaker rhythm with 100% capture and 100% sensing. The underlying atrial rhythm is fibrillation as there are no P waves visible.

❍ What is the interpretation of the ECG shown below?

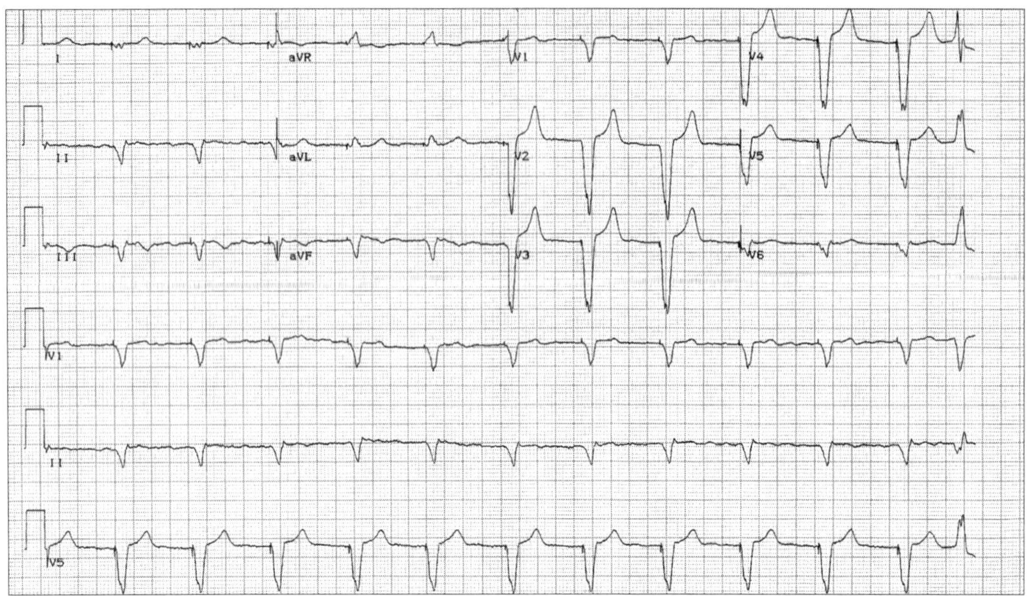

Single chamber ventricular pacemaker rhythm with 100% capture. The underlying atrial rhythm is fibrillation. This pacemaker is in VVI mode.

❍ What is the interpretation of the ECG shown below?

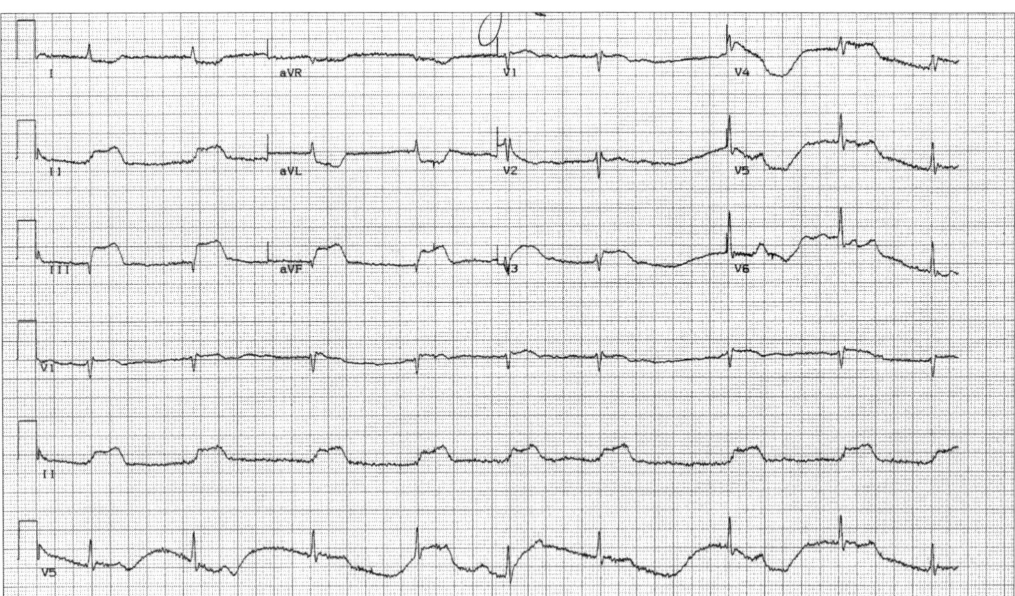

Acute inferior myocardial infarction with posterior wall involvement, atrial fibrillation with slow ventricular rate.

❍ What is the interpretation of the ECG shown below?

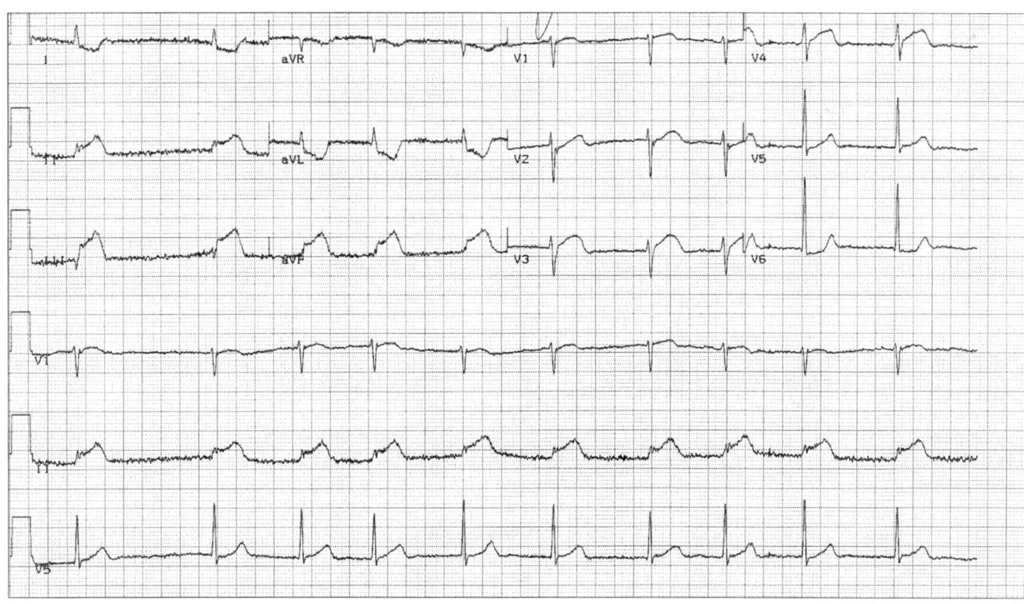

Acute inferior myocardial infarction, atrial fibrillation with slow ventricular rate.

❍ In the above ECG, does this patient absolutely have myocardial ischemia?

Not necessarily. Patients with supraventricular tachycardia of any type with ST depression can have "ischemic" appearing ST depression without having myocardial ischemia. The ST depression can be as a result of abnormal repolarization that occurs in any tachyarrhythmia. Nonetheless, it would be incorrect to automatically assume that this patient's ST depression is not due to myocardial ischemia.

❍ What is the interpretation of the ECG shown below?

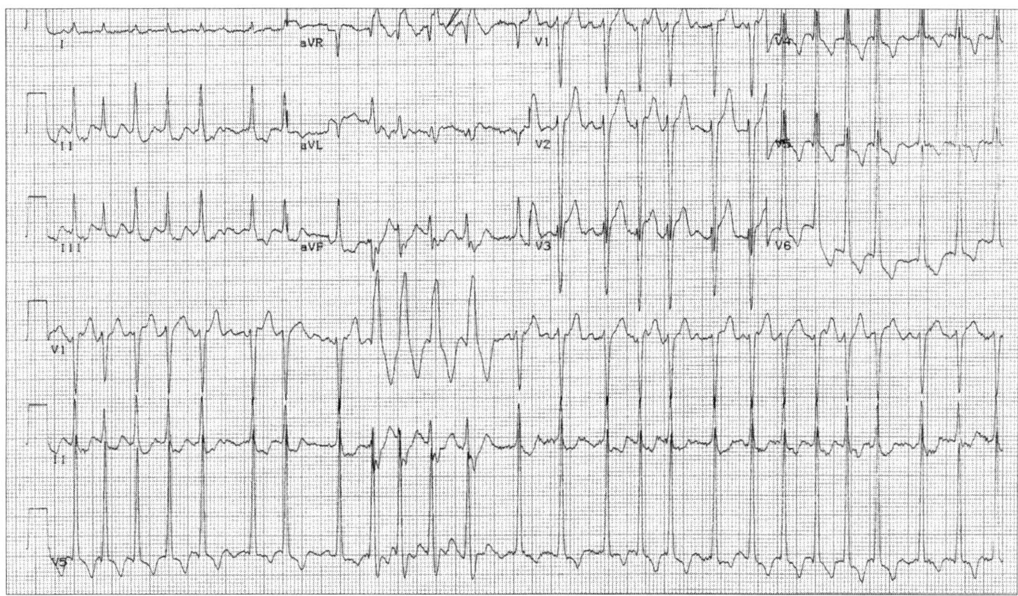

Atrial fibrillation with rapid ventricular rate of 155, LVH, and ischemic-type ST depression in the inferior and lateral leads.

❍ **What is the interpretation of the ECG shown below?**

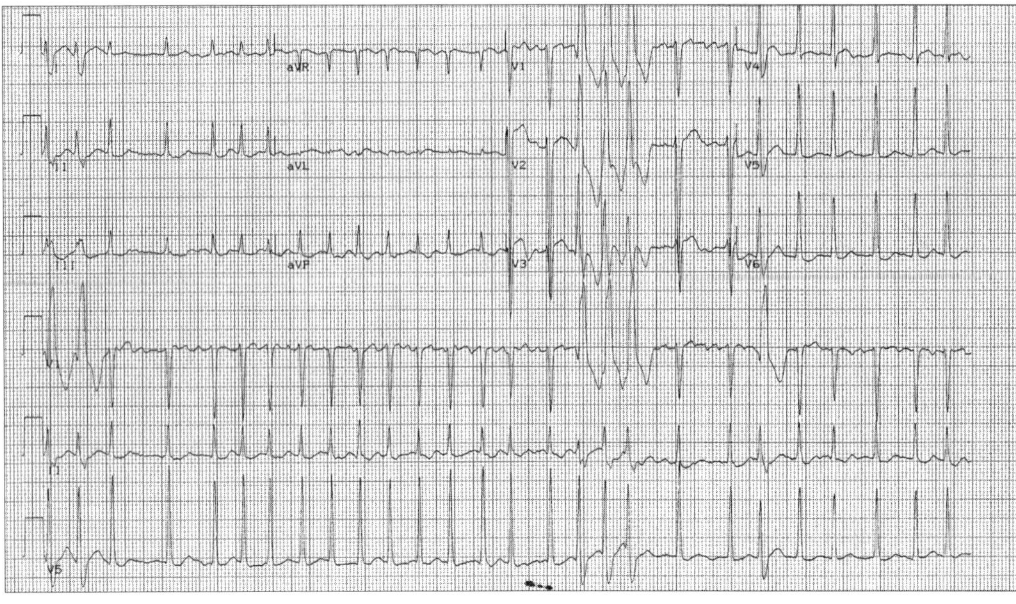

Atrial fibrillation with rapid ventricular rate, and classic example of Ashman's phenomenon. The aberrantly conducted wide-QRS complexes are not ventricular tachycardia, but aberrantly conducted impulses from the atrial fibrillation. Note the long-short-long R-R interval just preceding the Ashman's beats, a hallmark of Ashman's phenomenon.

❍ **Based on the ECG shown below, does this patient have a single chamber pacemaker or a dual chamber pacemaker?**

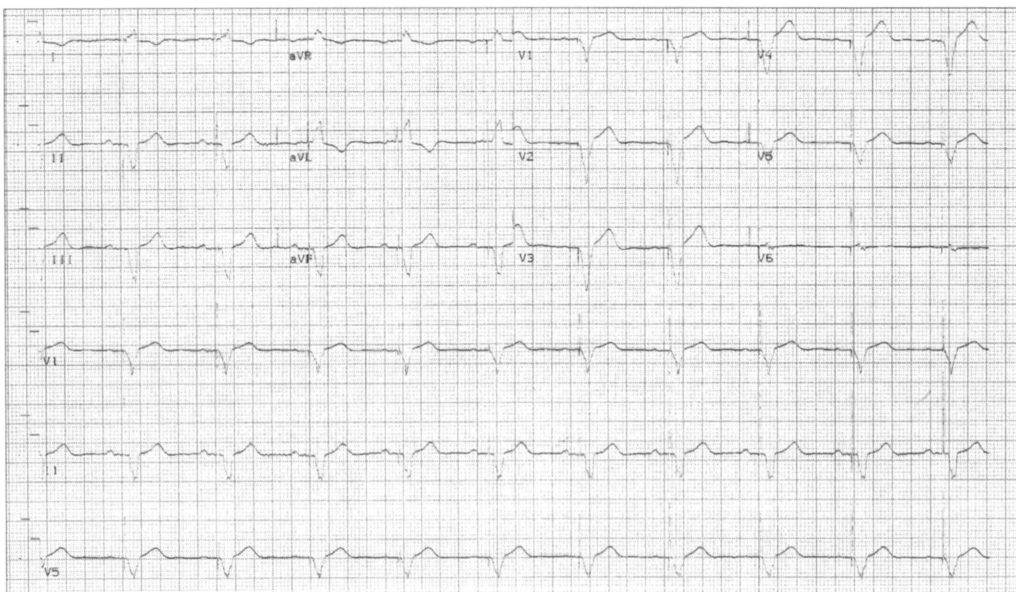

Dual chamber. Note the P waves preceding the ventricular pacer spikes and the constant P-R interval, thereby signifying a sensing of the native atrial impulses and pacing of the ventricle. A single chamber ventricular pacemaker would show AV dissociation in a patient with sinus rhythm.

❍ What is the interpretation of the ECG shown below?

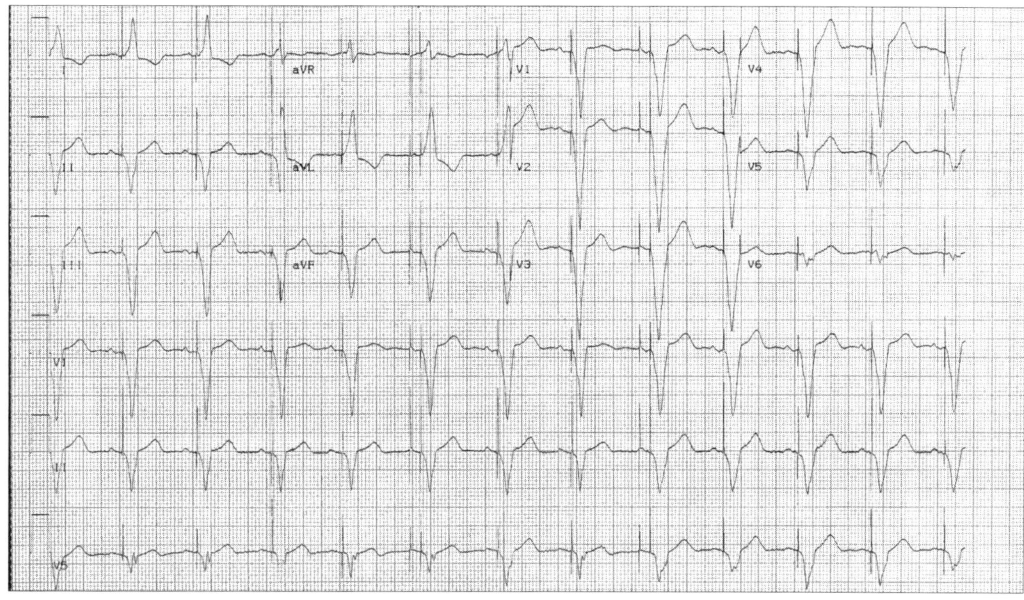

Dual chamber pacemaker in DDD mode with alternating AV sequential and AV synchronous pacing. Note the atrial sensing in the complexes without a preceding P spike prior to the P wave. The ventricle is 100% paced.

❍ What is the most likely underlying conduction abnormality in a patient with the ECG shown in the preceding question?

Complete AV block (3rd degree).

❍ What is the interpretation of the ECG shown below?

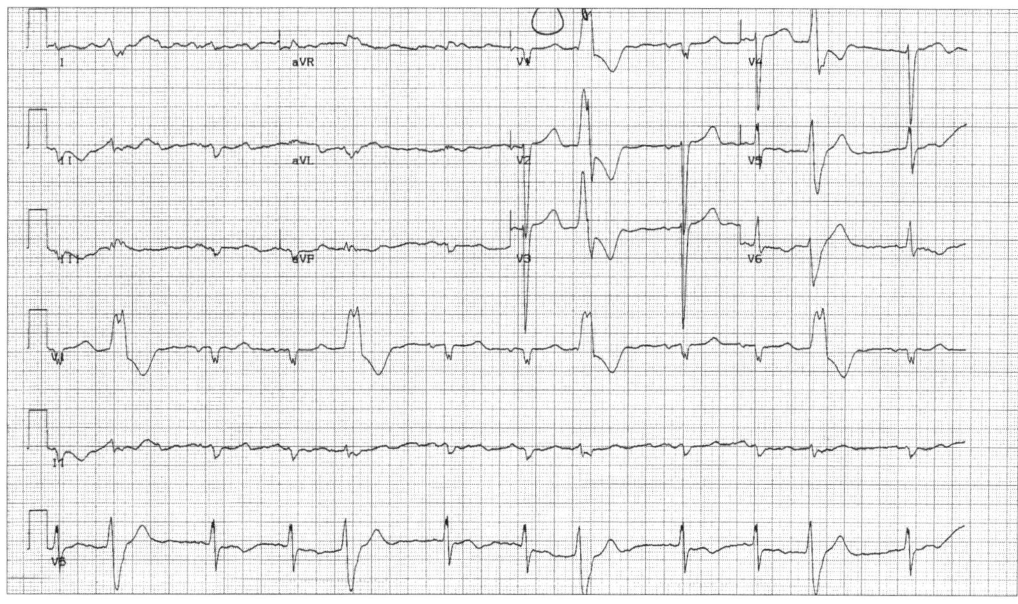

Normal sinus rhythm, left anterior fascicular block, multiple polymorphic PVC's, low voltage in the limb leads, left atrial enlargement and LVH.

❍ **What is the interpretation of the ECG shown below?**

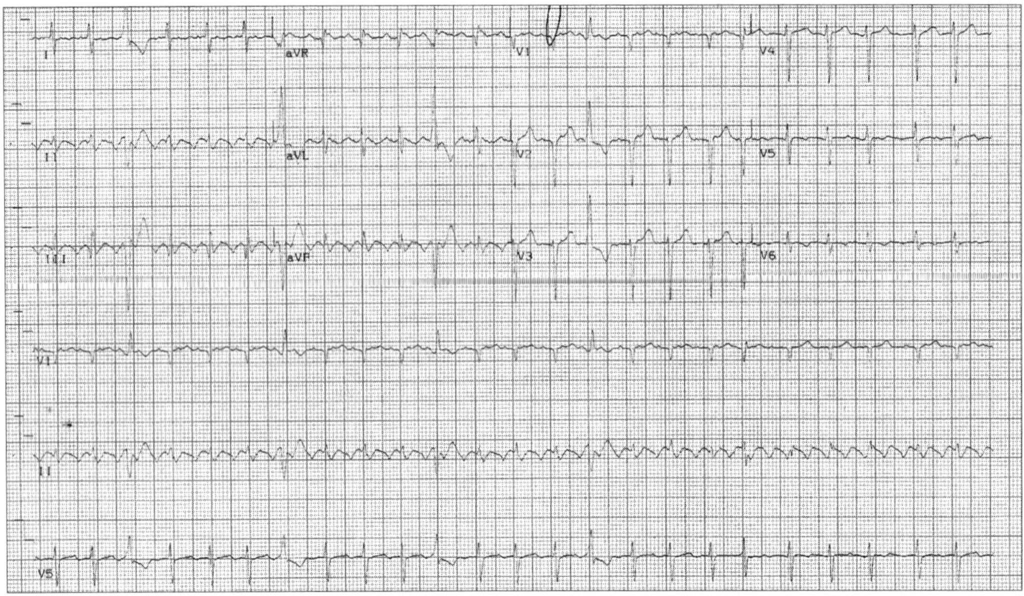

Atrial flutter with 2:1 block with aberrantly conducted complexes, old anteroseptal infarct and non-specific ST abnormality.

❍ **What is the interpretation of the ECG shown below?**

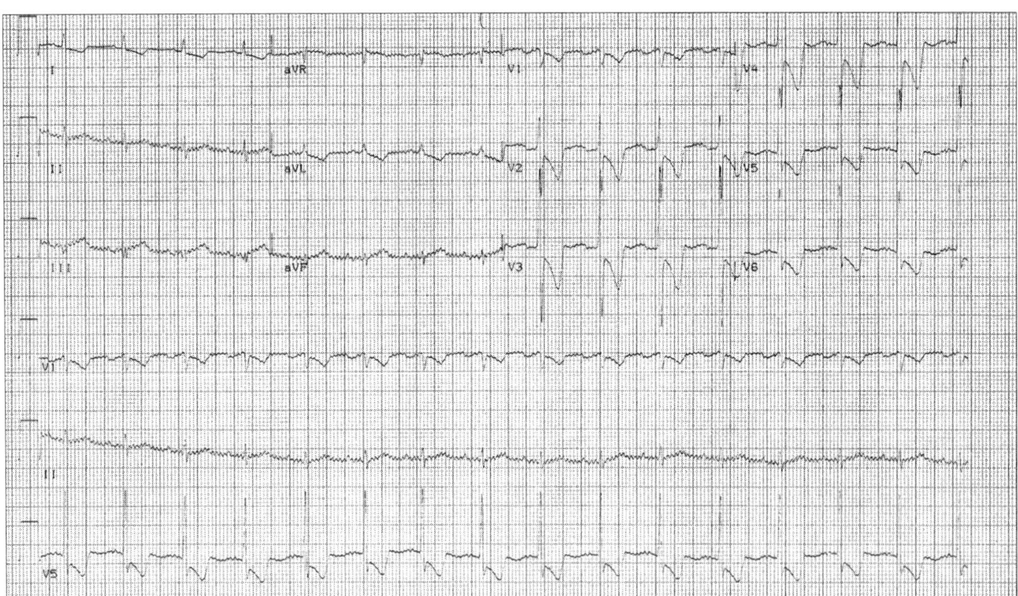

Normal sinus rhythm and profound anterolateral ST depression with T inversion, highly suggestive of a non-Q wave myocardial infarction.

What is the interpretation of the ECG seen below?

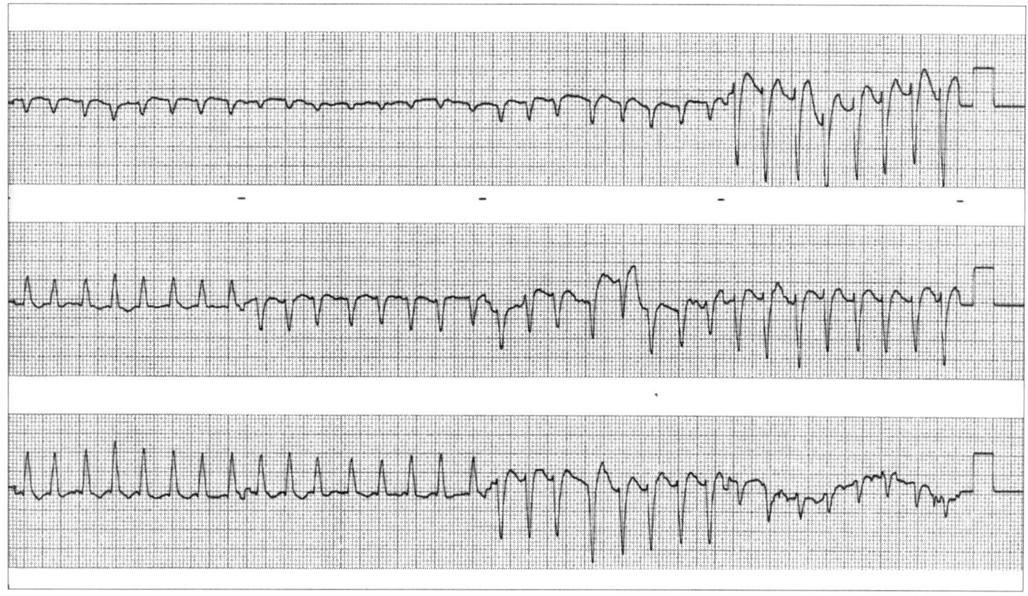

Supraventricular tachycardia.

What is the interpretation of the ECG shown below?

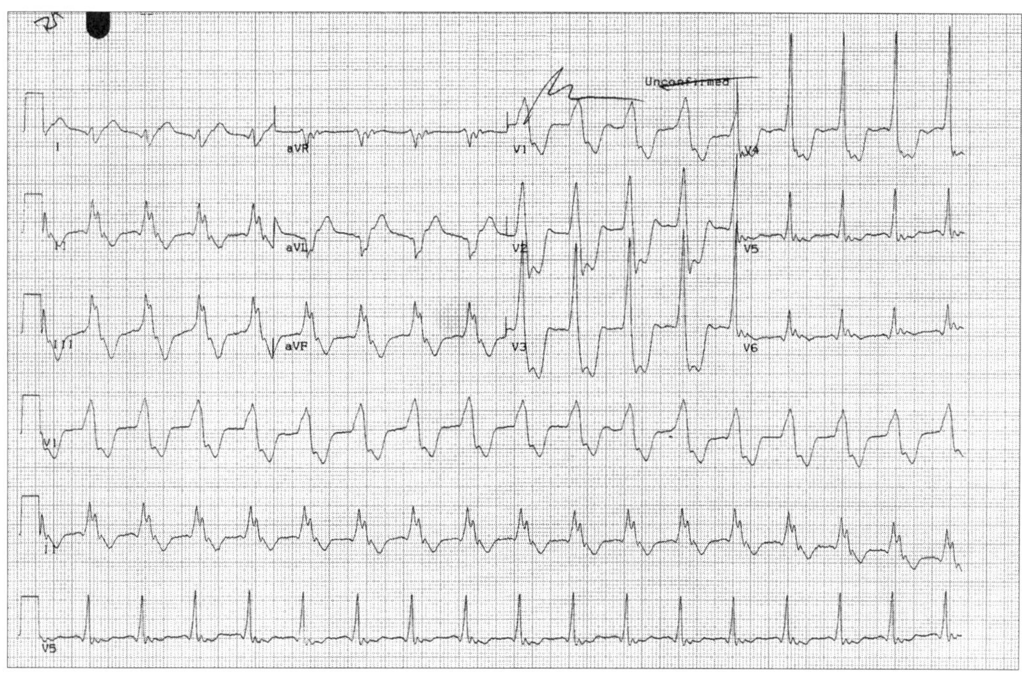

Ventricular tachycardia with a ventricular rate of 103. Note the VA conduction evidenced by the retrograde P waves, which occur in the early part of the ST segment.

❍ What is the interpretation of the ECG shown below?

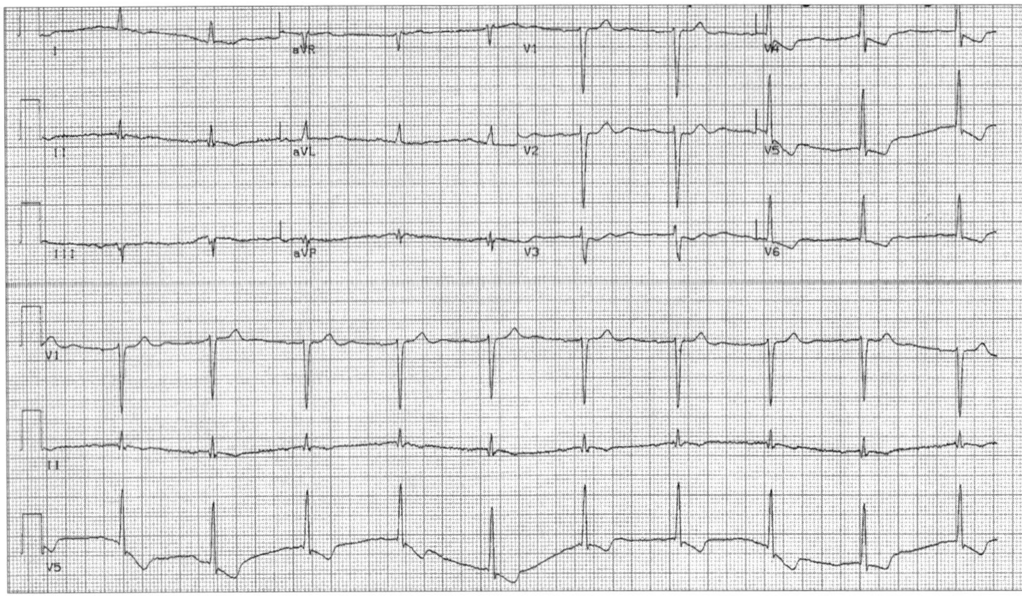

Atrial ectopic rhythm, old inferior myocardial infarction and non-specific ST-T abnormalities in the lateral leads. Note the inverted or biphasic P waves in the inferior leads.

❍ What is the interpretation of the ECG shown below?

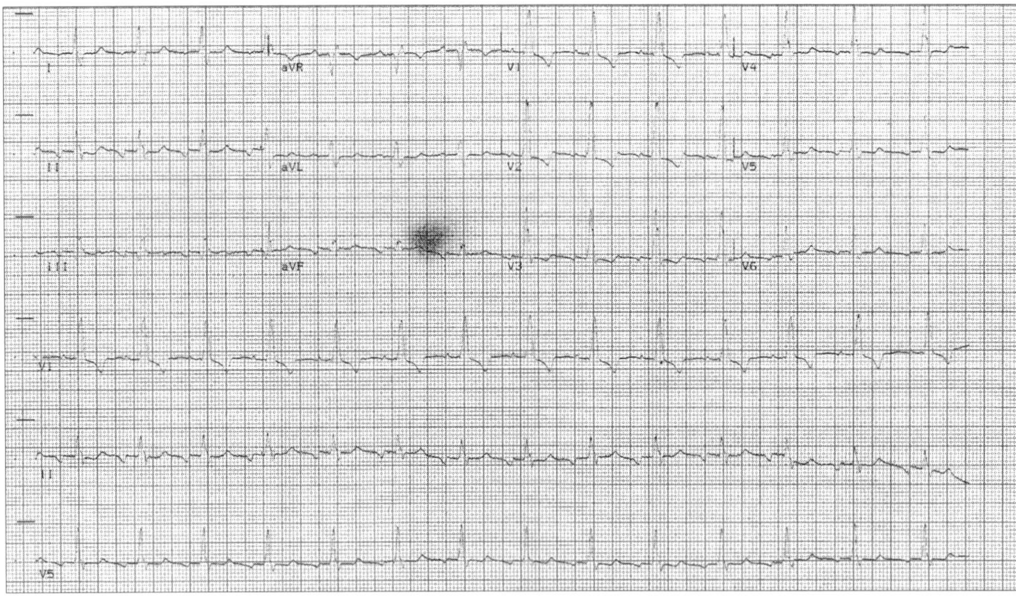

Atrial ectopic rhythm and RBBB.

❍ **What is the interpretation of the ECG shown below?**

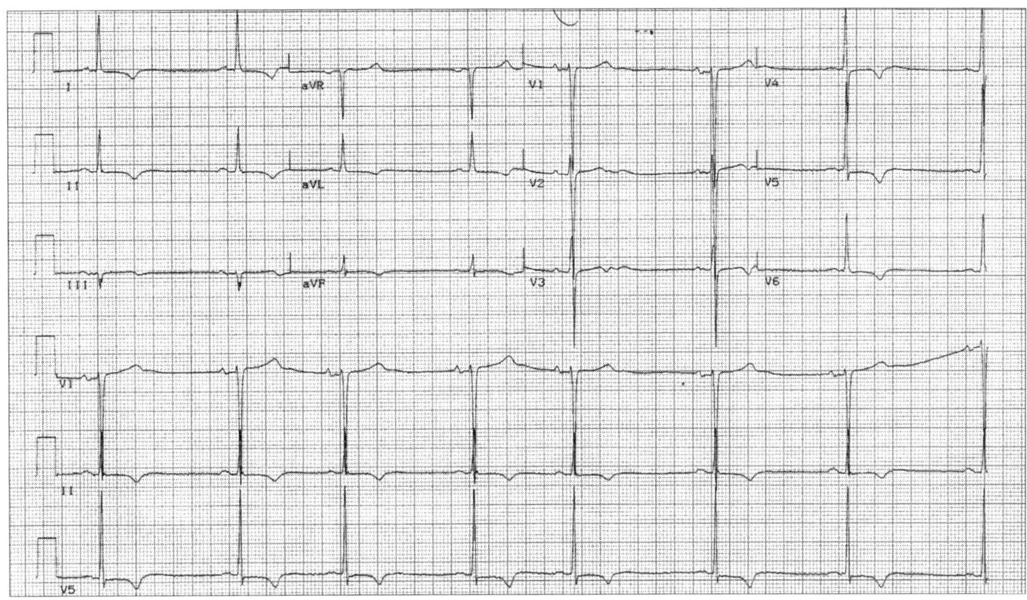

Sinus arrhythmia, a non-conducted PAC, and LVH with repolarization abnormalities. Note the P wave in the early part of the QRS of complex #5, followed by a U wave, followed by a pause.

❍ **What is the interpretation of the ECG shown below?**

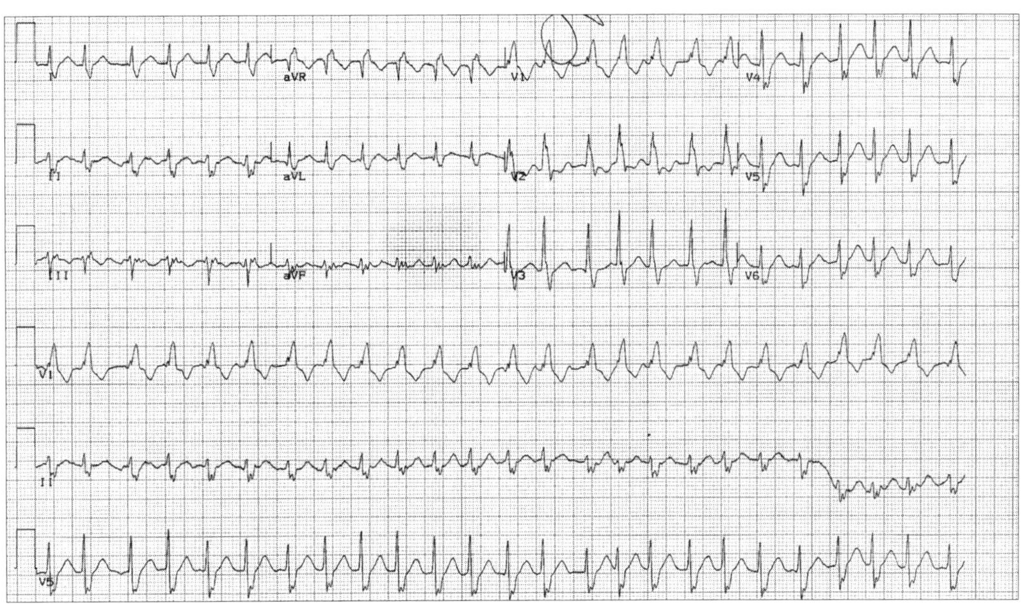

Normal sinus rhythm, RBBB and left anterior fascicular block (bifascicular block).

❍ **What is the interpretation of the ECG shown below?**

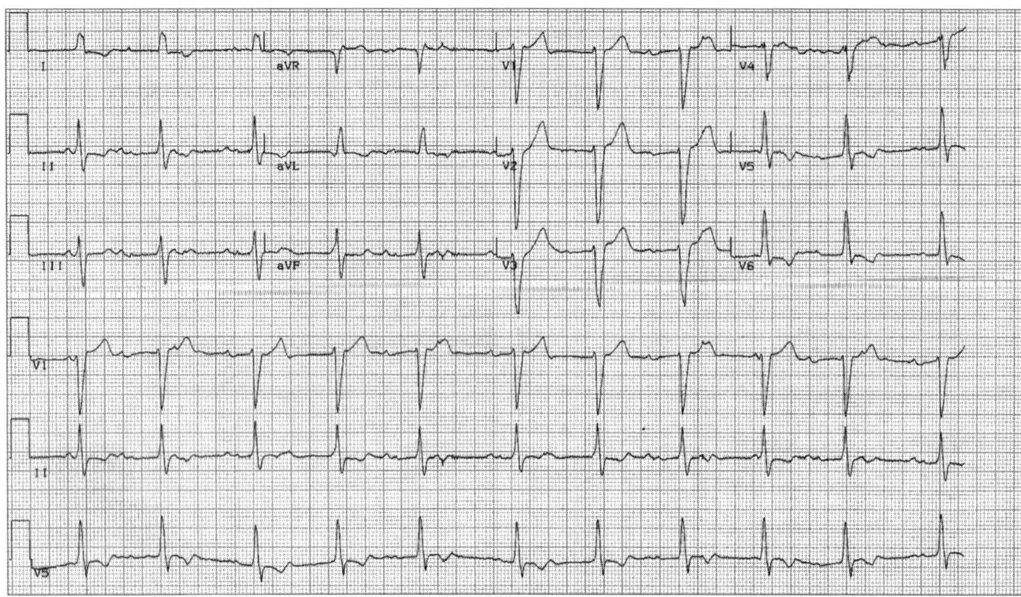

Normal sinus rhythm, 3rd degree AV block with accelerated ventricular rate.

❍ **What is the interpretation of the ECG shown below?**

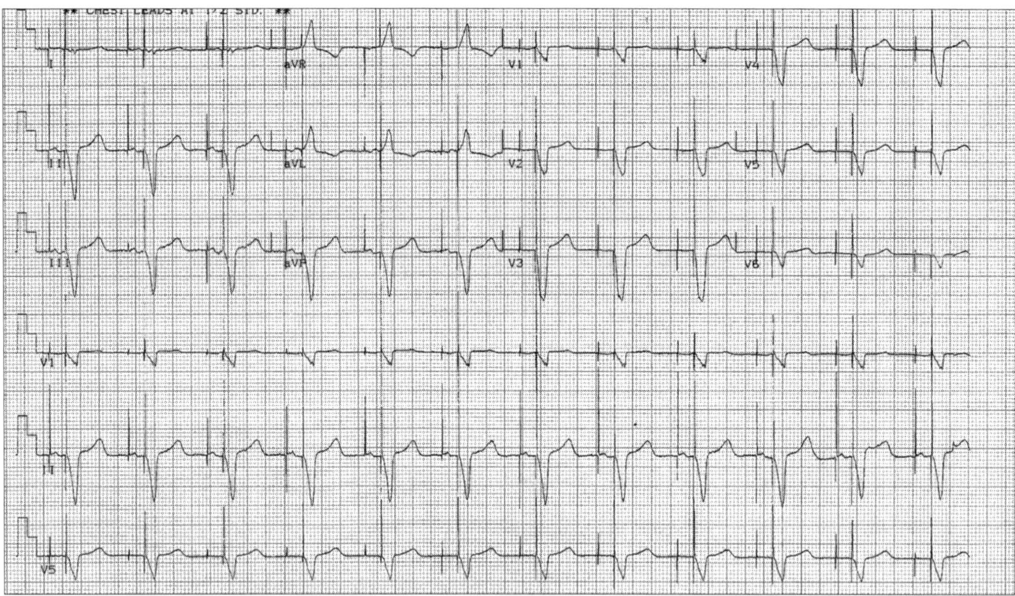

Dual chamber pacemaker rhythm with 100% pacing of both the atrium and ventricle.

❍ What is the interpretation of the ECG shown below?

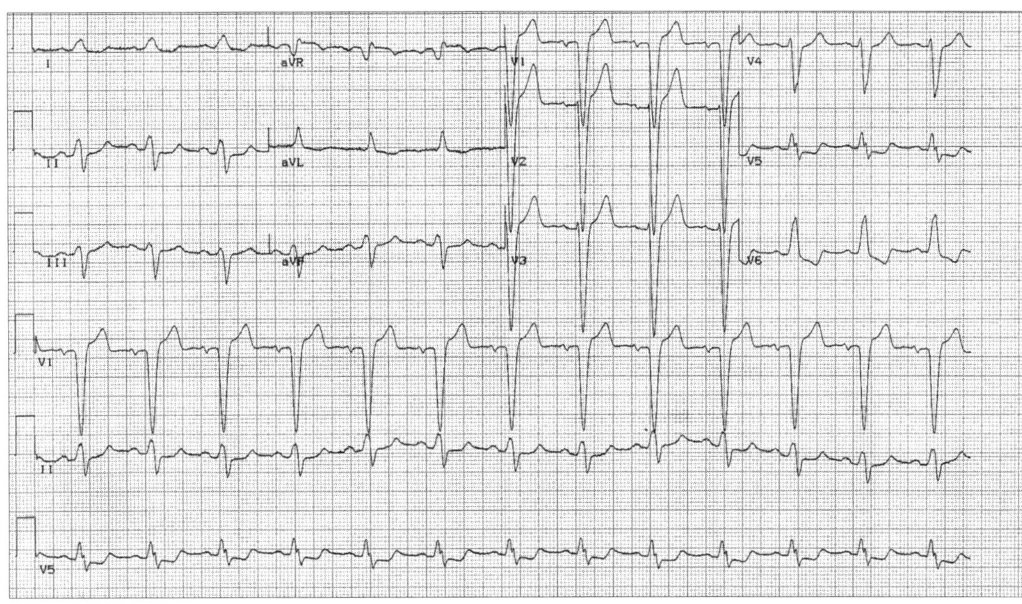

Normal sinus rhythm and LBBB with repolarization abnormalities. Note the very deep S wave in V2, measuring 33 mm, but this is 2 mm short of calling it LVH.

❍ What is the interpretation of the ECG shown below?

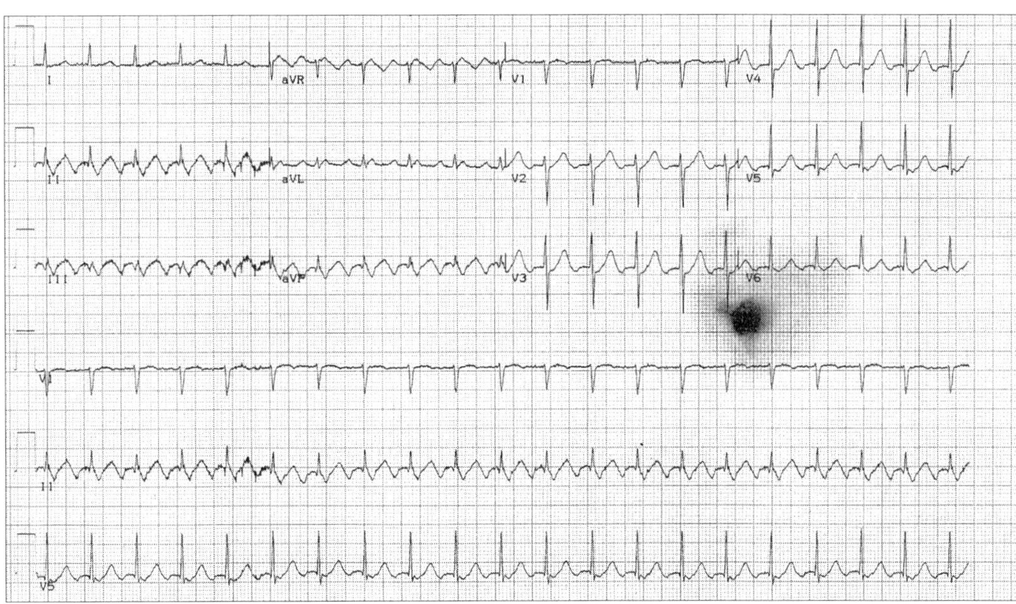

Atrial flutter with 2:1 conduction.

○ What is the interpretation of the ECG shown below?

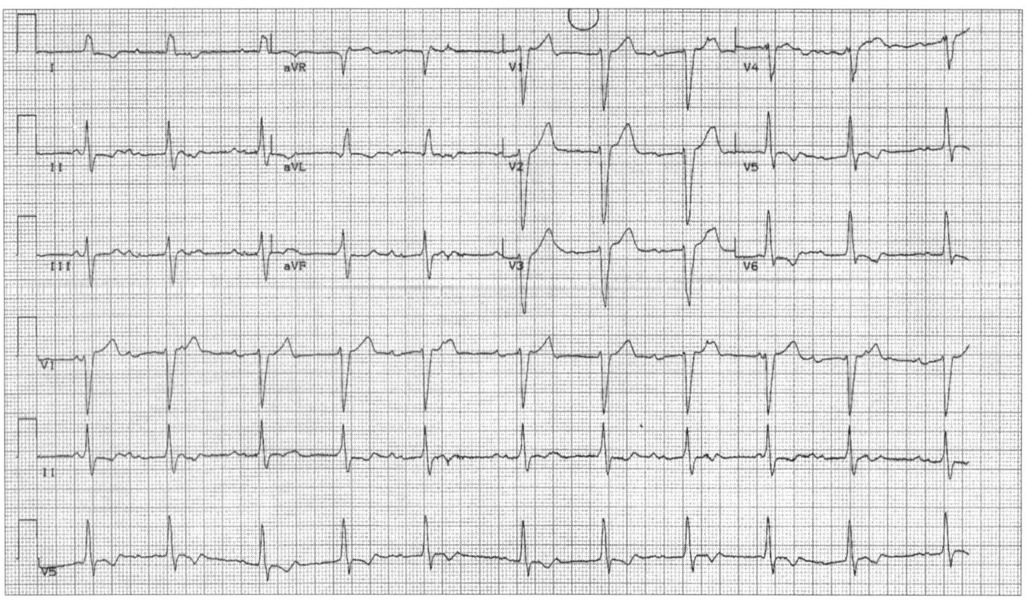

Complete heart block with left bundle branch type ventricular complexes.

○ What is the abnormality in the M-mode echocardiogram shown below?

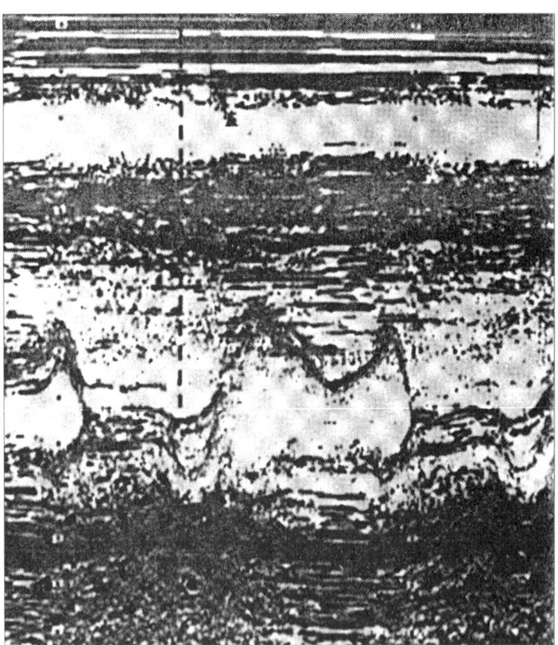

Prolapse of the posterior leaflet of the mitral valve.

- **What is the abnormality in the echocardiogram shown below?**

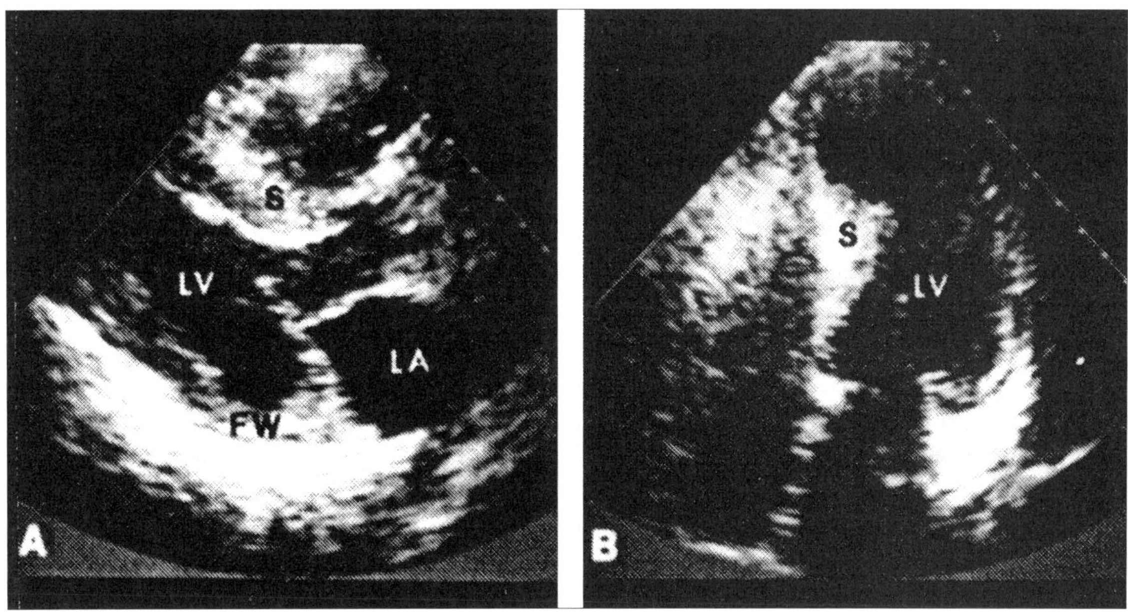

Hypertrophic cardiomyopathy. Note the very thickened septum and anterior systolic motion of the mitral valve.

- **What is the interpretation of the ECG seen below?**

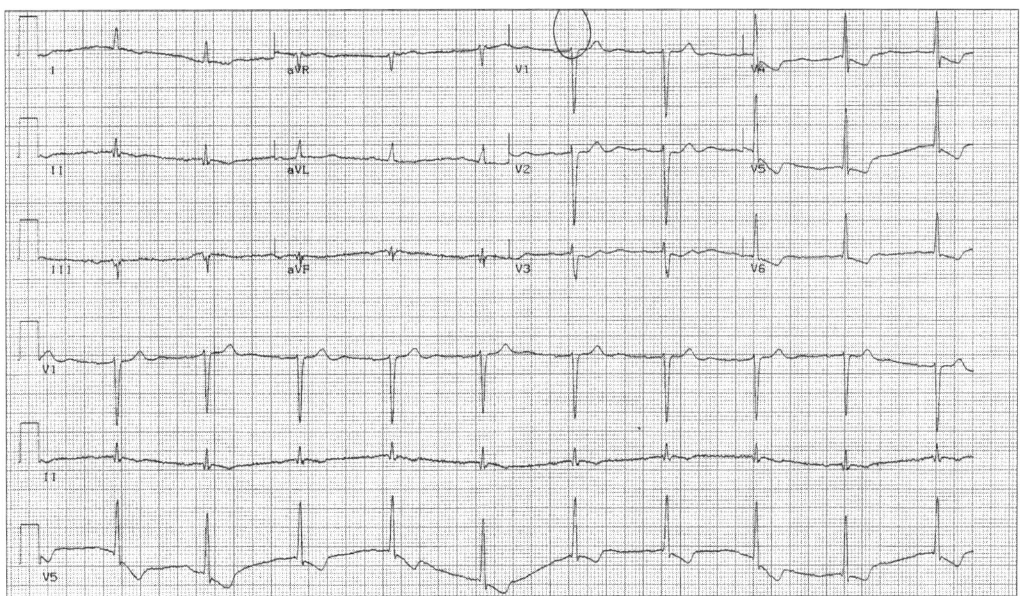

Ectopic atrial rhythm with an old inferior infarction and non-specific ST-T abnormality.

❍ **What is the interpretation of the ECG seen below?**

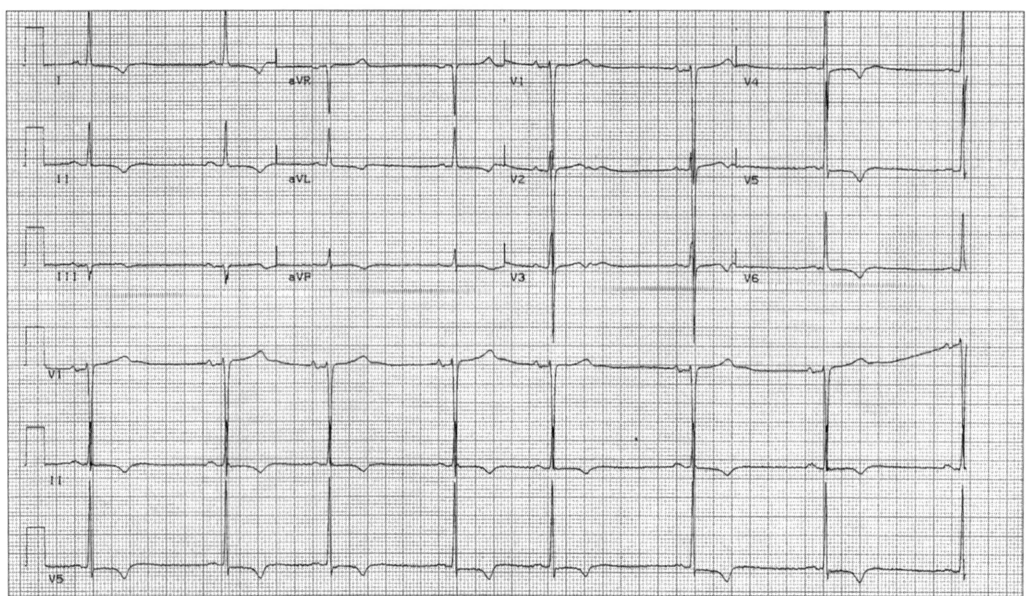

Marked sinus bradycardia with a non-conducted PAC, LVH with ST-T repolarization abnormality.

❍ **What is the interpretation of the ECG seen below?**

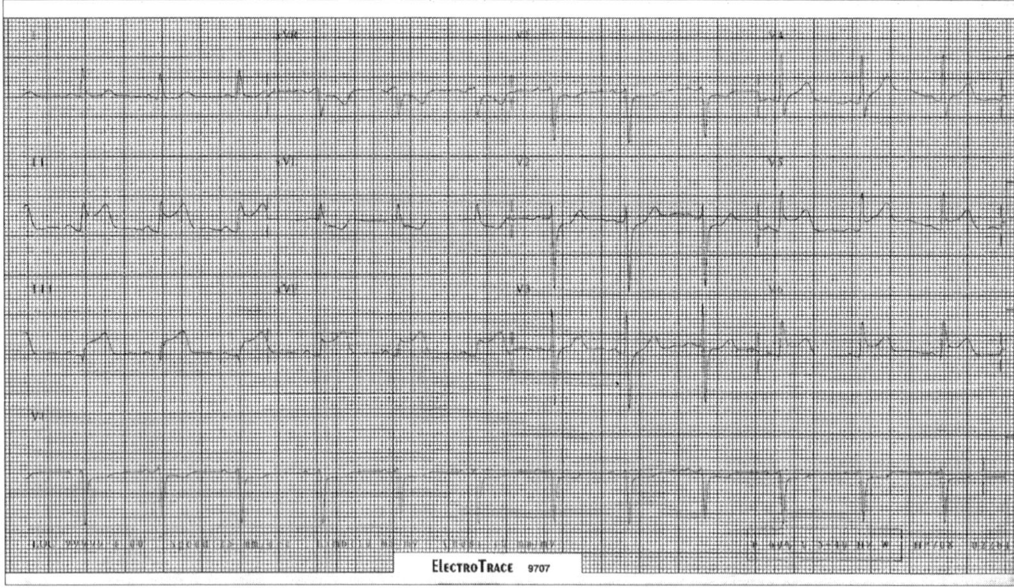

Normal sinus rhythm with an acute inferior wall myocardial infarction.

❍ **What is the interpretation of the ECG seen below?**

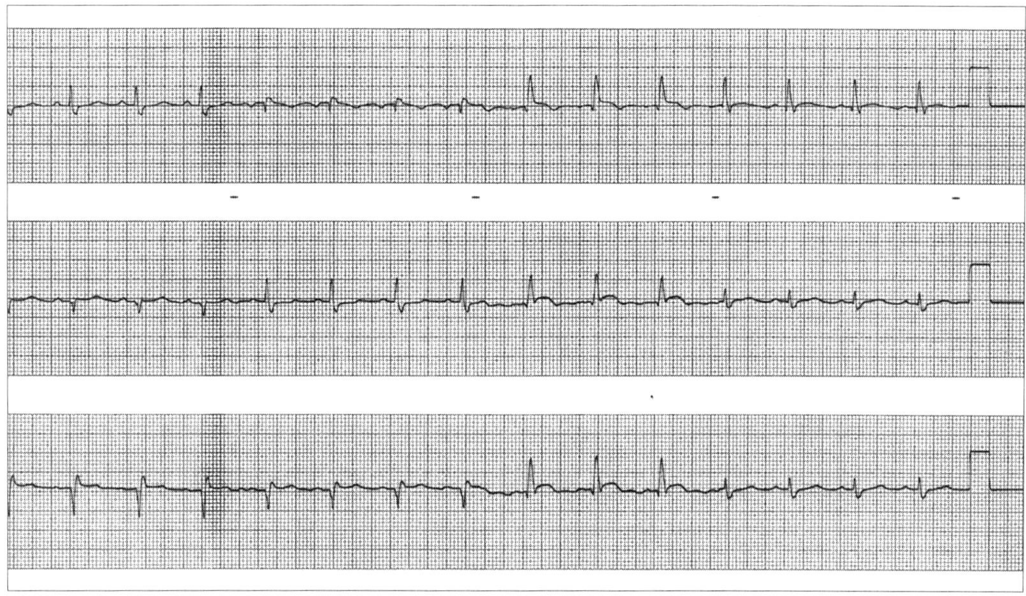

Normal sinus rhythm, RBBB, left anterior fascicular block and an acute anterior myocardial infarction.

❍ **What is the interpretation of the ECG seen below?**

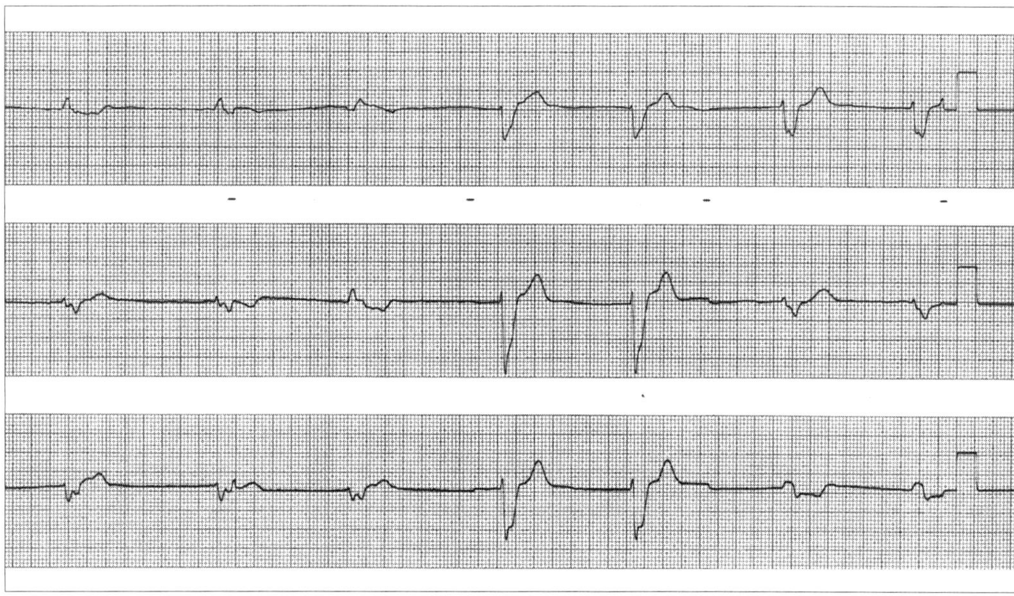

Idioventricular rhythm, rate of 40/min.

O What is the interpretation of the ECG seen below?

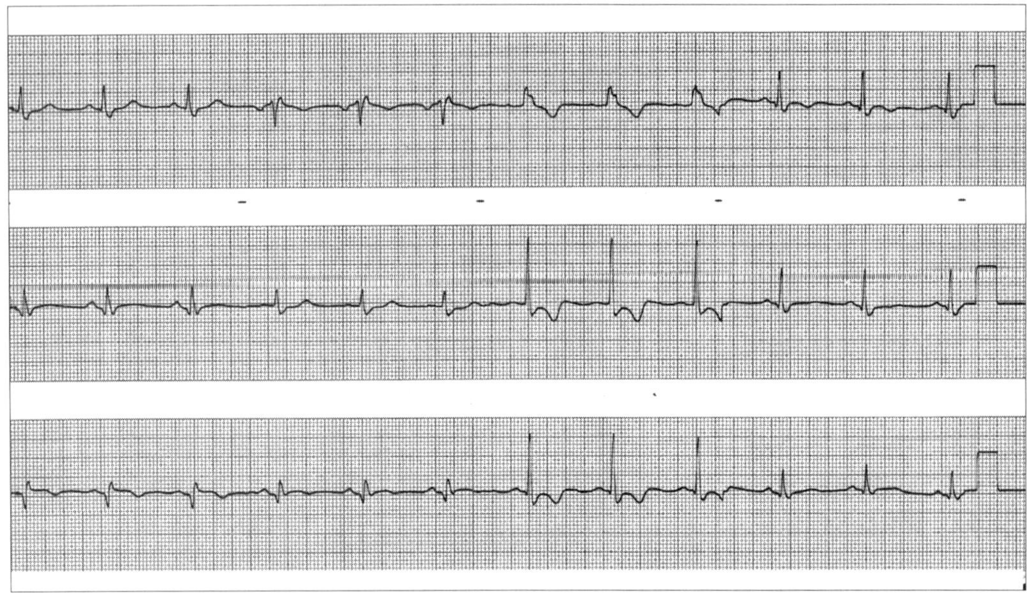

Normal sinus rhythm, RBBB and acute inferior infarction with posterior extension.

O What is the interpretation of the ECG seen below?

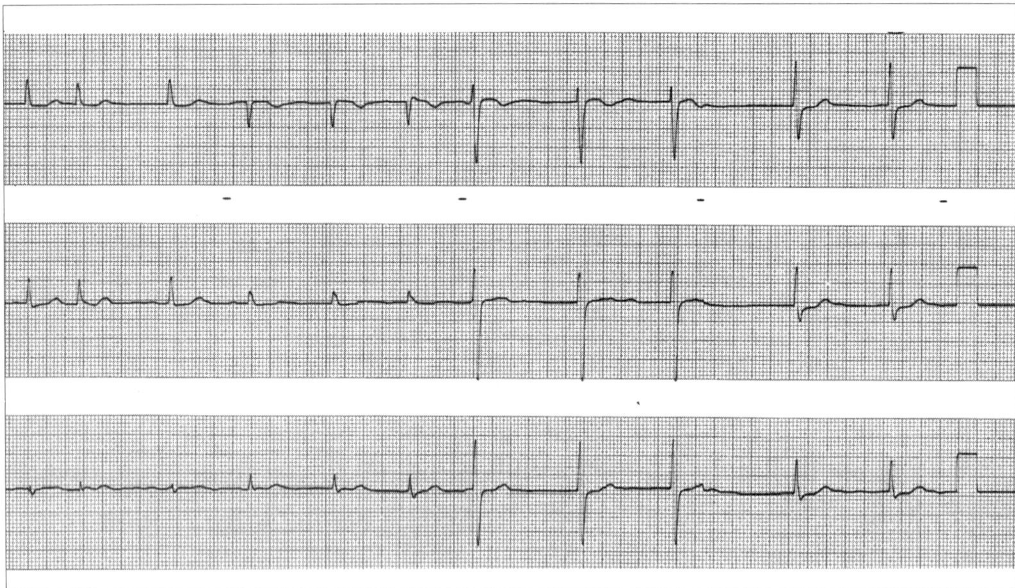

Atrial fibrillation, ventricular rate of 68/min.

BIBLIOGRAPHY

ACCP Critical Care Board Review, 2004.

Advanced Cardiac Life Support. Dallas: American Heart Association; 2000.

Advanced Trauma Life Support. Chicago: American College of Surgeons; 1995.

Albert, DM. *Clinical Practice Principles and Practice of Ophthalmology,* Vol. 2. Philadelphia: W.B. Saunders Co.; 1994.

Anderson, JE. *Grant's Atlas of Anatomy,* 8th ed. Baltimore: Williams & Wilkins; 1983.

Arieff, A. & Defronzo, R. *Fluid, Electrolyte and Acid Base Disorders*, 2nd ed. New York: Churchill Livingstone; 1995.

Auerbach, PS. *Management of Wilderness and Environmental Emergencies,* 4th ed. St. Louis: CV Mosby Company; 2001.

Avunduk, Canan, *Manual of Gastroenterology*, Lippincott Williams and Wilkins, 2002.

Bakerman, S. *ABCs of Interpretive Laboratory Data,* 2nd ed. Greenville: Interpretive Laboratory Data, Inc; 1984.

Baum's Textbook of Pulmonary Diseases, Lippincott, 2003.

Barash PG, Cullen BF, Stoelting RK (eds): *Clinical Anesthesia*, 4th ed. Philadelphia: Lippincott-Raven; 2000.

Barie PS, Shires GT (eds): *Surgical Intensive Care*. Boston: Little, Brown and Co.; 1993.

Berkow, R. *The Merck Manual,* 15th ed. Rahway: Merck Sharp & Dohme Research Laboratories; 1987.

Blomquist, IK & Bayer, AS. Life-threatening deep fascial space infections of the head and neck. *Infect Dis Clin N America.* 1988; 2 (1):237.

Bone LB, Johnson KD, Weigelt J, et al: Early versus delayed stabilization of femoral fractures: a prospective randomized study. *J Bone Joint Surg.* 1989; 71;336.

Bone, RC (ed): *Pulmonary and Critical Care Medicine*. 1993.

Bouachour G, Tirot P, Varache N, Gouello JP, Harr P, Alquier P. Hemodynamic changes in acute adrenal insufficiency. *Intensive Care Med.* 1994; 20:138-41.

Bracken MB, Shepard MJ, Collins WF, et al: A randomized, controlled trial of methylprednisolone or naloxone in the treatment of acute spinal cord injury: results of the Second National Acute Spinal Cord Injury Study. *N Engl J Med.* 1990; 322:1405-11.

Bradley, WG. *Neurology in Clinical Practice,* 4th ed. Newtown: Butterworth-Heineman; 2003.

Braverman LE & Utiger RD, eds: *The Thyroid*, 7th ed. Philadelphia: Lippincott-Raven; 1996:286-296.

Butcher, Graham, *Gastroenterology*, Churchill Livingstone, 2002.

Cahill, BC & Ingbar, DH. Massive hemoptysis. *Clinics in Chest Medicine*. 1994; 15:147.

Calleja, GA & Barkin, JS. Acute Pancreatitis. *Med Clin North Am*. 1993; 77:1037-1056.

Civetta JM, Taylor RW, Kirby RR. *Critical Care,* 3rd ed. New York: Lippincott-Raven Publishers; 1997.

Claussen MS, Landercasper J, Cogbill THE. Acute adrenal insufficiency presenting as shock after trauma and surgery: Three cases and review of the literature. *J Trauma*. 1992; 32:94-100.

Current Diagnosis & Treatment in Pulmonary Medicine, McGraw-Hill/Appleton & Lange; 1 edition (October 17, 2003)

Chronic Obstructive Pulmonary Disease, Oxford University Press, 2003.

Critical Care Transport, Jones & Bartlett, 2003.

Cynober, L, *Nutrition and Critical Care*, Ag Med & Sci, 2003.

DeGowin, EL. *Bedside Diagnostic Examination,* 4th ed. New York: Macmillan Publishing Co. Inc; 1981.

Diepenbrock, Nancy, *Quick Reference to Critical Care*, Lippincott Williams and Wilkins, 2003.

Dignass, *A, Topical Steroids in Gastroenterology and Hepatology*, Kluwer Academic Publisher, 2004.

Doods, Chris, *Anaesthesia and Critical Care*, Churchill Livingstone, 2003.

Edelstein, PH. Legionnaire's disease. *Clin Infect Dis*. 1993; 16:741.

Edwards, Zenia, *Gastroenterology at a Glance*, McGraw-Hill, 2004.
Ellenhorn, MJ. *Ellenhorn's Medical Toxicology: Diagnosis and Treatment of Human Poisoning,* 2nd ed. Baltimore: Williams & Wilkins; 1997.

Farb, Daniel, *Basic Critical Care,* Atlasbooks, 2004.

Farwell, AP. Sick euthyroid syndrome. *J Intens Care Med*. vol. 12: 5:249-260.

Fauci, AS & Braunwald, E. *Harrison's Principles of Internal Medicine*, 14th ed. New York: McGraw-Hill; 1998.

Feliciano DV, Moore EE, Mattox KL (eds): *Trauma*, 3rd ed. Stamford: Appleton & Lange; 1996.

Fishman, AP. *Fishman's Pulmonary Diseases and Disorders*, 3rd ed. New York: McGraw-Hill; 1998.

Forrester JS, Diamond G, Chatterjee K, Swan JC. Medical therapy of acute myocardial infarction by application of hemodynamic subsets (parts 1 and 2). *N Engl J Med*. 1976; 295, 1356-1362 & 1204-1213.

Flomenbaum, N. *Emergency Diagnostic Testing,* 2nd ed. St. Louis: Mosby-Year Book, Inc.; 1995.

Friedman, Scott, *Current Diagnosis and Treatment in Gastroenterology*, McGraw-Hill, 2002.

Goldfrank, LR, et al: *Goldfrank's Toxicologic Emergencies*, 6th ed. Stamford: Appleton & Lange; 1998.

Greenfield, LJ. *Surgery Scientific Principles and Practice*. Philadelphia: J.B. Lippincott Company; 1993.

Guyton, AC. *Textbook of Medical Physiology.* 10th ed. Philadelphia: W.B. Saunders Co.; 2000.

Hall JB, Schmidt GA, Wood LDH. *Principles of Critical Care*, 3rd ed. New York: McGraw Hill; 2005.

Harris, JH. *The Radiology of Emergency Medicine,* 2nd ed. Baltimore: Williams and Wilkins; 1981.

Harrison, TR. *Principles of Internal Medicine,* 16th ed. New York: McGraw-Hill Book Company; 2004.

Harwood-Nuss, A. *The Clinical Practice of Emergency Medicine,* 3rd ed. Philadelphia: JB Lippincott Company; 2001.

Hauser, Stephen, *Mayo Clinic Gastroenterology and Hepatology Board Review*, 2003.

Holland, JF. *Cancer Medicine,* 6th ed. Baltimore: Williams & Wilkins; 2003.

Hoppenfeld, S. *Physical Examination of the Spine and Extremities.* Norwalk: Appleton-Century-Crofts; 1976.

International Consensus Conference: Clinical Investigation of Ventilator-Associated Pneumonia. *Chest.* Nov 1992; vol. 102; 5: 1.

International Study Group, The. In-hospital mortality and clinical course of 20,891 patients with suspected acute myocardial infarction randomized between alteplase and streptokinase with and without heparin. *Lancet.* 1990; 336: 71-75.

International Consensus Conference: Clinical Investigation of Ventilator-Associated Pneumonia. *Chest.* Nov 1992; vol. 102; 5: 1.

Ivatury, RR & Cayten, CG (eds): *The Textbook of Penetrating Trauma.* Philadelphia: Williams & Wilkins; 1996: 319-332.

Jenison, S & Hejelle, B. Hantavirus pulmonary syndrome; clinical, diagnostic and virologic aspects. *Seminars in Respiratory Infections*. December 1995; vol. 10; 4: 259 – 269.

Johnson D & Cunha, B. Drug Fever. *Infectious Disease Clinics of North America.* March 1996; vol 10; 1: 85-91.

Kelley, WN. *Textbook of Internal Medicine*, 3rd ed. Lippincott-Raven; 1997.

Kelly C, Pothoulakis C, LaMont J. Clostridium difficile colitis. *NEJM.* January 1994; vol. 330; 4: 257-261.

Koenig, K. *Clinical Emergency Medicine.* New York: McGraw-Hill; 1996.

Leach, Richard, *Critical Care Medicine at a Glance,* Blackwell, 2004.

Levin, DL & Morris, FC. *Essentials of Pediatric Intensive Care.* Quality Medical Publishing, Inc.; 1990.

Linden, BE & Aguilar, EA. Sinusitis in the nasotracheally intubated patient. *Arch Otolaryngol Head Neck Surg*. August 1988; vol. 114: 860-861.

Mandell, D & B. *Principles and Practice of Infectious Diseases*, 5th ed. WB Saunders; 2000.

Marino, P. *The ICU Book*, 2nd ed. Baltimore: Williams and Wilkins; 1998.

Marrie, TJ. Community-acquired pneumonia. *Clin Infect Dis*. 1994; 18:501.

Marriott, HJL. *Practical Electrocardiography,* 10th ed. Baltimore: Williams and Wilkins; 2001.

Marshall JB. Acute Pancreatitis. A review with an emphasis on new developments. *Arch Int Med.* 1993;153:1185-1198.

MayoSmith MF, Hirsch PJ, Wodzinski SF, Schiffman FP: Acute epiglottitis in adults. An eight-year experience in the state of Rhode Island. *N Engl J Med.* 1986; 314(18): 1133.

Meduri, GU. Diagnosis of ventilator-associated pneumonia. *Infect Dis clin North Am.* 1993; 7:295.

Miller, RD (ed): *Anesthesia*, 5th ed. New York: Churchill Livingstone; 2000.

Mittman, Bradley, *Frontrunner's Internal Medicine Board Revew*, Frontrunners, 2004.

Mirvis, Stuart, *Imaging in Trauma and Critical Care*, Elsevier Science Health, 2003.

Molitoris, Bruce, *Critical Care Nephrology,* Remedica, 2003.

Montaner JS, Lawson LM, Levitt N, Belzber A, Schechrer,MT, Ruedy J. Corticosteroids prevent early deterioration in patients with moderately sever Pneumocystitis carinii pneumonia and the acquired immunodeficiency syndrome. *Ann Intern Med.* 1990; 113:14-20.

Moore, KL. *Clinically Oriented Anatomy.* 4th ed. Baltimore: Williams & Wilkins; 1999.

Murray, JF and Nadel, JA (ed): *Textbook of Respiratory Medicine*, 3rd ed. Philadelphia: WB Saunders; 2004.

Musher, DM: Infections caused by Streptococcus pneumoniae: Clinical spectrum, pathogenesis, immunity and treatment. *Clin Infect Dis*. 1992;14:801.

Nelson, W.E. *Textbook of Pediatrics.* 17th ed. Philadelphia: W.B. Saunders Company; 2004.

Niederman MS et al.: Guidelines for the initial management of adults with community-acquired pneumonia: Diagnosis, assessment of severity and initial antimicrobial therapy. *Am Rev Respir Dis*. 1993; 148:1418.

Oelkers, W. Adrenal Insufficiency. *N Engl J Med.* 1996; 335:1206-1212.

Owings JT, Kennedy JP, Blaisdell. FW. *Injuries to the Extremities*. Surgery, Scientific American; 1997.

Peitzman AB, Rhodes M, Schwab CW, Yealy DM (eds): *The Trauma Manual*. 2nd ed. Philadelphia: Lippincott-Raven; 2002.

Physicians' Desk Reference, 50th ed. Oradell: Medical Economics Company Inc; 1996.

Plantz, SH. *Emergency Medicine PreTest, Self-Assessment and Review.* McGraw-Hill; 1990.

Plantz, SH. *Emergency Medicine.* Baltimore: Williams & Wilkins; 1998.

Plantz, SH. *Emergency Medicine Pearls of Wisdom,* 6th ed. McGraw-Hill, 2005.

Practical Pulmonary Pathology: A Diagnostic Approach, Churchill Livingstone, 2004.

Prasad, Priyajit, *Gastroenterology*, Greenwich Medical Media, 2002.

Principles of Pulmonary Medicine, W.B. Saunders Company, 4th Edition, 2003.

Reddy PS, Curtiss EL, O'Toole JD, Shaver JA. Cardiac tamponade: hemodynamic observations in man. *Circulation.* 1978; 58: 265-272.

Reese, RE & Betts, RF (eds): *A Practical Approach to Infectious Diseases*, 4th ed. Boston: Little, Brown and Company.

Robbins, SL. *Pathologic Basis of Disease,* 3rd ed. Philadelphia: WB Saunders Company; 1984.

Roland, L. *Merritt's Textbook of Neurology.* Williams & Wilkins; 1995.

Rosen, P. *Emergency Medicine Concepts and Clinical Practice,* 4th ed. St. Louis: Mosby Year Book; 1998.

Rosenow EC, Myers JL, Swenson SJ & Pisani RJ: Drug-Induced Pulmonary Disease. *Chest.* 1992; 102:239-250.

Rowe, RC. *The Harriet Lane Handbook: A Manual for Pediatric House Officiers,* 16th ed. C.V Mosby; 2002.

Sabiston, DC. *Textbook of Surgery; The Biologic Basis of Modern Surgical Practice*. 17th ed, Philadelphia: W.B. Saunders Co.; 2004.

Salit, IE. Diagnostic approaches to head and neck infections. *Infect Dis Clin N America.* 1988; 2 (1):35.

Savage EB. *Essentials of Basic Science in Surgery*. Philadelphia: J.B. Lippincott Company; 1993.

Schrier, RW & Gottschalk, CW. *Diseases of the Kidney and Urinary Tract*, 7th ed. Williams & Wilkins; 2001.

Shapiro BA, Kacmarek RM, Cane RD, et al: *Clinical Application of Respiratory Care,* 4th.ed. St. Louis: Mosby-Year Book, Inc.; 1991.

Shapiro BA, Peruzzi WT, Templin R. *Clinical Application of Blood Gases*, 5th ed. St. Louis: Mosby-Year Book, Inc.; 1994.

Simon, RR. *Orthopedics in Emergency Medicine: The Extremities,* 2nd ed. Norwalk: Appleton & Lange; 1992.

Simon, RR. *Emergency Procedures and Techniques,* 2nd ed. Baltimore: Williams and Wilkins; 1987.

Skelly, Meg, *Conscious Sedation in Gastroenterology*, Whurr Publishers, 2003.

Squire, LF. *Fundamentals of Radiology,* 6th ed. Cambridge: Harvard University Press; 2004.

Stedman, TL. *Illustrated Stedman's Medical Dictionary,* 24th ed. Baltimore: Williams & Wilkins; 1982.

Stewart, CE. *Environmental Emergencies.* Baltimore: Williams and Wilkins; 1990.

Suarez, Jose, *Crtical Care Neurology and Neurosurgery*, Humana Press, 2003.

Tietjen PA, Kaner, RJ and Quinn CE: Aspiration Emergencies. *Clinics in Chest Medicine* 1994;15:117-135.

Tintinalli, JE. *Emergency Medicine A Comprehensive Study Guide,* 6th ed. New York: McGraw-Hill, Inc; 2003.

Urokinase Pulmonary Embolization Trial Study Group. Urokinase Pulmonary embolism trial- Phase I results. *JAMA*. 1970; 214: 2163-2172.
Vance, ML. Hypopituitarism. *N Engl J Med*. 1994; 330:1651-62 (Erratum, *N Engl J Med*. 1994; 331:487.)

Weigelt, JA & Lewis, FR (eds): *Surgical Critical Care*. Philadelphia: WB Saunders Co.; 1996.

Weiner, HL. *Neurology for the House Officer,* 7th ed. Baltimore: Williams & Wilkins; 2004.

Werber, SS & Ober, KP. Acute adrenal insufficiency. *Endocrinol Metab Clin North Am*. 1993; 22:303-28.

West, JB. *Respiratory Physiology: The Essentials*, 6th ed. Baltimore: Williams & Wilkins; 2000.

Whitley, RJ. Viral Encephalitis. *NEJM*. July 1990; 242 – 248.

Williams, RD & Larsen, PR. *Williams Textbook of Endocrinology*, 10th ed. Philadelphia: W.B. Saunders; 2002.

Wilson, R & Walt, A. *Management of Trauma: Pitfalls and Practice*, 2nd ed. Philadelphia: Williams & Wilkins; 1996.

Yamada, Tadataka, *Textbook of Gastroenterology*, Lippincott Williams and Wilkins, 2003.

Yoshikawa, TT & Quinn, W. The aching head: intracranial suppuration due to head and neck infections. *Infect Dis Clin N America.* 1988; 2 (1):265,

Youmans, JR. *Neurological Surgery,* 5th ed. Philadelphia: W.B. Saunders; 2003.

Zevitz, M. *Cardiovascular Pearls of Wisdom*. McGraw-Hill, 2005.

Zevitz, M. *Internal Medicine Pearls of Wisdom*. McGraw-Hill, 2005.